ANNALS OF THE NEW YORK ACADEMY OF SCIENCES

Volume 1009

EDITORIAL STAFF

Director, Publishing and New Media
SARAH GREENE

Managing Editor
JUSTINE CULLINAN

The New York Academy of Sciences
2 East 63rd Street
New York, New York 10021

THE NEW YORK ACADEMY OF SCIENCES
(Founded in 1817)

BOARD OF GOVERNORS, September 2003 – September 2004

TORSTEN N. WIESEL, *Chairman of the Board*
GERALD D. FISCHBACH, *Vice Chairman*
JOHN T. MORGAN, *Treasurer*
ELLIS RUBINSTEIN, *Chief Executive Officer* [ex officio]

Honorary Life Governors
WILLIAM T. GOLDEN   JOSHUA LEDERBERG

Governors

KAREN E. BURKE	PETER B. CORR	R. BRIAN FERGUSON
RONALD L. GRAHAM	MARNIE IMHOFF	WENDY EVANS JOSEPH
JACQUELINE LEO	RODERT W. LUCKY	PAUL MARKS
BRUCE McEWEN	RONAY MENSCHEL	JOHN F. NIBLACK
SANDRA PANEM	PETER RINGROSE	DAVID D. SABATINI
	LEE G. VANCE	DEBORAH WILEY

VICTORIA BJORKLUND, *Counsel* [ex officio]   LARRY R. SMITH, *Secretary* [ex officio]

AGMATINE AND IMIDAZOLINES

THEIR NOVEL RECEPTORS AND ENZYMES

ANNALS OF THE NEW YORK ACADEMY OF SCIENCES
Volume 1009

AGMATINE AND IMIDAZOLINES

THEIR NOVEL RECEPTORS AND ENZYMES

Edited by
John E. Piletz, Soundar Regunathan, and Paul Ernsberger

The New York Academy of Sciences
New York, New York
2003

Copyright © 2003 by the New York Academy of Sciences. All rights reserved. Under the provisions of the United States Copyright Act of 1976, individual readers of the Annals are permitted to make fair use of the material in them for teaching or research. Permission is granted to quote from the Annals provided that the customary acknowledgment is made of the source. Material in the Annals may be republished only by permission of the Academy. Address inquiries to the Permissions Department (editorial@nyas.org) at the New York Academy of Sciences.

Copying fees: For each copy of an article made beyond the free copying permitted under Section 107 or 108 of the 1976 Copyright Act, a fee should be paid through the Copyright Clearance Center, Inc., 222 Rosewood Drive, Danvers, MA 01923 (www.copyright.com).

∞ The paper used in this publication meets the minimum requirements of the American National Standard for Information Sciences—Permanence of Paper for Printed Library Materials, ANSI Z39.48-1984.

Library of Congress Cataloging-in-Publication Data

Agmatine and imidazolines : their novel receptors and enzymes / edited by John E. Piletz, Soundar Ragunathan, and Paul Ernsberger.
   p. ; cm. — (Annals of the New York Academy of Sciences ; v. 1009)
"This volume is the result of a conference entitled Fourth International Symposium on Agmatine and Imidazoline Systems (in memory of Donald J. Reis) held on April 9–11, 2003 in San Diego, California" — Contents p.
Includes bibliographical references and index.
   ISBN 1-57331-498-6 (cloth : alk. paper) — ISBN 1-57331-499-4 (pbk. : alk. paper) 1. Agmatine—Receptors — Congresses. 2. Imidazoline — Receptors — Congresses. 3. Neurotransmitters — Receptors — Congresses.
   [DNLM: 1. Agmatine—pharmacology—Congresses. 2. Arginine—pharmacology—Congresses. 3. Harmine—analogs & derivatives--Congresses. 4. Imidazoles—pharmacology—Congresses. 5. Receptors, Drug—Congresses. QU 61 I614a 2003] I. Piletz, John E. II. Ragunathan, Soundar. III. Ernsberger, Paul. IV. International Symposium on Agmatine and Imidazoline Systems. V. Title. VI. Series.
   Q11.N5 vol. 1009
   [QP563.A38]
   500 s—dc22
   [615/.
2003025207

Asterisk/CCP
Printed in the United States of America
ISBN 1-57331-498-6 (cloth)
ISBN 1-57331-499-4 (paper)
ISSN 0077-8923

ANNALS OF THE NEW YORK ACADEMY OF SCIENCES

Volume 1009
December 2003

AGMATINE AND IMIDAZOLINES
THEIR NOVEL RECEPTORS AND ENZYMES

Editors
JOHN E. PILETZ, SOUNDAR REGUNATHAN, AND PAUL ERNSBERGER

Conference Organizers
JOHN E. PILETZ, SOUNDAR REGUNATHAN, PAUL ERNSBERGER,
ANGELOS HALARIS, AND SANDRA ROERIG

Advisory Board
PASCAL BOUSQUET (*France*), MANFRED GÖTHERT (*Germany*),
PAUL INSEL (*USA*), JIN LI (*China*), NOEL G. MORGAN (*UK*),
ANGELO PARINI (*France*), PHIL SKOLNICK (*USA*),
GEORGE WILCOX (*USA*), ANTON BESPALOV (*Russia*),
JESUS GARCIA-SEVILLA (*Spain*), GEOFFREY A. HEAD (*Australia*),
STEVEN LANIER (*USA*), DUANE MILLER (*USA*), DAVID J. NUTT (*UK*),
JOSEPH SATRIANO (*USA*), SOLOMON SNYDER (*USA*),
AND PAUL M. VANHOUTTE (*France*)

This volume comprises the proceedings of the Fourth International Symposium on Agmatine and Imidazoline Systems (in memory of Donald J. Reis) held on April 9–11, 2003 in San Diego, California.

CONTENTS

In Memoriam: Donald J. Reis	xiii
Preface. *By* the Editors	xv
Keynote address: Relevance of Imidazoline Receptors and Agmatine to Psychiatry: A Decade of Progress. *By* A. HALARIS AND J.E. PILETZ	1

Part I. Agmatine: Basic and Molecular Aspects

Regulation of Inducible Nitric Oxide Synthase and Agmatine Synthesis in Macrophages and Astrocytes. *By* SOUNDAR REGUNATHAN AND JOHN E. PILETZ	20
Vertebrate Agmatinases: What Role Do They Play in Agmatine Catabolism? *By* SIDNEY M. MORRIS, JR.	30

Agmatine: At the Crossroads of the Arginine Pathways. *By* JOSEPH SATRIANO 34

Gastrointestinal Uptake of Agmatine: Distribution in Tissues and Organs and Pathophysiologic Relevance. *By* GERHARD J. MOLDERINGS, ANJA HEINEN, SIGRID MENZEL, FRIEDRICH LÜBBECKE, JÜRGEN HOMANN, AND MANFRED GÖTHERT 44

Structure-Activity Analysis of Guanidine Group in Agmatine for Brain Agmatinase. *By* M.-J. HUANG, S. REGUNATHAN, M. BOTTA, K. LEE, E. MCCLENDON, G.B. YI, M.L. PEDERSEN, D.B. BERKOWITZ, G. WANG, M. TRAVAGLI, AND J.E. PILETZ 52

Agmatine Crosses the Blood–Brain Barrier. *By* J.E. PILETZ, P.J. MAY, G. WANG, AND H. ZHU 64

Identification and Pharmacological Characterization of a Specific Agmatine Transport System in Human Tumor Cell Lines. *By* GERHARD J. MOLDERINGS, MICHAEL BRÜSS, HEINZ BÖNISCH, AND MANFRED GÖTHERT 75

Part II. Agmatine: Function and Pre-Clinical Aspects

Neuropharmacokinetic and Dynamic Studies of Agmatine (Decarboxylated Arginine). *By* H. OANH X. NGUYEN, CORY J. GORACKE-POSTLE, LORI L. KAMINSKI, AARON C. OVERLAND, ANDREW D. MORGAN, AND CAROLYN A. FAIRBANKS 82

Effect of Agmatine on Acute and Mononeuropathic Pain. *By* FEYZA ARICIOGLU, EYLEM KORCEGEZ, AYHAN BOZKURT, AND SULEYMAN OZYALCIN 106

Spinal and Supraspinal Agmatine Activate Different Receptors to Enhance Spinal Morphine Antinociception. *By* SANDRA C. ROERIG 116

Is Agmatine an Endogenous Factor Against Stress? *By* FEYZA ARICIOGLU, SOUNDAR REGUNATHAN, AND JOHN E. PILETZ 127

Agmatine-Morphine Interaction on Nociception in Mice. *By* EDUARDO RUIZ-DURÁNTEZ, JAVIER LLORENTE, ISABEL ULIBARRI, JOSEBA PINEDA, AND LUISA UGEDO 133

Is Agmatine an Endogenous Anxiolytic/Antidepressant Agent? *By* FEYZA ARICIOGLU AND HALE ALTUNBAS 136

Effect of Agmatine on Electrically and Chemically Induced Seizures in Mice. *By* FEYZA ARICIOGLU, BILGE KAN, OKAN YILLAR, EYLEM KORCEGEZ, AND KEMAL BERKMAN 141

Agmatine Inhibits Naloxone-Induced Contractions in Morphine-Dependent Guinea Pig Ileum. *By* FEYZA ARICIOGLU, ESER ERCIL, AND GUL DULGER .. 147

Effect of Agmatine on the Time Course of Brain Inflammatory Cytokines After Injury in Rat Pups. *By* YANGZHENG FENG AND MICHAEL H. LEBLANC 152

Part III. Other Endogenous Ligands for Imidazoline Receptors

Endogenous β-Carbolines as Clonidine-Displacing Substances. *By* E.S.J. ROBINSON, N.J. ANDERSON, J. CROSBY, D.J. NUTT, AND A.L. HUDSON 157

Comparative Effects of Efaroxan and β-Carbolines on the Secretory Activity of Rodent and Human β Cells. *By* NOEL G. MORGAN, E. JANE COOPER, PAUL E. SQUIRES, CLAIRE E. HILLS, CHRISTINE A. PARKER, AND ALAN L. HUDSON 167

Characterization of [^{3}H]Harmane Binding to Rat Whole Brain Membranes.
By N.J. ANDERSON, E.S.J. ROBINSON, S.M. HUSBANDS, P. DELAGRANGE,
D.J. NUTT, AND A.L. HUDSON 175

Effect of Harmane on Mononeuropathic Pain in Rats. *By* FEYZA ARICIOGLU,
EYLEM KORCEGEZ, AND SULEYMAN OZYALCIN 180

Inhibitory Effect of Harmane on Morphine-Dependent Guinea Pig Ileum.
By FEYZA ARICIOGLU AND TIJEN UTKAN 185

Effect of Harmane on the Convulsive Threshold in Epilepsy Models in Mice.
By FEYZA ARICIOGLU, OKAN YILLAR, EYLEM KORCEGEZ,
AND KEMAL BERKMAN 190

Harmane Induces Anxiolysis and Antidepressant-Like Effects in Rats.
By FEYZA ARICIOGLU AND HALE ALTUNBAS 196

No Evidence for Activation of α_2-Adrenoceptors by Methanolic Extracts of Bovine
Brain and Lung Containing Clonidine-Displacing Substance. *By* D. PINTHONG,
D.A. KENDALL, S.J. MACLENNAN, R.M. EGLEN, AND V.G.WILSON 201

Complex Interaction of α_2-Adrenoceptor Binding Sites with Bovine Brain and
Lung Extracts Containing Clonidine-Displacing Substance. *By* D. PINTHONG,
D.A. KENDALL, AND V.G. WILSON 216

Endogenous Imidazoline Receptor Ligands Relax Rat Aorta by an
Endothelium-Dependent Mechanism. *By* IAN F. MUSGRAVE,
ANDREA VAN DER ZYPP, MATHEW GRIGG, AND COLIN J. BARROW 222

Part IV. I-1 Imidazoline Receptors

I_1 Imidazoline Receptors Involved in Cardiovascular Regulation: Where Are
We and Where Are We Going? *By* P. BOUSQUET, H. GRENEY, V. BRUBAN,
S. SCHANN, J. D. EHRHARDT, L. MONASSIER, AND J. FELDMAN 228

Are Centrally Acting Imidazoline Agents Appropriate Therapy for Renovascular
Hypertension? *By* GEOFFREY A. HEAD AND SANDRA L. BURKE 234

Cardiac Effects of Moxonidine in Spontaneously Hypertensive Obese Rats.
By S. MUKADDAM-DAHER, A. MENAOUAR, R. EL-AYOUBI, J. GUTKOWSKA,
M. JANKOWSKI, R.A. VELLIQUETTE, AND P. ERNSBERGER 244

The Role of I_1-Imidazoline Receptors and α_2-Adrenergic Receptors in the Modulation
of Glucose and Lipid Metabolism in the SHROB Model of Metabolic
Syndrome X. *By* RICHARD J. KOLETSKY, RODNEY A. VELLIQUETTE,
AND PAUL ERNSBERGER 251

Involvement of Forebrain Imidazoline and α_2-Adrenergic Receptors in the
Antidipsogenic Response to Moxonidine. *By* CARINA A.F. ANDRADE,
LISANDRA B. OLIVEIRA, GIZELE MARTINEZ, DANIELA C.F. SILVA,
LAURIVAL A. DE LUCA, JR., AND JOSÉ V. MENANI 262

Moxonidine Displays a Presynaptic Alpha-2-Adrenoceptor-Dependent Synergistic
Sympathoinhibitory Action at Imidazoline-1 Receptors. *By* ULRICH SCHÄFER,
CHRISTOF BURGDORF, ASTRID ENGELHARDT, WALTER RAASCH,
THOMAS KURZ, AND GERT RICHARDT 265

Norepinephrine Release Is Reduced by I_1-Receptors in Addition to α_2-Adrenoceptors.
By WALTER RAASCH, BRITTA JUNGBLUTH, ULRICH SCHÄFER,
WALTER HÄUSER AND PETER DOMINIAK 270

Normalization of Up-Regulated Cardiac Imidazoline I_1-Receptors and Natriuretic Peptides by Chronic Treatment with Moxonidine in Spontaneously Hypertensive Rats. *By* R. EL-AYOUBI, A. MENAOUAR, J. GUTKOWSKA, AND S. MUKADDAM-DAHER 274

Alpha$_{2A}$-Adrenergic versus Imidazoline Receptor Controversy in Rilmenidine's Action: Alpha$_{2A}$-Antagonism in Humans versus Alpha$_{2A}$-Agonism in Rabbits. *By* GERHARD J. MOLDERINGS, HEINZ BÖNISCH, MICHAEL BRÜSS, AND MANFRED GÖTHERT 279

BU98008, a Highly Selective Imidazoline$_1$-Receptor Ligand. *By* E.S.J. ROBINSON, R.E. PRICE, D.J. NUTT, AND A.L. HUDSON 283

Apparent Absence of a Direct Renal Effect of Imidazoline Receptor Agonists. *By* D.D. SMYTH, D. PIRNAT, B. FORZLEY, AND S.B. PENNER 288

Atypical [^{3}H]Clonidine Binding Sites in Human Caudate and Platelets on Cryostat-cut Sections. *By* H. ZHU, A. HALARIS, AND J.E. PILETZ 296

Part V. I-2/I-3 Imidazoline Receptors

Novel Ligands for the Investigation of Imidazoline Receptors and Their Binding Proteins. *By* A.L. HUDSON, R.J. TYACKE, M.D. LALIES, N. DAVIES, D.P. FINN, O. MARTÍ, E. ROBINSON, S. HUSBANDS, M.C.W. MINCHIN, A. KIMURA, AND D.J. NUTT 302

The Effects of Chronic Administration of Inhibitors of Flavin and Quinone Amine Oxidases on Imidazoline I_1 Receptor Density in Rat Whole Brain. *By* ANDREW HOLT, KATHRYN G. TODD, AND GLEN B. BAKER 309

In Vivo Effects of the I_2–Alkylating Agent BU99006 on the Immunodensity of Imidazoline Receptor Proteins in the Mouse Brain. *By* JESUS A. GARCIA-SEVILLA AND MARCEL FERRER-ALCON 323

Restoration of First-Phase Insulin Secretion by the Imidazoline Compound LY374284 in Pancreatic Islets of Diabetic db/db Mice. *By* M.B. BRENNER, J. GROMADA, A.M. EFANOV, K. BOKVIST, AND H.-J. MEST 332

Effect of Postmortem Delay on Imidazoline Receptor-Binding Proteins in Human and Mouse Brain. *By* JOHN K. MA, HE ZHU, AND JOHN E. PILETZ 341

Association Between I_2 Binding Sites and Monoamine Oxidase-B Activity in Platelets. *By* H. ZHU AND J.E. PILETZ 347

Relationship Between Imidazoline$_2$ Sites and Monoamine Oxidase. *By* L.M. PATERSON, R.J. TYACKE, D.J. NUTT, AND A.L. HUDSON 353

Initial Evaluation of Novel Selective Ligands for Imidazoline$_2$ Receptors in Rat Whole Brain. *By* R.J. TYACKE, F. SĄCZEWSKI, P. TABIN, J. SĄCZEWSKI, D.J. NUTT, AND A.L. HUDSON 357

Investigation of the Affinities of Two New β-Carbolines for Rat Brain Imidazoline$_2$ Receptors. *By* R.J. TYACKE, A. LAU, B. GRELLA, R.A. GLENNON, D.J. NUTT, AND A.L. HUDSON 361

Identification of an I_2 Binding Protein From Rabbit Brain. *By* A. KIMURA, R.J. TYACKE, M.C.W. MINCHIN, D.J. NUTT, AND A.L. HUDSON 364

In Vivo Estimation of Imidazoline$_2$ Binding Site Turnover. *By* L.M. PATERSON, E.S.J. ROBINSON, D.J. NUTT, AND A.L. HUDSON 367

Specificity of Nonadrenergic Imidazoline Binding Sites in Insulin-Secreting Cells and Relation to the Block of ATP-Sensitive K^+ Channels. *By* TIMM GROSSE-LACKMANN, BERND J. ZÜNKLER, AND INGO RUSTENBECK 371

Part VI. IRAS Candidate Imidazoline Receptor

Moxonidine, a Mixed α_2-Adrenergic and Imidazoline Receptor Agonist, Identifies a Novel Adrenergic Target for Spinal Analgesia. *By* LAURA S. STONE, CAROLYN A. FAIRBANKS, AND GEORGE L. WILCOX 378

Evidence for Nonadrenoceptor Responses to Imidazoline Derivatives in the Porcine Isolated Rectal Artery. *By* MINYAN WANG, W.R. DUNN, S.L. CHAN, B. GARFIELD, AND V.G. WILSON 386

Cell Signaling by Imidazoline-1 Receptor Candidate, IRAS, and the Nischarin Homologue. *By* J.E. PILETZ, G. WANG, AND H. ZHU 392

IRAS Is an Anti-Apoptotic Protein. *By* MONIQUE DONTENWILL, JOHN E. PILETZ, MICHAEL CHEN, JAMES BALDWIN, GÉRALDINE PASCAL, PHILIPPE RONDÉ, LAURENCE DUPUY, HUGUES GRENEY, KEN TAKEDA, AND PASCAL BOUSQUET 400

Assembly of PRR-Containing Receptors on Scaffolds: A Model for Imidazoline I_1-Receptor Action. *By* I.F. MUSGRAVE, F.C. DEHLE, AND J. PILETZ 413

IRAS Splice Variants. *By* J.E. PILETZ, W. DELEERSNIJDER, B.L. ROTH, P. ERNSBERGER, H. ZHU, AND D. ZIEGLER 419

Intracellular Effect of Imidazoline Receptor on α_{2A}-Noradrenergic Receptor. *By* MICHAEL J. CHEN, HE ZHU, AND JOHN E. PILETZ 427

Relationship between Platelet Imidazoline Receptor-Binding Peptides and Candidate Imidazoline-1 Receptor, IRAS. *By* HE ZHU, JONATHAN HAYES, MICHAEL CHEN, JAMES BALDWIN, AND JOHN E. PILETZ 439

Index of Contributors 447

Financial support was provided by:

- AMERICAN RADIOLABELED CHEMICALS, INC.
- AMERICAN SOCIETY FOR PHARMACOLOGY AND EXPERIMENTAL THERAPEUTICS
- AVENTIS PHARMACEUTICALS
- MRS. CORNELIA REIS
- SOLVAY PHARMACEUTICALS

The New York Academy of Sciences believes it has a responsibility to provide an open forum for discussion of scientific questions. The positions taken by the participants in the reported conferences are their own and not necessarily those of the Academy. The Academy has no intent to influence legislation by providing such forums.

AGMATINE AND IMIDAZOLINES

THEIR NOVEL RECEPTORS
AND ENZYMES

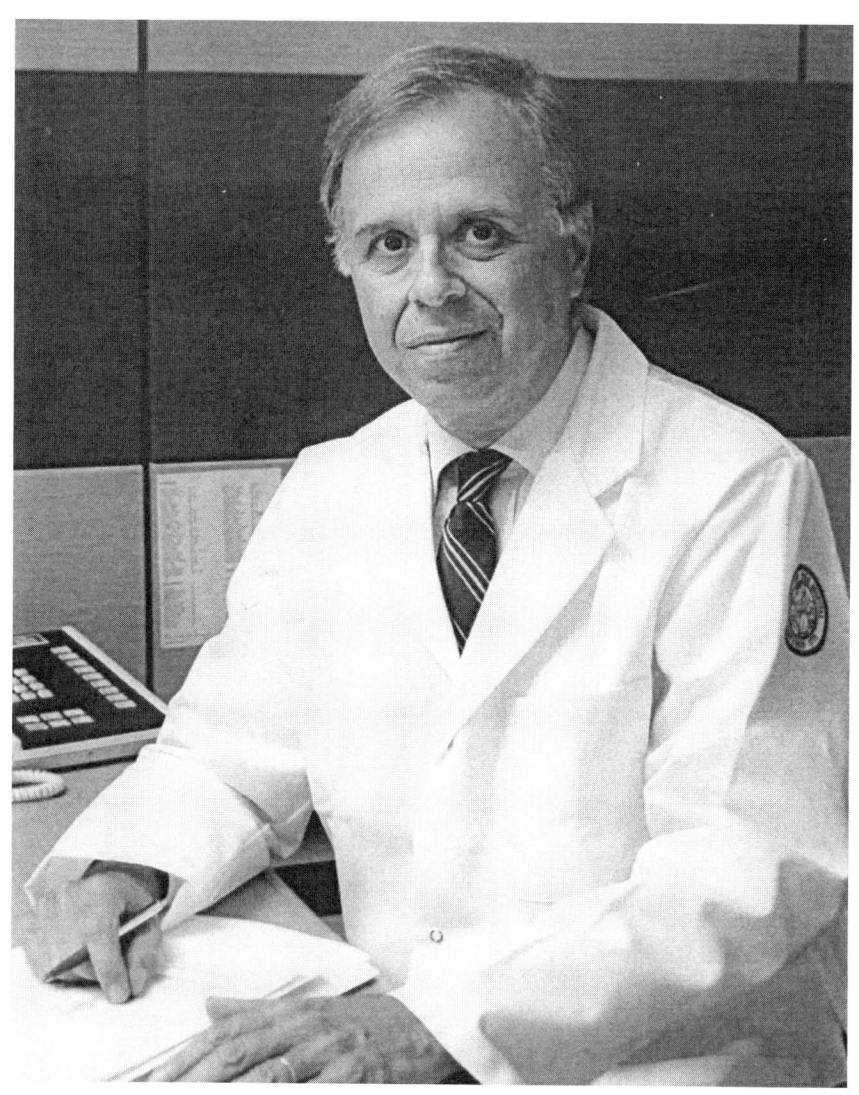

Donald J. Reis, M.D.
(1931–2000)

In Memoriam: Donald J. Reis

The entire scientific community, but especially scientists working on imidazoline receptors and agmatine, lost a great friend and stimulating leader in November 2000. Donald Reis' tireless dedication to research was truly inspirational, even during his intense personal battle with cancer. Don was still working vigorously in the laboratory until just before his death during surgery. One of Don's major scientific interests was the neural control of blood circulation, which he attacked from every available angle with every available tool. Don played a pivotal role in the inception of our field. In 1984, he returned from a meeting where he heard Pascal Bousquet report that imidazolines but not catecholamine α_2-adrenergic agonists, acted in the ventral brainstem to lower blood pressure. He also heard Daphne Atlas relate the discovery of an unknown substance that displaced ligands from α_2-adrenergic receptors, but was not a catecholamine. He asked many questions: "How is this possible? Are these two findings somehow related?" Then he heard from a new postdoc, one of the editors of the current volume, about a laboratory curiosity ignored up until that point: binding sites for imidazoline radioligands not displaced by catecholamines. Don's keen insight connected these disparate observations. He persuaded the reluctant postdoc to drop everything and work exclusively on imidazoline recognition sites. Don's intuition back in 1984 that great discoveries lay ahead has led us down a long road, culminating now in this third volume on the subject published by the New York Academy of Sciences.

Don's team accomplished a number of breakthroughs, culminating in the purification of an imidazoline binding protein and development of an antiserum against it, and the isolation of agmatine, a new neuromodulator hitherto not recognized to occur in mammals. This work provided the basis for many future studies that have linked imidazoline receptors and agmatine to a variety of cardiovascular and stress-related disorders, as well as leading to the cloning of a novel gene encoding an imidazoline binding protein. Thus, contributions from Don Reis and his laboratory, first reported in 1986 and 1987 and continuing up until his untimely death, left an indelible mark on the field of imidazoline and agmatine research. The editors hope that this volume of the proceedings of the IV International Symposium on Agmatine and Imidazoline Systems is a fitting tribute to Donald J. Reis for his enormous contributions to making our field of research possible, and we dedicate this volume to his memory.

Preface

The IV International Symposium on Agmatine and Imidazoline Systems was held in San Diego, California, from April 9–11, 2003. The opening keynote address focused on the emerging role for imidazoline receptors and agmatine in the cause and/or treatment of mood disorders. This was followed by oral presentations and poster sessions. This volume of the *Annals of the New York Academy of Sciences* includes representative manuscripts from most of the attendees. The range of topics covered is expansive, and the reader is pointed to some key discoveries (e.g., of the endogenous imidazoline receptor agonist, imidazoleacetic acid-ribotide, and the cloning of agmatine's synthetic enzyme) that will appear in other journals. This volume contains discussions of new molecular studies with IRAS and mammalian agmatinase, cell signaling effects of imidazolines on monoamine systems, a pharmacological characterization of agmatine-related agents on enzymes of arginine metabolism, animal behavioral studies of imidazolines and agmatine, human patient studies, a monkey study, and brain autopsy studies related to human diseases.

Since 1998, when the previous international symposium on imidazoline receptors was held in Bonn, Germany, this field has witnessed major developments in the areas of molecular cloning, cell signaling, synthesis of specific ligands, and purification of endogenous ligands (to name but a few topics of interest). For a while it appeared the concept of imidazoline receptors had waned, with reports that transgenic mice with mutant inactivated α_{2A}-adrenergic receptors failed to respond to imidazolines put into the circulation. However, our understanding of the molecular nature of imidazoline binding proteins and related enzymes has greatly expanded in the past five years. In the case of imidazoline-1 receptors, *in vivo* studies have revealed the need for microinjections directly to the brain in order to reveal imidazoline receptor effects in α_2-adrenergic receptor knockouts. Other data, including transfection studies with IRAS cDNA, have revealed a modulatory role for imidazoline receptors on coincidently activated receptors in the same cell, including the α_{2A}-adrenergic and fibronectin receptors. In the case of agmatine, this guanidine-aliphatic-amine seems to be either an endogenous antagonist or inverse agonist at imidazoline receptors, but also has major effects on NMDA receptors and neuronal nitric oxide synthase. Agmatine acts as a neuroprotective agent in brain trauma studies as well as an agent capable of alleviating chronic pain, drug withdrawal syndromes, and inflammatory responses. Furthermore, the potential clinical application of these agents has broadened from the field's earlier focus on hypertension to also now include evidence for treatments of diabetes and related metabolic syndromes, psychiatric stress disorders, neurodegenerative disorders, drug addiction, and neuropathic pain. The recent discoveries and characterization of two more endogenous ligands for imidazoline receptors (harmane, and imidazoleacetic acid-ribotide) have also pointed to the potential therapeutic value of these agents in unexpected areas like brain trauma and neurogenesis. It is hoped that this volume of the *Annals* will serve as a guidepost to further develop the field, much as Volumes 763 and 881 did before it. We are pleased to also announce that the newly elected President of the Imidazoline Receptor Society, Dr. David Nutt, is already planning the next international symposium, to take place in Bristol, England in 2006.

—JOHN E. PILETZ
—SOUNDAR REGUNATHAN
—PAUL ERNSBERGER

Relevance of Imidazoline Receptors and Agmatine to Psychiatry

A Decade of Progress

A. HALARIS[a,b] AND J.E. PILETZ[a,c]

[a]*University of Mississippi Medical Center, Jackson, Mississippi 39216, USA*
[b]*Loyola University Chicago Stitch School of Medicine, Chicago, Illinois 60153, USA*
[c]*Jackson State University, Jackson, Mississippi 39217, USA*

ABSTRACT: The cardiovascular relevance of imidazoline receptors (IR) has received tremendous attention since their discovery in 1984. However, evidence also has accumulated for the relevance of IR and an endogenous ligand, agmatine, to psychiatric disease. Emphasis has been placed on altered levels of the I_1-imidazoline site on human platelets and in human postmortem brain tissue from depressed patients. Attempts at exploring the molecular nature of the I_1 protein have led to the cloning of a protein, IRAS. Based on transfection studies, IRAS seems to be involved in neuronal plasticity events. The I_2 site also appears linked to psychiatric research since some of these sites are localized to a specific domain on monoamine oxidases. Different peptides have been identified by means of an imidazoline-receptor-binding-protein (IRBP) antiserum, and these peptides, some of which appear to be fragments derived from IRAS, undergo changes in platelets and brain commensurate with altered mood states of the subject, notably depressive symptomatology. The search for an endogenous ligand for imidazoline receptor(s) also has led to agmatine, a decarboxylated derivative of arginine. Research on agmatine has mushroomed over the past several years and its measurement in the blood and brain has opened new research opportunities. This novel neurotransmitter interacts with a variety of receptors and has been implicated in mediation of stress responses, analgesia, drug addiction and withdrawal, convulsions, and neuroprotection. Given that IR and agmatine appear involved in a multitude of neurophysiologic and pathologic functions, the potential for new drug development is intriguing.

KEYWORDS: imidazoline receptor platelets; depression; IRAS; P-selectin; agmatine

INTRODUCTION

Bousquet and colleagues[1] were the first to hypothesize the existence of imidazoline receptors (IR). This family of receptors has high affinity for imidazoline-class

Address for correspondence: John E. Piletz, Ph.D., Department of Psychiatry, University of Mississippi Medical Center, 2500 North State Street, Jackson, MS 39216-4505, USA. Voice: 601-982-5898.
e-mail: johnpiletz@yahoo.com

α_2-adrenergic agents but low affinity for known biogenic amines. Imidazoline binding sites (I_1 and I_2 sites) have been characterized in many tissues using radiolabeled imidazoline compounds under conditions that mask α_2-adrenoceptors (α_2AR).[2] The distinction between I_1 and I_2 sites is based on differences in their pharmacology, subcellular localization, and regional distribution.[2] Classical I_1 sites possess high affinity for centrally active antihypertensive drugs, which include clonidine, moxonidine, and rilmenidine.[2] These non-adrenergic clonidine-preferring sites are enriched in plasma membrane preparations.[2,3] I_1 sites are regionally distributed throughout the brain and numerous tissues.[2,4] By comparison, the I_2 site possesses high affinity for idazoxan and its analogues, relative to clonidine-like agents.[5,6] I_2 sites have been shown to reside on monoamine oxidases (MAOs), which are localized to the outer mitochondrial membrane.[7] Three endogenous neurotransmitter candidates have been identified and shown to possess varying affinities for I_1 and I_2 sites. They are a decarboxylated metabolite of arginine, agmatine[8]; a beta-carboline, harmane[9]; and a histamine derivative, imidazole-4-acetic acid-ribotide (Prell *et al.*, presented at this meeting).

Since the inception of the imidazoline receptor field, concerted efforts have been made to separate IR from α_2AR effects in the area of cardiovascular control. Focus has centered on brainstem IR in hopes of circumventing the undesirable side effects of α_2AR-mediated sedation through alternative neural circuits. In support of this hypothesis, the rank-order of antihypertensive potency of clonidine-related drugs is closely correlated with their affinity profile for I_1 binding sites in the rostroventral lateral medulla (RVLM), whereas no such correlation exists between the potencies of these drugs and their affinities at α_2AR sites.[10] Nonetheless, genetic manipulation of the α_{2A}-adrenergic receptor subtype in mice has revealed this subtype's predominant role in numerous responses to imidazolines, including agonist-induced hypotension and sedation.[11] Intriguingly, α_2-agonist treatments of mice heterozygous for an α_{2A}AR knockout mutation (α_2AR +/–) have shown lowered blood pressure without sedation.[12] One interpretation for this finding was that partial activation of α_{2A}AR in wild-type (+/+) animals might be key to the success of certain imidazoline compounds (i.e., agents with partial ability to couple α_{2A}AR occupancy to effector activation might elicit hypotension without sedation). Another interpretation, which most other studies favor,[13,14] is that IR mechanisms depend to some degree on α_2AR activation, but the sole effect of IR activation is best unmasked in heterozygous (α_2AR +/–) mice. Several manuscripts in this volume support an interactive concept for α_2AR and IR. Indeed, studies with α_2AR knockout mice have also revealed a protective role for α_{2A}AR in models of depression and anxiety and that the antidepressant effects of imipramine may be mediated by the α_{2A}AR.[15] Thus, evidence for an interaction between IR and α_2AR is an evolving story.

This review focuses on the role of I_1 and I_2 proteins in mood disorders. It includes a discussion of binding sites as well as related immunoreactive peptides and the endogenous ligands of I_1 and I_2 sites. For instance, one of the more I_1-selective compounds, moxonidine, exerts non-adrenergic behavioral properties in mice consistent with anxiolysis.[16] A number of additional central nervous system (CNS) functions have been suggested for I_1R, the most notable a brainstem role in the modulation of sympathetic outflow.[2,14] Brainstem I_1R may play a role in depression also because altered sympathetic overflow is a manifestation of this disease.[17] Likewise, idazoxan and other I_2 selective compounds have been reported to exhibit antidepressant properties.[18] The antidepressant-like effects of I_2 agents may relate to inhibition of

MAO,[18] which was the first discovered mechanism of antidepressant action. It also should be kept in mind that multiple subforms of I_1 and I_2 sites exist as well as an I_3 subtype identified by pharmacological techniques. A review of the literature indicates the existence of at least three affinity-defined I_1 sites: the classical moxonidine-sensitive I_1 site that may be encoded by IRAS[2,19]; a cirazoline/clonidine-sensitive I-site that exists in kidney, platelets, and brain[20] (Zhu et al. in this volume); and a rilmenidine-sensitive I-site.[21] There are two subclasses of I_2 sites that differ in affinity for amiloride: I_{2A} and I_{2B}.[22] These two subclasses of I_2 sites may correlate with MAO subtypes or with other types of oxidases.[22] Additionally, an I_3 site is found in pancreas, and is insulinotropic.[23] I_3 sites are closely related to the adenosine 5′-triphosphate (ATP)-sensitive potassium channel, Kir6.2.[23] The diverse family of imidazoline binding sites provides fertile ground for new drug discovery.

Recent progress also has been made into the molecular nature of an I_1R protein. A protein named IRAS was cloned[19,24] from a human hippocampal cDNA expression library using antisera directed against a partially purified imidazoline-receptor binding protein (IRBP antiserum).[25] Transfection of IRAS cDNA led to the appearance of I_1-like binding sites in some, but not all, cell lines.[19] Additional studies suggested that formation of classical I_1 sites may require the association of IRAS with another subunit protein.[19] There are currently two candidates for this second subunit of I_1 sites: α-5 integrin[26] and an insulin receptor substrate protein.[27] Indeed, the discovery of these associated proteins of IRAS has led to our current model of I_1R (Piletz in this volume), which is an intrinsically active protein that is modifiable by binding imidazoline and other ligands. Full-length human IRAS migrates as a 170 kD protein under the denaturing conditions of sodium dodecyl sulfate-polyacrylamide gel electrophoresis (SDS-PAGE). The amino acid sequence of IRAS is unique to protein databases and almost certainly not a G-protein coupled receptor.[19] IRAS peptide-specific (anti-epitopic) antisera have been generated in rabbits (Hays et al. in this volume) and shown to mainly detect proteins of 85 kD size and smaller in Western blots of native tissue homogenates.[19] Likewise, IRBP antiserum detects similar proteins of ≤85 kD in native tissues.[28,29] A series of protease protection studies[28,30] (Ma et al. in this volume) also have led to the suggestion that the lower molecular weight peptides of IRAS may constitute normal/active forms of the protein and/or that IRAS exhibits a relatively rapid fragmentation rate. IRBP antiserum has been shown by two independent research teams to identify disease-specific changes in protein levels of Western blot bands from brains[31,32] and platelets of depressed patients.[31,33] These details will be important to remember in the following review of I_1/IRAS in psychiatry.

PLATELET STUDIES OF I-SITES IN DEPRESSION

Human platelets are a readily available, peripheral cell type sharing biochemical properties with CNS serotonergic neurons. Platelets therefore have been studied extensively in depression and other psychiatric conditions. Early studies using platelet preparations in the study of depressive illness focused on $α_2AR$.[34] Presynaptic $α_2AR$ modulate the release of norepinephrine (NE), serotonin (5HT), and other neurotransmitters and are therefore potential targets for antidepressant and anxiolytic drug development. Human platelets also possess I_1 and I_2 subtypes of imidazoline binding sites[3,35] as well as immuno-related 33 kD and 45 kD proteins.[30,31] Our group published the first studies of I_1 binding sites in platelets from depressed patients and compared their binding density and affinity to that of matched healthy control subjects.[36–38] We determined that the density of I_1 binding sites on the plasma membranes of platelets of depressed patients is elevated compared with healthy control subjects. An equally robust finding in those early studies of I_1 sites in depression was their normalization (i.e., down-regulation) following treatment with either of two structurally and pharmacodynamically different antidepressants, namely, desipramine[36,37] and fluoxetine.[38] In a related study, Garcia-Sevilla and colleagues[31] utilized IRBP antiserum to demonstrate an elevation in immunodensity of IR on Western blots from platelets of unipolar depressed patients and from cortical autopsy samples of depressed suicide victims. Platelets from euthymic bipolar patients stabilized on lithium were studied also and shown to exhibit normal IRBP-immunodensities.[39] In one study, treatment with citalopram, clomipramine, or imipramine down-regulated IRBP-immunodensity on platelet membranes of depressed patients.[40] In our follow-up study, bupropion also down-regulated IRBP-immunodensity on platelet membranes of depressed patients after six weeks of treatment.[33] The consistency of these findings with I-sites contrasts with numerous studies of the platelet $\alpha_{2A}AR$ in depression[41] wherein α_2AR density was either unchanged or lower in depressed patients than in matched controls[42] (with the exception of agonist-induced state changes in α_2AR that respond to only the tricyclic class of antidepressants[38,42]). Thus, alterations in platelet I_1 sites and IRBP immunoreactivity are among the most consistent findings of all platelet markers studied thus far in depressed patients.

In one of our detailed studies of platelet I-sites in depression,[33] we chose bupropion as the antidepressant because it is structurally and pharmacodynamically different from all other known antidepressants. We were interested in determining whether the down-regulatory effects observed with the more traditional antidepressants could be replicated with a structurally different antidepressant using the immunodensity assay of platelet I_1 sites. In this way, we sought to establish whether the down-regulation of platelet I_1 sites is a class-specific pharmacological effect or related to clinical antidepressant efficacy. IRBP antiserum was used to quantify I-sites on Western blots of platelet plasma membranes from unipolar depressed subjects before and after 6 weeks of treatment with bupropion.[33] Western blots revealed an increase in IRBP-immunodensity in a 33 kD band in 21 untreated depressed patients as compared to 17 healthy control subjects.[33] The 33 kD band has previously been correlated with I_1 binding sites on platelets.[30] After 6 weeks of bupropion treatment, IRBP-immunodensity was down-regulated in the total group, but the effect was much more pronounced in the subset of treatment responders ($P = 0.005$). Patients nonresponsive to bupropion ($n = 5$) were significantly different from responders by exhibiting no elevation in IRBP-immunodensity at pretreatment and no down-regulation of the 33 kD band after treatment.[33] These results thus provided support to the hypothesis that up-regulation of I_1 receptor sites in untreated unipolar depression and down-regulation upon successful antidepressant treatment may be a state marker for this mood disorder.

In a second study with bupropion,[43] we sought to determine relationships between dosing and timing of the antidepressant agent with down-regulation of platelet I_1 binding sites in depressed patients. We compared two regimens of bupropion—a lower dose and a higher dose—and the patients were treated for 6 or 8 weeks, respectively.[43] The increase in I_1 density on platelet plasma membranes was confirmed at pretreatment.[43] Interestingly, the highest I_1 densities (B_{max}) at pretreatment were found in those patients that subsequently responded worst to treatment (mostly treatment drop-outs). Comparing this finding with our previous study of nonresponders[33] suggests that both abnormally high and low levels of I-sites may be clinically relevant: indicative of intolerance to treatment versus nonresponsivity, respectively. However, the lower regimen of bupropion failed to produce down-regulation even though most patients responded therapeutically.[43] Only the higher bupropion dose (450 mg/day) over an 8-week treatment period led to the expected down-regulation of platelet I_1 sites. Post-treatment I_1 B_{max} values were closely correlated with the plasma bupropion concentrations in the patients. A likely explanation for discrepant results between these two regimens is that at the lower dose of bupropion (300 mg/day) the therapeutic response may have been insufficiently consolidated to elicit the expected platelet I_1 down-regulation. These results have led to the suggestion that the antidepressant-induced down-regulation of platelet I_1 sites probably is a multistep process that lags behind therapeutic response even if the patient already may show a clear antidepressant mood response. We currently are exploring the possibility that platelet I_1 down-regulation may be viewed as a marker of "consolidated" response to treatment and thereby be a marker of reduced likelihood of relapse.

Throughout these studies there always has been concern about the specificity of the platelet I_1 up-regulation, whether it is unique to depressive illness or whether other primary disease entities with or without depressive symptoms also may display an I_1 up-regulation. A similar elevation in platelet I_1 sites has been described in untreated women with dysphoric premenstrual syndrome (PMS).[44] In a follow-up study with newly post-menopausal women, we studied platelet I_1 sites before and after 60 days' treatment with 0.1 mg estradiol transdermal patches.[45] These women were recruited through a psychiatric women's health clinic and were experiencing "change of life" issues (though they did not meet criteria for a mood disorder). Platelet I_1 sites were higher in the postmenopausal women compared to women of reproductive age, and estrogen replacement therapy down-regulated them. The platelet I_1 down-regulatory effect of transdermal estrogen for 60 days[45] was of approximately the same size as in our study of depressed patients using the higher dose of bupropion.[43] Thus, the specificity of the platelet I_1 up-regulatory finding in depression appears to "spillover" to agitated states in women experiencing dysphoric PMS and change of life. However, in another study of patients with generalized anxiety disorder we failed to find an elevation in platelet I_1 sites compared to matched control subjects.[37] Thus, depression and agitation, but not anxiety, are aligned with an elevation in platelet I_1 sites. To our knowledge, there are no other studies with different psychiatric conditions that support or refute the specificity of the I_1 up-regulatory phenomenon in the acute phase of depressive illness.

Another approach to the question of I_1 specificity in depression has been to expose healthy adult volunteers to antidepressant treatment. We conducted a preliminary study with 10 healthy adults. Desipramine was given over 6 weeks to simulate the dosing parameters and conditions used conventionally to treat depressed subjects and to be comparable to our earlier studies of depression.[36,38] Desipramine administration to healthy non-depressed subjects failed to produce down-regulation of platelet I_1 sites after a standard 6-week exposure (unpublished findings). The subjects remained euthymic throughout the course of desipramine treatment, although they did experience some of the side effects (i.e., anticholinergic) of this agent. By comparison to our two earlier studies that showed I_1 down-regulation after desipramine treatment of depressed patients,[36,38] the likely explanation is that platelet I_1 down-regulation is not primarily a pharmacological effect but also requires mood state improvement. Interestingly, platelet α_2AR binding was down-regulated by desipramine during the same course of treatment in the same healthy volunteers (same unpublished study). Thus, an elevation in platelet membrane I_1 sites follows the expectations of a state maker of depression, while the platelet α_2AR seems more like a pharmacologically regulated site, only by the tricyclic class of antidepressants.

By comparison to I_1 research, we could find only two reports[31,41] using clinical patients to study I_2 sites. This is surprising since I_2 sites now are accepted as being allosteric sites on MAOs.[46] Perhaps a reason for the dirth of studies on platelet I_2 sites is that platelet MAO-B activity already has been studied extensively in various types of psychiatric patients without positive findings. Yet, I_2 sites are known to exist in far less than 1:1 ratio with MAO protein amount, and this dichotomy is particularly pronounced in platelets.[47] Therefore, it seems that more than two studies should exist on platelet I_2 sites in depressed patients. In a small study of nine depressed patients, we reported[41] a lower-than-control level of [^{3}H]-idazoxan binding to the platelet I_2 site at pretreatment, which was up-regulated after antidepressant therapy.[41] However, Garcia-Sevilla *et al.* have reported[31] that a 45 kD IRBP band associated with I_2 sites is up-regulated in depressed patients at pretreatment and down-regulated after treatment. Thus, the only two clinical studies on I_2 sites in platelets stand at odds. More clarification of the role of I_2 sites in psychiatry will be mentioned below.

In summary, platelet studies to date have yielded considerable evidence for an elevation in membranous I_1 sites being linked with the state of depression. However, little information exists about whether the reported changes are specific for one subtype or another of the affective disorders, or, for that matter, for one or more specific symptoms of the affective symptomatology spectrum. However, we did present a preliminary report on significant correlations between the endogenomorphic and psychomotor retardation clusters of depression extracted from the Hamilton Depression Rating Scale, which correlated with platelet $I_1R\ B_{max}$ and platelet 33 kD IRBP immunodensity in one of our patient studies.[48] The question of specificity remains an area of active study.

IMIDAZOLINE-1 RECEPTORS IN BRAIN

Although platelet studies are a valuable tool to assess peripheral receptor function in relation to clinical symptoms, there always is concern about engaging in unfounded extrapolations to the human brain. We therefore were interested in transferring the same methodology we had developed for platelet I-sites to human postmortem brain obtained from individuals who died by suicide and had a documented history of depression. The hippocampus was of primary interest to us because this limbic structure is thought to be involved in mood, learning, and memory. A precedent study of prefrontal cortex (PFC) from depressed suicide patients existed before we began our study.[31] That study showed that the immunodensity of IRBP bands is altered in the

PFC of depressed suicide victims. From that study, we hypothesized that hippocampal proteins on Western blots also might contain a 29/30 kD IRBP cluster of bands with decreased immunoreactivity in MDD subjects relative to controls, and a 45 kD IRBP band that would be increased in MDD subjects compared to controls.

We next conducted a study of human hippocampi to compare Western blots from subjects with depression versus subjects without depression at the time of death, using IRBP antiserum.[32] Toxicological findings revealed no antidepressants or antipsychotic compounds in the blood, urine, or bile of any subjects in our study. Postmortem diagnoses were obtained also for all subjects, yielding 17 cases with Axis I Major Depressive Disorder (MDD) and 17 cases without any evidence of Axis I psychopathology (controls). Hippocampal samples then were sectioned from anatomically defined brain regions. These were assessed histologically to ensure identical levels of the brain between subjects. Adjacent sections then were scraped from the slides for Western blotting. Subjects were paired for postmortem delay and age throughout the entire procedure; that is, each MDD sample was paired for SDS-PAGE and Western blotting with a control sample based on nearly identical life spans and postmortem delays. The first finding was that the expected 29/30 kD cluster of bands reported in PFC[31] was not seen. Instead, a triad of IRBP bands of 40 to 50 kD was detected in all hippocampi. Our main finding was that MDD subjects showed significantly lower immunodensity of the 40 to 50 kD IRBP bands compared to controls ($P = 0.01$).[32] This finding agrees with lowered 29/30 kD bands in the PFC of depressed suicide victims,[31,41] although the hippocampal IRBP cluster is of higher molecular weight than the 29/30 kD cluster reported in PFC. Considering that these IRBP bands are likely all breakdown products of IRAS (Ma *et al.* in this volume), it is conceivable that the same parent protein (IRAS) was under study in PFC and hippocampus in the two studies, except that they were fragmented differently. Therefore, we believe the results from these two studies generally agree in showing lower than normal IRBP in brains from depressed patients.[31,32] The findings are, of course, opposite to other findings of elevated IRBP in platelets of depressed patients. Two possible explanations for this paradox may lie in the differing pathophysiologic milieu that platelets and brain are exposed to in depressed patients as well as in the nature of IRAS itself (elaborated below).

Of course, it is one thing to establish that levels of I_1/IRAS vary with the high and low mood swings of subjects, and it is another thing to speculate whether such proteins actually participate in the neuronal modulation of an affective disorder. Insight into this question may be derived from animal studies on the behavioral properties of imidazoline agents. Moxonidine is a centrally active imidazoline compound with preferential affinity for I_1R over α_2AR.[49] Vandergriff and coworkers reported[50] that moxonidine selectively suppresses acoustic startle responses in rats during ethanol withdrawal by acting in an I_1R selective manner. Injection of clonidine at doses threefold higher than moxonidine did not elicit a similar suppression of the acoustic startle response associated with ethanol withdrawal.[50] Their interpretation was that preferential I_1R activation by moxonidine, over clonidine, suppresses the startle response. Clinically, moxonidine is advantageous for treating hypertension over clonidine and pure α_2-adrenergic agonists (i.e., guanabenz) due to its lowered incidence of sedative side effects. Guanabenz is a non-imidazoline α_2-agonist that crosses the blood brain barrier and lowers blood pressure, but with profound sedation. We recently reported[16] divergent behavioral effects of low doses of moxonidine and guanabenz in C57Bl/6 mice placed in an exploratory arena. Low-dose moxonidine (0.05 mg/kg i.p.) elicited an increase in novel object contacts (+36%) and more movement into open space (+56%; $P < 0.01$) compared to saline-injected controls By contrast, guanabenz induced only dose-responsive sedative-like behaviors in the same paradigm. Importantly, these two agonists were indistinguishable in terms of blood pressure changes over a similar dose-response range (0.025 to 0.1 mg/kg i.p.) in consciously free-moving C57Bl/6 mice (Δ mean ± SEM = –12.3 ± 3.2 mm Hg for moxonidine vs. –13.5 ± 1.9 mm Hg for guanabenz). As expected of α_2AR involvement, the sedative-like effects of guanabenz were completely blocked by pretreatment with the non-imidazoline α_2-antagonist, SKF86466 (0.5 or 1.0 mg/kg i.p.). However, the pro-exploratory effects of two low doses of moxonidine (0.05 or 0.1 mg/kg) were not antagonized by SKF86466. These results suggest that moxonidine acts preferentially through a non-adrenergic mechanism, possibly I_1R, to elicit pro-exploratory behavior. Moxonidine's ability to induce ventures into the central area of an exploratory arena could be interpreted as anxiolytic.

VISUALIZATION OF IMIDAZOLINE RECEPTOR SITES IN BRAIN

De Vos and coworkers were first to visualize the binding of [^{3}H]-clonidine to I_1–like sites in the brain by means of autoradiography.[51] In their study of human brain, clear-cut regional and affinity differences were apparent between the non-adrenergic I-sites labeled by [^{3}H]-clonidine and I_2 sites labeled by [^{3}H]-idazoxan. Their study further delineated the difference between these I-sites and adrenergic sites labeled with an α_2AR-selective [^{3}H]-antagonist, RX821002. A modification of the De Vos method then was developed by our group to ensure differentiation from a possible agonist-induced sub-state of the α_2AR that also binds [^{3}H]-clonidine.[52] Using our slight modification of the De Vos method, we compared by autoradiography the distribution of adrenergic agonist sites versus non-adrenergic sites for [^{3}H]-clonidine across 27 brain regions. Special attention was given to the hippocampus because our postmortem study of depressed subjects had revealed a decrease in IR immunodensity by Western blotting.[32] Pharmacological rank ordering of affinities was performed also for the I-sites labeled by [^{3}H]-clonidine in caudate sections. Our first finding was that the localization of [^{3}H]-clonidine-labeled I-sites in the human hippocampus was not representative of an agonist state of the α_2-adrenergic receptor family. Our second finding was that this unique I-site could not qualify completely as a classical I_1 site.[52] Instead, this site corresponded to the [^{3}H]-cirazoline I-site described by Angel and coworkers.[20] Much more information on the possible interrelationship of this clonidine/cirazoline-preferring I-site with classical I_1 sites can be found in this volume of the *Annals* (Zhu *et al.*).

Having established the autoradiographic technique, we were next interested in determining whether the [^{3}H]-clonidine-labeled I-sites visualized in brain autoradiograms could provide more information about the previously seen deficiency of IRBP bands reported in hippocampi[32] and in prefrontal cortices[31] of depressed suicide victims. We therefore undertook a second imaging study to apply our modified autoradiographic technique with [^{3}H]-clonidine to characterize differentially α_2AR and I-sites in two brain regions of depressed subjects versus matched controls.[53] In this study, left orbitofrontal cortex (OFC) from the Brodmann's area[47] and right amygdala were obtained from depressed victims of suicide versus matched controls. The choice of amygdala was based on an earlier report[54] showing reciprocal alterations between the amygdala and OFC in terms of resting blood flow and glucose metabolism in mood disorders. We first observed that the amounts of binding of [^{3}H]-clonidine to α_2AR (OFC > amygdala) and I-sites (amygdala > OFC) were reciprocal between the two brain regions regardless of depressed or control subject groups. This difference between OFC and amygdala seems to fit a concept of reciprocity of activity between opposite ends of a cortical-limbic circuit, as described by other investigators and noted earlier in this article. The second finding was a tendency across L1-L6 OFC layers for α_2AR sites to be lower and I-sites to be higher in depressed subjects compared to controls. This resulted in a very clear result ($P = 0.007$) of a reduced ratio of α_2AR: I-sites in the OFC of depressed subjects versus controls. In fact, the α_2AR: I-site ratios of the depressed subject group was nearly half that of the control subjects in all six layers of the OFC. This finding also was regionally specific since no changes in the α_2AR:I-site ratio were noted in the amygdala of depressed subjects. We have interpreted these findings to indicate that alterations occur in both α_2AR and I-sites in depression, and that the two receptors in some manner might be expressed reciprocally. At the same time, we did not confirm our expectation that I-sites under autoradiographic scrutiny would be decreased in brains of depressed suicide victims, just as reports of IRBP immunodensity have shown.[31,32] The reason for this is unclear.

Taken together, the findings of our group and those described by other investigators[31] provide ample evidence for I_1R alterations in mood disorders, at least in the primary major unipolar type of depressive illness. If platelets are a suitable model, the fact that the rise in IR density observed at baseline (untreated-depressed state) is reversible with successful antidepressant therapy suggests that level changes in I_1R in depression are probably state-dependent effects.

BRAIN I_2 SITES

I_2 sites are of interest to psychiatry because they are encoded by MAO-A and MAO-B. An I_2 binding site was localized within a 73 amino acid sequence of MAO-B.[7] This I_2 site lies outside the catalytic domain proposed for MAO-B enzymatic inhibition, but a point mutation within the same region causes complete loss of MAO-B activity.[55] Most currently available I_2-selective ligands have been shown to act as allosteric inhibitors of both MAO isozymes,[46] a known antidepressant mechanism. Accordingly, Nutt and coworkers have reported[18] that the I_2-selective agent, 2-BFI, has a similar antidepressant effect as desipramine in the rat forced swim test. They also reported that idazoxan and 2BFI—but not selective alpha$_2$ antagonists—will increase food intake in nonfood-deprived rats.[18] The currently available I_2 ligands nonetheless may not reach development as antidepressants in humans because they require μmol/L range concentrations to achieve MAO inhibition.[46] More potent I_2 ligands therefore must be developed for antidepressant trials.

There is additional evidence that I_2 sites are linked to depression. Chronic treatment of naïve rats, in vivo, with any of the "irreversible" MAO inhibitors, phenelzine, isocarboxazid, clorgyline, or tranylcypromine, markedly reduces the density of I_2 sites in rat brain and liver as measured by non-adrenergic [^{3}H]-idazoxan binding.[56] Similarly, the tricyclic antidepressant, imipramine, up-regulated I_2 sites in rat brain after chronic administration.[57] These findings indicate that I_2 sites are regulated under antidepressant treatments.

To understand fully the postmortem studies of I_2 sites, it should be realized that not all I_2 sites are consistent with MAO-A or MAO-B molecules. MAO proteins have molecular weights around 55 kD. However, some I_2 sites have been associated with a 29/30 kD IRBP cluster in brain.[58] Correlations have been established between the immuno-intensities of the 29/30 kD IRBP bands versus B_{max} values for I_2 sites across several rat and human tissues and after different regulatory conditions.[58] Furthermore, a 70 kD non-adrenergic protein from bovine adrenal chromaffin cell membranes has been partially purified by binding to idazoxan affinity columns,[59] which also appears to be a non-MAO I_2 protein. By contrast, 33, 45, and 85 kD bands detected by IRBP antiserum have been correlated with I_1 sites in human tissues.[28,60] Thus, there is still some uncertainty about the molecular nature of these I_2 sites. Nonetheless, studies have shown that I_2 sites labeled by [^{3}H]-idazoxan are decreased in frontal cortices of depressed suicide victims.[61] This is the same as the 29/30 kD cluster of IRBP immunodensity, which also is decreased in frontal cortices of depressed suicide victims.[31,60,61]

INTEGRINS, IMIDAZOLINE RECEPTORS, AND PLATELET ACTIVATION

Extracellular matrix proteins (EMP) and their receptors, the integrins, actively participate in the control of many fundamental cellular functions in platelets and in the developing nervous system. EMP-integrin interactions regulate cell migration, differentiation, and survival and the control of neurite outgrowth. After development, integrin signaling in the nervous system has commonly been misconstrued to be a static system of little importance to regulation of neuronal function. However, it has been demonstrated recently that integrins and their ligands are actually capable of rapid neuromodulatory actions in mature neurons.[62] Wildering and coworkers[62] showed that integrin ligands can alter neuronal pacemaker properties, intracellular free Ca^{2+} levels, and voltage-gated Ca^{2+} currents in a matter of minutes. The discovery that the murine form of IRAS, named Nischarin, interacts with the integrin alpha5 protein[26] might not be viewed as a mere curiosity far removed from I_1R function, since IRAS also binds to imidazoline agents.[19]

The purview of this article does not permit a full discussion of Nischarin, the murine form of IRAS.[26] Suffice it to say that Nischarin is anchored to the intracellular side of the plasma membrane by binding to the cytoplasmic tail of the integrin alpha5 subunit of the fibronectin receptor. It is known also that the interaction of Nischarin with the integrin alpha5 protein mediates cell shape change.[26] We believe these findings apply directly to IRAS because the two species homologues are 100% identical in amino acid sequence over the domain identified to bind the integrin alpha5 protein.[26] This finding has been seminal in our understanding of IRAS, and based on it we have recently hypothesized that IRAS is an intrinsically active protein that mediates integrin signaling in a manner that is modifiable by imidazolines and other ligands (Musgrave *et al.* in this volume). Furthermore, the discovery that IRAS binds to a subunit of the fibronectin receptor (the alpha5 integrin subunit) has caused us to rethink the earlier findings of altered levels of IRBP in platelets and brains from depressed subjects.[31–33] IRBP antiserum led to the cloning of IRAS, and at least some IRBP bands are derived from IRAS. The platelet fibronectin receptor, known also as glycoprotein GPIc-IIa (alpha 5-beta 1), is involved in platelet adhesion and thrombus growth on damaged subendothelium through interactions with fibronectin, fibrinogen, von Willebrand factor, and other adhesive proteins.[63,64] Thus, IRAS probably is functionally important to platelet adhesion and thrombus growth. From this understanding, we began to wonder if the elevation in plasma membrane-bound IRBP in depressed patients might reflect heightened platelet activation in depression.

We chose to investigate platelet p-selectin as a possible marker in our studies of depression because this protein is a procoagulant platelet marker. p-selectin also is known as CD62 protein, GMP140, or PADGEM. p-selectin translocates to the plasma membrane after activation-dependent alpha granule release (i.e., platelet degranulation). Thus, p-selectin measured on platelet plasma membranes is an index of platelet activation.[65] In platelet research, another intrinsic membrane protein known as β3-integrin immunoreactivity (antigen CD61) often is used as a reference because it is not activation-dependent.[66] By calculating the ratio of these two proteins (CD62:CD61) on platelet plasma membranes, one obtains an index of platelet activation. Musselman and colleagues[67,68] were first to use monoclonal antibodies to these proteins (as well as other markers) to identify changes in platelet procoagulant state in depressed patients. There are compelling reports in the literature linking ischemic heart disease (IHD) and cardiac mortality to depressive illness.[69–72] Threefold higher mortality rates have been reported for heart attack patients who became depressed in the immediate post-myocardial infarction period, compared to patients who did not experience clinical depression after their myocardial infarction.[73] A common denominator in IHD and depression may be stress and associated changes in stress hormones that render platelets procoagulant in both conditions.[74] It is well accepted that stressful life events and the onset of major depression are correlated, depressed subjects experience higher amounts of stress due to their illness, and myocardial infarction patients undergo severe stress due to loss of health, limitations in normal activity, and a potentially fatal outcome. Thus, we sought to replicate the findings of Musselman et al.[67,68]

As an ancillary study to our earlier study of platelet I-sites in depressed patients treated with bupropion (described earlier in this article[33,43]), we examined p-selectin immunoreactivity. The choice of bupropion was important because this antidepressant does not appreciably alter plasma concentrations of NE or 5HT, both of which can induce platelet degranulation. We found that p-selectin was increased significantly in platelet plasma membrane fractions from depressed patients analyzed by Western blotting.[75] The elevation in p-selectin also remained significantly higher than in untreated control subjects after 6 to 8 weeks of bupropion treatment.[75] Moreover, the elevation in p-selectin was significant whether or not the patient had responded to treatment.[75] By contrast, no changes were noted in the amount of β3-integrin (CD61) in the same samples compared to controls. It was concluded that platelets are more procoagulant in depression. Furthermore, the elevation in platelet p-selectin behaved as a *trait* marker of depression. Of particular importance will be to establish whether normalization of the p-selectin elevation in depression lags behind mood improvement as did the normalization of I_1 binding sites.[43] It also will be necessary to determine if other antidepressants fail to induce normalization of the elevation in platelet p-selectin in patients treated for depression. In any case, these results give credence to the possibility that an elevation in platelet IRBP may be related to a heightened state of platelet activation in depression.

AGMATINE: A NOVEL NEUROTRANSMITTER

Agmatine (1-amino-4-guanidinobutane) is derived from the enzymatic decarboxylation of arginine. While attempting to isolate an endogenous "clonidine-displacing substance" for imidazoline receptors, the formation of agmatine was discovered as an alternative pathway for arginine metabolism in the brain.[8] The enzyme responsible for the formation of agmatine is arginine decarboxylase (ADC), and it is found in significant amounts in the rat and bovine brain. Agmatine is widely, yet unevenly, distributed in many tissues.[76,77] ADC resides on mitochondrial membranes and functions in direct competition for substrate (arginine) with enzymes that produce nitric oxide (NO) and polyamines in the brain. Yet, agmatine is more than an alternative to NO on at least three counts: (1) Agmatine at micromolar concentrations irreversibly inhibits nitric oxide synthase (NOS) as demonstrated by in vitro[78] and in vivo studies.[79] (2) Agmatine is packaged into and released from synaptic vesicles whereby it interacts with *trans*membrane receptors.[80] At the receptor level, agmatine acts as an antagonist at least at NMDA-glutamatergic receptors.[81,82] A proposed antagonistic effect of agmatine at imidazoline receptors[83] prompted us to investigate its possible relevance to the pathophysiology of depression (described below). (3) Agmatine is hydrolyzed by the enzyme agmatinase (agmatine uryl hydrolase) to form putrescine, a polyamine and precursor of the growth-promoting polyamines. Rat brain and macrophages express agmatinase, revealing an additional pathway for mammalian polyamine biosynthesis.[84]

It now is accepted that agmatine meets most of the conventional criteria for neurotransmitter status.[80] What, then, is its predominant physiological role in normal brain function? This question remains unclear because there are no pharmacological tools to manipulate its endogenous levels. However, based on studies with the exogenous administration of agmatine, a number of functions have been connected with agmatine that point to potential therapeutic actions of this compound. They are:

(1) Ligand channel blocker: Agmatine can act as antagonist at certain ligand-gated Ca^{++} channels, such as the nicotinic cholinergic and $5-HT_3$ channels.[85,86]
(2) Hormone secretagogue: Agmatine facilitates the release of catecholamines from adrenal chromaffin cells,[8] insulin from pancreatic β cells,[87] and luteinizing hormone releasing hormone from hypothalamus.[88] Agmatine also inhibits the release of NE from presynaptic terminals.[89]
(3) Anti-inflammatory agent: Agmatine can inhibit the induction of inducible NOS (iNOS) by inflammatory stimuli.[90,91]

Based on the findings summarized above—and this is by no means an exhaustive review of the pertinent literature—agmatine appears to have relevance to neurological, and possibly psychiatric, disorders. In particular, agmatine administration may have therapeutic value in the following conditions:

(1) Neuroprotection: Administered intrathecally or even systemically, agmatine reduces neuronal loss produced by ischemia[92–94] or by excitotoxins.[81] The exact mechanism for this neuroprotective effect still eludes us, but it may relate to agmatine's ability to inhibit iNOS and to block the NMDA receptor and also voltage-dependent Ca^{++} channels, since blockade of these signaling proteins is neuroprotective.

(2) Pain control and morphine tolerance: Agmatine has been shown to be analgesic in chronic pain models. Intrathecally administered agmatine can relieve experimentally induced chronic pain.[95] Agmatine also will block the development of morphine tolerance and naloxone-precipitated signs of morphine withdrawal.[96,97] These effects may relate to agmatine's antagonism of NOS and/or NMDA receptors in neurons.[98]

(3) Drug withdrawal: Aricioglu-Kartal and Uzbay[96] demonstrated that single injections of agmatine into adult rats can attenuate all signs of naloxone-precipitated abstinence symptoms after morphine implantation. Li et al.[99] reported similar findings in mice. Uzbay et al.[100] obtained impressive attenuation of the withdrawal effects of alcohol with a single agmatine dose given to rats fed a liquid ethanol diet for 21 days. It was concluded that peripheral injections of agmatine dose-dependently attenuated drug withdrawal symptoms in animals. To our knowledge, these findings have not been tested in human subjects.

(4) Stress reduction: An "anti-stress effect" of agmatine was first reported by Stewart and McKay.[101] These investigators determined that peripheral injection of agmatine to rats prior to contextual fear conditioning impaired the acquisition of contextual fear, which was measured as defensive freezing 26 hours later. The data of Stewart and McKay suggested that low endogenous agmatine concentrations, probably in the hippocampus, might be permissive for acquisition of and/or consolidation of contextual fear stimuli. More recently, a report by Zomkoski et al.[102] showed that agmatine administration to mice produced "antidepressant-like effects" in two stress models of mice. The effects were dose-dependent and without accompanying changes in ambulation in an open field test. Antidepressant-like effects of agmatine were observed also in a forced swim test following intracerebroventricular administration of agmatine. In that same study, agmatine co-administered with a known antidepressant (imipramine) enhanced the anti-immobility effect of imipramine. While one could deduce a synergistic effect of agmatine along with imipramine, the precise mechanism by which agmatine produces these anti-anxiety and/or antidepressant-like effects still eludes us.

PLASMA AGMATINE IN DEPRESSION

Our laboratory developed a high-performance liquid chromatographic assay for the measurement of plasma agmatine.[76] This method was then applied to the measurement of agmatine in plasma of depressed patients who participated in our study with bupropion.[103] We were only able to obtain plasma from patients on the lower regimen of bupropion (300 mg/day), as described above. Plasma concentrations of agmatine were elevated significantly in depressed patients as compared to healthy subjects; mean plasma concentrations were 38.5 ± 5.4 ng/mL in healthy controls compared to 70.6 ± 6.5 ng/mL in depressed subjects ($P = 0.004$).[103] Following bupropion treatment, plasma agmatine concentrations were reduced to a mean value of 57.0 ± 6.7 ng/mL. This represented a decline of 19%, but the difference between post-treatment and pre-treatment values did not reach statistical significance ($P = 0.17$). Compared to plasma agmatine concentrations in the healthy control group, the post-bupropion agmatine levels in the depressed patient group remained marginally higher ($P = 0.065$). It is possible that if the bupropion regimen had been of a higher dose (450 mg/day) or had been extended longer than 6 weeks, then post-treatment agmatine values might have been identical to those of the healthy controls. Also noteworthy were two nonresponders to bupropion treatment who had plasma agmatine concentrations of 83.8 to 84.4 ng/mL at pre-treatment, compared to post-treatment values of 36.2 to 55.4 ng/mL. Thus, bupropion led to a normalization of plasma agmatine levels even when it did not relieve depressive symptoms. An additional finding was no correlation between plasma bupropion concentrations and plasma agmatine concentrations, or between plasma bupropion concentrations and change scores from pre- to post-treatment for plasma agmatine. To our knowledge, this is the only clinical study published on agmatine levels. If the study can be replicated, the results would indicate that plasma agmatine is elevated in depression and that, following acute treatment with an antidepressant, agmatine concentrations return to normal.

CONCLUSIONS

This article provides a summary of psychiatrically relevant research on imidazoline receptor sites and agmatine in brain and platelets conducted over the past 10 years. In animal studies, administration of imidazoline-selective agents and agmatine has uncovered unique behavioral effects that hopefully will lead to further drug development. In postmortem studies, I_2- and I_1-like sites have been visualized in areas of the brain involved in mood regulation. Clinical studies have been fairly reproducible in showing changes in I_1R regulation occurring in brain and platelets of depressed patients. Based on platelet measurements before and after antidepressant treatments, the changing levels of an I_1 site—and possibly an I_2 site—appear to fulfill state marker criteria for the unipolar subtype of depression. However, there remain a number of unresolved questions pertaining to the relationship among various IRBP bands that have been identified in platelets and brain. We have drawn attention to the use of IRBP antiserum to clone an I_1 binding protein, IRAS; and in so doing, attempted to interpret the literature on IRBP as literature on various peptide fragments of IRAS. IRBP bands have been found altered in depressed patients, in many cases in a manner that parallels changes in their related I_1 and I_2 binding sites. The fact that IRAS is linked to fibronectin signaling further suggests that elevations in platelet I_1 sites and IRBP in depressed patients may be linked to the known susceptibility these patients have for coronary artery disease. The potential for a rise in platelet p-selectin to become a vulnerability marker for depression also merits further exploration. In the brain, changes in IRBP/IRAS may relate to integrin-mediated neuroplasticity effects. Clearly, more work remains to establish the range of mood disorders that lead to up-regulation in platelets and brain of IRBP and I_1 density. In summary, the potential for imidazoline receptor sites to serve as a state marker for at least the unipolar subtype of depression looks rather promising. Finally, agmatine appears to hold great promise as a therapeutic agent for eliciting neuroprotection and for minimizing drug withdrawal, stress-related symptoms, chronic pain, and morphine tolerance. The therapeutic potential of agmatine is just beginning to be assessed.

ACKNOWLEDGMENT

This research was supported by federal grants MH49248 and MH57601.

REFERENCES

1. BOUSQUET, P., J. FELDMAN & J. SCHWARTZ. 1984. Central cardiovascular effects of alpha-adrenergic drugs: differences between catecholamines and imidazolines. J. Pharmacol. Exp. Ther. **230:** 232–236.
2. ERNSBERGER, P., M.E. GRAVES, L.M. GRAFF, et al. 1995. I1-Imidazoline receptors: Definition, characterization, distribution and transmembrane signaling. Ann. N. Y. Acad. Sci. **763:** 22–42.
3. PILETZ, J.E. & K. SLETTEN. 1993. Nonadrenergic imidazoline binding sites on human platelets. J. Pharmacol. Exp. Ther. **267:** 1493–1502.
4. PILETZ, J.E., J.C. JONES, H. ZHU, et al. 1999. Imidazoline receptor antisera-selected cDNA clone and mRNA distribution. Ann. N. Y. Acad. Sci. **881:** 1–7.
5. PARINI, A., C.G. MOUDANOS, N. PIZZINAT, et al. 1996. The elusive family of imidazoline binding sites. Trends Pharmacol. Sci. **17:** 13–16.
6. TESSON, F., I. LIMON-BOULEZ, P. URBAN, et al. 1995. Localization of I2-imidazoline binding sites on monoamine oxidases. J. Biol. Chem. **270:** 9856–9861.
7. RADDATZ, R., A. PARINI & S.M. LANIER. 1997. Localization of the imidazoline binding domain on monoamine oxidase B. Mol. Pharmacol. **52:** 549–553.
8. LI, G., S. REGUNATHAN, C.J. BARROW, et al. 1994. Agmatine: an endogenous clonidine-displacing substance in the brain. Science **263:** 966–969.
9. HUDSON, A., R. PRICE, R.J. TYACKE, et al. 1999. Harmane, norharmane and tetrahydro beta-carboline have high affinity for rat imidazoline binding sites. Br. J. Pharmacol. **126:** 2P.
10. ERNSBERGER, P., R. GIULIANO, R.N. WILLETTE, et al. 1990. Role of imidazole receptors in the vasodepressor response to clonidine analogs in the rostral ventrolateral medulla. J. Pharmacol. Exp. Ther. **253:** 408–418.
11. MACMILLAN, L.B., L. HEIN, M.S. SMITH, et al. 1996. Central hypotensive effects of the alpha-2A adrenergic receptor subtype. Science **273:** 801–803.
12. TAN, C.M., M.H. WILSON, L.B. MACMILLAN, et al. 2002. Heterozygous alpha 2A-adrenergic receptor mice unveil unique therapeutic benefits of partial agonists. Proc. Natl. Acad. Sci. U. S. A. **99:** 12471–12476.
13. HEAD, G.A., S.L. BURKE & F.J. SANNAJUST. 2001. Involvement of imidazoline receptors in the baroreflex effects of rilmenidine in conscious rabbits. J. Hypertens. **19:** 1615–1624.
14. BRUBAN, V., V. ESTATO, S. SCHANN, et al. 2002. Evidence for synergy between alpha(2)-adrenergic and nonadrenergic mechanisms in central blood pressure regulation. Circulation **105:** 1116–1121.
15. SCHRAMM, N.L., M.P. MCDONALD & L.E. LIMBIRD. 2001. The alpha(2A)-adrenergic receptor plays a protective role in mouse behavioral models of depression and anxiety. J. Neurosci. **21:** 4875–4882.
16. ZHU, H., I.A. PAUL, D.E. STEC, et al. 2003. Non-adrenergic exploratory behavior induced by moxonidine at mildly hypotensive doses. Brain Res. **964:** 9–20.
17. PILETZ, J.E., M. ANDREW, H. ZHU, et al. 1998. Alpha 2-adrenoceptors and I1-imidazoline binding sites: relationship with catecholamines in women of reproductive age. J. Psychiatr. Res. **32:** 55–64.

18. NUTT, D.J., N. FRENCH, S. HANDLEY, et al. 1995. Functional studies of specific imidazoline-2 receptor ligands. Ann. N. Y. Acad. Sci. **763:** 125–139.
19. PILETZ, J.E., T.R. IVANOV, J.D. SHARP, et al. 2000. Imidazoline receptor antisera-selected (IRAS) cDNA: cloning and characterization. DNA Cell Biol. **19:** 319–329.
20. ANGEL, I., M. LE ROUZIC, C. PIMOULE, et al. 1995. [^{3}H]cirazoline as a tool for the characterization of imidazoline sites. Ann. N. Y. Acad. Sci. **763:** 112–124.
21. HOSSEINI, A.R., G.P. JACKMAN, P.R. KING, et al. 1998. Pharmacology and subcellular distribution of [^{3}H]rilmenidine binding sites in rat brain. J. Auton. Nervous Sys. **72:** 129–136.
22. OLMOS, G., R. ALEMANY, M.A. BORONAT, et al. 1999. Pharmacologic and molecular discrimination of I2-imidazoline receptor subtypes. Ann. N. Y. Acad. Sci. **881:** 144–160.
23. MONKS, L.K., K.E. COSGROVE, M.J. DUNNE, et al. 1999. Affinity isolation of imidazoline binding proteins from rat brain using 5-amino-efaroxan as a ligand. FEBS Lett. **447:** 61–64.
24. IVANOV, T.R., J.C. JONES, M. DONTENWILL, et al. 1998. Characterization of a partial cDNA clone detected by imidazoline receptor-selective antisera. J. Auton. Nerv. Syst. **72:** 98–110.
25. WANG, H., S. REGUNATHAN, D.A. RUGGIERO, et al. 1993. Production and characterization of antibodies specific for the imidazoline receptor protein. Mol. Pharmacol. **43:** 509–515.
26. ALAHARI, S.K., J.W. LEE & R.L. JULIANO. 2000. Nischarin, a novel protein that interacts with the integrin alpha5 subunit and inhibits cell migration. J. Cell Biol. **151:** 1141–1154.
27. SANO, H., S.C. LIU, W.S. LANE, et al. 2002. Insulin receptor substrate 4 associates with the protein IRAS. J. Biol. Chem. **23:** 23–33.
28. IVANOV, T.R., H. ZHU, S. REGUNATHAN, et al. 1998. Co-detection by two imidazoline receptor protein antisera of a novel 85 kilodalton protein. Biochem. Pharmacol. **55:** 649–655.
29. ESCRIBA, P.V., A. OZAITA & J.A. GARCIA-SEVILLA. 1999. Pharmacologic characterization of imidazoline receptor proteins identified by immunologic techniques and other methods. Ann. N. Y. Acad. Sci. **881:** 8–25.
30. IVANOV, T.R., Y. FENG, H. WANG, et al. 1998. Imidazoline receptor proteins are regulated in platelet-precursor MEG-01 cells by agonists and antagonists. J. Psychiatr. Res. **32:** 65–79.
31. GARCIA-SEVILLA, J.A., P.V. ESCRIBA, M. SASTRE, et al. 1996. Immunodetection and quantitation of imidazoline receptor proteins in platelets of patients with major depression and in brains of suicide victims. Arch. Gen. Psychiatry **53:** 803–810.
32. PILETZ, J.E., H. ZHU, G. ORDWAY, et al. 2000. Imidazoline receptor proteins are decreased in the hippocampus of individuals with major depression. Biol. Psychiatry **48:** 910–919.
33. ZHU, H., A. HALARIS, S. MADAKASIRA, et al. 1999. Effect of bupropion on immunodensity of putative imidazoline receptors on platelets of depressed patients. J. Psychiatr. Res. **33:** 323–333.
34. GARCIA-SEVILLA, J.A., A.P. ZIS, P.J. HOLLINGSWORTH, et al. 1981. Platelet alpha-2 adrenergic receptors in major depressive disorder. Arch. Gen. Psychiatry **38:** 1327–1333.
35. PILETZ, J.E., A.C. ANDORN, J.R. UNNERSTALL, et al. 1991. Binding of [^{3}H]-p-aminoclonidine to a2-adrenoceptor states plus a non-adrenergic site on human platelet plasma membranes. Biochem. Pharmacol. **42:** 569–584.
36. PILETZ, J.E., A. HALARIS, A. SARAN, et al. 1991. Desipramine lowers [^{3}H]-para-aminoclonidine binding in platelets of depressed patients. Arch. Gen. Psychiatry **48:** 813–820.
37. PILETZ, J.E., A. HALARIS, J. NELSON, et al. 1996. Platelet I1-imidazoline binding sites are elevated in depression but not generalized anxiety disorder. J. Psychiatric Res. **30:** 147–168.
38. PILETZ, J.E., A.E. HALARIS, D. CHIKKALA, et al. 1996. Platelet I-1 imidazoline binding sites are decreased by two dissimilar antidepressant agents in depressed patients. J. Psychiatric Res. **30:** 169–184.

39. GARCIA-SEVILLA, J.A., P.V. ESCRIBA, A. OZAITA, et al. 1998. Density of imidazoline receptors in platelets of euthymic patients with bipolar affective disorder and in brains of lithium-treated rats. Biol. Psychiatry **43:** 616–618.
40. GARCIA-SEVILLA, J.A., P.V. ESCRIBA, X. BUSQUETS, et al. 1996. Platelet imidazoline receptors and regulatory G proteins in patients with major depression. Neuroreport **8:** 169–172.
41. PILETZ, J.E., A. HALARIS & P.R. ERNSBERGER. 1994. Psychopharmacology of imidazoline and alpha 2-adrenergic receptors: implications for depression. Crit. Rev. Neurobiol. **9:** 29–66.
42. MAES, M., A. VAN GASTEL, L. DELMEIRE, et al. 1999. Decreased platelet alpha-2 adrenoceptor density in major depression: effects of tricyclic antidepressants and fluoxetine. Biol. Psychiatry **45:** 278–284.
43. HALARIS, A., H. ZHU, J. ALI, et al. 2002. Down-regulation of platelet imidazoline-1 binding sites after bupropion treatment. Int. J. Neuropsychopharm. **5:** 37–46.
44. HALBREICH, U., J.E. PILETZ, S. CARSON, et al. 1993. Increased imidazoline and alpha 2 adrenergic binding in platelets of women with dysphoric premenstrual syndromes. Biol. Psychiatry **34:** 676–686.
45. PILETZ, J.E. & U. HALBREICH. 2000. Imidazoline and alpha(2A)-adrenoceptor binding sites in postmenopausal women before and after estrogen replacement therapy. Biol. Psychiatry **48:** 932–939.
46. LALIES, M., A. HIBELL, A. HUDSON, et al. 1999. Inhibition of central monoamine oxidase by imidazoline-2 site-selective ligands. Ann. N.Y. Acad. Sci. **881:** 114–117.
47. RADDATZ, R., A. PARINI & S.M. LANIER. 1995. Imidazoline/guanidinium binding domains on monoamine oxidases. Relationship to subtypes of imidazoline-binding proteins and tissue-specific interaction of imidazoline ligands with monoamine oxidase-B. J. Biol. Chem. **270:** 27961–27968.
48. HALARIS, A., J.E. PILETZ, S. MADAKASIRA, et al. 2000. Imidazoline receptors: new candidates for affective modulation? In Progress in Differentiated Psychopathology. E. Franzek, G.S. Ungvari, E. Ruther, H. Beckmann, Eds.: 113–120. International Wernicke-Kleist-Leonhard Society. Wursburg, Germany.
49. ERNSBERGER, P., T.H. DAMON, L. GRAFF, et al. 1993. Moxonidine, a centrally-acting antihypertensive agent, is a selective ligand for I1-Imidazoline sites. J. Pharmacol. Exper. Ther. **264:** 172–182.
50. VANDERGRIFF, J., M.J. KALLMAN & K. RASMUSSEN. 2000. Moxonidine, a selective imidazoline-1 receptor agonist, suppresses the effects of ethanol withdrawal on the acoustic startle response in rats. Biol. Psychiatry **47:** 874–879.
51. DE VOS, H., G. BRICCA, J. DE KEYSER, et al. 1994. Imidazoline receptors, non-adrenergic idazoxan binding sites and alpha 2-adrenoceptors in the human central nervous system. Neuroscience **59:** 589–598.
52. PILETZ, J.E., G.A. ORDWAY, H. ZHU, et al. 2000. Autoradiographic comparison of [^{3}H]-clonidine binding to non-adrenergic sitres and alpha2-adrenergic receptors in human brain. Neuropsychopharmacology **23:** 697–708.
53. PILETZ, J., G. ORDWAY, G. RAJKOWSKA, et al. 2003. Differential expression of alpha(2)-adrenoceptor vs. imidazoline binding sites in postmortem orbitofrontal cortex and amygdala of depressed subjects. J. Psychiatr. Res. **37:** 399–409.
54. DAVIDSON, R.J. 2002. Anxiety and affective style: role of prefrontal cortex and amygdala. Biol. Psychiatry **51:** 68–80.
55. CESURA, A.M., J. GOTTOWIK, H.-W. LAHM, et al. 1996. Investigation on the structure of the active site of monoamine oxidase B by affinity labelling with the selective inhibitor lazabemide and by site-directed mutagenesis. Eur. J. Biochem. **236:** 996–1002.
56. ALEMANY, R., G. OLMOS & J.A. GARCIA-SEVILLA. 1995. The effects of phenelzine and other monoamine oxidase inhibitor antidepressants on brain and liver I2 imidazoline-preferring receptors. Br. J. Pharmacol. **114:** 837–845.
57. ZHU, H., I.A. PAUL, M. MCNAMARA, et al. 1997. Chronic imipramine treatment upregulates I2-imidazoline receptive sites in rat brain. Neurochem. Int. **30:** 101–107.
58. ESCRIBA, P.V., R. ALEMANY, M. SASTRE, et al. 1996. Pharmacological modulation of immunoreactive imidazoline receptor proteins in rat brain: relationship with non-adrenoceptor [^{3}H]-idazoxan binding sites. Br. J. Pharmacol. **118:** 2029–2036.

59. WANG, H., S. REGUNATHAN, M.P. MEELEY, et al. 1992. Isolation and characterization of imidazoline receptor protein from bovine adrenal chromaffin cells. Mol. Pharmacol. **42:** 792–801.
60. GARCIA-SEVILLA, J., P. ESCRIBA & J. GUIMON. 1999. Imidazoline receptors and human brain disorders. Ann. N. Y. Acad. Sci. **881:** 392–409.
61. SASTRE, M. & J.A. GARCIA-SEVILLA. 1997. Densities of I2-imidazoline receptors, alpha-2 adrenoceptors and monoamine oxidase B in brains of suicide victims. Neurochem. Int. **30:** 63–72.
62. WILDERING, W.C., P.M. HERMANN & A.G. BULLOCH. 2002. Rapid neuromodulatory actions of integrin ligands. J. Neurosci. **22:** 2419–2426.
63. GOODMAN, S.L., S.L. COOPER & R.M. ALBRECHT. 1993. Integrin receptors and platelet adhesion to synthetic surfaces. J. Biomed. Mater. Res. **27:** 683–695.
64. SUEHIRO, K., J. GAILIT & E.F. PLOW. 1997. Fibrinogen is a ligand for integrin alpha5beta1 on endothelial cells. J. Biol. Chem. **272:** 5360–5366.
65. HSU-LIN, S., C.L. BERMAN, B.C. FURIE, et al. 1984. A platelet membrane protein expressed during platelet activation and secretion. Studies using a monoclonal antibody specific for thrombin-activated platelets. J. Biol. Chem. **259:** 9121–9126.
66. METZELAAR, M.J., J. KORTEWEG, J.J. SIXMA, et al. 1991. Biochemical characterization of PECAM-1 (CD31 antigen) on human platelets. Thromb. Haemost. **66:** 700–707.
67. MUSSELMAN, D.L., A. TOMER, A.K. MANATUNGA, et al. 1996. Exaggerated platelet reactivity in major depression. Am. J. Psychiatry **153:** 1313–1317.
68. MUSSELMAN, D.L., U.M. MARZEC, A. MANATUNGA, et al. 2002. Platelet reactivity in depressed patients treated with paroxetine: preliminary findings. Arch. Gen. Psychiatry **57:** 875–882.
69. ANDA, R., D. WILLIAMSON, D. JONES, et al. 1993. Depressed affect, hopelessness, and the risk of ischemic heart disease in a cohort of U.S. adults. Epidemiology **4:** 285–294.
70. WASSERTHEIL-SMOLLER, S., W.B. APPLEGATE, K. BERGE, et al. 1996. Change in depression as a precursor of cardiovascular events. SHEP Cooperative Research Group (Systoloc Hypertension in the elderly). Arch. Intern. Med. **156:** 553–561.
71. FORD, D.E., L.A. MEAD, P.P. CHANG, et al. 1998. Depression is a risk factor for coronary artery disease in men: the precursors study. Arch. Intern. Med. **158:** 1422–1426.
72. WULSIN, L.R., G.E. VAILLANT & V.E. WELLS. 1999. A systematic review of the mortality of depression. Psychosom. Med. **61:** 6–17.
73. FRASURE-SMITH, N., F. LESPERANCE, G. GRAVEL, et al. 2000. Social support, depression, and mortality during the first year after myocardial infarction. Circulation **101:** 1919–1924.
74. MARKOVITZ, J.H., K.A. MATTHEWS, J. KISS, et al. 1996. Effects of hostility on platelet reactivity to psychological stress in coronary heart disease patients and in healthy controls. Psychosom. Med. **58:** 143–149.
75. PILETZ, J.E., H. ZHU, S. MADAKASIRA, et al. 2000. Elevated p-selectin on platelets in depression: response to bupropion. J. Psychiatric Res. **34:** 397–404.
76. FENG, Y., A.E. HALARIS & J.E. PILETZ. 1997. Determination of agmatine in brain and plasma using high-performance liquid chromatography with fluorescence detection. J. Chromatogr. B. Biomed. Appl. **691:** 277–282.
77. OTAKE, K., D.A. RUGGIERO, S. REGUNATHAN, et al. 1998. Regional localization of agmatine in the rat brain: an immunocytochemical study. Brain Res. **787:** 1–14.
78. DEMADY, D.R., S. JIANMONGKOL, J.L. VULETICH, et al. 2001. Agmatine enhances the NADPH oxidase activity of neuronal NO synthase and leads to oxidative inactivation of the enzyme. Mol. Pharmacol. **59:** 24–29.
79. GALEA, E., S. REGUNATHAN, V. ELIOPOULOS, et al. 1996. Inhibition of mammalian nitric oxide synthases by agmatine, an endogenous polyamine formed by decarboxylation of arginine. Biochem. J. **316:** 247–249.
80. REIS, D.J. & S. REGUNATHAN. 2000. Is agmatine a novel neurotransmitter in brain? Trends Pharmacol. Sci. **21:** 187–193.
81. OLMOS, G., N. DEGREGORIO-ROCASOLANO, M. PAZ REGALADO, et al. 1999. Protection by imidazol(ine) drugs and agmatine of glutamate-induced neurotoxicity in cultured cerebellar granule cells through blockade of NMDA receptor. Br. J. Pharmacol. **127:** 1317–1326.

82. YANG, X.C. & D.J. REIS. 1999. Agmatine selectively blocks the N-methyl-D-aspartate subclass of glutamate receptor channels in rat hippocampal neurons. J. Pharmacol. Exp. Ther. **288:** 544–549.
83. PILETZ, J.E., D.N. CHIKKALA & P. ERNSBERGER. 1995. Comparison of the properties of agmatine and endogenous clonidine-displacing substance at imidazoline and alpha-2 adrenergic receptors. J. Pharmacol. Exp. Ther. **272:** 581–587.
84. SASTRE, M., S. REGUNATHAN, E. GALEA, et al. 1996. Agmatinase activity in rat brain: a metabolic pathway for the degradation of agmatine. J. Neurochem. **67:** 1761–1765.
85. LORING, R.H. 1990. Agmatine acts as an antagonist of neuronal nicotinic receptors. Br. J. Pharmacol. **99:** 207–211.
86. MOLDERINGS, G.J., K. SCHMIDT, H. BONISCH, et al. 1996. Inhibition of 5-HT3 receptor function by imidazolines in mouse neuroblastoma cells: potential involvement of sigma 2 binding sites. Naunyn Schmiedebergs Arch. Pharmacol. **354:** 245–252.
87. SENER, A., P. LEBRUN, F. BLACHIER, et al. 1989. Stimulus-secretion coupling of arginine-induced insulin release. Insulinotropic action of agmatine. Biochem. Pharmacol. **38:** 327–330.
88. KALRA, S.P., E. PEARSON, A. SAHU, et al. 1995. Agmatine, a novel hypothalamic amine, stimulates pituitary luteinizing hormone release in vivo and hypothalamic luteinizing hormone-releasing hormone release in vitro. Neurosci. Lett. **194:** 165–168.
89. MOLDERINGS, G.J. & M. GOTHERT. 1995. Inhibitory presynaptic imidazoline receptors on sympathetic nerves in the rabbit aorta differ from I1- and I2-imidazoline binding sites. Naunyn Schmiedebergs Arch. Pharmacol. **351:** 507–516.
90. REGUNATHAN, S., FEINSTEIN, D.L. & D. J. REIS. 1999. Anti-proliferative and anti-inflammatory actions of imidazoline agents. Are imidazoline receptors involved? Ann. N.Y. Acad. Sci. **881:** 410–419.
91. ABE, K., Y. ABE & H. SAITO. 2000. Agmatine suppresses nitric oxide production in microglia. Brain Res. **872:** 141–148.
92. GILAD, G.M., K. SALAME, J.M. RABEY, et al. 1996. Agmatine treatment is neuroprotective in rodent brain injury models. Life Sci. **58:** 41–46.
93. GILAD, G.M. & V.H. GILAD. 2000. Accelerated functional recovery and neuroprotection by agmatine after spinal cord ischemia in rats. Neurosci. Lett. **296:** 97–100.
94. FENG, Y., J.E. PILETZ & M.H. LEBLANC. 2002. Agmatine suppresses nitric oxide production and attenuates hypoxic-ischemic brain injury in neonatal rats. Pediatr. Res. **52:** 606–611.
95. FAIRBANKS, C.A., K.L. SCHREIBER, K.L. BREWER, et al. 2000. Agmatine reverses pain induced by inflammation, neuropathy, and spinal cord injury. Proc. Natl. Acad. Sci. U. S. A. **97:** 10584–10589.
96. ARICIOGLU-KARTAL, F. & I.T. UZBAY. 1997. Inhibitory effect of agmatine on naloxone-precipitated abstinence syndrome in morphine dependent rats. Life Sci. **61:** 1775–1781.
97. LI, J., X. LI, G. PEI, et al. 1999. Analgesic effect of agmatine and its enhancement on morphine analgesia in mice and rats. Chung Kuo Yao Li Hsueh Pao **20:** 81–85.
98. MACHELSKA, H., D. LABUZ, R. PRZEWLOCKI, et al. 1997. Inhibition of nitric oxide synthase enhances antinociception mediated by mu, delta and kappa opioid receptors in acute and prolonged pain in the rat spinal cord. J. Pharmacol. Exp. Ther. **282:** 977–984.
99. LI, J., X. LI, G. PEI, et al. 1999. Effects of agmatine on tolerance to and substance dependence on morphine in mice. Chung Kuo Yao Li Hsueh Pao **20:** 232–238.
100. UZBAY, I.T., O. YESILYURT, T. CELIK, et al. 2000. Effects of agmatine on ethanol withdrawal syndrome in rats. Behav. Brain Res. **107:** 153–159.
101. STEWART, L.S. & B.E. MCKAY. 2000. Acquisition deficit and time-dependent retrograde amnesia for contextual fear conditioning in agmatine-treated rats. Behav. Pharmacol. **11:** 93–97.
102. ZOMKOWSKI, A.D., L. HAMMES, J. LIN, et al. 2002. Agmatine produces antidepressant-like effects in two models of depression in mice. Neuroreport **13:** 387–391.
103. HALARIS, A., H. ZHU, Y. FENG, et al. 1999. Plasma agmatine and platelet imidazoline receptors in depression. Ann. N.Y. Acad. Sci. **881:** 445–451.

Regulation of Inducible Nitric Oxide Synthase and Agmatine Synthesis in Macrophages and Astrocytes

SOUNDAR REGUNATHAN AND JOHN E. PILETZ

Department of Psychiatry and Human Behavior, Division of Neurobiology and Behavior Research, University of Mississippi Medical Center, Jackson, Mississippi 39216, USA

ABSTRACT: Agmatine is a novel endogenous guanido amine synthesized from arginine by arginine decarboxylase. Among several biologic effects, the ability of agmatine to protect against ischemic injury and chronic neuropathic pain is particularly interesting. Because inflammation is a common contributor to these conditions, we sought to determine if agmatine acts by decreasing the production of proinflammatory molecules such as nitric oxide and if agmatine synthesis is regulated by inflammatory stimuli. We tested whether agmatine affects astroglial and macrophage (RAW 264.7 cell line) nitric oxide synthase-2 (NOS-2) expression. NOS-2 was induced in these cells by incubation with lipopolysaccharide (LPS) plus three cytokines for astrocytes and LPS alone for RAW 264.7 cells in the presence and absence of varying concentrations of agmatine. NOS-2 activity was assessed after 24 hours by nitrite accumulation in the culture media. Agmatine dose-dependently inhibited nitrite accumulation, and shorter incubation with agmatine (1 and 4 hours) also caused significant reduction. Agmatine decreased the expression of NOS-2 activity and NOS-2 protein as determined by immunoblot analysis. Incubation of astrocytes and RAW 264.7 cells with LPS/cytokines for 2 hours resulted in an increase in arginine decarboxylase (ADC) activity, whereas longer-term incubation (12–17 hours) lowered ADC activity. Agmatine levels in these cells are increased after 6-hour incubation with LPS/cytokines. These results show that agmatine inhibits the production of nitric oxide by decreasing the activity of NOS-2 in macrophages and astroglial cells by decreasing the levels of NOS-2 protein. These findings provide a molecular basis for the neuroprotective and anti-inflammatory actions of agmatine.

KEYWORDS: agmatine; arginine decarboxylase; nitric oxide synthase; arginine; inflammation

INTRODUCTION

Agmatine is an amine and an organic cation formed by the decarboxylation of L-arginine by the enzyme arginine decarboxylase (ADC).[1] Although long known

---

Address for correspondence: Dr. Soundar Regunathan, Ph.D., Department of Psychiatry and Human Behavior, Division of Neurobiology and Behavior Research, University of Mississippi Medical Center, 2500 North State Street, Jackson, MS 39216, USA. Voice: 601-984-5471; fax: 601-984-5899.
e-mail: sregunathan@psychiatry.umsmed.edu

to be synthesized and stored in plants, bacteria, and invertebrates, agmatine and its biosynthetic enzyme were recently discovered in mammals, originally in rat brain,[2] and later in other tissues and serum.[3–5] Agmatine binds to imidazoline and α_2-adrenergic receptors and is proposed to be an endogenous ligand for imidazoline receptors.[2,6,7] Subsequently agmatine has been shown to have several biologic actions in brain and in the periphery.[8–14] Of particular interest among the actions of agmatine is its ability to offer protection against ischemic injury and chronic neuropathic pain.[15–18] A common mechanism that contributes to these two conditions is the increased production of proinflammatory molecules including inducible nitric oxide synthase (NOS-2). We demonstrated earlier that the potent NOS-2 inducer, the bacterial endotoxin lipopolysaccharide (LPS), reduced the activity of ADC in macrophages,[19] and conversely that agmatine could inhibit the catalytic activity of all three NOS isoforms.[20] Because agmatine and nitric oxide are derived from the same substrate, arginine, and because these two products have opposite effects on inflammation, we hypothesized that the enzymes that produce these molecules could be regulated in a opposite manner. Recent reports confirms that agmatine decreases the production of nitric oxide (NO) in microglia[21] as well as during hypoxia in vivo,[22] suggesting that agmatine protects neurons by blocking the production of NO in brain.

Because agmatine is produced by the decarboxylation of arginine, which is also the substrate for NOS, we sought to determine whether agmatine regulates the production of NO and the expression of NOS-2 during inflammatory stimuli and whether such stimuli could also regulate the production of agmatine and expression of ADC activity. Our present results, using macrophages (RAW 264.7) and primary rat cortical astrocytes, demonstrate that agmatine reduces the production of NO and the expression of NOS-2 activity after inflammatory stimuli, whereas such stimuli increase ADC activity and the levels of agmatine.

MATERIALS AND METHODS

Reagents

Cell culture reagents, Dulbecco's modified Eagle medium (DMEM), antibiotic agents, and LPS (*Salmonella typhimurium*) were obtained from Sigma (St. Louis, MO, USA). Fetal calf serum (FCS) was obtained from Atlanta Biological (Norcross, GA, USA). Cytokines such as interleukin 1-β (IL1-β), interferon-γ (IFN-γ) and tumor necrosis factor-α (TNF-α) were obtained from Sigma Chemicals (St Louis, MO, USA). Peroxidase conjugated goat secondary antibodies were obtained from Vector Labs (Burlingame, CA, USA), and enhanced chemiluminescence reagents were obtained from Amersham Pharmacia Biotech (Piscataway, NJ, USA).

Cell Culture

Primary astrocytes were prepared from cerebral cortices of postnatal day 1 Sprague-Dawley rats.[23] These cultures consist of more than 95% astrocytes, as determined with antibodies to the astrocyte-specific marker glial fibillary acidic protein (GFAP), and between 1% and 3% microglial cells. The mouse macrophage RAW 264.7 cell line was obtained from American Type Culture Collection (ATCC) and was maintained in DMEM with 10% FCS.

NOS-2 Induction Protocol

The growth medium was removed, the cells were washed once in serum-free medium, and NOS-2 inducers in fresh serum-free medium were added. For RAW 264.7 cells, LPS-dependent induction was done with 1 µg/mL LPS; for astrocytes, induction was done with 1 µg/mL LPS plus 20 units/mL IFN-γ because LPS alone is insufficient to induce NOS-2 in these cells. For both cell types, cytokine induction is done with a three-cytokine mixture (CM) consisting of IFN-γ (20 units/mL), IL1-β (2 ng/mL), and TNF-α (10 ng/mL). Incubations were carried out for 24 hours for nitrite, NOS activity, and immunoblot analysis and for 4 hours for mRNA analysis.

Nitrite Production

NOS-2 activity was indirectly assessed by accumulation of NO_2 in the cell culture medium, 18 to 24 hours after addition of inducers. An aliquot of the medium (100 µL) was mixed with 50 µL of Griess reagent, incubated for 5 minutes at room temperature, and the absorbance at 546 nm determined. Solutions of $NaNO_2$ diluted in DMEM served as standards. The absorbance readings caused by incubation of cells in DMEM alone were subtracted from sample values. Activity is calculated as nmoles of NO_2 accumulated per 24 hours per mg of total cellular protein.

NOS-2 Activity Assay and Immunoblot Analysis

The activity of NOS-2 was directly measured by the conversion of $1\,^{14}C$-arginine to $1\,^{14}C$-citrulline.[23] After cells were incubated for 24 hours with drugs, cell lysates were prepared from RAW 264.7 or astrocytes by homogenization in 50 mM Tris-HCl (pH 7.5). Assays were carried out in the presence of all cofactors (nicotinamide adenine dinucleotide phosphate [NADPH], flavin mononucleotide [FMN], flavin adenine dinucleotide [FAD], and tetrahydrobiopterin), 10 µM arginine, and 2 mM ethylene glycol tetraacetic acid (EGTA) to inhibit any calcium-dependent enzyme activity. The activity is expressed as pmol/hour/mg protein. The analysis of NOS-2 protein was carried out by Western blot as described earlier using specific NOS-2 antibody.[23] After incubating overnight with stimulating agents and agmatine, cells were harvested in phosphate-buffered saline (PBS), and cellular protein was prepared by sonication in 8 M urea. Samples were diluted in 2% sodium dodecyl sulfate (SDS), 62 mM Tris-HCl (pH 6.8), 10% 2-mercaptoethanol, and 25% glycerol, boiled and used for separation of proteins by 7.5% polyacrylamide gels. The proteins were electrotransferred to polyvinylidene difluoride membranes, blocked with 5% dry milk, and incubated overnight with primary antibody (1:2000 dilution of rabbit anti-NOS-2 antibody, Chemicon, Temecula, CA). The membranes were washed, exposed to horseradish peroxidase (HRP)-labeled anti-rabbit IgG, and bands were visualized with enhanced chemiluminescence reagents.

Measurement of Agmatine

Agmatine levels were measured by high-pressure liquid chromatography (HPLC) as described extensively in our earlier papers.[4,5] Briefly, harvested cells were homogenized in phosphate buffer containing internal standard and 10% trichloroacetic acid (TCA) and centrifuged at 16,000 × gravity to precipitate proteins. The supernatant was mixed with o-pthalaldehyde (OPA) and injected into the HPLC system with C18 column and detected by fluorescence detector (excitation, 338 nm; emission 425 nm). The concentration of agmatine was calculated using external standard and expressed as ng/10^6 cells.

Measurement of ADC Activity

Activity of ADC was measured in cell membrane fractions as described earlier[2,12] based on the release of $^{14}CO_2$ from 1 ^{14}C-arginine. Briefly, cell pellets were resuspended in Tris EDTA buffer (pH 7.4), sonicated, and centrifuged at 27,000 × gravity for 20 minutes. The membrane pellet was washed once by sonication and recentrifugation in Tris-HCl buffer and resuspended in the incubation buffer. The membrane suspension (500 µL) was incubated for 1 hour at 25°C in 20 mM Tris-HCl buffer (pH 8.25), containing 1 mM MgSO4, 0.5 mM dithiothreitol, 0.5 mM phenylmethane sulfonyl fluoride (PMSF), 0.2 mM EDTA, 0.1 mM L-arginine, and 7.28 µM L[1-^{14}C] arginine. Release of $^{14}CO_2$ from 1 ^{14}C-arginine was measured by trapping the $^{14}CO_2$ in filter-paper wicks saturated with benzethonium hydroxide. The reaction was stopped by the injection of 40% TCA into the reaction chamber. The filters were transferred to minivials containing 5 mL CytoScint cocktail (ICN Biomedicals, Aurora, OH) and were counted for radioactivity by liquid scintillation spectrometry (Beckman model LS 5801, Beckman Instruments, Fullerton, CA).

RESULTS

Effect of Agmatine on the Induction of NOS-2 Activity

In initial experiments, we tested the effect of agmatine and idazoxan on LPS-induced nitrite accumulation in astrocytes and RAW 264.7 cells (macrophage cell line). When these cells were incubated with LPS for 24 hours, a large increase in the accumulation of nitrite in the medium was observed because of the induction of NOS-2 activity. When these cells were exposed to agmatine along with LPS, a marked

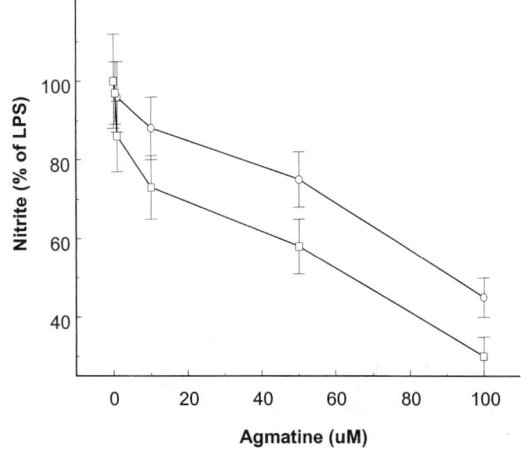

FIGURE 1. Effect of agmatine on LPS-induced accumulation of nitrite in astrocytes (○—○) and RAW 264.7 cells (□—□). Cells were incubated with LPS (RAW 264.7 cell) or LPS + CM (astrocytes) in the presence of various concentrations of agmatine for 24 hours. The nitrite accumulation in the medium was measured and expressed as nmol nitrite/mg cell protein. Values are from three different cell preparations, carried out in triplicate and expressed as percent of LPS group (100%).

decrease in nitrite production was observed. The effect of agmatine was dose-dependent in all the three cell types, and the effect was most potent in RAW 264.7 cells, with IC_{50}s ranging from 50 to 100 µM (FIG. 1). Agmatine, even at higher concentrations (1 mM), has no toxic effects on these cells as measured by medium lactate dehydrogenase (LDH) (data not shown) and thus the effect is not caused by a lower number of cells resulting from cell death.

Although the initial experiments were carried out by incubating the cells with agmatine and LPS for 24 hours, it is important to understand whether agmatine can initiate events as soon as it is added or whether long-term incubation is needed to block the increase in NO production. To address this question, cells were incubated for a short term with agmatine and changed to agmatine-free medium. In these experiments, RAW 264.7 cells were incubated with different concentrations of agmatine and LPS for various time periods (1 hour and 4 hours). After the incubation the medium was removed, the cells were washed once with medium, the medium was replaced with medium containing LPS until next day (total incubation time of 24 hours), and the accumulation of nitrite was measured in the medium. As shown in FIGURE 2, the accumulation of nitrite was significantly reduced in the medium of cells incubated with agmatine (50 µM and 100 µM) for 4 hours, whereas only 100 µM agmatine showed significant effect with 1-hour incubation. Although this effect was smaller than that seen with the continuous incubation with agmatine for 24 hours, significant reduction in nitrite accumulation suggests that agmatine might block an early event in the induction of NOS-2 activity by LPS.

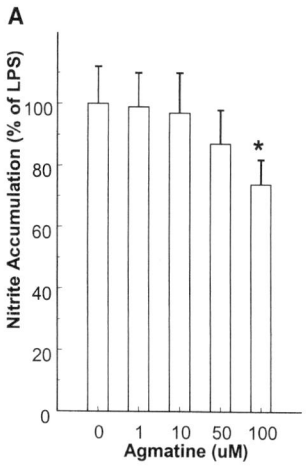
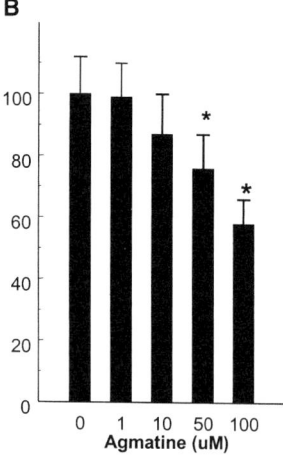

FIGURE 2. Effect of short-term incubation with agmatine on LPS-induced nitrite accumulation in RAW 264.7 cells. Cells were incubated with LPS in the presence of various concentrations of agmatine for 1 hour (**A**) or 4 hours (**B**), and the medium was replaced with medium containing only LPS. The nitrite accumulation in the medium was measured after 24 hours and expressed as nmol nitrite/mg cell protein. Values are from three different cell preparations, carried out in triplicate and expressed as percent of LPS group (100%).

TABLE 1. Effect of agmatine on NOS-2 activity in LPS-treated astrocytes and RAW 264.7 cells

Treatment	Astrocytes	RAW 264.7
Control	28 ± 3.8	67 ± 5.7
LPS	117 ± 17*	875 ± 32*
LPS + agmatine (10 µM)	106 ± 15	576 ± 28**
LPS + agmatine (100 µM)	74 ± 11**	16 ± 14**

Cells were treated with LPS (LPS + CM for astrocytes) for 24 hours with or without agmatine, and cell lysates were prepared. NOS-2 activity was measured by the conversion of ^{14}C-arginine to ^{14}C-citrulline, and the results are expressed as pmol/hour/mg protein. CM, three-cytokine mixture; LPS, lipopolysaccharide; NOS, nitric oxide synthase.
* $P < 0.01$ compared with control.
** $P < 0.01$ compared with LPS group.

Effect of Agmatine on the Expression of NOS-2 Protein

Although agmatine potently reduced the accumulation of nitrite induced in the medium by LPS, it would be necessary to show that this effect results from reduced NOS-2 enzyme activity, because lower nitrite production could result from decreased substrate or cofactor availability for the enzyme activity. Therefore, the activity of NOS-2 was determined in RAW 264.7 and astrocyte cell lysates prepared from cells incubated with LPS (RAW 264.7) or LPS with CM (astrocytes) in the presence and absence of agmatine by measuring the conversion of L-arginine to L-citrulline, as described earlier. As shown in TABLE 1, although the control cells had small NOS activity, cells treated with LPS showed an approximate 15-fold increase in the enzyme activity in RAW 264.7 cells and an approximate fivefold increase in astrocytes. In the presence of agmatine, the NOS activity was significantly reduced compared with LPS-treated cells. The effect of agmatine was significant at 100 µM in both RAW 264.7 and astrocytes, whereas 10 µM agmatine was effective only in RAW 264.7 cells. These findings clearly indicated the ability of agmatine to reduce NOS-2 activity induced by inflammatory stimuli. To determine whether such reversal actually

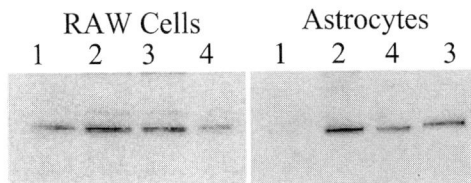

FIGURE 3. Effect of agmatine on the expression of NOS-2 protein as measured by immunoblot analysis. After incubation with LPS in the presence and absence of agmatine for 24 hours, cell lysates were used for immunoblot analysis using specific antibodies to NOS-2 protein. Lanes are: (1) control; (2) LPS (LPS + CM for astrocytes); (3) LPS plus agmatine (10 µM); (4) LPS + agmatine (100 µM). This figure is a representative blot; similar results were obtained from three different cell preparations.

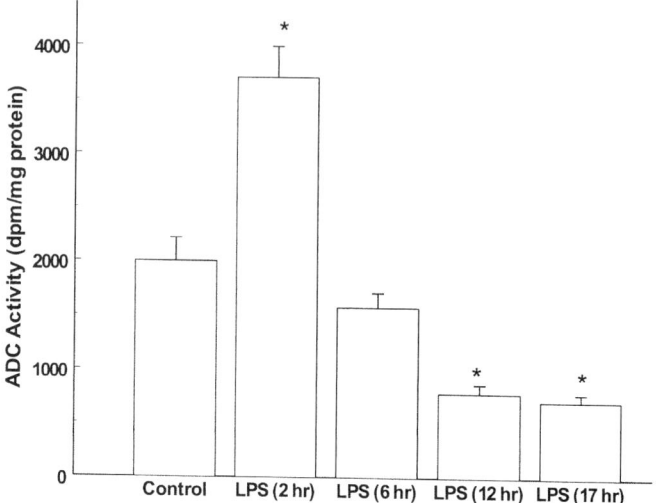

FIGURE 4. Effect of LPS on ADC activity in RAW 264.7 cells. Cells were incubated with LPS (1 µg/mL), and ADC activity was measured in cell membranes after specified time. Values are mean ± SE from three experiments, each done in triplicate. * $P < 0.001$ compared with control cells.

results from the decreased expression of the enzyme protein, we used immunoblot analysis to investigate the expression of NOS-2 enzyme using specific antibodies. As shown in FIGURE 3, NOS-2 protein was expressed only in LPS-treated RAW 264.7 and astrocytes, and agmatine largely reduced the NOS-2 protein levels.

Effect of LPS/Cytokines on ADC Activity

The previous studies demonstrated the inhibitory effects of exogenously applied agmatine on NO production and the induction of NOS-2. The next question was to determine whether the synthesis of endogenous agmatine is altered during inflammatory condition. We measured the activity of ADC in cultured RAW 264.7 cells after incubation with LPS/cytokines for various time periods. As shown in FIGURE 4, ADC activity changes in a biphasic manner, increasing in the early stages of treatment (2 hours) and decreasing after 12 hours compared with control levels.

Effect of LPS/Cytokines on Agmatine Levels

To determine whether changes in ADC activity result in corresponding changes in cellular agmatine levels, we measured the levels of agmatine in RAW 264.7 and astrocytes after exposure to LPS/cytokines. As shown in FIGURE 5, agmatine levels are increased 6 hours after exposure to LPS/cytokines in astrocytes and RAW 264.7 cells, and longer treatment (12 hours and 24 hours) resulted in the levels not significantly different from control levels (data not shown).

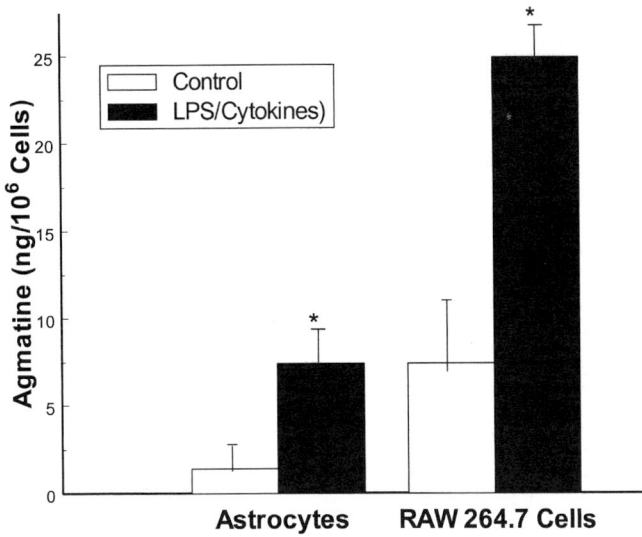

FIGURE 5. Effect of LPS/cytokines on agmatine levels in RAW 264.7 cells and astrocytes. Cells were incubated with LPS plus cytokines for 6 hours, and agmatine levels were measured in cell lysates by HPLC. Values mean ± SE from three experiments, each done in triplicate. * $P < 0.001$ compared with control cells.

DISCUSSION

In this study, we have demonstrated that incubation of cortical astrocytes or mouse macrophage cell line, RAW 264.7, with agmatine significantly reduces the induction of NOS-2 by bacterial endotoxin, LPS, and cytokines as measured by the accumulation of nitrite in the medium. This reduction in nitrite accumulation is consistent with lower NOS-2 activity in agmatine-treated cells as measured by the conversion of L-arginine to L-citrulline. The decreased NOS-2 enzyme activity was paralleled by decreased NOS-2 protein as determined by immunoblot analysis. The effect was more potent in RAW 264.7 cells than in astrocytes. This finding is in contrast to that observed with imidazoline drug, idazoxan, which was more potent in astrocytes.[23] These results raise the issue whether the effects of agmatine or idazoxan are mediated by imidazoline receptors.[24] Our preliminary binding studies using ^{3}H-idazoxan revealed no specific binding in RAW 264.7 cell membranes (data not shown), indicating the absence of imidazoline receptors in macrophages. Although the effects of idazoxan in astrocytes may be mediated by imidazoline receptors,[23] the effect of agmatine on the suppression of NOS-2 activity in RAW 264.7 is clearly not mediated by imidazoline receptors.

The mechanism by which agmatine blocks the induction of NOS-2 is not clear at present, but our results indicate that the continuous presence of agmatine for 24 hours is not required to show the effect. This finding suggests that agmatine may block an initial step in the pathway that induces or stabilizes NOS-2 after LPS/cytokine stimulation. One intriguing observation is that the NOS-2 mRNA is not reduced but rather is increased after agmatine exposure, whereas NOS-2 enzyme activity and protein levels are markedly decreased. Agmatine clearly decreases the production of NO and the activity and protein levels of NOS-2, as reported here and in reports from other laboratories.[20,21,25,26] This result would be expected because NO is an important proinflammatory agent, and agmatine exhibits anti-inflammatory properties in in vivo animal models.[17,18] A previous report showed that agmatine reduces neuronal NOS activity by inducing NADPH oxidase leading to oxidative inactivation of the enzyme,[27] and such a mechanism could also explain the lower NOS-2 activity in glia and macrophages after agmatine exposure. Administration of agmatine in animal models markedly reduces the pain induced by inflammation, neuropathy, and spinal cord injury.[18,28,29] Agmatine also reverses the lesion induced by ischemic injury and spinal cord injury.[15,16,30] The protective mechanism for the action of agmatine in these conditions may be related to its ability to block the production of NO.

The biosynthesis of agmatine is also regulated by inflammatory stimuli in both RAW 264.7 cells and astrocytes. The early increase in ADC activity after exposure to LPS/cytokines could be part of a homeostatic mechanism to increase agmatine levels in the cells. The higher ADC activity is not sustainable, however, and the activity returns to lower levels after longer exposure.[19] These findings indicate that the biosynthesis of agmatine and NO could be regulated in opposite manner during inflammation.

To conclude, we have shown that agmatine inhibits the production of NO, stimulated by inflammatory cytokines and LPS, and that this effect results from decreased NOS-2 activity and protein levels in astroglia and macrophages, providing evidence for the molecular basis of the anti-inflammatory and neuroprotective actions of agmatine in brain and peripheral tissues. We have also shown that endogenous agmatine levels and ADC activity are regulated as a protective mechanism against inflammatory response.

ACKNOWLEDGMENT

This work was supported by NIH grant NS 39445 to S.R.

REFERENCES

1. TABOR, C.W. & H. TABOR. 1984. Polyamines. Ann. Rev. Biochem. **53:** 749–790.
2. LI, G., S. REGUNATHAN, C.J. BARROW, *et al.* 1994. Agmatine: an endogenous clonidine-displacing substance in the brain. Science **263:** 966–969.
3. LORTIE, M.J., *et al.* 1996. Agmatine, a bioactive metabolite of arginine. J. Clin. Invest. **97:** 413–420.
4. RAASCH, W., *et al.* 1995. Agmatine, the bacterial amine, is widely distributed in mammalian tissues. Life Sci. **56:** 2319–2330.
5. FENG, Y., *et al.* 1997. Determination of agmatine in brain and plasma using high-performance liquid chromatography with fluorescence detection. J. Chromatogr. **691:** 277–286.
6. PILETZ, J.E., *et al.* 1995. Comparison of the properties of agmatine and endogenous clonidine-displacing substance at imidazoline and alpha-2 adrenergic receptors J. Pharmacol. Exp. Ther. **272:** 581–587.
7. PINTHONG, D., *et al.* 1995. Agmatine recognizes alpha 2-adrenoceptor binding sites but neither activates nor inhibits alpha 2-adrenoceptors. Naunyn Schmiedeberg's Arch. Pharmacol. **351:** 10–16.

8. KALRA, S.P., et al. 1995. Agmatine, a novel hypothalamic amine, stimulates pituitary luteinizing hormone release in vivo and hypothalamic luteinizing hormone-releasing hormone release in vitro. Neurosci. Lett. **194:** 165–168.
9. KOLESNIKOV, Y., S. JAIN & G.W. PASTERNAK. 1996. Modulation of opioid analgesia by agmatine. Eur. J. Pharmacol. **296:** 17–22.
10. GONZALEZ, C., et al. 1996. Agmatine is an endogenous modulator of noradrenergic neurotransmission in the rat tail artery. Br. J. Pharmacol. **119:** 677–684.
11. JURKIEWICZ, N.H., et al. 1996. Functional properties of agmatine in rat vas deferens. Eur. J. Pharmacol. **307:** 299–304.
12. REGUNATHAN, S., et al. 1996. Imidazoline receptors and agmatine in blood vessels: a novel system inhibiting vascular smooth muscle proliferation. J. Pharmacol. Exp. Ther. **276:** 1272–1282.
13. SATRIANO, J., et al. 1998. Agmatine suppresses proliferation by frameshift induction of antienzyme and attenuation of cellular polyamine levels. J. Biol. Chem. **273:** 15313–15316.
14. GREENBERG, G.S., et al. 2001. The effect of agmatine administration on ischemic-reperfused isolated rat heart. J. Cardiovasc. Pharmacol. Ther. **6:** 37–45.
15. GILAD, G.M., et al. 1996. Agmatine treatment is neuroprotective in rodent brain injury models. Life Sci. **58:** PL41–46.
16. GILAD, G.M. & V.H. GILAD. 2000. Accelerated functional recovery and neuroprotection by agmatine after spinal cord ischemia in rats. Neurosci. Lett. **296:** 97–100.
17. ONAL, A. & N. SOYKAN. 2001. Agmatine produces antinociception in tonic pain in mice. Pharmacol. Biochem. Behav. **69:** 93–97.
18. FAIRBANKS, C.A., et al. 2000. Agmatine reverses pain induced by inflammation, neuropathy, and spinal cord injury. Proc. Natl. Acad. Sci. U. S. A. **97:** 10584–10589.
19. SASTRE, M., et al. 1998. Metabolism of agmatine in macrophages: modulation by lipopolysacharides and inhibitory cytokines. Biochem. J. **330:** 1405–1409.
20. GALEA, E., et al. 1996. Inhibition of mammalian nitric oxide synthases by agmatine, an endogenous polyamine formed by decarboxylation of arginine. Biochem. J. **316:** 247–249.
21. ABE, K., Y. Abe & H. SAITO. 2000. Agmatine suppresses nitric oxide production in microglia. Brain Res. **872:** 141–148.
22. FENG, Y., J.E. PILETZ & M.H. LEBLANC. 2002. Agmatine suppresses nitric oxide production and attenuates hypoxic-ischemic brain injury in neonatal rats. Pediatr. Res. **52:** 606–611.
23. FEINSTEIN, D.L., D.J. REIS & S. REGUNATHAN. 1999. Inhibition of astroglial nitric oxide synthase type 2 expression by idazoxan. Mol. Pharmacol. **55:** 306–308.
24. REGUNATHAN, S., D.L. FEINSTEIN & D.J. REIS. 1999. Anti-proliferative and anti-inflammatory actions of imidazoline agents: are imidazoline receptors involved? Ann. N. Y. Acad. Sci. **881:** 410–419.
25. SCHWARTZ, D., et al. 1997. Agmatine effects glomerular filtration via a nitric oxide synthase-dependent mechanism. Am. J. Physiol. **272:** F597–F601.
26. SATRIANO, J.S. Suppression of inducible nitric oxide generation by agmatine aldehyde: beneficial effects in sepsis. J. Cell. Physiol. **188:** 313–320.
27. DEMADY, D.R., et al. 2001. Agmatine enhances the NADPH oxidase activity of neuronal NO synthase and leads to oxidative inactivation of the enzyme. Mol. Pharmacol. **59:** 24–29.
28. YU, C.G., et al. 2000. Agmatine improves locomotor function and reduces tissue damage following spinal cord injury. Neuroreport **11:** 3203–3207.
29. HORVATH G.K., et al. 1999. Effect of intrathecal agmatine on inflammation-induced thermal hyperalgesia in rats. Eur. J. Pharmacol. **368:** 197–204.
30. FAIRBANKS, C.A., et al. 1998. The behavioral and neuroprotective effects of agmatine in different models of pain and neuronal injury in rodents. Abstr. Soc. Neurosci. **24:** 1253.

Vertebrate Agmatinases: What Role Do They Play in Agmatine Catabolism?

SIDNEY M. MORRIS, JR.

Department of Molecular Genetics and Biochemistry, University of Pittsburgh School of Medicine, Pittsburgh, Pennsylvania 15261, USA

ABSTRACT: Whereas agmatine in vertebrates may be derived from multiple sources such as the diet, endogenous synthesis via arginine decarboxylase, and possibly also from enteric bacteria, agmatinase is the only enzyme specific for agmatine catabolism. As it hydrolyzes a guanidino group within agmatine and also contains signature amino acid residues that act as ligand binding sites for the Mn^{++} cofactor, agmatinase is classified as a member of the arginase superfamily. Very little information is available regarding how much agmatine in vertebrate species is catabolized by agmatinase versus other enzymes such as diamine and amine oxidases. Moreover, comparisons of primary sequences of several vertebrate agmatinases demonstrate that several residues essential for catalytic activity are not conserved in the mouse. This leads to the prediction that the agmatinase protein in mouse has little or no catalytic activity, not only raising questions about the physiologic routes of agmatine disposal in this organism, but also suggesting the existence of species-specific differences in mechanisms for regulating agmatine levels.

KEYWORDS: agmatine; catabolism; mammalian agmatinases; arginine superfamily

Agmatine is produced from L-arginine by arginine decarboxylase and can be catabolized by agmatinase (agmatine ureohydrolase; EC 3.5.3.11) to produce urea and putrescine. Thus, these enzymes can provide an alternative to arginase and ornithine decarboxylase as a route to synthesis of polyamines from L-arginine. Within the past 10 years, metabolism of agmatine was demonstrated to occur in mammals, due in large part to pioneering studies by Donald Reis and his colleagues.[1,2] This has resulted in efforts to clone and characterize mammalian arginine decarboxylase and agmatinase in order to provide tools to investigate the localization and regulation of agmatine metabolism.

Because agmatine has a wide range of biological effects, there is considerable interest in understanding the physiologic mechanisms by which agmatine levels are regulated. One critical piece of information is the identification of the potential metabolic routes by which agmatine can be metabolized in mammals. Although not strictly a polyamine itself, agmatine can be used as a substrate by diamine or amine

Address for correspondence: Sidney M. Morris, Jr., Department of Molecular Genetics and Biochemistry University of Pittsburgh School of Medicine, Pittsburgh, PA 15261, USA. Voice: 412-648-9338; fax: 412-624-1401.
e-mail: smorris@pitt.edu

oxidases.[3–5] Unfortunately, however, there is very little information on the extent to which agmatine is catabolized by agmatinase, relative to its catabolism by other enzymes in mammalian cells. One exception is a recent study that analyzed agmatine metabolism by cultured hepatocytes.[4] Even though the highest levels of agmatinase mRNA are found in liver,[6] agmatinase did not represent the major route by which agmatine was catabolized in these cells. Instead, the major route of catabolism was via

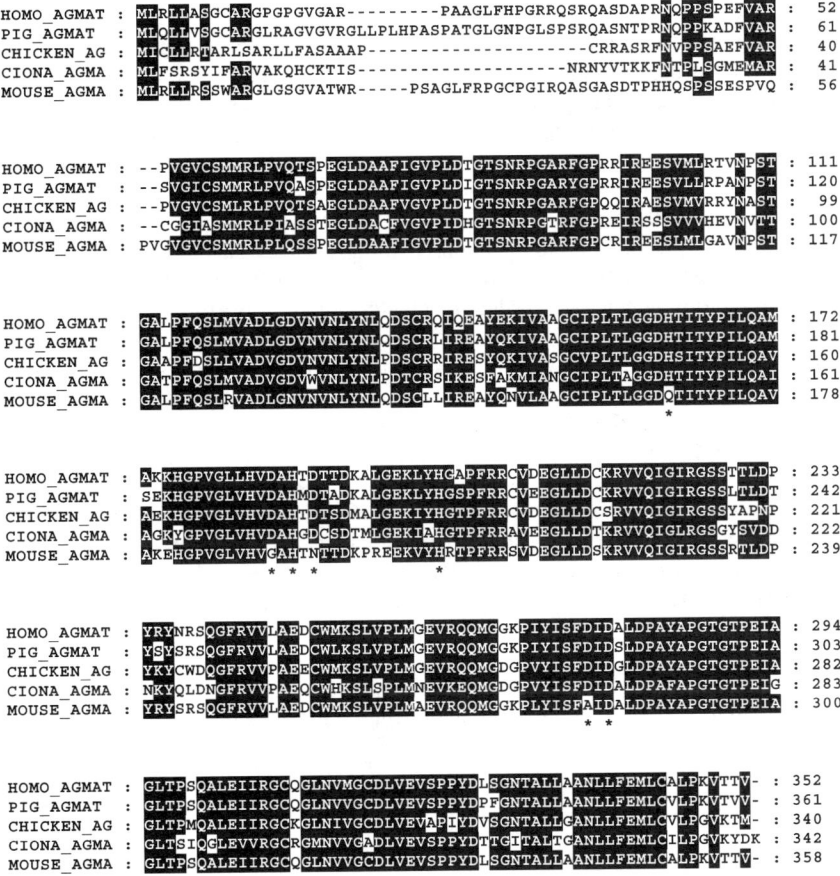

FIGURE 1. Alignment of chordate agmatinases. Sequences were aligned by ClustalW 1.8 (http://searchlauncher.bcm.tmc.edu/multi-align/multi-align.html) and displayed using the GeneDoc utility (http://www.psc.edu/biomed/genedoc/). Identical residues and conservative substitutions present in at least four of the five sequences are shaded. Locations of the seven histidine and aspartate residues required for metal ligand binding and enzymatic activity that are conserved in members of the arginase superfamily[8] are indicated by the asterisks below the alignment. Sequences of agmatinases for *Homo sapiens*,[6] chicken,[6] and mouse (GenBank accession number XM_131722) were obtained from the indicated sources; agmatinase sequences for pig and *Ciona intestinalis* were deduced from EST sequences in GenBank (S.M. Morris, unpublished results).

oxidases. Thus, agmatinase does not represent the sole—or perhaps even the major—route for catabolism of agmatine in mammals.

Characterization of the enzymes that produce or degrade agmatine would represent a major step in understanding how levels of agmatine are regulated. Cloning of human agmatinase by ourselves and another group was reported in 2002,[6,7] and an initial report of the cloning of human arginine decarboxylase by Soundar Regunathan and his colleagues is presented elsewhere in this volume. However, the enzymatic properties of mammalian agmatinases or arginine decarboxylases remain to be rigorously determined.

As comparative studies of enzymes from different species often can provide clues to important structural and functional features, an initial comparison was conducted by aligning sequences of agmatinases from five chordate species (FIG. 1). This alignment revealed a very high degree of sequence conservation over almost the entire molecule. The greatest sequence diversity was in the N-terminal segment, corresponding to the region that probably represents the mitochondrial targeting sequence. For most species, the alignment also identified seven histidine and aspartate residues that are virtually invariant among members of the arginase superfamily from a wide range of eukaryotic and prokaryotic species.[8,9] A key feature of this family of enzymes is a requirement for a divalent metal cofactor such as Mn^{++} at the active site. As revealed by the x-ray structures of arginases from rat liver[10] and *B. caldovelox*[11] and of proclavaminic acid hydrolase,[12] six of the invariant residues are involved in binding the Mn^{++} cofactor (FIG. 2A). A seventh histidine residue is not directly involved in binding the cofactor but is required for robust enzymatic activity in arginase[13] and *E. coli* agmatinase.[14] Remarkably, four of the six ligand-binding residues are not conserved in murine agmatinase, despite the very high degree of sequence conservation overall (FIG. 1). These amino acid substitutions in murine agmatinase are predicted to drastically reduce or abolish the affinity of the enzyme for the Mn^{++} cofactor (FIG. 2), thus rendering the enzyme virtually inactive. Though obviously important, the actual effects of these amino acid substitutions are unknown because no enzymatic studies have been reported for purified agmatinase from any vertebrate.

The primary goal of this brief presentation has been to emphasize the considerable deficits in our basic knowledge about mammalian agmatinases and their function. The

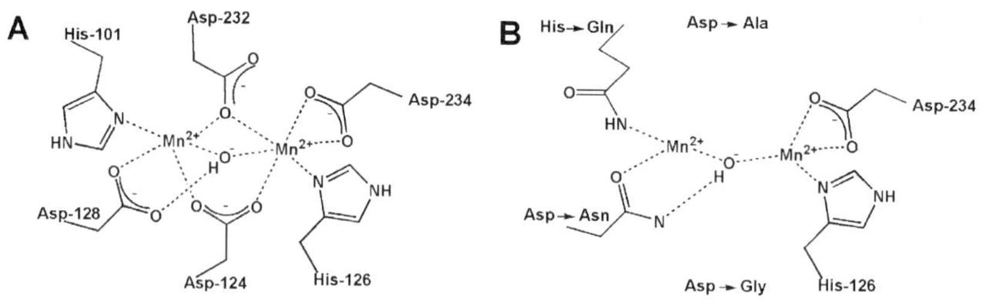

FIGURE 2. Roles of conserved residues in binding Mn^{++} in arginase superfamily (**A**) and predicted consequences of nonconservative substitutions in murine agmatinase (Fig. 1) on ligand binding (**B**). Binding interactions and numbering of residues in (**A**) are based on the x-ray structure of rat liver arginase.[10]

available information indicates not only that agmatinase may not be the major enzyme involved in catabolism of agmatine, but also that its enzymatic properties may vary significantly among mammals. In particular, the mouse may be an inappropriate experimental model for understanding agmatine metabolism in other mammals, including humans.

ACKNOWLEDGMENT

This work was supported in part by NIH grant GM57384.

REFERENCES

1. LI, G., et al. 1994. Agmatine: An endogenous clonidine-displacing substance in the brain. Science **263**: 966–969.
2. SASTRE, M., et al. 1996. Agmatinase activity in rat brain: a metabolic pathway for the degradation of agmatine. J. Neurochem. **67**: 1761–1765.
3. HOLT, A. & G.B. BAKER. 1995. Metabolism of agmatine (clonidine-displacing substance) by diamine oxidase and the possible implications for studies of imidazoline receptors. Prog. Brain Res. **106**: 187–197.
4. CABELLA, C., et al. 2001. Transport and metabolism of agmatine in rat hepatocyte cultures. Eur. J. Biochem. **268**: 940–947.
5. ASCENZI, P. et al. 2002. Agmatine oxidation by copper amine oxidase. Eur. J. Biochem. **269**: 884–892.
6. MISTRY, S.K., et al. 2002. Cloning of human agmatinase. An alternate path for polyamine synthesis induced in liver by hepatitis B virus. Am. J. Physiol. **282**: G375–G381.
7. IYER, R.K., et al. 2002. Cloning and characterization of human agmatinase. Molec. Genet. Metab. **75**: 209–218.
8. PEROZICH, J., J. HEMPEL & S.M. MORRIS JR. 1998. Roles of conserved residues in the arginase family. Biochim. Biophys. Acta. **1382**: 23–37.
9. SEKOWSKA, A., A. DANCHIN & J.-L. RISLER. 2000. Phylogeny of related functions: the case of polyamine biosynthetic enzymes. Microbiology **146**: 1815–1828.
10. KANYO, Z.F., et al. 1996. Structure of a unique binuclear manganese cluster in arginase. Nature **383**: 554–557.
11. BEWLEY, M.C., et al. 1999. Crystal structures of Bacillus caldovelox arginase in complex with substrate and inhibitors reveal new insights into activation, inhibition and catalysis in the arginase superfamily. Structure **7**: 435–448.
12. ELKINS, J.M., et al. 2002. Oligomeric structure of proclavaminic acid amidino hydrolase: evolution of a hydrolytic enzyme in clavulanic acid biosynthesis. Biochem J. **366**: 423–434.
13. CAVALLI, R.C., et al. 1994. Mutagenesis of rat liver arginase expressed in *Escherichia coli*: role of conserved histidines. Biochemistry **33**: 10652–10657.
14. CARVAJAL, N., et al. 1999. Evidence that histidine-163 is critical for catalytic activity, but not for substrate binding to *Escherichia coli* agmatinase. Biochem. Biophys. Res. Commun. **264**: 196–200.

Agmatine: At the Crossroads of the Arginine Pathways

JOSEPH SATRIANO

University of California, San Diego, Department of Medicine, Division of Nephrology-Hypertension, the Stein Institute for Research on Aging, and the Veterans Administration San Diego Healthcare System, San Diego, California 92161, USA

> ABSTRACT: In acute inflammatory responses, such as wound healing and glomerulonephritis, arginine is the precursor for production of the cytostatic molecule nitric oxide (NO) and the pro-proliferative polyamines. NO is an early phase response whereas increased generation of polyamines is requisite for the later, repair phase response. The temporal switch of arginine as a substrate for the inducible nitric oxide synthase (iNOS)/NO axis to arginase/ornithine decarboxylase (ODC)/polyamine axis is subject to regulation by inflammatory cytokines as well as interregulation by the arginine metabolites themselves. Herein we describe the capacity of another arginine pathway, the metabolism of arginine to agmatine by arginine decarboxylase (ADC), to aid in this interregulation. Agmatine is an antiproliferative molecule due to its suppressive effects on intracellular polyamine levels, whereas the aldehyde metabolite of agmatine is a potent inhibitor of iNOS. We propose that the catabolism of agmatine to its aldehyde metabolite may act as a gating mechanism at the transition from the iNOS/NO axis to the arginase/ODC/polyamine axis. Thus, agmatine has the potential to serve in the coordination of the early and repair phase pathways of arginine in inflammation.
>
> KEYWORDS: agmatine; arginine; nitric oxide; polyamines

INTRODUCTION

In mammals arginine synthesis is primarily a function of the kidney and the liver. The liver does not contribute significantly to plasma arginine levels as most liver arginine is consumed within the urea cycle. The maintenance of plasma arginine levels is primarily dependent upon its synthesis in the kidney, and dietary intake. In addition to its role as a component of proteins, arginine is a precursor for the synthesis of other molecules including nitric oxide (NO), citrulline, agmatine, urea and ornithine. Dietary arginine is required for optimal growth in animals, and becomes "essential" in conditions of starvation, injury or stress.[1] Arginine supplementation is beneficial in animal and human models of wound healing as well as lymphocyte responses and mitogenesis.[1–4]

In 1980 Furchgott and Zawadzki discovered acetylcholine-mediated vasorelaxation requires a substance derived from endothelial cells.[5] This substance, termed

---

Address for correspondence: Joseph Satriano, UCSD and VASDHS, 3350 La Jolla Village Dr. (9111H), San Diego, CA 92161, USA. Voice: 858-552-8585 x6167; fax: 858-552-7549.
e-mail: jsatriano@ucsd.edu

Ann. N.Y. Acad. Sci. 1009: 34–43 (2003). © 2003 New York Academy of Sciences.
doi: 10.1196/annals.1304.004

endothelium-dependent relaxing factor, was later identified as the molecule nitric oxide (NO).[6–9] NO has evolved into a unique bioregulatory molecule involved in diverse physiologic, pathologic, pharmacologic, and toxicologic processes.[10] NO is synthesized from arginine by a family of nitric oxide synthase (NOS) isozymes.[7,9,11] There are three distinct mammalian NOS isoforms. The first isolated NOS was localized to peripheral neurons, and was thus denoted neuronal or nNOS, and is sometimes referred to as brain derived or bNOS.[12] Similarly, eNOS was first localized to the membrane fraction of endothelial cells.[13,14] The third isoform, inducible or iNOS, whose activation is induced by certain cytokines or microbial products was first purified and cloned from a macrophage cell line. This "high-output" form of NOS evokes protective actions in mammalian tissues due, in part, to its cytostatic/bactericidal activity towards certain pathogens.

Juxtaposed to the cytostatic effects of NO are the pro-proliferative effects of the polyamines. Polyamines (putrescine, spermidine, and spermine) are small ubiquitous cationic molecules required for cell growth and homeostasis.[15,16] The first and rate-limiting enzyme of polyamine biosynthesis, ornithine decarboxylase (ODC), metabolizes ornithine to putrescine (FIG. 1). ODC has a very short half-life and is one of the most highly regulated eukaryotic enzymes. Its expression and activity are transiently induced by a number of factors, including all growth factors, to elicit a complex yet coordinated series of responses. Transformation, whether oncogenic, carcinogenic or viral, constitutively induces ODC activity. ODC is a proto-oncogene.

Intracellular polyamine concentrations are autoregulated by the induction of the

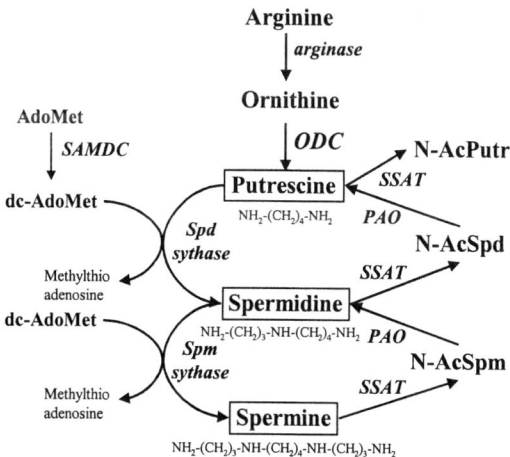

FIGURE 1. Polyamine interconversion pathways. Enzymes involved in the formation of polyamines include arginase and arginase/ornithine decarboxylase (ODC). Enzymes for the forward conversion of polyamines include S-adenosylmethionine decarboxylase (SAMDC), spermidine synthase, and spermine synthase. Enzymes involved in back conversion from higher to lower order polyamines include acetyl CoA:Spd/Spm N-acetyltransferase (SSAT) and polyamine oxidase (PAO). Abbreviations: AdoMet, S-adenosylmethionine; dc-AdoMet, decarboxylated S-adenosylmethionine; N-Ac, N-acetylated; Putr, putrescine; Spd, spermidine; Spm, spermine.

protein antizyme.[17] Induction of antizyme is by a programmed +1 ribosomal frameshift.[17] This novel mechanism of induction affords rapid modulation in response to intracellular polyamine concentrations. However, the cell is required to constitutively maintain levels of antizyme mRNA requisite for this response, which underscores the importance of this system. Antizyme is the only known endogenous protein that binds to ODC, inhibiting its activity and accelerating its degradation in an ubiquitin independent process catalyzed by the 26S proteasome.[18] In addition to inhibiting polyamine biosynthesis, antizyme also suppresses polyamine transporters,[19,20] and increases polyamine export.[21] This unique negative feedback system is effective in limiting intracellular polyamine levels. Previous studies support the view that induction of antizyme may prove to be a viable method of attenuating neoplastic growth.[22–25] Antizyme is considered a tumor suppressor.

THE TEMPORAL REGULATION OF NO AND POLYAMINE PATHWAYS

Two well-described pathways of L-arginine metabolism in inflammation include the conversion of arginine to NO and citrulline by NOS, and the breakdown of arginine to urea and ornithine by arginase. These pathways are temporally regulated in inflammatory models including wound healing and glomerulonephritis.[26–28] Induction of iNOS expression and a marked generation of NO characterize an early phase response. High output NO generation from iNOS during periods of cellular stress is known to exert cytostatic/cytotoxic effects.[29–36] This is followed by the production of ornithine, which initiates the later repair phase. Ornithine is converted to polyamines via ODC, required for growth, and to proline via ornithine aminotransferase (OAT), a constituent of extracellular matrix.[37] The production of ornithine and its metabolism to polyamines and proline are important elements of the repair phase.

Arginine, but not ornithine, deprivation induces compensatory polyamine transport.[38] This observation supports the position that arginine is at the crux of polyamine synthesis as well as NO generation. Furthermore, inhibiting NOS by L-NMMA administration in experimental glomerulonephritis increases both the magnitude and onset of the repair phase response.[27] NOS may inhibit arginase by competing for substrate, or by the generation of an intermediate in the production of NO, N^G-hydroxy-L-arginine (NOHA).[39] However, in experimental glomerulonephritis the cells that employ arginine for NO generation (macrophage cells) are different than those that utilize arginine for the repair functions of polyamine and proline synthesis (mesangial cells).[27,40] Thus, the NO intermediate NOHA would need to exhibit paracrine effects. The effectiveness of NOHA in such a setting in vivo is yet to be determined, although NOHA levels increase in lipopolysaccharide (LPS)-treated rats.[41] Furthermore, NOHA induced caspase-3 activity and apoptosis in a breast cancer cell line, but depletion of polyamines decreased caspase-3 activity and did not induce apoptosis.[42] These results imply other effects of NOHA beyond suppressing the arginase/ODC/polyamine axis.

NO, however, does have a direct effect on ODC. We and others have shown NO can directly nitrosylate and inhibit ODC activity.[43,44] This process is readily reversible, depending upon the oxidative state of the cell. For example, low glutathione under conditions of oxidative stress could promote and maintain, whereas high glutathione levels typical of unstressed cells could reverse, nitrosylation. In the rat aortic smooth muscle model, inhibition of cellular proliferation by NO was due to inactivation of ODC.[45]

There are numerous examples of arginase inhibiting NOS activity by competing for substrate, arginine.[46–51] Conversely, up-regulation or overexpression of arginase increases polyamine synthesis and growth.[50,52–56] Furthermore, whereas T helper 1 (Th1) cells generate interferon-γ and induction of iNOS, Th2 cells generate interleukin (IL)-4 and IL-10 with resultant induction of arginase and suppression of iNOS.[57]

AGMATINE

The conversion of arginine to agmatine by arginine decarboxylase (ADC) is a third arginine pathway that will be discussed within the context of interregulation of arginine pathways. Constitutive ADC activity is most prevalent in the kidney and the liver,[58,59] as is arginine synthesis. In normal kidney, production of labeled agmatine is second only to the conversion of arginine to ornithine, and in large excess to the conversion of arginine to citrulline.[58] Agmatine concentrations in plasma and tissues by HPLC in early reports were markedly underestimated due to the lability of agmatine in the derivatization process, a problem that has not been entirely eradicated. Recently, the intracellular level of agmatine in the rat kidney was reported approximating 430 μmol/L, with plasma concentrations of 2.8 μmol/L.[60] Agmatine, like arginine, is widely distributed by the plasma and can be selectively concentrated in several organs that do not maintain ADC activity, some at several-fold higher levels than the kidney itself.[58,61] Many of the organs that retain high levels of agmatine are prone to environmental insult.[61] So, "Why does the kidney constitutively produce agmatine, and why would it maintain, and many other organs/tissues obtain, agmatine at such high intracellular levels? What is it doing?" In several prokaryotes agmatine is a precursor to polyamine synthesis. But that function has, as has the ADC enzyme itself,[62] evolved substantially in mammals to what we believe is a regulatory role.

Agmatine has apparent vasodilatory effects. Our laboratory observed an increase in glomerular filtration rate (GFR) when agmatine was microperfused into the urinary space of surface glomeruli of the rat.[58] This effect was inhibited by co-administration of a NOS inhibitor, suggesting that the effects of agmatine on glomerular ultrafiltration are by a NOS-dependent mechanism. Vasodilatory effects of agmatine noted by others include a decrease in systemic arterial pressure in rats, and vasorelaxation in rat aortic rings preparations.[63,64] In the latter proposal, administration of either a NOS inhibitor or endothelium denudation abolished these effects. Furthermore, agmatine increases NO endproduct formation in endothelial cells, purportedly via an increase in intracellular Ca^{++} transients.[65] More recent data demonstrate that NO and agmatine may act synergistically to induce ryanodine receptor mediated Ca^{++} release in cells in culture (unpublished data). Together, these results support NOS involvement in agmatine-mediated vasodilation. In apparent contradiction to these findings, agmatine was shown to inhibit NOS.[66,67] However, others using highly purified enzyme preparations have demonstrated that agmatine itself is neither a substrate for, nor inhibitor of, NOS.[68–71] We have demonstrated that the inhibitory effects of agmatine on iNOS generation of NO is primarily by the aldehyde metabolite of agmatine, rather than agmatine itself.[72] Although this point at first glance may seem trivial, it would explain the aforementioned contradictory effects on NO generation, and is fundamental for the model system we will propose (FIG. 2).

We demonstrated the capacity of agmatine to directly induce antizyme via a +1 ribosomal frameshift with a resultant suppression of polyamine biosynthesis and transport.[73] Prior to this finding, induction of antizyme was thought to be exclusively in response to intracellular polyamine accumulation. Agmatine is the only known endogenous molecule, other than the canonical polyamines themselves, with the ability to induce full length, active antizyme. In accord with these observations, transformed kidney proximal tubule epithelial cells, MCT, display a reduction in ODC activity

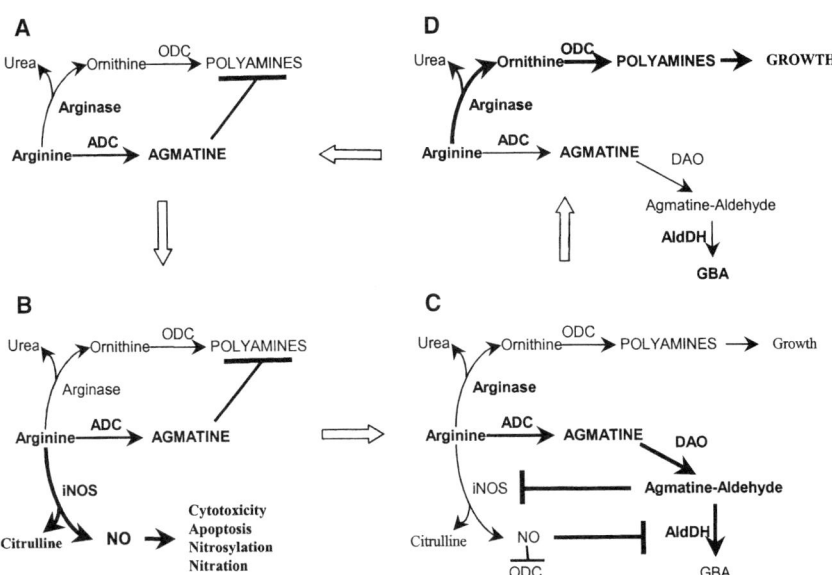

FIGURE 2. Proposed interregulation of arginine pathways by ADC metabolites. In inflammatory models, arginine to NO production is an early phase response whereas the production of ornithine and polyamines is a later repair phase response. (**A**) Agmatine induction of antizyme and SSAT can aid in the regulation of intracellular polyamine levels in normal cell homeostasis, in part by adding to the free polyamine pool. (**B**) The early phase of an acute inflammatory response: induction of iNOS and NO mediated events. (**C**) Suppression of iNOS via agmatine aldehyde comprises the transition phase: DAO induction agmatine metabolizes to an aldehyde. Nitrosylation by NO inhibits AldDH activity and suppresses the further metabolism of agmatine aldehyde. Suppression of iNOS can occur by several other factors released during inflammation, such as cytokines. (**D**) The metabolism of agmatine shifts its repression away from the polyamines. This shift is permissive for growth and supports the repair phase. Activation of AldDH occurs after suppression of iNOS allowing metabolism of the aldehydes. Resetting to (A) occurs when AO returns to normal levels. Bars represent negative regulation. Abbreviations: ODC, ornithine decarboxylase; ADC, arginine decarboxylase; NO, nitric oxide; iNOS, inducible nitric oxide synthase; DAO, diamine oxidase; AldDH, aldehyde dehydrogenase; GBA, guanidinobutyric acid.

(antizyme dependent), polyamine content, [^{3}H] thymidine incorporation and growth in response to agmatine.[73] In addition, agmatine suppresses ODC activity by greater than 70% in all immortalized and transformed cell lines examined.[73] Agmatine also can reduce intracellular polyamines by up-regulation of SSAT, an enzyme involved in the back conversion of polyamines, that is, to a lower charged molecule (FIG. 1).[74] The resultant lower order and acetyl polyamines are more readily exported from the cell. Agmatine-mediated polyamine depletion inhibits proliferation in transformed cell lines. We are currently looking further into the mode(s) of arrest mediated by agmatine.

The capacity of agmatine to modulate intracellular polyamine levels and curb proliferation was evaluated in the model of experimental glomerulonephritis. In this model monoclonal anti-Thy-1 antibody is administered to rats. This antibody binds to the Thy-1 antigen expressed on the glomerular mesangial cell membrane and targets these cells for attack by the immune system. At day 1 there is a peak in NO levels that corresponds with mesangiolysis. Mesangial cell proliferation and extracellular matrix deposition signal an active repair phase by day 4, and by day 7 the glomeruli become congested and dysfunctional due to hypercellularity and fibrosis. A marked decrease in GFR accompanies these events. In this model, agmatine administration normalized GFR and markedly reduced hypercellularity and fibrosis at day 7.[75]

PROPOSED MODEL: THE AGMATINE PENDULUM

We believe in a normal physiologic state that agmatine would act as a guardian against aberrant proliferation. It would be complimentary, that is, additive, to the endogenous polyamine pool and would thereby effectively lower the threshold levels of "free" intracellular polyamine required to bring about the induction of antizyme. It also could perform these duties by other means such as increasing SSAT activity.[74] As such, agmatine has the capacity to suppress intracellular polyamine levels required for growth (FIG. 2A).[73]

In inflammatory conditions agmatine aldehyde could exert beneficial constraining influences on iNOS. We envision this potential feedback loop in a pendulum-like manner (FIG. 2). An acute inflammatory response would be set into motion by the transient up-regulation of iNOS and generation of NO. NO would promote cytostatic/bactericidal effects, as well as the nitrosylation and nitration of several proteins and enzymes (FIG. 2B). One enzyme inactivated by NO mediated nitrosylation is aldehyde dehydrogenase (AldDH).[76,77] The end of the NO phase and advent of the repair phase would be marked by increased diamine oxidase (DAO) activity. DAO metabolizes agmatine to agmatine aldehyde,[78] and its activity correlates with disease activity in numerous inflammatory states.[79–81] This would shift the effects of agmatine away from polyamine regulation, and thus be permissive for growth. The aldehyde metabolite of agmatine formed would be sustained longer than normal as NO inactivates AldDH, the enzyme that converts the aldehyde into a stable acid. Increased levels of agmatine aldehyde could suppress NO generation (FIG. 2C). Lower NO relieves inhibition of AldDH allowing metabolism of agmatine aldehyde (FIG. 2D). Resetting occurs with DAO returning to normal levels. Although hypothetical, in accord with this model we observed beneficial effects of agmatine administration in the LPS model of sepsis and Thy-1 mediated glomerulonephritis.[72,75] The LPS model of sepsis is particularly noteworthy as we observe indistinguishable results with agmatine as with a selective iNOS inhibitor, but different results from that of general (non-selective) NOS inhibition.[72,82] That agmatine is neuroprotective in ischemic neuronal injury may also be attributed to its effects on the arginine pathways.[83–86]

Thus, the products of a third arginine metabolic pathway, via ADC, pose the potential to coordinate regulation of both the NO and repair phase pathways of arginine.

ACKNOWLEDGMENTS

Supported in part by NIH grants DK02920 and DK28602, the American Cancer Society, UCSD Cancer Center, the Stein Institute for Research on Aging, and funds supplied by the Research Service of the Department of Veterans Affairs.

REFERENCES

1. BARBUL, A. 1986. Arginine: biochemistry, physiology, and therapeutic implications. JPEN. J. Parenter. Enteral Nutr. **10:** 227–238.
2. BARBUL, A., et al. 1990. Arginine enhances wound healing and lymphocyte immune responses in humans. Surgery **108:** 331–336; discussion 336–337.
3. NIRGIOTIS, J.G., P.J. HENNESSEY & R.J. ANDRASSY. 1991. The effects of an arginine-free enteral diet on wound healing and immune function in the postsurgical rat. J. Pediatr. Surg. **26:** 936–941.
4. SEIFTER, E., et al. 1978. Arginine: an essential amino acid for injured rats. Surgery **84:** 224–230.
5. FURCHGOTT, R.F. & J.V. ZAWADZKI. 1980. The obligatory role of endothelial cells in the relaxation of arterial smooth muscle by acetylcholine. Nature **288:** 373–376.
6. IGNARRO, L.J., et al. 1987. Endothelium-derived relaxing factor produced and released from artery and vein is nitric oxide. Proc. Natl. Acad. Sci. U. S. A. **84:** 9265–9269.
7. PALMER, R.M., D.S. ASHTON & S. MONCADA. 1988. Vascular endothelial cells synthesize nitric oxide from L-arginine. Nature **333:** 664–666.
8. PALMER, R.M., A.G. FERRIGE & S. MONCADA. 1987. Nitric oxide release accounts for the biological activity of endothelium-derived relaxing factor. Nature **327:** 524–526.
9. SAKUMA, I., et al. 1988. Identification of arginine as a precursor of endothelium-derived relaxing factor. Proc. Natl. Acad. Sci. U. S. A. **85:** 8664–8667.
10. NATHAN, C. & Q.W. XIE. 1994. Nitric oxide synthases: roles, tolls, and controls. Cell **78:** 915–918.
11. MONCADA, S. & E.A. HIGGS. 1995. Molecular mechanisms and therapeutic strategies related to nitric oxide. FASEB. J. **9:** 1319–1330.
12. BREDT, D.S., et al. 1991. Nitric oxide synthase protein and mRNA are discretely localized in neuronal populations of the mammalian CNS together with NADPH diaphorase. Neuron. **7:** 615–624.
13. MICHEL, T., G.K. LI & L. BUSCONI. 1993. Phosphorylation and subcellular translocation of endothelial nitric oxide synthase. Proc. Natl. Acad. Sci. U. S. A. **90:** 6252–6256.
14. BUSCONI, L. & T. MICHEL. 1993. Endothelial nitric oxide synthase. N-terminal myristoylation determines subcellular localization. J. Biol. Chem. **268:** 8410–8413.
15. TABOR, C.W. & H. TABOR. 1984. Polyamines. Annu. Rev. Biochem. **53:** 749–790.
16. PEGG, A.E. & P.P. MCCANN. 1982. Polyamine metabolism and function. Am. J. Physiol. **243:** C212–C221.
17. MATSUFUJI, S., et al. 1995. Autoregulatory frameshifting in decoding mammalian ornithine decarboxylase antizyme. Cell **80:** 51–60.
18. HAYASHI, S., Y. MURAKAMI & S. MATSUFUJI. 1996. Ornithine decarboxylase antizyme: a novel type of regulatory protein. Trends Biochem. Sci. **21:** 27–30.

19. MITCHELL, J.L., et al. 1994. Feedback repression of polyamine transport is mediated by antizyme in mammalian tissue-culture cells. Biochem. J. **299**: 19–22.
20. SUZUKI, T., et al. 1994. Antizyme protects against abnormal accumulation and toxicity of polyamines in ornithine decarboxylase-overproducing cells. Proc. Natl. Acad. Sci. U. S. A. **91**: 8930–8934.
21. SAKATA, K., K. KASHIWAGI & K. IGARASHI. 2000. Properties of a polyamine transporter regulated by antizyme. Biochem. J. **347**(Pt 1): 297–303.
22. KOIKE, C., D.T. CHAO & B.R. ZETTER. 1999. Sensitivity to polyamine-induced growth arrest correlates with antizyme induction in prostate carcinoma cells. Cancer Res. **59**: 6109–6112.
23. FEITH, D.J., L.M. SHANTZ & A.E. PEGG. 2001. Targeted antizyme expression in the skin of transgenic mice reduces tumor promoter induction of ornithine decarboxylase and decreases sensitivity to chemical carcinogenesis. Cancer Res. **61**: 6073–6081.
24. PEGG, A.E., et al. 2003. Transgenic mouse models for studies of the role of polyamines in normal, hypertrophic and neoplastic growth. Biochem. Soc. Trans. **31**: 356–360.
25. IWATA, S., et al. 1999. Anti-tumor activity of antizyme which targets the ornithine decarboxylase (ODC) required for cell growth and transformation. Oncogene **18**: 165–172.
26. ALBINA, J.E., et al. 1990. Temporal expression of different pathways of l-arginine metabolism in healing wounds. J. Immunol. **144**: 3877–3880.
27. COOK, H.T., et al. 1994. Arginine metabolism in experimental glomerulonephritis: interaction between nitric oxide synthase and arginase. Am. J. Physiol. **267**: F646–F653.
28. KETTELER, M., W.A. BORDER & N.A. NOBLE. 1994. Cytokines and L-arginine in renal injury and repair. [editorial] Am. J. Physiol. **267**: F197–F207.
29. ALBINA, J.E. & W.L. HENRY JR. 1991. Suppression of lymphocyte proliferation through the nitric oxide synthesizing pathway. J. Surg. Res. **50**: 403–409.
30. DE GROOTE, M.A. & F.C. FANG. 1995. NO inhibitions: antimicrobial properties of nitric oxide. Clin. Infect. Dis. **21**(Suppl 2): S162–S165.
31. DE GROOTE, M.A., et al. 1995. Genetic and redox determinants of nitric oxide cytotoxicity in a Salmonella typhimurium model. Proc. Natl. Acad. Sci. U. S. A. **92**: 6399–6403.
32. KURATA, S., M. MATSUMOTO & U. YAMASHITA. 1996. Concomitant transcriptional activation of nitric oxide synthase and heme oxygenase genes during nitric oxide-mediated macrophage cytostasis. J. Biochem. (Tokyo). **120**: 49–52.
33. PEUNOVA, N. & G. ENIKOLOPOV. 1995. Nitric oxide triggers a switch to growth arrest during differentiation of neuronal cells. Nature **375**: 68–73.
34. STEIN, C.S., et al. 1995. Involvement of nitric oxide in IFN-gamma-mediated reduction of microvessel smooth muscle cell proliferation. Mol. Immunol. **32**: 965–973.
35. STUEHR, D.J. & C.F. NATHAN. 1989. Nitric oxide. A macrophage product responsible for cytostasis and respiratory inhibition in tumor target cells. J. Exp. Med. **169**: 1543–1555.
36. VINCENDEAU, P. & S. DAULOUEDE. 1991. Macrophage cytostatic effect on Trypanosoma musculi involves an L-arginine-dependent mechanism. J. Immunol. **146**: 4338–4343.
37. KETTELER, M., et al. 1996. L-arginine metabolism in immune-mediated glomerulonephritis in the rat. Am. J. Kidney Dis. **28**: 878–887.
38. BOGLE, R.G., et al. 1994. Endothelial polyamine uptake: selective stimulation by L-arginine deprivation or polyamine depletion. Am. J. Physiol. **266**: C776–C783.
39. BUGA, G.M., et al. 1998. N^G-hydroxy-L-arginine and nitric oxide inhibit Caco-2 tumor cell proliferation by distinct mechanisms. Am. J. Physiol. **275**: R1256–R1264.
40. JANSEN, A., et al. 1994. Induction of nitric oxide synthase in rat immune complex glomerulonephritis. Kidney Int. **45**: 1215–1219.
41. HECKER, M., et al. 1995. Inhibition of arginase by N^G-hydroxy-L-arginine in alveolar macrophages: implications for the utilization of L-arginine for nitric oxide synthesis. FEBS. Lett. **359**: 251–254.
42. SINGH, R., et al. 2001. Activation of caspase-3 activity and apoptosis in MDA-MB-468 cells by N(omega)-hydroxy-L-arginine, an inhibitor of arginase, is not solely dependent on reduction in intracellular polyamines. Carcinogenesis **22**: 1863–1869.

43. SATRIANO, J., et al. 1999. Regulation of intracellular polyamine biosynthesis and transport by NO and cytokines TNF-alpha and IFN-gamma. Am. J. Physiol. **276:** C892–C899.
44. BAUER, P.M., et al. 2001. Nitric oxide inhibits ornithine decarboxylase via S-nitrosylation of cysteine 360 in the active site of the enzyme. J. Biol. Chem. **276:** 34458–34464.
45. IGNARRO, L.J., et al. 2001. Role of the arginine-nitric oxide pathway in the regulation of vascular smooth muscle cell proliferation. Proc. Natl. Acad. Sci. U. S. A. **98:** 4202–4208.
46. GOBERT, A.P., et al. 2001. Helicobacter pylori arginase inhibits nitric oxide production by eukaryotic cells: a strategy for bacterial survival. Proc. Natl. Acad. Sci. U. S. A. **98:** 13844–13849.
47. MORI, M. & T. GOTOH. 2000. Regulation of nitric oxide production by arginine metabolic enzymes. Biochem. Biophys. Res. Commun. **275:** 715–719.
48. WADDINGTON, S.N. & V. CATTELL. 2000. Arginase in glomerulonephritis. Exp. Nephrol. **8:** 128–134.
49. MODOLELL, M., et al. 1995. Reciprocal regulation of the nitric oxide synthase/arginase balance in mouse bone marrow-derived macrophages by TH1 and TH2 cytokines. Eur. J. Immunol. **25:** 1101–1104.
50. LI, H., et al. 2001. Regulatory role of arginase I and II in nitric oxide, polyamine, and proline syntheses in endothelial cells. Am. J. Physiol. **280:** E75–E82.
51. BRUCH-GERHARZ, D., et al. 2003. Arginase 1 overexpression in psoriasis: limitation of inducible nitric oxide synthase activity as a molecular mechanism for keratinocyte hyperproliferation. Am. J. Pathol. **162:** 203–211.
52. KEPKA-LENHART, D., et al. 2000. Arginase I: a limiting factor for nitric oxide and polyamine synthesis by activated macrophages? Am. J. Physiol. **279:** R2237–R2242.
53. DURANTE, W., et al. 2001. Transforming growth factor-beta(1) stimulates L-arginine transport and metabolism in vascular smooth muscle cells: role in polyamine and collagen synthesis. Circulation **103:** 1121–1127.
54. CAI, D., et al. 2002. Arginase I and polyamines act downstream from cyclic AMP in overcoming inhibition of axonal growth MAG and myelin in vitro. Neuron. **35:** 711–719.
55. DAVEL, L.E., et al. 2002. Arginine metabolic pathways involved in the modulation of tumor-induced angiogenesis by macrophages. FEBS. Lett. **532:** 216–220.
56. WITTE, M.B., et al. 2002. Upregulation of arginase expression in wound-derived fibroblasts. J. Surg. Res. **105:** 35–42.
57. MUNDER, M., et al. 1999. Th1/Th2-regulated expression of arginase isoforms in murine macrophages and dendritic cells. J. Immunol. **163:** 3771–3777.
58. LORTIE, M.J., et al. 1996. Agmatine, a bioactive metabolite of arginine. Production, degradation, and functional effects in the kidney of the rat. J. Clin. Invest. **97:** 413–420.
59. MORRISSEY, J., et al. 1995. Partial cloning and characterization of an arginine decarboxylase in the kidney. Kidney Int. **47:** 1458–1461.
60. LORTIE, M.J., et al. 2000. Bioactive products of arginine in sepsis: tissue and plasma composition after LPS and iNOS blockade. Am. J. Physiol. **278:** C1191–C1199.
61. RAASCH, W., et al. 1995. Agmatine, the bacterial amine, is widely distributed in mammalian tissues. Life Sci. **56:** 2319–2330.
62. REIS, D.J. & S. REGUNATHAN. 2000. Is agmatine a novel neurotransmitter in brain? Trends Pharmacol. Sci. **21:** 187–193.
63. ISHIKAWA, T., et al. 1995. N omega-hydroxyagmatine: a novel substance causing endothelium-dependent vasorelaxation. Biochem. Biophys. Res. Commun. **214:** 145–151.
64. GAO, Y., et al. 1995. Agmatine: a novel endogenous vasodilator substance. Life Sci. **57:** L83–L86.
65. MORRISSEY, J.J. & S. KLAHR. 1997. Agmatine activation of nitric oxide synthase in endothelial cells. Proc. Assoc. Am. Physicians **109:** 51–57.
66. GALEA, E., et al. 1996. Inhibition of mammalian nitric oxide synthases by agmatine, an endogenous polyamine formed by decarboxylation of arginine. Biochem. J. **316:** 247–249.
67. AUGUET, M., et al. 1995. Selective inhibition of inducible nitric oxide synthase by agmatine. Jpn. J. Pharmacol. **69:** 285–287.

68. STUEHR, D.J., et al. 1991. N omega-hydroxy-L-arginine is an intermediate in the biosynthesis of nitric oxide from L-arginine. J. Biol. Chem. **266:** 6259–6263.
69. YOKOI, I., et al. 1994. Structure-activity relationships of arginine analogues on nitric oxide synthase activity in the rat brain. Neuropharmacology **33:** 1261–1265.
70. KOMORI, Y., G.C. WALLACE & J.M. FUKUTO. 1994. Inhibition of purified nitric oxide synthase from rat cerebellum and macrophage by L-arginine analogs. Arch. Biochem. Biophys. **315:** 213–218.
71. SENNEQUIER, N. & D.J. STUEHR. 1996. Analysis of substrate-induced electronic, catalytic, and structural changes in inducible NO synthase. Biochemistry **35:** 5883–5892.
72. SATRIANO, J., et al. 2001. Suppression of inducible nitric oxide generation by agmatine aldehyde: Beneficial effects in sepsis. J. Cell. Physiol. **188:** 313–320.
73. SATRIANO, J., et al. 1998. Agmatine suppresses proliferation by frameshift induction of antizyme and attenuation of cellular polyamine levels. J. Biol. Chem. **273:** 15313–15316.
74. VARGIU, C., et al. 1999. Agmatine modulates polyamine content in hepatocytes by inducing spermidine/spermine acetyltransferase. Eur. J. Biochem. **259:** 933–938.
75. ISHIZUKA, S., et al. 2000. Agmatine inhibits cell proliferation and improves renal function in anti-thy-1 glomerulonephritis. J. Am. Soc. Nephrol. **11:** 2256–2264.
76. MCDONALD, L.J. & J. MOSS. 1993. Nitric oxide-independent, thiol-associated ADP-ribosylation inactivates aldehyde dehydrogenase. J. Biol. Chem. **268:** 17878–17882.
77. DEMASTER, E.G., et al. 1997. Mechanism for the inhibition of aldehyde dehydrogenase by nitric oxide. Alcohol **14:** 181–189.
78. HOLT, A. & G.B. BAKER. 1995. Metabolism of agmatine (clonidine-displacing substance) by diamine oxidase and the possible implications for studies of imidazoline receptors. Prog. Brain Res. **106:** 187–197.
79. HERMAN, J.J. 1982. Eosinophil diamine oxidase activity in acute inflammation in humans. Agents Actions **12:** 46–48.
80. TACHIBANA, T., et al. 1986. Histimine metabolism in the arthus reaction. Exp. Mol. Pathol. **44:** 76–82.
81. KUSCHE, J., R. MENNIGEN & K. ERPENBACH. 1988. The intestinal diamine oxidase activity under the influence of adaptive proliferation of the intestinal mucosa—a proliferation terminating principle? Agents Actions **23:** 354–356.
82. SCHWARTZ, D., et al. 1997. Inhibition of constitutive nitric oxide synthase (NOS) by nitric oxide generated by inducible NOS after lipopolysaccharide administration provokes renal dysfunction in rats. J. Clin. Invest. **100:** 439–448.
83. FENG, Y., J.E. PILETZ & M.H. LEBLANC. 2002. Agmatine suppresses nitric oxide production and attenuates hypoxic-ischemic brain injury in neonatal rats. Pediatr. Res. **52:** 606–611.
84. FAIRBANKS, C.A., et al. 2000. Agmatine reverses pain induced by inflammation, neuropathy, and spinal cord injury. Proc. Natl. Acad. Sci. U. S. A. **97:** 10584–10589.
85. YU, C.G., et al. 2000. Agmatine improves locomotor function and reduces tissue damage following spinal cord injury. Neuroreport **11:** 3203–3207.
86. GILAD, G.M. & V.H. GILAD. 2000. Accelerated functional recovery and neuroprotection by agmatine after spinal cord ischemia in rats. Neurosci. Lett. **296:** 97–100.

Gastrointestinal Uptake of Agmatine

Distribution in Tissues and Organs and Pathophysiologic Relevance

GERHARD J. MOLDERINGS,[a] ANJA HEINEN,[a] SIGRID MENZEL,[a]
FRIEDRICH LÜBBECKE,[b] JÜRGEN HOMANN,[c] AND MANFRED GÖTHERT[a]

[a]*Institute of Pharmacology and Toxicology, University of Bonn, Bonn, Germany*
[b]*Department of Internal Medicine, Kreiskrankenhaus Uelzen, Uelzen, Germany*
[c]*Department of Internal Medicine, Evangelisches Krankenhaus, Bonn, Germany*

ABSTRACT: The authors report on (1) the absorption of agmatine from the gastrointestinal tract as an important source of this polycation in the organism, (2) its organ distribution, and (3) its putative role in liver regeneration. When rats received 0.5 µCi [^{14}C]agmatine contained in 5 grams of standard rat chow after a fasting period of 24 hours, radioactivity was recovered in all organs investigated, in blood, and in urine. In the liver 67% ± 7% of administered radioactivity was found. After partial (two-thirds) hepatectomy, administration of 250 mg and 500 mg agmatine by gavage for 6 days reduced liver regeneration at day 7 by 20% and 22%, respectively, compared with animals that received no agmatine. Agmatine is absorbed from the gastrointestinal tract, probably by means of a specific transporter. It is likely that agmatine in the chyme of the gut represents an essential source of agmatine in the tissues of the organism. An increase in the availability of gastrointestinal agmatine for absorption impairs liver regeneration and may contribute to the development of liver diseases.

KEYWORDS: agmatine distribution; agmatine uptake; agmatine transporter; liver regeneration

INTRODUCTION

The organic polycation agmatine is enzymatically formed from L-arginine by arginine decarboxylase. Although arginine decarboxylase has been found in several mammalian tissues, its organ distribution in rats differs from that of its product agmatine, pointing to another source of this compound in addition to its local biosynthesis (for review, see Ref. 1). Moreover, the activity of mammalian arginine decarboxylase seems to be low,[2] confirming that only a fraction of agmatine found in the mammalian tissues is probably formed by endogenous enzymatic de novo synthesis. A substantial portion is assumed to be caused by uptake by a specific high-capacity carrier

Address for correspondence: Gerhard J. Molderings, Institute of Pharmacology and Toxicology, University of Bonn, Reuterstr. 2b D-53113, Bonn, Germany. Voice: (+49) 228-735421; fax: (+49) 228-735404.
e-mail: molderings@uni-bonn.de

Ann. N.Y. Acad. Sci. 1009: 44–51 (2003). © 2003 New York Academy of Sciences.
doi: 10.1196/annals.1304.005

from the lumen of the gastrointestinal tract which contains a high amount of agmatine.[1,3] The high content of agmatine in the lumen of the gastrointestinal tract stems from three sources: (1) Agmatine is formed and released at high amounts by bacteria of the physiological gut microflora (e.g., *E. coli*[4]) as well as by pathogens such as *Helicobacter pylori*[3]; (2) ingested food may contain variable amounts of agmatine (TABLE 1); (3) luminal agmatine may also be derived from desquamated gastrointestinal epithelial cells, although this source seems to be of minor significance as suggested by its limited importance for the luminal content of polyamines.[5]

TABLE 1. Agmatine content of food

Food	Agmatine Content	Food	Agmatine Content
Starchy food		Dried common file fish	112 mg/kg
Rice, polished	n.d.	Other dried fish	n.d.
Corn	n.d.	Preserved albacore	n.d.
Wheat flour	0.5–82 mg/kg	Preserved anchovies	62 mg/kg
Potato	n.d.	Preserved sardines	80 mg/kg
Vegetables		Shellfish and fish products	
Spinach	≤1 mg/kg	Salted squid	650 mg/kg
Carrot	n.d.	Shells, fresh	2–224 mg/kg
Tomato	n.d.	Alaska pollack roe, fresh	73 mg/kg
Eggplant	n.d.		
Soybean, dried	n.d.	Milk and egg products	
Mushrooms, various	n.d.	Egg (hen)	n.d.
Fruits		Milk (cow)	≤0.2 mg/kg
Orange	n.d.	Yogurt	≤0.4 mg/kg
Apple	n.d.	Cheese (young)	n.d.
Meat		Cheese (old)	≤30 mg/kg
Pork	≤1.5 mg/kg	Alcoholic beverages	
Beef	≤2.5 mg/kg	Liquor, distilled	n.d.
Chicken	≤7 mg/kg	Beer	≤15 mg/L
Cured meat products (ham, sausage)	≤10 mg/kg	Sake	114 mg/L
Fish		Nonalcoholic beverages	
Fresh fish (various)	≤20 mg/kg	Tea	n.d.
Salted dried herring	217 mg/kg	Protein drink	0.5 µg/kg

ABBREVIATIONS: n.d., not detectable.
SOURCE: Data are compiled from Kawabata *et al.*,[28] Okamoto *et al.*,[29] Erkan *et al.*,[30] and from the authors' unpublished experiments.

Although agmatine exerts various effects in vivo and in vitro, the biologic significance is under debate because, as reviewed by Raasch et al.,[1] the concentrations at which those effects occur (1–1000 µM) are much higher than those so far determined in blood and most tissues (3.5 nM–1 µM). Recent data, however, suggest that the contents of agmatine summarized in that article might have been underestimated because a loss of agmatine by metabolic degradation during the extraction procedure was not sufficiently taken into account. Experiments on isolated cells have shown that agmatine is degraded by the enzymes diamine oxidase (DAO), which converts agmatine to guanidinobutyraldehyde,[6] and agmatinase, which splits agmatine to urea and putrescine.[7–9] Recently, the metabolism of [^{14}C]agmatine in rat hepatocyte cultures has been investigated in detail.[10] About 30% of the total radioactivity was found as unchanged labeled agmatine; 1% to 3% was converted to [^{14}C]GABA; 10% was transformed to the polyamines putrescine, spermidine, and N^1-acetylspermidine, but 50% was transformed into guanidinobutyraldehyde by DAO. This metabolite cannot be derivatized with o-phthalaldehyde and, hence, cannot be detected by the analytic procedure for agmatine detection.[11] In agreement with those results we found that only about 30% to 50% of agmatine in standard solutions added to liver suspensions was recovered after derivatization with o-phthalaldehyde by the HPLC method (results not shown). The observation that circulating plasma levels of agmatine in rat increased twofold after DAO inhibition[6] further emphasized the importance of DAO as a metabolic pathway for agmatine. The fate of agmatine in the tissues is highly dependent on the organ under study. In rat liver and kidney, for example, the conversion of agmatine to the aldehyde by DAO seems to be the main pathway, whereas the DAO pathway seems to be without importance in rat brain.[12]

To elucidate the source of tissue agmatine, further experiments were carried out in our laboratory (Ref.13 and unpublished results). We examined whether exogenous agmatine may contribute to the organ content of this polycation in addition to the amount formed enzymatically in the organism by arginine decarboxylase. Second, we investigated the effect of agmatine on proliferation of rat and human liver cells in vitro and in vivo to examine whether alterations in intracellular agmatine content might be of relevance for serious liver diseases.

RESULTS AND DISCUSSION

Absorption of Agmatine from the Gastrointestinal Tract

Considerable activity of luminal arginine decarboxylase, besides that found in the colon, has been detected only in the stomach.[14] Thus, the stomach seems to be a physiologic site of absorption of agmatine in rats, and the existence of a carrier for agmatine in rat stomach was therefore postulated. In fact, our experiments with isolated rat stomach demonstrated that [^{14}C]agmatine was temperature-dependently accumulated in the wall of the isolated organ by an agmatine-specific transport mechanism.[13] This transport shares essential pharmacologic properties with the agmatine carrier identified in human glioma and Caco2 cells because it was inhibited by phentolamine and putrescine (see Molderings et al., in this volume). A substantial contribution of an influx of [^{14}C]agmatine through activated nicotinic cation channels[15,16] to the accumulation of radioactivity in the isolated stomach wall was ruled out by the failure of the agonist at nicotinic acetylcholine receptors, DMPP, to increase ^{14}C accumulation.

The potential contribution of exogenous agmatine to the intracellular agmatine pool in the various tissues of rats in vivo was investigated by determining the accumulation of radioactivity in organs and tissues after [^{14}C]agmatine ingestion.[13] Radioactivity was absorbed from the stomach and distributed unevenly among the organs; by far highest accumulation of radioactivity occurred in the liver (67% ± 7%). Putrescine dose-dependently reduced accumulation of radioactivity, at least in liver, spleen, and lung, and probably also in the central nervous system. This finding is consistent with the involvement of a specific agmatine carrier possessing the pharmacologic properties of that found in rat stomach in vitro and in other tissues and cell lines.[10,17–21]

Although the concentration of radioactivity in blood was relatively low, [^{14}C]-agmatine must have been distributed into the organs through the circulation. This assumption is supported by the high ^{14}C content in the urine, which must result from the removal of ^{14}C from the blood by glomerular filtration in the kidney. The low amount of radioactivity detected in the blood probably results from the operation of the highly effective agmatine carrier in the various tissues. In this context it is interesting to note that agmatine concentration in rat plasma varies considerably. In our study the concentration ranged from below the detection limit of 0.1 ng/mL to 5.8 ng/mL with a median value of 0.33 ng/mL (n = 38). Others have reported concentrations of 0.45 ng/mL[11] and 91.1 ng/mL.[6] These differences in concentration might be caused by inter-individual differences (1) in the gastrointestinal luminal agmatine content, (2) in the kinetics of agmatine uptake by the various tissues, and (3) in the activity of the agmatine carrier present in erythrocytes. Therefore, agmatine concentration in whole blood, serum, or plasma cannot be expected to be correlated with intestinal agmatine absorption or agmatine concentrations in the tissues and, hence, cannot be used to monitor gastrointestinal agmatine uptake and tissue content in vivo.

As a consequence of the 24-hour fasting period before ingestion of the standard chow containing [^{14}C]agmatine and the well-known physiologic storage of food in the gastric lumen of rats for several hours, the jejunal lumen did not contain any macroscopically visible chyme. Nonetheless, the ileum and colon were not empty after the 3-hour digestion period, and radioactivity was detected in the luminal content of these segments of the gut. Again, luminal radioactivity in ileum and colon was decreased when putrescine ingestion preceded the agmatine administration, suggesting the involvement of the agmatine carrier. Because [^{14}C]agmatine-containing stomach content was not transported into the ileum and colon, the radioactivity detected in the latter must be assumed to be caused by secretion either by intestinal mucosa cells or into the pancreaticobiliary fluid. The latter possibility is supported by analogous findings with putrescine.[14] Therefore it seems likely that agmatine is subject to enterohepatic circulation.

Effect of Agmatine in Liver Cell Proliferation

In view of the pronounced accumulation of exogenous agmatine in the liver, a substantial involvement of agmatine in the liver cell homeostasis is conceivable, in particular when considering that agmatine interacts with the polyamine pathway in cells by multiple mechanisms. Thus it suppresses the activity of the rate-limiting, polyamine-forming enzyme ornithine decarboxylase, it reduces the uptake of polyamines, and it increases the activity of spermidine/spermine N^1-acetyltransferase and S-adenosylmethionine decarboxylase. This multi-target action of agmatine results in an inhibition of proliferation of tumor and non-tumor cells (for review, see Molderings et al., in this volume).

Therefore, we investigated whether agmatine inhibits proliferation of the rat and human hepatocarcinoma cells McRH7777 and HepG2, respectively. In fact, the proliferation of both cell types was reduced in proportion to the agmatine concentration, with mean $IC_{50\%}$ values (concentrations causing 50% inhibition of cell growth) of 223 mM and 626 mM for McRH7777 and HepG2 cells, respectively (unpublished results).

On the basis of these results, we investigated whether this inhibition in vitro was reflected by alterations in liver function in vivo. A suitable animal model to study the interference of agmatine with polyamine-regulated liver functions in vivo is the investigation of rat liver regeneration after two-thirds hepatectomy. In rat the original liver mass is restored in about 1 week by proliferation of all existing mature cell populations composing the intact organ (for review, see Ref. 22). Polyamines, in particular spermidine, are specifically required for the initiation of rat liver regeneration.[23,24] Putrescine seems to serve as a precursor for spermidine, whereas spermine seems to be a deposit used for back-conversion into spermidine.[24] Because liver weight is closely correlated to body weight, the relative liver weight (i.e., the ratio of liver wet weight to body weight) can be used to monitor the regeneration process. After two-thirds hepatectomy, daily administration of 250 mg or 500 mg of agmatine to rats for 6 days by gavage significantly reduced weight gain of the remnant liver at day 7, by 19.5% and 22.3%, respectively, when compared with the weight gain of control animals (unpublished results). This delay in regeneration was associated with an approximately 13- to 15-fold increase of agmatine content in the liver compared with the basal value before surgery, whereas the agmatine content in the liver of the control group remained unchanged.

Relevance of Luminal Intestinal Agmatine in Humans

If agmatine taken up from the gut were substantially involved in the regulation of liver function in man, therapeutic interventions that are known to improve or disturb liver function should be accompanied by changes in agmatine homeostasis. Because direct investigation of agmatine effects in patients is not possible, we tried to unravel a modulatory role of agmatine on liver function indirectly. If agmatine inhibits regenerative processes in human liver cells in vivo, a reduction of the enteral availability of agmatine as a substantial source for the organism should be accompanied by an improvement of hepatic encephalopathy in patients with decompensated liver cirrhosis. It is well known that oral administration of lactulose can diminish the signs of hepatic encephalopathy. This beneficial effect of lactulose has been ascribed to changes in the composition of the physiologic bacterial flora, which are assumed to result in a decreased ammonia concentration in blood. Because a firm correlation between the ammonia concentration in blood and the occurrence of hepatic encephalopathy has not yet been demonstrated, however (for review, see Refs. 25 and 26), other mechanisms may come into play. In our study we were able to show for the first time that treatment of hepatic encephalopathy with oral lactulose was signifi-

TABLE 2. Agmatine concentrations before and after successful treatment with lactulose[a]

	Feces weight pre-treatment[b]	Feces weight post-treatment[b]	Plasma pre-treatment[c]	Plasma post-treatment[c]	Erythrocytes pre-treatment[d]	Erythrocytes post-treatment[d]
Median	123.0	54.0*	6.73	3.70	38.30	12.20
Minimum	14.7	3.4	1.10	0	3.28	0.61
Maximum	15760.0	144.4	31.00	160.50	100.00	244.7

[a] Data from nine patients with signs of hepatic encephalopathy before and after successful treatment with lactulose (10 g/day for 4–7 days).
[b] In ng/g pellet weight.
[c] In ng/mL.
[d] In ng/g wet weight.
* Significantly different from value before lactulose treatment.

cantly associated with a decrease of fecal agmatine content by $73\% \pm 8\%$ ($P < 0.004$, Wilcoxon signed rank test; n = 9; for range of agmatine content in feces, see TABLE 2). This change was not paralleled by consistent changes of agmatine concentration in blood, irrespective of whether plasma or erythrocytes were analyzed (TABLE 2). This result is probably a consequence of the rapid clearance of agmatine (half-life of injected agmatine in rat blood: 5 minutes[27]) either by uptake into the tissues or by degradation by diamine oxidase.[6,12] The decrease in luminal agmatine content is unlikely to result from dietary modification (which is an accompanying therapeutic principle in the treatment of hepatic encephalopathy), because food contributes to the content of agmatine in chyme only marginally, if at all (see TABLE 1). It is also unlikely that this decrease is the result of a dilution by the lactulose-induced increase in stool volume, because agmatine concentration was calculated on the basis of the pellet weight of the respective feces specimen. Therefore, it seems justified to assume that the content of agmatine in the chyme of the gut, which is mainly caused by agmatine production by the bacteria of the physiologic intestinal flora (e.g., *E. coli*, as reviewed in Ref. 4), decreased because lactulose induced a change in the composition of the bacterial microflora towards bacteria with a reduced ability to produce agmatine. The coincidence of a decreased agmatine content in the chyme of the gut after lactulose therapy and the improvement of hepatic encephalopathy may be interpreted as a lactulose-induced reduced availability of agmatine for uptake from the intestinal lumen. In turn, this reduced availability of agmatine would lead to a decrease of agmatine concentration in the liver cells[13] and, hence, to a reduction of its noxious action on hepatocytes. Thus, the reduction of enteral agmatine content might, beside other possible effects of lactulose, contribute to the beneficial outcome of this therapy.

Conclusions

Taken together, our data are compatible with the view that agmatine can be absorbed from the stomach and the gut by means of an energy-dependent specific agmatine-transport mechanism. Agmatine itself or its degradation products, which also have the potential to be pharmacologically active, are unevenly distributed among the organs and probably undergo an enterohepatic circulation. In view of the high intraluminal concentration of agmatine in the gastrointestinal tract and the operation of an agmatine transporter, it is rather likely that agmatine in the chyme of the gut represents an important source for agmatine which is functionally active in the tissues of the organism, in particular in the liver.

ACKNOWLEDGMENT

The technical assistance of Marlies Hartwig and Regina Müller is gratefully acknowledged. This study was supported by grants from the Deutsche Forschungsgemeinschaft and the Wilhelm-Sander-Stiftung.

REFERENCES

1. RAASCH, W., U. SCHÄFER, J. CHUN, et al. 2001. Biological significance of agmatine, an endogenous ligand at imidazoline binding sites. Br. J. Pharmacol. **133:** 755–780.
2. PENAFIEL, R., C. RUZOFA, E. PEDRENO, et al. 1998. Agmatine metabolism in rodent tissues. In Biogenically Active Amines in Food, Vol. 2. S. A. Bardoczs, G. White, G. Hajos, Eds.: 79–85. European Communities. Brussels, Belgium.
3. MOLDERINGS, G.J., M. BURIAN, J. HOMANN, et al. 1999. Potential relevance of agmatine as a virulence factor of Helicobacter pylori. Dig. Dis. Sci. **44:** 2397–2404.
4. TABOR, C.W. & H. TABOR. 1984. Polyamines. Ann. Res. Biochem. **53:** 749–790.
5. BENAMOUZIG, R., S. MAHÉ, C. LUENGO, et al. 1997. Fasting and postprandial polyamine concentrations in the human digestive lumen. Am. J. Clin. Nutr. **65:** 766–770.
6. LORTIE, M.J., W.F. NOVOTNY, O.W. PETERSON, et al. 1996. Agmatine, a bioactive metabolite of arginine. J. Clin. Invest. **97:** 413–420.
7. GILAD, G.M., Y. WOLLAM, A. IAINE, et al. 1996. Metabolism of agmatine into urea but not into nitric oxide in rat brain. Neuroreport **7:** 1730–1732.
8. SASTRE, M., S. REGUNATHAN, E. GALEA, et al. 1996. Agmatinase activity in rat brain: a metabolic pathway for the degradation of agmatine. J. Neurochem. **67:** 1761–1765.
9. SASTRE, M., E. GALEA, D. FEINSTEIN, et al. 1998. Metabolism of agmatine in macrophages: modulation by lipopolysaccharide and inhibitory cytokines. Biochem. J. **330:** 1405–1409.
10. CABELLA, C., G. GARDINI, D. CORPILLO, et al. 2001. Transport and metabolism of agmatine in rat hepatocyte cultures. Eur. J. Biochem. **268:** 940–947.
11. RAASCH, W., S. REGUNATHAN, et al. 1995. Agmatine, the bacterial amine, is widely distributed in mammalian tissues. Life Sci. **56:** 2319–2330.
12. HOLT, A. & G.B. BAKER. 1995. Metabolism of agmatine (clonidine-displacing substance) by diamine oxidase and the possible implications for studies of imidazoline receptors. Progress Brain Res. **106:** 187–197.
13. MOLDERINGS, G.J., A. HEINEN, S. MENZEL, et al. 2002. Exposure of rat isolated stomach and rats in vivo to [^{14}C]agmatine: accumulation in the stomach wall and distribution in various tissues. Fundam. Clin. Pharmacol. **16:** 219–225.
14. OSBORNE, D.L. & E.R. SEIDEL. 1990. Gastrointestinal luminal polyamines: cellular accumulation and enterohepatic circulation. Am. J. Physiol. **258:** G576–G584.
15. YOSHIKAMI, P. 1981. Transmitter sensitivity of neurons assayed by autoradiography. Science **212:** 929–930.
16. QUIK, M. 1985. Inhibition of nicotinic receptor mediated ion fluxes in rat sympathetic ganglia by BGT II-S1 a potent phospholipase. Brain Res. **325:** 79–88.
17. BABAL, P., M. RUCHKO, J.W. OLSON, et al. 2000. Interactions between agmatine and polyamine uptake pathways in rat pulmonary artery endothelial cells. Gen. Pharmacol. **34:** 255–261.

18. DEL VALLE, A.E., J.C. PAZ, F. SANCHEZ-JIMENEZ, et al. 2000. Agmatine uptake by cultured hamster kidney cells. Biochem. Biophys. Res. Commun. **280:** 307–311.
19. MOLDERINGS, G.J., H. BÖNISCH, M. GÖTHERT, et al. 2001. Agmatine and putrescine uptake in the human glioma cell line SK-MG-1. Naunyn-Schmiedeberg's Arch. Pharmacol. **363:** 671–679.
20. SATRIANO, J., M. ISOME, R.A. CASERO, et al. 2001. Polyamine transport system mediates agmatine transport in mammalian cells. Am. J. Physiol. Cell. Physiol. **281:** C329–C334.
21. HEINEN, A., M. BRÜSS, H. BÖNISCH, et al. 2003. Pharmacological characteristics of the specific transporter for the endogenous cell growth inhibitor agmatine in six tumor cell lines. Int. J. Colorectal Dis. **18:** 314–319.
22. MICHALOPOULOS, G.K. & M.C. DEFRANCES. 1997. Liver regeneration. Science **276:** 60–66.
23. HIGAKI, I., I. MATSUI-YUASA, K. HIROHASHI, et al. 1999. The role of polyamines in growth factor induced DNA synthesis in cultured rat hepatocytes. Hepatogastroenterology **46:** 1874–1879.
24. ALHONEN, L., T.L. RÄSÄNEN, R. SINERVIRTA, et al. 2002. Polyamines are required for the initiation of rat liver regeneration. Biochem. J. **362:** 149–153.
25. BUTTERWORTH, R.F. 2002. Complications of cirrhosis. III. Hepatic encephalopathy. J Hepatology **32**(Suppl. 1): 171–180.
26. GERBER, T. & H. SCHOMERUS. 2000. Hepatic encephalopathy in liver cirrhosis. Drugs **60:** 1353–1370.
27. RAASCH, W., U. SCHÄFER, F. QADRI, et al. 2002. Agmatine, an endogenous ligand at imidazoline binding sites, does not antagonize the clonidine-mediated blood pressure reaction. Br. J. Pharmacol. **135:** 663–672.
28. KAWABATA, T., H. OHSHIMA, M. INO. 1978. Occurrence of methylguanidine and agmatine in foods. IARC Sci. Publ. **19:** 415–423.
29. OKAMOTO, A., E. SUGI, Y. KOIZUMI, et al. 1997. Polyamine content of ordinary foodstuffs and various fermented foods. Biosci. Biotech. Biochem. **61:** 1582–1584.
30. ERKAN, N., N. HELLE, Ö. ÖZDEN. 2001. Determination of biogenic amines in canned fish of the Turkish market. Berl. Munch. Tierarztl. Wochenschr. **114:** 241–245.

Structure-Activity Analysis of Guanidine Group in Agmatine for Brain Agmatinase

M.-J. HUANG,[a] S. REGUNATHAN,[b] M. BOTTA,[c] K. LEE,[a] E. McCLENDON,[a] G.B. YI,[b] M.L. PEDERSEN,[d] D.B. BERKOWITZ,[d] G. WANG,[b] M. TRAVAGLI,[c] AND J.E. PILETZ[a,b]

[a]*Department of Chemistry, Jackson State University, Jackson, Mississippi, USA*

[b]*University of Mississippi Medical Center, Jackson, Mississippi, USA*

[c]*Dipartimento Farmaco Chimico Technologico, Universita degli Studi di Seina, Italy*

[d]*Department of Chemistry, University of Nebraska-Lincoln, Nebraska, USA*

ABSTRACT: To identify a selective inhibitor of mammalian agmatinase, screening was performed on four analogues of agmatine with modifications directly to the guanidine group, six analogues with modifications to the carbon-amine chain, and one analogue with modifications at both ends of the molecule. Control compounds were aminoguanidine and 7-nitroindazole, known inhibitors of the three isoforms (i, e, n) of nitric oxide synthase (NOS), and arcaine, a known inhibitor of the glutamate NMDA receptor. These compounds were compared for inhibition of rat agmatinase and arginine decarboxylase (ADC) activities. Results were studied by *ab initio* Hartee-Fock descriptors based on optimized geometries and van der Waals radii. Linear correlations were obtained using various geometric and electronic descriptors of the carbon (C), nitrogen (N), and hydrogen (H) atoms in the guanidine moiety. The best fit equation for percent activity remaining of rat agmatinase was = 0.3225 D + 72.76 D1916 + 64.97 D1920 − 192.58 H21 − 253.09 (r = 0.89), where D is the calculated dipole moment, D1916 and D1920 are the N19-N16 and N19-N20 distances, respectively, and H21 is the charge on H21. This agmatinase equation is distinct from the equations fit for ADC, the three NOS isoforms, and inhibition of NMDA receptor binding.

KEYWORDS: agmatine; guanidine; agmatinase; nitric oxide synthase; NMDA receptor; arginine decarboxylase

INTRODUCTION

Agmatine is an endogenous amine and four carbon guanidine cation that is synthesized following decarboxylation of L-arginine by arginine decarboxylase (ADC; EC 4.1.1.19).[1] Recent evidence suggests that brain agmatine is more than a mere metabolic intermediate in a pathway leading to polyamine synthesis.[2] Animal studies have revealed agmatine's beneficial effects in idiopathic pain,[3] convulsions,[4] and

---

Address for correspondence: Ming-Ju Huang, Ph.D., Department of Chemistry, P.O. Box 17910, 1400 J.R. Lynch Street, Jackson State University, Jackson MS 39217-0510, USA. Voice: 601-979-3492; fax: 601-979-3674.

e-mail: mhuang@chem.jsums.edu

stress-mediated behaviors.[5,6] Exogenously applied agmatine also exerts complex interactive effects with morphine: enhancing the analgesia of,[7] blocking tolerance and substance dependence to,[8] and attenuating the withdrawal symptoms from[9] morphine. Agmatine treatments also are neuroprotective if given in the early stages of ischemic brain injury.[10] Although originally identified in the brain as an endogenous neurotransmitter for imidazoline receptors,[1] agmatine's effects have mostly been ascribed to inhibition of nitric oxide synthase (NOS)[11] or blockade of glutamate NMDA receptor channels and other ligand-gated cationic channels.[12] Agmatinase is the predominant enzyme that regulates the half-life of agmatine in the brain.[13] Therefore, a selective inhibitor of brain agmatinase has been sought. In this study we have attempted to determine the characteristics expected of a selective inhibitor of rat brain agmatinase by comparing chemical derivatives of agmatine across a battery of six assays: rat brain agmatinase, ADC, iNOS, eNOS, nNOS, and competition binding at the NMDA receptor.

MATERIALS AND METHODS

Agmatine sulfate, aminoguanidine, arcaine sulfate, and 7-nitroindazole were purchased from Sigma Chemical Co. (St. Louis, MO, USA). Other agmatine analogues were obtained from a variety of sources. A racemic mixture of alpha-vinylarginine was synthesized by D. Berkowitz.[14] Compounds CS51, R74, TRV187, TRV162, G3, and RO5 were from M. Botta.[15] Three compounds were synthesized locally by K. Lee and G.B.Yi at Jackson State University using commercially available reagents: The synthesis of 3-aminopropylguanidine (KL-1) and trans-4-aminocyclohexylguanidine (KL-2) started with an aqueous solution of cyanamide added drop-wise to a boiling solution of 1,3-diaminopropane in concentrated hydrochloric solution. The mixture was refluxed for 1 hour, and then an aqueous solution of NaOH was added. The white precipitate was isolated and ^{1}H NMR spectrum was obtained to confirm the structures. The synthesis of Bis(3-(N-Iminomethyl)-aminopropyl)amine (GY) is described elsewhere.

Nitric Oxide Synthase

NOS activity was measured by monitoring the conversion of [^{3}H]arginine to [^{3}H]citrulline[16] from three commercially available isoforms of rat NOS: nNOS (602 units/mL, 14.9 mg/mL), iNOS (249.7 units/mL, 21.1 mg/ml) and eNOS (30 units/mL, 14.6 mg/mL) (Cayman, Ann Arbor, MI, USA). Neuronal NOS and iNOS were diluted 1:10; eNOS was used directly without dilution. Unless otherwise indicated, each tube was incubated at 37°C for 60 minutes. Assay buffer contained 50 mM Tris-HCl pH 7.4, 2 mM $CaCl_2$, 1 mM nicotinamide adenine dinucleotide phosphate (NADPH), 10 mM BH_4, 5 mM flavin adenine dinucleotide (FAD), 5 mM flavin mononucleotide (FMN), and 10 mg/mL calmodulin plus radioactive precursor. After incubation, the assay reaction was halted by addition of 400 μL of buffer containing 5 mM ethylenediaminetetraacetic acid (EDTA) and 50 mM HEPES. Equilibrated resin (200 mL, Dowex AG50WX-8 (Na^+ form) was added, and the reaction mixture was transferred to spin cups and into cup holders. The mixture was passed through the Dowex AG50WX-8 resin and the filtrate was collected in a spin cup. NOS activity was determined by counting the radioactivity in the flow-through (unbound) fraction. Each assay was measured in triplicate.

Agmatinase Activity

Agmatinase activity was measured by the method of Satishchandran and Boyle (1986) as detailed in an earlier publication.[13] The assay is based on the hydrolysis of [guanido ^{14}C]agmatine to [^{14}C]urea and putrescine, and subsequent trapping of [^{14}C]O_2 released from [^{14}C]urea by addition of urease. Assays were carried out for 30 minutes at 37°C in 300 μL of sample containing 100 mM HEPES pH 7.8, 4 mM $MgSO_4$, 1 mM dithiothreitol, 10 mM L-agmatine, 7 μM [^{14}C]agmatine, and 0.06 units of urease. Release of [^{14}C]O_2 from [^{14}C]urea was measured by trapping the [^{14}C]O_2 in filter-paper wicks saturated with benzethonium hydroxide. The reaction was stopped by injection of 40% trichloroacetic acid (TCA) into the reaction chamber, and the filters were transferred to minivials containing 5 ml CytoScint cocktail (ICN Biomedicals, Irvine, CA), and counted for radioactivity by liquid scintillation spectrometry (Beckman model LS 5801; Beckman/Coulter Inc., Fullerton, CA).

Arginine Decarboxylase Activity

Activity of ADC was measured in cell membrane fractions as described earlier,[17] based on the release of [^{14}C]O_2 from [1-^{14}C]arginine. Cell pellets were resuspended in Tris-HCl, EDTA buffer (pH 7.4), sonicated, and centrifuged at 27,000 × gravity for 20 minutes. The membrane pellet was washed once by sonication and recentrifugation in Tris-HCl buffer and resuspended in the incubation buffer. The membrane suspension (500 μl) was incubated for 1 hour at 25°C in 20 mM Tris-HCl buffer (pH 8.25), containing 1 mM $MgSO4$, 0.5 mM dithiothreitol, 0.5 mM polymethylsulfonylfluoride (PMSF), 0.2 mM EDTA, 0.1 mM L-arginine, and 7.28 μM L[1-^{14}C] arginine. Release of [^{14}C]O_2 from L[1-^{14}C]arginine was measured by trapping the [^{14}C]O_2 in filter-paper wicks saturated with benzethonium hydroxide. The reaction was stopped by the injection of 40% TCA into the reaction chamber, the filters were transferred to minivials containing 5 mL CytoScint cocktail (ICN Biomedicals), and counted for radioactivity by liquid scintillation spectrometry.

[^3H]MK801 Binding

The binding of [^3H]MK801 to NMDA receptors was measured in rat brain membranes as described previously.[18] Briefly, the membranes were incubated in HEPES buffer (pH 7.4) containing 0.4 nM [^3H]MK801, 100 μM glutamate, and 30 μM glycine for 1 hour at 25°C. The binding was terminated by rapid filtration over glass fiber filters, and radioactivity was counted. Nonspecific binding was defined by using 50 μM unlabelled MK801.

Quantitative Structure-Activity Relationships

Quantitative structure-activity relationships (QSARs) were studied by ab initio Hartree-Fock calculations with the Gaussion 94 computer program (Gaussian, Inc., Pittsburgh, PA, USA).[19] Based on the optimized geometry and van der Waals radius of each atom, calculations were performed with BlogP and BlogW programs[20–22] to determine molecular surfaces, volumes, ovalities, partition coefficients, and water solubilities. Linear combinations of these calculated descriptors were then fitted to the observed enzyme activities. The observed activities were the remaining percentage of rat agmatinase activity at 0.5 mM of each compound, the remaining percentage of rat NOS isozyme activity at 1 mM of each compound, and the remaining percentage of rat brain NMDA receptor binding at 0.1 mM of each compound.

RESULTS

Fourteen agmatine analogues (FIG. 1) were tested for inhibition of rat agmatinase, ADC, NOS isozymes, and the NMDA receptor. Data for inhibition of rat agmatinase, rat NOS isoforms, and competitive binding at the rat brain NMDA receptor are listed in TABLES 1, 2, and 3, respectively. No single compound was found with pure selectivity as a mammalian agmatinase inhibitor without also inhibiting to some degree the NOS isozymes and/or the NMDA receptor. Moreover, none of the compounds noticeably inhibited mammalian ADC (note: the experiments with CS51 were not interpretable for ADC and agmatinase).

QSAR analysis of the guanidine group in each compound allows certain predictions about the types of compounds that might be selective for agmatinase. The atom-numbering scheme of the guanidine group is shown in FIGURE 2. The best correlation for activity remaining (percentage not inhibited) of rat agmatinase was

$$\text{Activity remaining} = 0.3225 \, D + 72.76 \, D1916 + 64.97 \, D1920 - 192.58 \, H21 - 253.09$$
$$(n = 12, F = 6.8033, r = 0.8919, SD = 0.13199)$$

where n is the number of compounds submitted to the regression; r is the correlation coefficient; SD is the standard derivation; and F is the Fisher's variance ratio. The D in the equation is the calculated dipole moment of the compound. The D1916 and D1920 are the distances between N19 and N16 and between N19 and N20 respectively, and H21 is the charge on H21 (see FIG. 2).

According to this equation, the experimental and calculated activities of the analogues on rat agmatinase are shown in FIGURE 3. This QSAR analysis suggested that the smaller the dipole moment, the smaller the N19 and N16 distance, and the smaller the N19 and N20 distance, the greater the charge on H21 of the compound, and the less the percentage of remaining activity (more potent inhibitor).

Similar QSAR calculations were performed for nNOS. The best correlation for the activity remaining (percentage not inhibited) of rat nNOS was

$$\text{Activity remaining} = -0.0882 \, DNN19 - 99.890 \, D1921 + 26.073 \, D1620 + 40.970$$
$$(n = 13, F = 18.1157, r = 0.9262, SD = 0.10607)$$

where DNN19, D1921, and D1620 are the distances between N (the unlabelled nitrogen in FIG. 2) and N19, between N19 and H21, and between N16 and N20, respectively.

According to this equation, the experimental and calculated activities of the analogues on rat nNOS are shown in FIGURE 4. It is suggested that the greater the

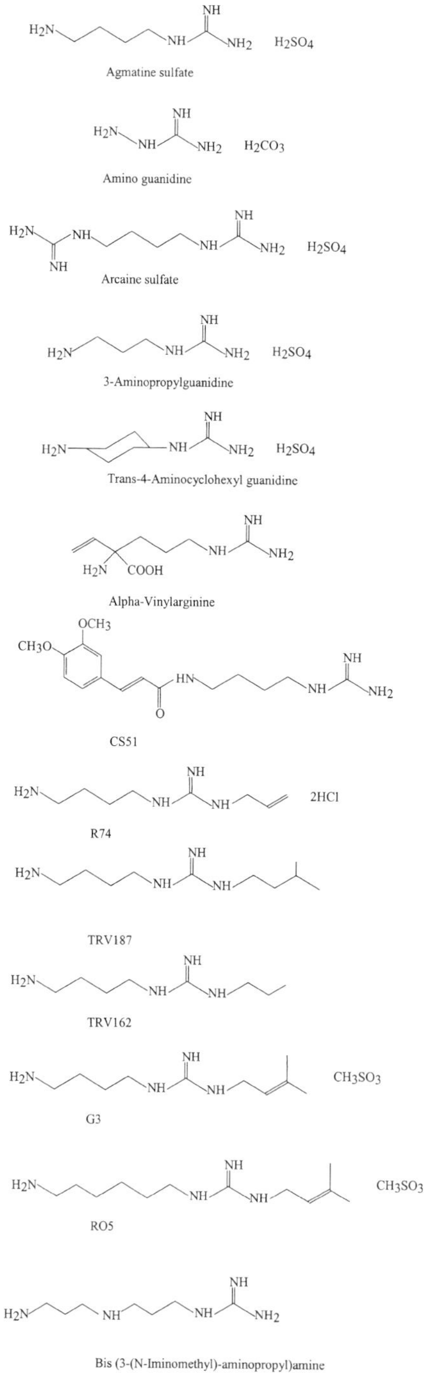

FIGURE 1. Chemical structures of the thirteen studied compounds.

TABLE 1. Results for inhibition by agmatine analogues of rat agmatinase

	Compounds	Agmatinase Activity Remaining (%) (Concentration = 0.5 mM)
1	Agmatine sulfate	37
2	Amino guanidine	53
3	Arcaine sulfate	29.5
4	3-Aminopropylguanidine	3.1
5	Trans-4-aminocyclohexyl guanidine	97.0
6	Alpha-vinylarginine	52.0
7	CS51	Not interpretable*
8	R74	15.3
9	TRV187	66.0
10	TRV162	98.0
11	G3	35.0
12	RO5	30.0
13	Bis(3-(N-iminomethyl)-aminopropyl)amine	38.0

* Methanol had to be used to solubilize CS51, and even the lowest concentration of methanol in the assay was inhibitory by itself.

TABLE 2. Results for rat NOS inhibition by agmatine analogues

	Compounds	Activity Remaining (%) (Conc = 1 mM) nNOS	Activity Remaining (%) (Conc = 1 mM) iNOS	Activity Remaining (%) (Conc = 1 mM) eNOS
1	Agmatine sulfate	32.5	35.2	97.4
2	Amino guanidine	20.0	1.0	30.0
3	Arcaine sulfate	9.8	37.8	83.4
4	3-Aminopropylguanidine	6.9	5.1	60.8
5	Trans-4-aminocyclohexyl guanidine	42.5	99.6	69.4
6	Alpha-vinylarginine	4.2	7.0	67.4
7	CS51	95.0	94.0	84.9
8	R74	2.1	9.6	90.5
9	TRV187	2.6	70.2	75.9
10	TRV162	57.0	92.7	95.6
11	G3	0.1	7.2	3.9
12	RO5	0.24	76.2	4.3
13	Bis(3-(N-iminomethyl)-aminopropyl)amine	23.5	65.2	88.7
14	7-Nitroindazole	1.0	1.0	0

TABLE 3. Results of competitive binding by agmatine analogues on rat brain NMDA receptors using [^{3}H]MK801

	Compounds	^{3}H-MK801 Binding Remaining (%) (Conc = 0.1mM)
1	Agmatine sulfate	93.8
2	Amino guanidine	90.6
3	Arcaine sulfate	45.1
4	3-Aminopropylguanidine	93.9
5	Trans-4-aminocyclohexyl guanidine	97.3
6	Alpha-vinylarginine	99.7
7	CS51	99.7
8	R74	99.7
9	TRV187	93.2
10	TRV162	99.4
11	G3	89.3
12	RO5	48.9
13	Bis(3-(N-iminomethyl)-aminopropyl)amine	99.7

distance between N and N19, the greater the distance between N19 and H21, and the smaller the distance between N16 and N20, the less the percentage of remaining activity (more potent nNOS inhibitor).

Similar QSAR calculations were next performed on iNOS. The best correlation for the activity remaining (percentage not inhibited) of rat iNOS was

$$\text{Activity remaining} = 17.559 \text{ LUMO} + 165.71 \text{ D1921} + 0.039287 \text{ V} - 13.152 \text{ O} - 155.38$$
$$(n = 13, F = 13.7018, r = 0.9341, SD = 0.13612)$$

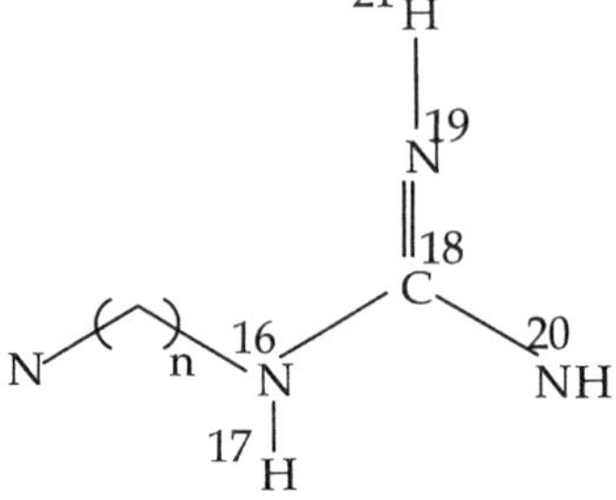

FIGURE 2. The general molecular structure of tested analogs and the numbering system.

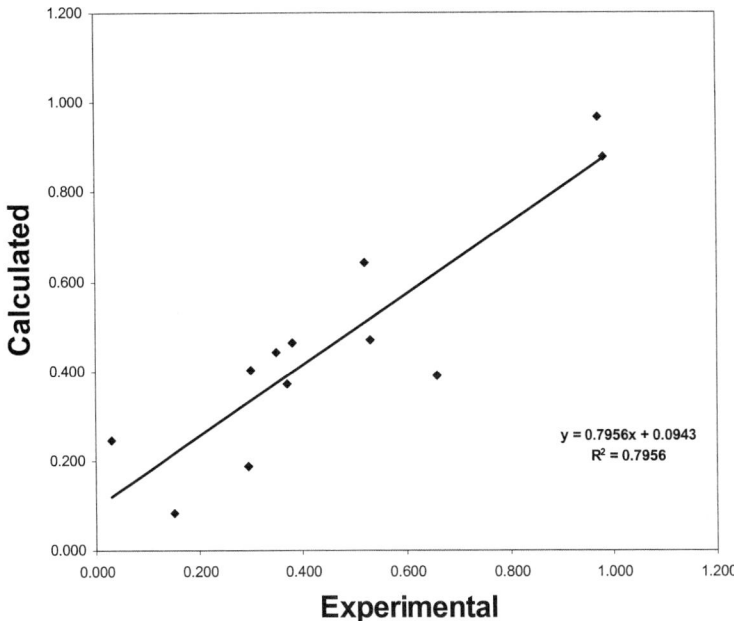

FIGURE 3. The calculated versus experimental activity remaining percentage of rat agmatinase of analogues.

where LUMO is the lowest unoccupied molecular orbital energy, D1921 is the bond length of N19 and H21, V is the volume of the compound, and O is the ovality of the compound.

According to this equation, the experimental and calculated activities of the analogues on rat iNOS are shown in FIGURE 5. It is suggested that the lower the LUMO energy, the smaller the bond length of N19 and H21, the smaller the molecular volume and the higher the ovality of the compound, the less the percentage of remaining activity (more potent iNOS inhibitor).

Similar QSAR calculations were next performed for eNOS. The best correlation for the activity remaining percentage-wise of rat eNOS was

$$\text{Activity remaining} = 41.468\, D1820 + 57.345\, N19 - 359.848\, D1617 + 351.56$$
$$(n = 13, F = 18.3879, r = 0.9272, SD = 0.12200)$$

where D1820 and D1617 are the distances between C18 and N20 and between N16 and H17, respectively. N19 is the charge on N19.

According to this equation, the experimental and calculated activities of the analogues on rat eNOS are shown in FIGURE 6. It is suggested that the smaller the distance between C18 and N20, the lower the charge on N19, the greater the distance between N16 and H17, the less the percentage of remaining activity (more potent eNOS inhibitor).

Similar QSAR calculations were next performed for NMDA receptor binding inhibition. The best correlation for the binding remaining percentage-wise at the rat NMDA was

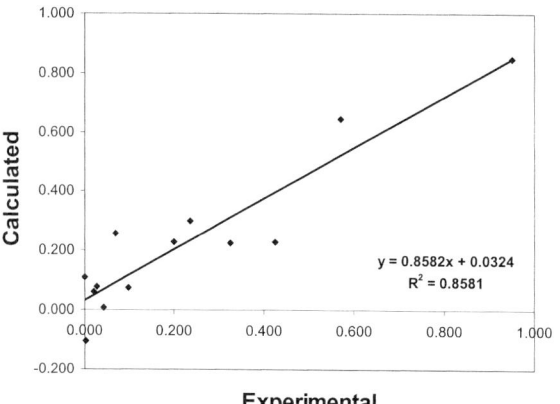

FIGURE 4. The calculated versus experimental activity remaining percentage of rat nNOS of analogues.

$$\text{Activity remaining} = 0.6715 - 0.2503 \text{ LOGP} - 0.3023 \text{ LOGW} + 0.1970 \text{ DNN19} - 0.2873 \text{ DNN20}$$
$$(n = 13, F = 9.64147, r = 0.9101, SD = 0.07786)$$

where LOGP is the calculated log of the partition coefficient of the compound, LOGW (logarithm of the water solubility, units of moles/liter) is the calculated log of the water solubility of the compound, and DNN20 is the distance between the N and N20.

Based on this equation, the experimental and calculated binding inhibition of the agmatine analogues at the rat NMDA are shown in FIGURE 7. It is suggested that the greater the partition coefficient of the compound, the greater the water solubility of the compound; the greater the distance between N and N20 and the smaller the

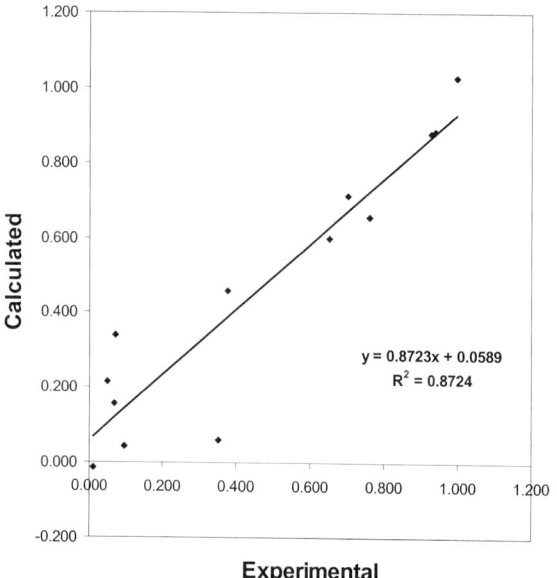

FIGURE 5. The calculated versus experimental activity remaining percentage of rat iNOS of analogues.

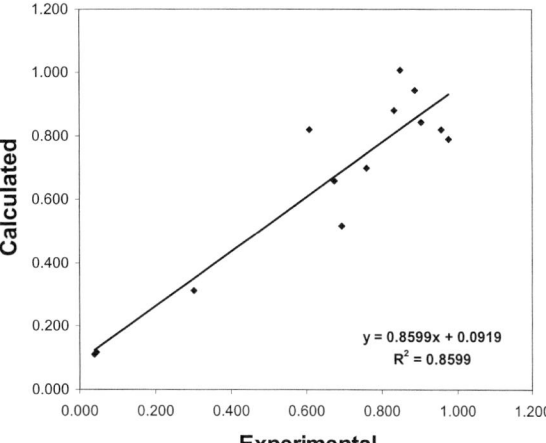

FIGURE 6. The calculated versus experimental activity remaining percentage of rat eNOS of analogues.

distance between N and N19, the less the percentage of remaining binding (more potent NMDA blockade).

DISCUSSION

None of the compounds in this study had selectivity as a mammalian agmatinase inhibitor because those effective at inhibiting agmatinase (i.e., KL-1 and R74) also inhibited NOS isozymes or NMDA receptor binding. The fact that QSAR predictions were distinct for each of the biologic targets suggests that it may be possible to synthesize compounds that are selective for mammalian agmatinase and ADC.

From the five QSAR correlations presented, we have developed mathematical equations that may predict the selective activities of novel compounds. With regard to agmatinase, chemical modifications to the guanidine group of agmatine could tend towards selectivity. Specifically, analogues that compact N19-N16 and N19-

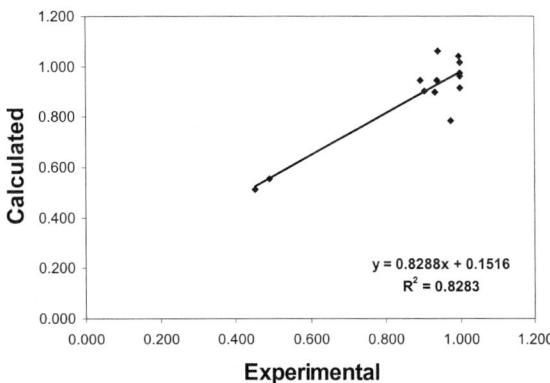

FIGURE 7. The calculated versus experimental activity remaining percentage of rat NMDA receptor analogues.

N20 distances and have a high positive charge on H21 would likely be selective for agmatinase inhibition. It is left for the synthetic chemists to produce new compounds that exploit these equations.

ACKNOWLEDGMENTS

Research was supported by grants from the National Science Foundation CREST program (HRD0125484) and the Italian MIUR (Cofin 2002, prot. 2002038577-002). Calculations were performed on facilities provided by the Army High-Performance Computing Research Center (AHPCRC). The content of this publication does not necessarily reflect the position or policy of the government, and no official endorsement should be inferred.

REFERENCES

1. LI, G., S. REGUNATHAN, C.J. BARROW, et al. 1994. Agmatine: an endogenous clonidine-displacing substance in the brain. Science **263:** 966–969.
2. REIS, D.J. & S. REGUNATHAN. 2000. Is agmatine a novel neurotransmitter in brain? Trends Pharmacol. Sci. **21:** 187–193.
3. FAIRBANKS, C.A., K.L. SCHREIBER, K.L. BREWER, et al. 2000. Agmatine reverses pain induced by inflammation, neuropathy, and spinal cord injury. Proc. Natl. Acad. Sci. U. S. A. **97:** 10584–10589.
4. DEMEHRI, S., H. HOMAYOUN, H. HONAR, et al. 2003. Agmatine exerts anticonvulsant effect in mice: modulation by alpha(2)-adrenoceptors and nitric oxide. Neuropharmacology **45:** 534–542.
5. ZOMKOWSKI, A.D., L. HAMMES, J. LIN, et al. 2002. Agmatine produces antidepressant-like effects in two models of depression in mice. Neuroreport **13:** 387–391.
6. LAVINSKY, D., N. ARTENI & C. NETTO. 2003. Agmatine induces anxiolysis in the elevated plus maze task in adult rats. Behav. Brain Res. **141:** 19–24.
7. KOLESNIKOV, Y., S. JAIN & G.W. PASTERNAK. 1996. Modulation of opioid analgesia by agmatine. Eur. J. Pharmacol. **296:** 17–22.
8. LI, J., X. LI, G. PEI, et al. 1999. Effects of agmatine on tolerance to and substance dependence on morphine in mice. Chung Kuo Yao Li Hsueh Pao **20:** 232–238.
9. ARICIOGLU-KARTAL, F. & I.T. UZBAY. 1997. Inhibitory effect of agmatine on naloxone-precipitated abstinence syndrome in morphine dependent rats. Life Sci. **61:** 1775–1781.
10. GILAD, G.M., K. SALAME, J.M. RABEY, et al. 1996. Agmatine treatment is neuroprotective in rodent brain injury models. Life Sci. **58:** 41–46.
11. DEMADY, D.R., S. JIANMONGKOL, J.L. VULETICH, et al. 2001. Agmatine enhances the NADPH oxidase activity of neuronal NO synthase and leads to oxidative inactivation of the enzyme. Mol. Pharmacol. **59:** 24–29.
12. YANG, X.C. & D.J. REIS. 1999. Agmatine selectively blocks the N-methyl-D-aspartate subclass of glutamate receptor channels in rat hippocampal neurons. J. Pharmacol. Exp. Ther. **288:** 544–549.
13. SASTRE, M., S. REGUNATHAN, E. GALEA, et al. 1996. Agmatinase activity in rat brain: a metabolic pathway for the degradation of agmatine. J. Neurochem. **67:** 1761–1765.
14. PEDERSEN, M.L. & D.B. BERKOWITZ. 1993. Formal alpha-vinylation of amino acids. use of a new benzeneselenolate equivalent. J. Org. Chem. **58:** 6966–6975.
15. CARMIGNANI, M., A.R. VOLPE, B. BOTTA, et al. 2001. Novel hypotensive agents from *Verbesina caracasana*. 8. Synthesis and pharmacology of (3,4-dimethoxycinnamoyl)-N(1)-agmatine and synthetic analogues (1). J. Med. Chem. **44:** 2950–2958.
16. BRET, D.S. & S.H. SNYDER. 1990. Isolation of nitric oxide synthetase, a calmodulin requiring enzyme. Proc. Natl. Acad. Sci. U. S. A. **87:** 682–685.

17. REGUNATHAN, S. & D.J. REIS. 2000. Characterization of arginine decarboxylase in rat brain and liver: distinction from ornithine decarboxylase. J. Neurochem. **74:** 2201–2208.
18. REYNOLDS, I.J. 1990. Arcaine is a competitive antagonist of the polyamine site on the NMDA receptor. Eur. J. Pharmacol. **177:** 215–216.
19. FRISCH, M.J., G.W. TRUCKS, H.B. SCHLEGEL, *et al.* 1995. Gaussian 94, Revision E.2. Gaussian, Inc. Pittsburgh, PA.
20. BODOR, N., Z. GABANYI & C.-K. WONG. 1989. A new method for estimation of partition coefficient. J. Am. Chem. Soc. **111:** 3783–3786.
21. BODOR, N. & M.-J. HUANG. 1992. An extended version of a novel method for the estimation of partition coefficients. J. Pharm. Sci. **81:** 272–281.
22. BODOR, N. & M.-J. HUANG. 1992. A new method for the estimation of the aqueous solubility of organic compounds. J. Pharm. Sci. **81:** 954–960.

Agmatine Crosses the Blood–Brain Barrier

J.E. PILETZ,[a,b] P.J. MAY,[a] G. WANG,[a,c] AND H. ZHU[a]

[a]*University of Mississippi Medical Center, Jackson, Mississippi 39216, USA*
[b]*Jackson State University, Jackson, Mississippi, USA*
[c]*Unit on Molecular Neurotherapeutics, National Institute of Mental Health, National Institutes of Health, Bethesda, Maryland, USA*

ABSTRACT: The question of whether agmatine crosses the blood–brain barrier has not been directly addressed, even though peripheral injection of this compound has produced behavioral responses in drug withdrawal, antidepressant, and anti-anxiety paradigms. Two models were used in this investigation. In the first, mice were injected intraperitoneally (i.p.) with agmatine (10, 50, or 300 mg/kg body weight) or arginine (600 mg/kg). After 1 or 3 hours, the animals were killed under gas anesthesia by perfusing their brains with ice-cold saline, and whole-brain agmatine was measured by HPLC. In parallel studies, a rhesus monkey was injected under gas anesthesia either intravenously (i.v.) with agmatine (30 mg/kg) or arginine (150 mg/kg), or intracerebroventricularly (i.c.v.) with agmatine (0.3 mg/kg i.c.v.). At varying times thereafter, cisterna magna cerebrospinal fluid (CSF) and blood plasma were collected and analyzed for agmatine levels. A rise in mouse brain agmatine was apparent after doses of 50 and 300 mg/kg i.p. Monkey CSF agmatine peaked in parallel with plasma agmatine 15 minutes following intravenous (i.v.) agmatine injection and at one sixth the level of the plasma peak. Monkey CSF agmatine peaked 43 minutes after i.v. arginine injection. The ventricular injection of agmatine resulted in a threefold sustained rise in blood plasma agmatine for at least 24 hours after injection. Therefore, agmatine and its precursor, arginine, cross the blood–brain barrier. CSF agmatine may be newly synthesized from peripherally injected arginine.

KEYWORDS: agmatine; arginine; blood–brain barrier; monkey; cerebrospinal fluid

INTRODUCTION

Agmatine is an endogenous amine and four-carbon guanidine compound formed by decarboxylation of arginine.[1] With the discovery in 1994 of a mitochondrial arginine decarboxylase (ADC; EC 4.1.1.19),[1,2] the production of agmatine was seen to compete for substrate (arginine) directly with two pivotal mediators of neuronal function: the enzymatic pathways that produce nitric oxide (NO) and polyamines.[3] Physiologically relevant concentrations (μM) of agmatine have also been shown to inhibit nitric oxide synthase (NOS) irreversibly.[4] Furthermore, agmatine is more

Address for correspondence: He Zhu, M.D., Department of Psychiatry, University of Mississippi Medical Center, 2500 North State Street, Jackson, MS 39216, USA. Voice: 601-984-5798; fax: 601-984-5899.
e-mail: HZhu@psychiatry.umsmed.edu

Ann. N.Y. Acad. Sci. 1009: 64–74 (2003). © 2003 New York Academy of Sciences.
doi: 10.1196/annals.1304.007

than a metabolic intermediate. Agmatine is known to be packaged into and released from synaptic vesicles,[5] to act on transmembrane receptors,[3] and to antagonize imidazoline and glutamatergic NMDA receptors.[6,7] In addition, agmatine levels are regulated by stress, because endogenous agmatine concentrations have been shown to be increased in the brains of rat pups by hypoxia[8] and in adult rats by cold-restraint (see Aricoglu et al., in this volume). In line with these findings, treatment studies have shown that exogenous agmatine acts as a neuroprotectant under conditions of high glutamate or cortisol levels[9] and also counteracts hypoxic ischemia in newborn rat pups.[8]

Herein, we have sought to determine the extent to which agmatine crosses the blood–brain barrier. This question is important, because agmatine administration may have clinical usefulness. Animal studies have already revealed agmatine's beneficial effects on hypoxic ischemia,[8,10] idiopathic pain,[11] morphine tolerance,[12] drug withdrawal,[13] and stress behaviors.[14,15]

MATERIALS AND METHODS

Mouse Study

Adult male Swiss Webster mice weighing 24 to 30 g (Harlan Inc., Indianapolis, IN, USA) were housed for at least 1 week before experimentation, six per cage under a 12-hour light/dark cycle, with food and water ad libitum. Three injection doses of agmatine (10, 50, and 300 mg/kg i.p.) were assessed in different groups. These doses are comparable with those previously shown to inhibit withdrawal symptoms in rats during naloxone-precipitated morphine withdrawal[16] and in ethanol addiction.[13] Other mice were injected with the ADC substrate, arginine (600 mg/kg i.p.). At 1 or 3 hours after injection, the mice were placed under gas anesthesia and rapidly killed by perfusion with ice-cold saline. Whole brains were rapidly excised and processed.

Monkey Study General Procedures

Protocols were approved by the Institutional Animal Care and Use Committee, which has an Animal Welfare Assurance on file (#A3275-01) with the Office for Protection from Research Risks. A healthy 8-year-old male rhesus monkey, of 12-kg weight, was donated (courtesy of Dr. William Woolverton, University of Mississippi Medical Center) after undergoing an 18-month hiatus from previous experiments which had involved low-dose administration of cocaine. The monkey was kept in its normal cage and room, with a 12-hour light/dark cycle. All procedures began after an overnight fast (water ad libitum). On the surgical implant day, and on day 1 of each experiment, 10 mg/kg ketamine-HCl was given intramuscularly (i.m.) as a preanesthetic. The monkey was moved to a sterile suite, where isoflurane anesthesia was administered through an endotracheal tube. Body temperature was maintained with a circulating-water heating pad and monitored with a rectal probe. Heart and respiratory rates were monitored continuously with dedicated circuitry. An intravenous drip ensured proper hydration. When sample collection was the only procedure undertaken, the anesthetic consisted of 10 mg/kg ketamine-HCl (i.m.) given in the cage.

The monkey was allowed to recover for 1 week after implant surgery before experiment 1 began. Subsequent experiments were performed on the same monkey 1 to 3 weeks apart under the same anesthetic conditions. At standardized times, blood was withdrawn by venipuncture from a groin vein. At the same times as the blood drawings, systolic and diastolic blood pressures (BP) were monitored on the arm with a cuff sized for a newborn human. After the final collections and measurements, the monkey was deeply anesthetized with pentobarbital (70 mg/kg i.p.), and perfused through the heart with cold, sterile PBS i.m. An Ommaya reservoir was removed and found to be intact.

Implant Surgery

The animal's head was placed in a stereotaxic frame. Besides the analgesics, atropine sulfate (0.05 mg/kg i.m.) was given to prevent choking, and dexamethasone (2.5 mg/kg i.v.) was given to prevent swelling. The atlanto-occipital membrane was revealed by tilting the head nose-down 20° and making a midline incision through the skin and then through the muscle at the back of the neck. The perforated tip of a catheter was inserted into the cisterna magna through a small hole made in the atlanto-occipital membrane and underlying dura. The catheter was stabilized by suturing to the muscles as they were reattached in layers at the midline. The other end of the catheter was attached firmly to a sterile Ommaya reservoir, which was ligated to muscle beneath the skin on the back of the neck. The Ommaya reservoir with Pundenz ventricular catheter was purchased from Medtronic Neurologic Technologies (Memphis, TN, USA). This reservoir was 28 mm wide × 8 mm high and held 1.1 mL. The catheter, which had an inner diameter of 1.2 mm and an outer diameter of 2.1 mm, had a perforated tip (1.6 cm) with four rows of eight holes 0.04 inches in diameter. To obtain baseline agmatine samples, 1 mL of cerebrospinal fluid (CSF) was withdrawn after discarding the known fore-volume in the reservoir of 1.1 mL of Dulbecco's PBS; at the same time, 2 mL of blood was collected by venipuncture from the groin. A second midline incision was then made at the top of the skull, and the temporalis muscle was moved laterally. A small craniotomy was drilled to allow access to the brain. Afterwards, the hole was filled with absorbable gelatin sponge to serve as a future injection port. Muscle layers and skin were then re-approximated and closed. The incisions were infused with bupivacaine (2.5% subcutaneously). Buprenorphine (0.01 mg/kg, i.v.) was then given as a postoperative analgesic. Neither the Ommaya reservoir, nor the catheter seemed to irritate the monkey during 5 weeks of study. CSF could be withdrawn repeatedly from the Ommaya reservoir without surgical trauma.

Monkey Experiment 1

After the monkey recovered from implantation, the goal of experiment 1 was to determine whether infusion of agmatine (30 mg/kg i.v. in 2 mL of sterile PBS given over 5 minutes) would elevate agmatine levels in blood or CSF and for what time period. The dose of agmatine was based on a study by Bradley and Healy[17] in which agmatine (25–200 mg/kg i.v.) was administered to alpha-chloralose–anesthetized rats. At the highest dose these investigators reported a drop in BP from 131 to 69 mm Hg (returning to normal levels by 14 minutes),[17] so we also monitored BP. Sedation with isoflurane began 10 minutes after the ketamine injection (at 9:30 hours), and the gas was maintained through five experimental times (0–196 minutes). Each collection consisted of 2 mL of blood and 1 mL of CSF, as described previously. CSF removed from the Ommaya reservoir was replaced each time with sterile PBS. The sample collection times were (1) pre-agmatine baseline after 10 minutes of isoflurane sedation; (2) 30 minutes later, which was 15 minutes after agmatine administration; (3) 43 minutes after agmatine administration; (4) 70 minutes after agmatine administration; (5) 196 minutes after agmatine administration. The animal was then awakened and returned to its home cage. The monkey received food and water ad libitum until 22:00 hours and then food was withheld overnight (water was provided ad libitum). The next day, the animal was re-anesthetized (10 mg/kg ketamine-HCl, i.m.). Twenty minutes later, we collected sample 6, the 24-hour post-agmatine blood and CSF collection.

Monkey Experiment 2

The goal of monkey experiment 2 was to determine whether an infusion of arginine (150 mg/kg i.v. in 2 mL of sterile PBS given over 5 minutes) would elevate the concentration of agmatine in blood or CSF and for what time period. The dose of arginine was chosen based on a study by Tangphao et al.[18] in which arginine (approximately 400 mg/kg i.v. in 300 mL over 30 minutes) was administered to 10 healthy humans. The investigators reported no significant effects on vital signs and no adverse reactions in humans.[18] The sampling procedure was identical to that in monkey experiment 1.

Monkey Experiment 3

The goal of monkey experiment 3 was to determine whether an injection of agmatine into the lateral ventricle (300 µg/kg in 0.3 mL of sterile PBS given over 5 minutes) would increase the concentration of agmatine within intracisternal CSF or blood and for what time period. The dose of agmatine was chosen to be less than the maximum intracerebroventricular (i.c.v.) dose (578 µg/kg agmatine i.c.v. in 5 µL) reported in the literature to be without detrimental effects in pentobarbitone-anesthetized normotensive rats.[19] Under anesthesia, the head of the monkey was placed in a stereotaxic device, and the scalp was opened to expose the small hole previously drilled in the skull during implant surgery. Injection was made into the lateral ventricle by use of a stereotaxically placed, blunt-ended Hamilton syringe. Blood collection times were identical to those in experiments 1 and 2, except they began 30 minutes after isoflurane sedation. Unfortunately, the cisternal catheter became clogged after the baseline CSF collection, and therefore only the post-196 minutes and 24-hour samples of CSF were collected directly from the cistern after agmatine i.c.v.

High-Pressure Liquid Chromatography Assay of Agmatine

Because agmatine has been found to be fairly unstable in biologic samples, we immediately placed the samples on ice after collection. These samples were then extracted within 10 minutes of collection into ice-cold trifluoroacetic acid.[20] Once extracted, agmatine is very stable.[20] The high-pressure liquid chromatography (HPLC) assay of agmatine by isocratic chromatography has already been described.[20] One methodologic advance was the use of a new internal standard: 1-(3-aminopropyl)2-pipecodine (0.8 ng per HPLC injection) (Sigma Chemical Co., St. Louis, MO, USA). Repeated measures coefficients of variation were less than 5%.

RESULTS

FIGURE 1 provides evidence that agmatine and arginine can enter the mouse brain. After i.p. injection of each compound, mice were killed under gaseous anesthesia while their brains were perfused with ice-cold sterile saline. Perfusion of the brain was performed to ensure that these compounds were not merely compartmentalized in the blood. Whole-brain agmatine concentrations were noted to be nonsignificantly elevated 3 hours after agmatine dosing at 10 and 50 mg/kg i.p. compared with saline-treated controls (FIG. 1, *stippled bars*). Agmatine administration at 300 mg/kg i.p. led to a clear rise after 3 hours in the concentration of whole-brain agmatine compared with saline-treated controls ($P \leq 0.001$) (FIG. 1). An arginine dose of 600 mg/kg i.p. also led to a significant rise in whole-brain agmatine ($P \leq 0.05$) (FIG. 1). Furthermore, brain agmatine concentrations following an injection of 50 mg/kg agmatine were higher after 1 hour (FIG. 1, *open bar*) than after 3 hours (FIG. 1, *stippled bar*). This finding suggested that exogenous agmatine rapidly entered the brain but was metabolized in, or otherwise cleared from, the mouse brain within 3 hours.

Monkey experiment 1 sought to determine whether agmatine crosses the blood-brain barrier in a primate (FIG. 2). Concentrations of agmatine in blood plasma and CSF were found to rise in parallel 15 minutes after injection of 30 mg/kg agmatine i.v. (FIG. 2). Concentrations of agmatine in blood plasma and CSF then declined in parallel between 43 and 70 minutes and attained baseline levels by 196 minutes after injection (FIG. 2). The highest molarities of agmatine, occurring at 15 minutes after i.v. injection, were calculated to be 70.2 µM in plasma (9,126 ng/mL plasma) and 11.3 µM in CSF (1,469 ng/mL CSF) (FIG. 2). These levels bracket the apparent dis-

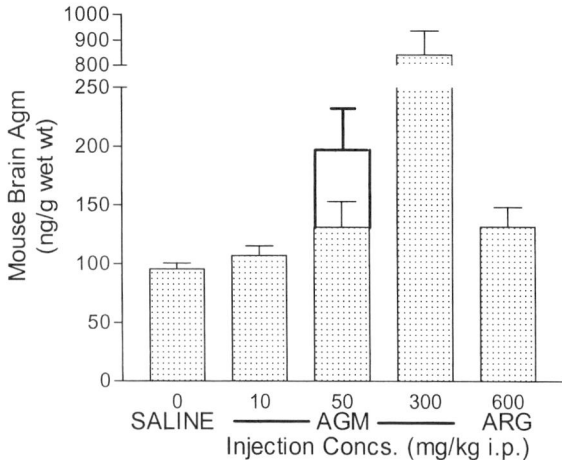

FIGURE 1. Agmatine crosses the blood–brain barrier in adult mice. Mice (n = 3–4/group) were injected with the indicated concentrations of agmatine (AGM, 0 saline, 10, 50, or 300 mg/kg body weight i.p.) or arginine (ARG, 600 mg/kg i.p.) After 1 h (*open bar*) or 3 h (*stippled bars*) the mice were killed by cervical dislocation and their brain rapidly perfused with saline. Brains were immediately excised and processed on ice for agmatine assay. Data represent the mean ± SEM.

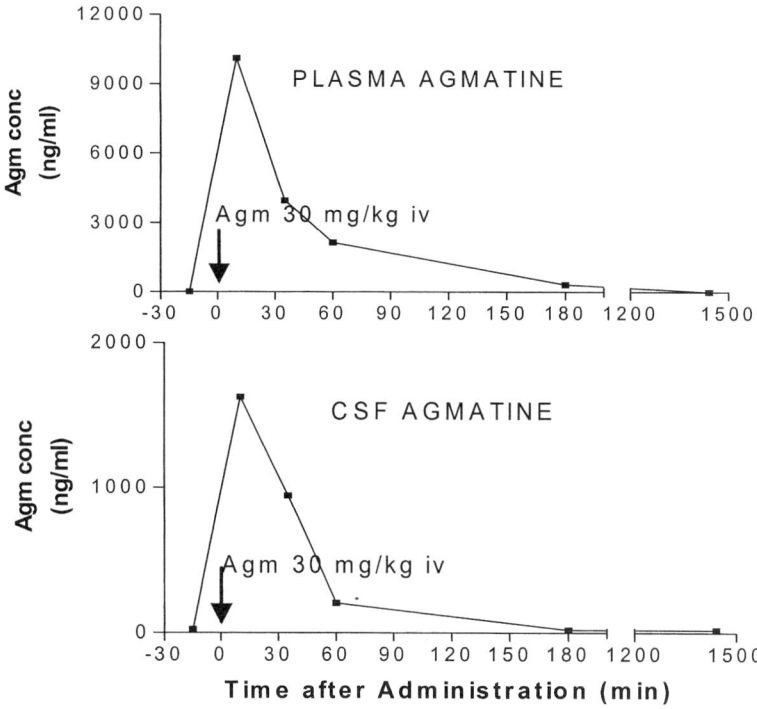

FIGURE 2. Experiment 1: Agmatine crosses the blood–brain barrier in monkey. Agmatine (30 mg/kg i.v.) was injected at time zero, and plasma and cerebrospinal fluid from the cisterna magnum were assayed thereafter by HPLC for concentration of agmatine. CSF, cerebrospinal fluid.

sociation constant of 29 μM reported[4] in vitro for agmatine to inactivate neuronal NOS irreversibly. By comparison, baseline concentrations of agmatine on four different days before the implant surgery and in experiments 1 through 3 ranged from 6.8 to 16.9 ng/mL in blood plasma and from 6.1 to 23.5 ng/mL in CSF of the monkey.

Experiment 2 sought to determine whether an i.v. injection of the ADC substrate, arginine (150 mg/kg i.v.), would lead to a rise in plasma or CSF agmatine levels. Arginine seemed more of a CSF precursor of agmatine than a blood precursor of agmatine (FIG. 3). CSF agmatine peaked 43 minutes after the i.v. injection of arginine, whereas the peak of blood plasma agmatine was 22-fold lower than in CSF and occurred 70 minutes after the i.v. injection of arginine (FIG. 3). The concentration of agmatine in CSF returned to its baseline level by 70 minute after arginine administration, and the concentration in plasma returned to baseline by 196 minutes after arginine administration (FIG. 3). The highest plasma concentration of agmatine (18.2 ng/mL), attained 70 minutes after arginine injection, was calculated to be 0.14 μM. The highest CSF concentration of agmatine (286 ng/mL), attained 43 minutes after arginine injection, was calculated to be 2.2 μM (FIG. 3).

Experiment 3 sought to determine whether an i.c.v. injection of agmatine (300 μg/kg i.c.v.) into the lateral ventricle would lead to a rise in intracisternal CSF

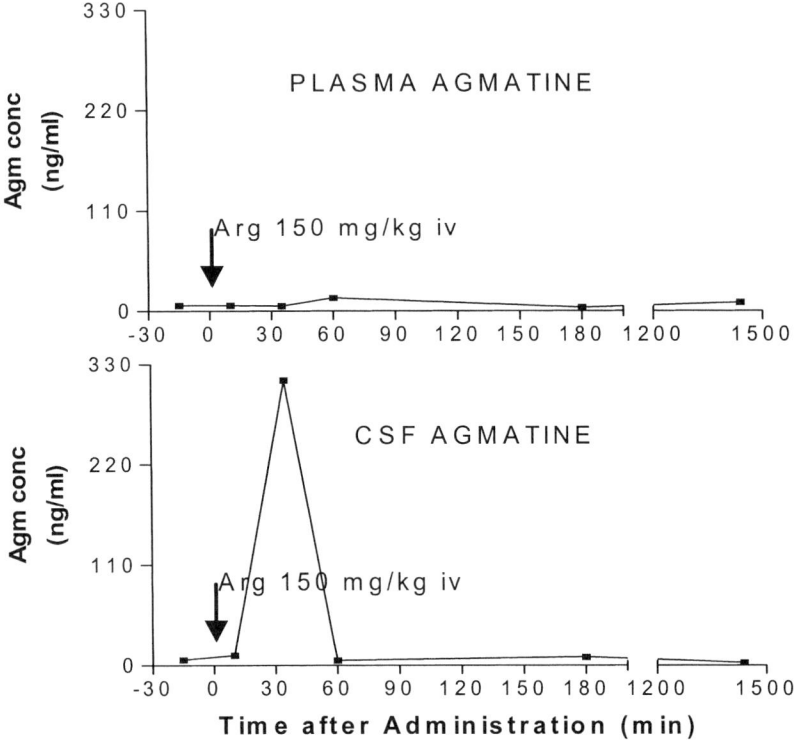

FIGURE 3. Experiment 2: Arginine leads to rise in agmatine in monkey. Arginine (150 mg/kg i.v.) was injected at time zero, and plasma and cerebrospinal fluid from the cisterna magnum were assayed thereafter by HPLC for concentration of agmatine. CSF, cerebrospinal fluid.

agmatine or blood plasma agmatine (FIG. 4). The concentration of agmatine in intracisternal CSF was very high 196 minutes after its i.c.v. injection and remained high for 24 hours (FIG. 4). The highest concentration of agmatine attained in the cisterna magnum (48,230 ng/mL) was equivalent to 371.0 µM (FIG. 4). The cisternal concentration of agmatine (12,272 ng/mL) 24 hours after i.cv. injection of agmatine was equivalent to 94.4 µM. In addition, the concentrations of agmatine in blood plasma also rose threefold from 60 minutes after its i.c.v. injection and remained at the same elevated level 24 hours after injection (FIG. 4). The highest concentration of agmatine attained in blood plasma (65 ng/mL) after i.c.v. agmatine was equivalent to 0.5 µM. Thus, agmatine was shown to enter the central nervous system (CNS) (see FIGS. 1 & 2) and also to traverse from the CNS to the periphery (FIG. 4).

In conjunction with the aforementioned pharmacokinetic studies of agmatine and arginine, a number of physiologic measurements were made. Both agmatine (i.v.) and arginine (i.v.) were found to be hypotensive and to lower heart rate in the monkey. Intravenous agmatine lowered systolic BP by an average of 23 mm Hg, with no consistent effect on diastolic BP, which was sustained from 15 to 70 minutes after injection.

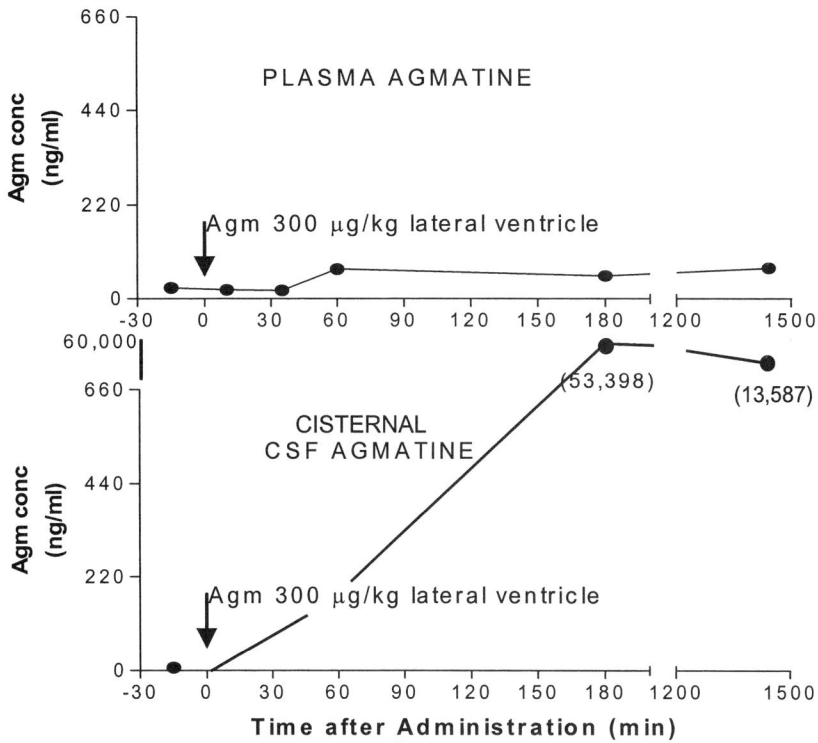

FIGURE 4. Experiment 3: Agmatine crosses from CSF to blood in monkey. Agmatine (300 μg/kg i.c.v.) was injected into the lateral ventricle at time zero, and plasma and cerebrospinal fluid from the cisterna magnum were assayed thereafter by HPLC for concentration of agmatine. Values in parentheses are ng/mL concentration. CSF, cerebrospinal fluid.

Likewise, heart rate declined from 136 beats per min (bpm) to an average of 113 bpm between 15 and 70 minutes after i.v. administration of agmatine. Arginine (i.v.) exerted similar although slightly lagging effects. Arginine (i.v.) lowered systolic BP by an average of 18.5 mm Hg, with a 6-mm drop in diastolic BP, which was sustained between 43 and 70 minutes after injection. Heart rate also declined from 134 bpm to an average of 114 bpm between 43 and 70 minutes after arginine (i.v). In contrast to these depressor effects, agmatine (i.c.v.) exerted a rapid rise in systolic BP by 9 mm Hg after 15 minutes, 17 mm Hg after 43 minutes, 20 mm Hg after 70 minutes, and 28 mm Hg after 196 minutes. No consistent effects of i.c.v. dosing of agmatine were noted on diastolic BP or heart rate.

For some days after each injection there was an apparent loss of appetite by the monkey. For about 3 days after each experiment the monkey ate roughly half as much food as before but remained adequately hydrated. This reduced intake led to an 8% body weight loss over the 5 weeks of our study. After experiment 2, a blood sample was collected, and evidence was found of a mild level of uremia. No other behavioral changes were observed in the monkey after any of the injections of agmatine or arginine.

DISCUSSION

Because agmatine is a polar cation, questions have remained about the extent to which it crosses the blood–brain barrier. In the present study, agmatine (i.p.) was observed to cross the blood–brain barrier in mice in a concentration-dependent manner (see FIG. 1). Furthermore, agmatine was observed to enter primate CSF within 15 minutes after i.v. injection (see FIG. 2). The kinetics of agmatine's passage into monkey CSF directly paralleled its rise and fall in blood plasma (FIG. 2). Taken together, these data indicate that agmatine readily crosses the blood–brain barrier.

Our present findings support the hypothesis that peripherally delivered agmatine enters the brain and has direct CNS effects. It has been realized for some time that the peripheral injection of agmatine can exert a variety of CNS-mediated effects.[8,10–15] From previous in vitro studies, it is also known that biologically relevant concentrations of agmatine should be in the µM range. For instance, µM concentrations of agmatine are required to inhibit neuronal NOS.[4] In our study, µM concentrations of agmatine were attained in the brains of mice and in the CSF of a monkey following peripheral injections of agmatine. Thus, we now know that biologically relevant concentrations of agmatine are attained in vivo following peripheral routes of delivery.

Another observation of our study was that agmatine passed from the primate's lateral ventricle into the blood by 70 minutes after i.c.v. injection (see FIG. 4). This finding indicates that agmatine can flow out of the CNS to the blood. Based on our CSF data, it seems that the rate at which agmatine enters the brain is faster than the rate at which it leaves the brain (compare FIGS. 2 & 4). This difference may be explained by the faster flow of blood to the brain, compared with the relatively slow flow of CSF from the lateral ventricle to its point of exit at the archnoid villi.

Another question we have only begun to address is the extent to which endogenous brain agmatine may contribute to agmatine in the blood. We now know that a contribution from the CNS is at least a possibility based on the inside-to-outside flow of agmatine (FIG. 4). Blood levels of agmatine have also been reported to be higher in depressed patients and to be normalized after therapy,[21] suggesting a CNS source. Attention might also be drawn to the sustained rise observed in blood plasma agmatine levels following the i.c.v. route of administration in the monkey (FIG. 4). FIGURE 4 indicates that blood plasma agmatine levels were sustained from 70 minutes to 24 hours after i.c.v. injection of agmatine (FIG. 4). This observation is unlikely to be artifactual because it parallels the high levels of agmatine in cisternal CSF over the same time period (FIG. 4). One explanation for this finding is that agmatine might be very stable in the CSF. This possibility is supported by another study showing agmatine's slow turnover rate in rat CSF (Fairbanks *et al.*, in this volume). If agmatine in CSF is very stable, it would also be expected to accumulate in the CSF to comparably high levels, especially under conditions where it is induced (i.e., stress).[8] If agmatine accumulates in the CSF, then CSF levels of agmatine might become high enough to constitute a major source of blood agmatine.

The present study also demonstrates that peripherally delivered arginine leads to an increase in agmatine concentration in the brain (see FIG.1) and CSF (see FIG. 3).

A partial surprise was that the CSF levels of agmatine were higher than the blood levels of agmatine after i.v. injection of arginine (FIG. 3). This finding could simply result from the conversion of arginine to agmatine, which is known to be more active in the brain than in the periphery.

It should be emphasized that this is a preliminary study. Only one monkey was available for this study, and it was a previously cocaine-treated subject. Secondly, the doses of agmatine and arginine that were given were not physiologic doses. Indeed, they may have been slightly toxic to the monkey, because agmatine (30 mg/kg i.v.) and arginine (150 mg/kg i.v.) produced a combined modest level of blood uremia. Obviously, further studies using physiologic doses are warranted before these findings can be generalized. This study, however, is the first to demonstrate clearly that agmatine crosses the blood–brain barrier.

ACKNOWLEDGMENTS

We appreciate the assistance of Dr. Andrew Grady and other competent veterinary staff for their help with the monkey surgery and collection procedures. Andrea Means and Jason Black are also thanked for their help with the laboratory procedures. This research was partially supported by NIH Grant MH57601.

REFERENCES

1. LI, G., S. REGUNATHAN, C.J. BARROW, et al. 1994. Agmatine: an endogenous clonidine-displacing substance in the brain. Science **263:** 966–969.
2. REGUNATHAN, S. & D.J. REIS. 2000. Characterization of arginine decarboxylase in rat brain and liver: distinction from ornithine decarboxylase. J. Neurochem. **74:** 2201–2208.
3. REIS, D.J. & S. REGUNATHAN. 2000. Is agmatine a novel neurotransmitter in brain? Trends Pharmacol. Sci. **21:** 187–193.
4. DEMADY, D.R., S. JIANMONGKOL, J.L. VULETICH, et al. 2001. Agmatine enhances the NADPH oxidase activity of neuronal NO synthase and leads to oxidative inactivation of the enzyme. Mol. Pharmacol. **59:** 24–29.
5. REIS, D.J., X.C. YANG & T.A. MILNER. 1998. Agmatine containing axon terminals in rat hippocampus form synapses on pyramidal cells. Neurosci. Lett. **250:** 185–188.
6. REIS, D.J. & S. REGUNATHAN. 1999. Agmatine: an endogenous ligand at imidazoline receptors is a novel neurotransmitter. Ann. N. Y. Acad. Sci. **881:** 65–80.
7. OLMOS, G., N. DEGREGORIO-ROCASOLANO, M. PAZ REGALADO, et al. 1999. Protection by imidazol(ine) drugs and agmatine of glutamate-induced neurotoxicity in cultured cerebellar granule cells through blockade of NMDA receptor. Br. J. Pharmacol. **127:** 1317–1326.
8. FENG, Y., J.E. PILETZ & M.H. LEBLANC. 2002. Agmatine suppresses nitric oxide production and attenuates hypoxic-ischemic brain injury in neonatal rats. Pediatr. Res. **52:** 606–611.
9. ZHU, M.-Y., J. PILETZ, A. HALARIS, et al. 2002. Effect of agmatine against cell death induced by NMDA and glutamate in neurons and PC 12 cell. Cell. Mol. Neurobiol. **23:** 865–872.
10. GILAD, G.M., K. SALAME, J.M. RABEY, et al. 1996. Agmatine treatment is neuroprotective in rodent brain injury models. Life Sci. **58:** 41–46.
11. FAIRBANKS, C.A., K.L. SCHREIBER, K.L. BREWER, et al. 2000. Agmatine reverses pain induced by inflammation, neuropathy, and spinal cord injury. Proc. Natl. Acad. Sci. U. S. A. **97:** 10584–10589.
12. KOLESNIKOV, Y., S. JAIN & G.W. PASTERNAK. 1996. Modulation of opioid analgesia by agmatine. Eur. J. Pharmacol. **296:** 17–22.

13. UZBAY, I.T., O. YESILYURT, T. CELIK, *et al.* 2000. Effects of agmatine on ethanol withdrawal syndrome in rats. Behav. Brain Res. **107:** 153–159.
14. STEWART, L.S. & B.E. MCKAY. 2000. Acquisition deficit and time-dependent retrograde amnesia for contextual fear conditioning in agmatine-treated rats. Behav. Pharmacol. **11:** 93–97.
15. ZOMKOWSKI, A.D., L. HAMMES, J. LIN, *et al.* 2002. Agmatine produces antidepressant-like effects in two models of depression in mice. Neuroreport **13:** 387–391.
16. ARICIOGLU-KARTAL, F. & I.T. UZBAY. 1997. Inhibitory effect of agmatine on naloxone-precipitated abstinence syndrome in morphine dependent rats. Life Sci. **61:** 1775–1781.
17. BRADLEY, K.J. & P.M. HEADLEY. 1997. Effect of agmatine on spinal nociceptive reflexes: lack of interaction with alpha2-adrenoceptor or mu-opioid receptor mechanisms. Eur. J. Pharmacol. **331:** 133–138.
18. TANGPHAO, O., M. GROSSMANN, S. CHALON, *et al.* 1999. Pharmacokinetics of intravenous and oral L-arginine in normal volunteers. Br. J. Clin. Pharmacol. **47:** 261–266.
19. PENNER, S.B. & D.D. SMYTH. 1996. Natriuresis following central and peripheral administration of agmatine in the rat. Pharmacology **53:** 160–169.
20. FENG, Y., A.E. HALARIS & J.E. PILETZ. 1997. Determination of agmatine in brain and plasma using high-performance liquid chromatography with fluorescence detection. Journal of Chromatography B: Biomedical Applications **691(2):** 277–282.
21. HALARIS, A., H. ZHU, Y. FENG, *et al.* 1999. Plasma agmatine and platelet imidazoline receptors in depression. Ann. N. Y. Acad. Sci. **881:** 445–451.

Identification and Pharmacological Characterization of a Specific Agmatine Transport System in Human Tumor Cell Lines

GERHARD J. MOLDERINGS, MICHAEL BRÜSS, HEINZ BÖNISCH, AND MANFRED GÖTHERT

Institute of Pharmacology and Toxicology, University of Bonn, Bonn, Germany

ABSTRACT: Specific accumulation of [^{14}C]agmatine in six human intestinal tumor cell lines and in the glioma cell line SK-MG-1 was inhibited by phentolamine, idazoxan, clonidine, 1,3-di-(2-tolyl)guanidine, histamine, putrescine, spermine and spermidine. Corticosterone, desipramine, O-methylisoprenaline, cirazoline, moxonidine, L-arginine, L-lysine, verapamil, nifedipine, $CdCl_2$, ondansetron, and L-carnitine failed to inhibit specific [^{14}C]agmatine accumulation, thus excluding that it is mediated by amino acid or monoamine carriers, by the putrescine carrier, by 5-HT$_3$ receptor channels, by Ca^{2+} channels or by the organic cation transporters OCT1, OCT2, OCT3, OCTN1, or OCTN2. This conclusion is supported by the finding that transfection of HEK293 cells with cDNA encoding either hOCT1, hOCT2, or hOCT3 did not enhance specific [^{14}C]agmatine accumulation compared to nontransfected cells. The data suggest that agmatine is accumulated by a specific agmatine transporter. Since incubation with exogenous agmatine for 24 hours increased intracellular agmatine content in all cell lines by a multiple of the basal endogenous content, the agmatine uptake system may be relevant for the regulation of the intra- and extracellular concentration of agmatine in humans.

KEYWORDS: agmatine transporter; intestinal tumor cell lines; SK-MG-1 cells; HEK293 cells; human organic cation transporters (hOCT); [^{14}C]agmatine uptake

PHARMACOLOGICAL CHARACTERIZATION OF THE AGMATINE UPTAKE PROCESS

A variety of effects has been demonstrated in response to agmatine in vitro and in vivo. The high concentrations at which those effects are induced (1 to 1000 µmol/L) can be achieved in the tissues in vivo by absorption of agmatine from the gut where it is formed and released at high amounts by bacteria of the physiological gut microflora.[1] As expected from its charged structure at physiologic pH, agmatine behaves as an organic cation and, hence, biological membranes are almost completely impermeable to agmatine in the absence of an uptake system. Therefore, absorption from the gut and accumulation in the tissues and cells must occur via a carrier mechanism.

Address for correspondence: Gerhard J. Molderings, Institute of Pharmacology and Toxicology, University of Bonn, Reuterstr. 2b D-53113, Bonn, Germany. Voice: (+49) 228-735421; fax (+49) 228-735404.
e-mail: molderings@uni-bonn.de

A selective uptake system for agmatine was first reported to exist in rat brain.[2] In addition, we have recently demonstrated the existence of a specific carrier-mediated agmatine uptake in the human glioblastoma cell line SK-MG-1,[3] in six intestinal carcinoma cell lines and in HEK293 cells.[4]

The detailed pharmacological characterization of the [^{14}C]agmatine uptake in SK-MG-1 and Caco-2 cells as representatives of tumor cells of different origin revealed that the agmatine carrier is not identical with the transporter for the structurally related amino acids arginine and lysine (system Y$^+$; SLC7A2), because neither L-arginine nor L-lysine affected [^{14}C]agmatine uptake (TABLE 1). Desipramine also had no effect on the uptake of [^{14}C]agmatine, indicating that the sodium-dependent norepinephrine transporter (SLC6A2) is not involved (TABLE 1). The failure of the 5-HT$_3$ receptor antagonist ondansetron to inhibit [^{14}C]agmatine uptake[3] ruled out an influx of the radiolabeled polycation through 5-HT$_3$ receptor channels that might be present in the cells investigated. The insensitivity of [^{14}C]agmatine uptake to the L-type Ca^{2+}-channel blockers nifedipine and verapamil as well as the nonselective Ca^{2+}-channel blocker CdCl$_2$ argues against the involvement of Ca^{2+}-channels in the uptake of [^{14}C]agmatine (TABLE 1). In addition, the failure of 100 μmol/L verapamil to inhibit uptake of [^{14}C]agmatine excludes an identity of the transporter with the P-glycoprotein transport process (MDR1; TABLE 1).

Comparison of the pharmacological profile of [^{14}C]putrescine uptake with that of [^{14}C]agmatine uptake clearly demonstrated that the agmatine transporter is not identical with the putrescine transporter.[3] The potency of certain imidazoline and guanidine derivatives, in particular of phentolamine, in inhibiting [^{14}C]agmatine uptake was clearly different from its potency as an inhibitor of [^{14}C]putrescine uptake (TABLE 1).[3] In addition, L-arginine and CdCl$_2$ inhibited [^{14}C]putrescine uptake, whereas they were without effect on [^{14}C]agmatine uptake (TABLE 1).[3]

The involvement of the organic cation transporters OCT1 (SLC22A1), OCT2 (SLC22A2), OCT3 (SLC22A3), OCTN1 (SLC22A4), and OCTN2 (SLC22A5) is very unlikely in view of the clear-cut differences in the pattern of effect of certain key drugs acting at those transporters and at the [^{14}C]agmatine uptake in SK-MG-1 cells (TABLE 1).[3] To confirm that hOCT1, hOCT2 or hOCT3 are not involved in the specific agmatine transport, agmatine accumulation in three stably transfected HEK293 cell lines expressing either hOCT1, hOCT2 or hOCT3 were studied.[4] In non-transfected HEK293 cells, a specific agmatine uptake similar to that in the intestinal cell lines and in SK-MG-1 cells was present. However, expression of hOCT1 and hOCT3 in HEK293 cells did not further increase uptake of agmatine,[4] thus ruling out the transport of agmatine by those organic cation transporters. Expression of hOCT2 even led to a reduced uptake of agmatine compared with non-transfected HEK293 cells. This observation probably indicates that in analogy to renal excretion of cations by the hOCT2,[5] this cation transporter might be able to produce an outward transport of agmatine from the cells.

Recently, Gründemann and coworkers[6] reported on an hOCT3-mediated agmatine uptake into HEK293 cells that had been stably transfected with this organic cation transporter. This hOCT3-related intracellular accumulation of agmatine exhibited a strong pH dependence and was maximal at pH 8.5, but only very weak at physiologic pH (Fig. 7 in reference 6). This finding is not contradictory to the results of our experiments that failed to demonstrate an uptake of agmatine by hOCT3 in stably transfected HEK 293 cells (see above), since our experiments were performed

TABLE 1. Functional characteristics of the selective [^{14}C]agmatine uptake in SK-MG-1 and Caco2 cells and comparison with eleven possible uptake mechanisms for organic cations

	Corticosterone ≤0.1 mmol/L	O-Methylisoprenaline ≤0.1 mmol/L	Desipramine ≤0.01 mmol/L	Phentolamine ≤3 mmol/L	Histamine ≤0.3 mmol/L	Verapamil 0.1 mmol/L	Nifedipine 0.1 mmol/L	CdCl$_2$ 1 mmol/L	Arginine 10 mmol/L	Lysine 1 mmol/L
Agmatine uptake	0	0	0	→	→	0	↑	0	0	0
Putrescine transporter	0	0	0	(↓)	→	0	0	→	→	0
hOCT1	(↓)	→	0		←					
hOCT2	→	(↓)	0		→					
hOCT3	→	→	0		→					
OCTN1			→			→				
OCTN2			→			→				
L-type Ca^{2+} channel						→	→	→		
Non-selective Ca^{2+} channel							→	→		
System Y$^+$						→			→	→
Norepinephrine transporter			→						→	
P-glycoprotein transport						→				

Data are from Molderings et al.[3] and Heinen et al.[4] including the references therein. Symbols are effect of the drugs on cation uptake by the respective uptake process: ↓ (inhibition); (↓) (small inhibition); ↑ (enhancement); 0 (no effect).

at a physiologic pH. The selective agmatine transport mechanism operative at physiologic conditions in our experiments is clearly not identical with hOCT3-mediated agmatine transport at alkaline pH conditions. Whether this uptake via hOCT3 significantly contributes to accumulation at physiologic pH in vivo remains to be investigated.

Since agmatine possesses structural similarity to L-carnitine, the possibility had to be considered that agmatine was taken up into the HEK293 cells by the carnitine transporter hOCTN2[7,8] that is endogenously expressed in HEK293 cells.[7] The failure of 500 μmol/L L-carnitine to inhibit [^{14}C]agmatine accumulation[4] makes an involvement of hOCTN2 in agmatine transport very unlikely. In accordance with this observation, desipramine and verapamil, which have been shown to inhibit the carnitine transporter, also failed to affect agmatine uptake in SK-MG-1 cells (TABLE 1).

The pharmacologic characteristics of the agmatine carrier, determined in the intestinal cell lines and the human glioma cell line SK-MG-1 (TABLE 1),[3,4] are similar to those of the selective agmatine transporters recently found in rat hepatocytes,[9] rat arterial smooth muscle cells,[10] hamster kidney cells,[11] and other mammalian cell lines.[12] Because of its unique pharmacologic properties, this agmatine carrier is not identical with any known organic cation transport systems thus far (TABLE 1) and it is also not identical with the uptake process initially described in rat brain synaptosomes[2] (detailed in reference 3).

MOLECULAR IDENTIFICATION OF THE AGMATINE TRANSPORTER: FIRST ATTEMPTS

On the basis of our working hypothesis that the agmatine carrier is an organic cation transporter, we used a consensus sequence derived from the sequences of hOCT1, hOCT2 and hOCT3 to search for homologous sequences in human genome databases. This search resulted in two full length cDNA sequences with the accession numbers NM_004794 (ORCTL4) and BC026358 (FLIPT1), respectively, for which the depositors assumed that they might code for organic cation transporter proteins. If the agmatine carrier would be encoded by one of the two sequences, corresponding mRNA had to be present in the six intestinal tumor cell lines and in HEK293 cells because each of these cell lines expresses the selective agmatine uptake mechanism. Therefore, reverse transcription-polymerase chain reaction (RT-PCR) analysis of mRNA of ORCTL4 (FIG. 1) and FLIPT1 (FIG. 2) was performed with RNA isolated from the seven cell lines. Total RNA from about 10^7 cells of each human cell line was isolated (RNeasy MiniKit, Qiagen, Germany) and primed with an Oligo (dT)$_{18}$ primer to synthesize the first strand cDNA using SuperScript II Reverse Transcriptase (Gibco, Life Technologies) according to the manufacturer's protocol. Amplification of ORCTL4 (646 bp; FIG. 1) and FLIPT1 (504 bp; FIG. 2) fragments was performed using primers (0.2 μmol/L each) deduced from the published sequences (ORCTL4: sense primer: 5′-GCCTCTGTCCTGGACTTCTG-3′; antisense primer: 5′-CATTCTT GGCCGCTTCCTCA-3′; FLIPT1: sense primer: 5′-GGTGAA CAGCCATTC CTTGTC-3′; antisense primer: 5′-CCAGAGGCATAAAAG ACG-3). PCR was performed with cDNA from the respective cell lines with the FailSafe PCR System (Biozym) using buffer G according to the manufacturer's protocol and the following temperature programs: 40 cycles at 94°C for 1 minute, 60°C (ORCTL4)

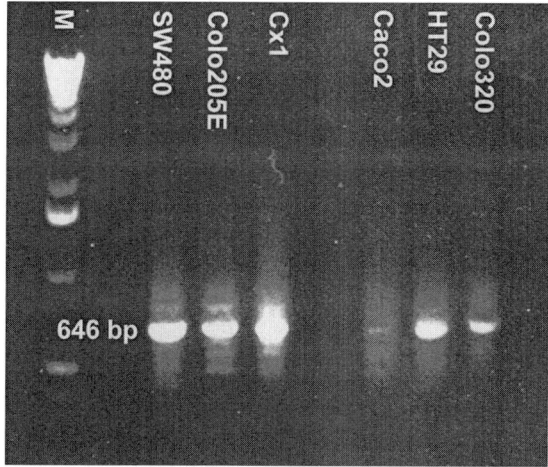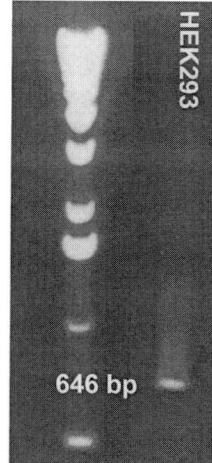

FIGURE 1. Agarose gel electrophoresis of a 646 bp fragment of NM_004803 in six human intestinal tumor cell lines (SW480, Colo205E, Cx1, Caco2, HT29, Colo320) and in HEK293 cells (stably transfected with the human 5-HT transporter). M: Gibco 1 kb DNA ladder. The ORCTL4-fragment is expressed in each cell line.

or 50°C (FLIPT1) for 1 minute, and 72°C for 1 minute. As shown in the Figures, both ORCTL4 (FIG. 1) and FLIPT1 (FIG. 2) were expressed in all cell lines examined. Hence, the results of these experiments were compatible with the possibility that one of the two sequences might code for the agmatine carrier.

To further investigate this possibility, we examined [^{14}C]agmatine uptake into

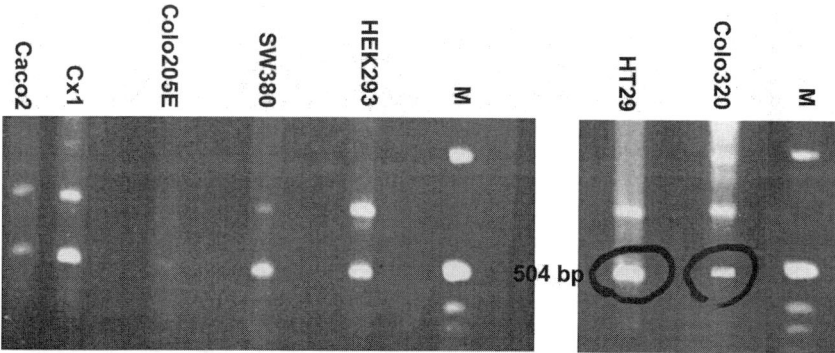

FIGURE 2. Agarose gel electrophoresis of a 504 bp fragment of FLIPT1 in six human intestinal tumor cell lines (SW480, Colo205E, Cx1, Caco2, HT29, Colo320) and in HEK293 cells (stably transfected with the human 5-HT transporter). M: Gibco 1 kb DNA ladder. The FLIPT1-fragment is expressed in each cell line.

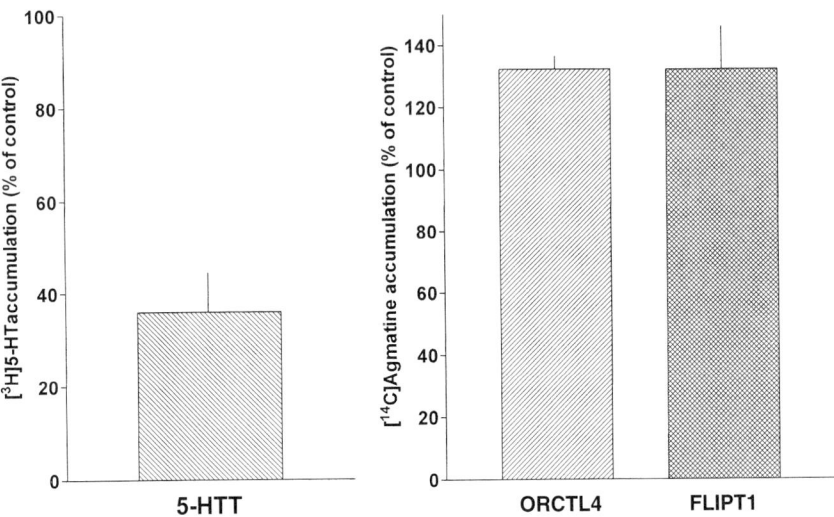

FIGURE 3. [³H]5-HT and [¹⁴C]agmatine accumulation into HEK293 cells (stably transfected with the human 5-HT transporter [5-HTT]) after incubation of the cells for 72 hours with short interference RNA targeting the mRNAs that either code for the 5-HT transporter protein or the putative organic cation transport proteins ORCTL4 and FLIPT1, respectively. Data are means ± SEM of 4 experiments in each series. 100% corresponds to 10.2 ± 4.4 nCi/mg protein in the case of [³H]5-HT accumulation and to 4.8 ± 1.8 nCi/mg protein in the case of [¹⁴C]agmatine accumulation. * $P < 0.05$ (compared to corresponding controls without short interference RNA during the incubation period).

HEK293 cells (stably transfected with the human 5-HT transporter; Brüss *et al.*, unpublished results) with and without incubation of the cells with 21-mer short interference (si) RNAs targeting the two cDNA sequences under study (transfection performed with Oligofectamine according to the manufacturer's protocol; Invitrogen, Germany). In our experiments neither incubation for 72 hours with siRNA targeting ORCTL4 (5'-AAGCAGGAUGACAAGUUUGCC-3') nor with that targeting FLIPT1 (5'-AAUCAGAGCCACGGUAACCAG-3') resulted in a decrease of [¹⁴C]-agmatine uptake into the HEK293 cells (FIG. 3), whereas in reference experiments performed in parallel, incubation for 72 hours with siRNA targeting the human 5-HT transporter (5'-AAGAUGGAGAAGAUUGUCAGG-3') led to a significant decrease of [³H]5-HT uptake (methods are in references 3 and 13) by about 64 ± 15% (FIG. 3). The decrease in [³H]5-HT uptake clearly indicates that transfection with the siRNA targeting the 5-HT transporter mRNA has been effective. Accordingly, it seems justified to assume that transfection with the siRNAs targeting the cDNAs putatively encoding the agmatine transporter, if present in the cells, also should have been effective. Hence, the failure to decrease [¹⁴C]agmatine uptake suggests that the selective agmatine carrier is neither encoded by ORCTL4 nor by FLIPT1. Further candidate cDNAs will be investigated by this procedure in future experiments.

CONCLUSIONS

Investigation of ^{14}C accumulation in six human intestinal tumor cell lines and in the glioma cell line SK-MG-1 provided functional evidence for the operation of a specific agmatine transporter in these cells. Its existence could not be confirmed by current molecular biological techniques, but the short interference RNA targeting technology appears to be a promising approach to its identification.

REFERENCES

1. MOLDERINGS, G.J., A. HEINEN, S. MENZEL, et al. 2002. Exposure of rat isolated stomach and rats in vivo to [^{14}C]agmatine: accumulation in the stomach wall and distribution in various tissues. Fund. Clin. Pharmacol. **16:** 219–225.
2. SASTRE, M., S. REGUNATHAN & D.J. REIS. 1997. Uptake of agmatine into rat brain synaptosomes: possible role of cation channels. J. Neurochem. **69:** 2421–2426.
3. MOLDERINGS, G.J., H. BÖNISCH, M. GÖTHERT, et al. 2001. Agmatine and putrescine uptake in the human glioma cell line SK-MG-1. Naunyn Schmiedeberg's Arch. Pharmacol. **363:** 671–679.
4. HEINEN, A., M. BRÜSS, H. BÖNISCH, et al. 2003. Pharmacological characteristics of the specific transporter for the endogenous cell growth inhibitor agmatine in six tumor cell lines. Int. J. Colorectal Dis. **18:** 314–319.
5. BARENDT, W.M. & S.H. WRIGHT. 2002. The human organic cation transporter (hOCT2) recognizes the degree of substrate ionization. J. Biol. Chem. **277:** 22491–22496.
6. GRÜNDEMANN, D., C. HAHNE, R. BERKELS, et al. 2003. Agmatine is efficiently transported by non-neuronal monoamine transporters extraneuronal monoamine transporter (EMT) and organic cation transporter 2 (OCT2). J. Pharmacol. Exp. Ther. **304:** 810–817.
7. TAMAI, I., R. OHASHI, J. NEZU, et al. 1998. Molecular and functional identification of sodium ion-dependent, high affinity human carnitine transporter OCTN2. J. Biol. Chem. **273:** 20378–20382.
8. WU, X., W. HUANG, P.D. PRASAD, et al. 1999. Functional characteristics and tissue distribution pattern of organic cation transporter 2 (OCTN2), an organic cation/carnitine transporter. J. Pharmacol. Exp. Ther. **290:** 1482–1492.
9. CABELLA, C., G. GARDINI, D. CORPILLO, et al. 2001. Transport and metabolism of agmatine in rat hepatocyte cultures. Eur. J. Biochem. **268:** 940–947.
10. BABAL, P., M. RUCHKO, J.W. OLSON, et al. 2000. Interactions between agmatine and polyamine uptake pathways in rat pulmonary artery endothelial cells. Gen. Pharmacol. **34:** 255–261.
11. DEL VALLE, A.E., J.C. PAZ, F. SANCHEZ-JIMENEZ, et al. 2000. Agmatine uptake by cultured hamster kidney cells. Biochem. Biophys. Res. Commun. **280:** 307–311.
12. SATRIANO, J., M. ISOME, R.A. CASERO, et al. 2001. Polyamine transport system mediates agmatine transport in mammalian cells. Am. J. Cell. Physiol. **281:** C329–C334.
13. BRYAN-LLUKA, L.J. & H. BÖNISCH. 1997. Lanthanides inhibit the human noradrenaline, 5-hydroxytryptamine and dopamine transporters. Naunyn-Schmiedeberg's Arch. Pharmacol. **355:** 699–706.

Neuropharmacokinetic and Dynamic Studies of Agmatine (Decarboxylated Arginine)

H. OANH X. NGUYEN,[a,b] CORY J. GORACKE-POSTLE,[a,c] LORI L. KAMINSKI,[a] AARON C. OVERLAND,[a,c] ANDREW D. MORGAN,[d] AND CAROLYN A. FAIRBANKS[a,b,c]

[a]*Department of Pharmaceutics, College of Pharmacy, University of Minnesota, Minneapolis, Minnesota 55455, USA*

[b]*Department of Pharmacology, Medical School, University of Minnesota, Minneapolis, Minnesota 55455, USA*

[c]*Department of Neuroscience, Medical School, University of Minnesota, Minneapolis, Minnesota 55455, USA*

[d]*Department of Psychiatry, Medical School, University of Minnesota, Minneapolis, Minnesota 55455, USA*

> ABSTRACT: Agmatine has been previously proposed to represent a novel neurotransmitter. One of the criteria required to test that hypothesis is that the exogenously administered chemical produces pharmacological effects similar to the physiological effects of the putative neurotransmitter. Since agmatine was first identified in brain, approximately sixty studies of the *in vivo* effects of exogenously administered agmatine have been reported. Despite the assertion that agmatine functions as a neuromodulator/neurotransmitter, the vast majority of experiments have administered agmatine through systemic (rather than central) routes of administration. Systemic delivery of agmatine for studies of centrally mediated phenomenona (e.g., pain, spinal cord injury, cardiovascular responses) relies on the presumption that agmatine (a polar compound) gains appreciable access to the CNS. The mechanism by which agmatine crosses the blood–brain barrier is not well understood. A number of studies have examined the *in vivo* effects of agmatine following central administration (e.g., intracerebroventricular and intrathecal). This paper summarizes and provides a comparison between the systemic versus central routes of administration for delivery of agmatine in experimental subjects.
>
> KEYWORDS: agmatine; central administration; spinal; intrathecal; epidural; pain

INTRODUCTION

The development of methods that permit direct delivery of compounds to the CNS has greatly furthered the scientific understanding of drug action in the CNS.

Through the use of central routes of administration, we have learned that a drug delivered in one location may not have the same physiologic effect when it is delivered in a different location. This finding is also true for systemic administration of drugs versus central administration of drugs. To appreciate fully the physiologic role and therapeutic potential of agmatine, it is imperative to consider the literature and future experimental results in terms of route of administration and site of action.

This review has several objectives. First, we illustrate the importance of considering the route of drug administration in experimental design and in interpretation of the literature. Second, we review the in vivo observations of agmatinergic function with specific attention to dose and route of administration. Third, we describe the value of including central routes of administration in designing experimental in vivo studies of agmatine. We hope to encourage more agmatinergic researchers to consider the use of central routes of administration in their experimental designs, at the very least for comparison with systemic routes of administration. Incorporation of such experiments may show more clearly the therapeutic usefulness of agmatine in a wide variety of in vivo models of neuronal adaptation.

ROUTE OF DRUG ADMINISTRATION

Drugs are delivered systemically by a number of routes (e.g., orally, intraperitoneally, subcutaneously, rectally, intravenously, and intranasally). The delivery of drug by these routes is not implicitly equivalent. The outcome of drug delivery by different routes can result in differential absorption, distribution, metabolism, and elimination. Therefore it is imperative to consider carefully the route of administration when designing experiments investigating drug delivery. Further, the site of delivery of a drug can dramatically affect the physiologic consequences of presentation of that drug to its target. This concept was nicely illustrated by the work of Roerig and colleagues.[1] These researchers showed that morphine delivered intracerebroventricularly (ICV) produced supra-additivity (or synergy) with morphine that was simultaneously delivered intrathecally. The proposed mechanism of this supra-additivity is that activating opioid receptors in the brain causes a concomitant release of norepinephrine in the spinal cord. This norepinephrine then becomes available to produce antinociceptive synergy with morphine (the term "antinociceptive" refers to the analgesia observed by an experimenter in an experimental non-human subject). Morphine delivered in the spinal cord does not cause release of norepinephrine. Therefore, receptors activated at different regions can result in different cellular or molecular responses that can affect the intended physiologic response in different ways.

In another example, Porreca and colleagues[2] showed another functional discrepancy between agonists delivered intrathecally and supraspinally. Both supraspinal and spinal delivery of delta opioid receptor (DOR)–targeted antisense oligonucleotides result in decreased production of the DOR. When the DOR-selective agonist[2] DPDPE is administered to those sites following antisense treatment, however, analgesia is reduced spinally but not supraspinally. This example shows that delivery of an agent to one CNS region to act on a particular receptor is not necessarily predictive of how that same agent will respond in a separate CNS region where those receptors may also be present.

We can also compare observations made between the peripheral and central cardiovascular and neuroendocrine effects induced by injection of agmatine in both anesthetized and pithed spontaneously hypertensive rats (SHRs). Agmatine injected intravenously in anesthetized SHRs showed a dose-dependent decrease in both blood pressure and heart rate.[3–5] Interestingly, ICV administration of agmatine resulted in increased blood pressure and had no effect on heart rate. A converse pattern of response was noted when agmatine was injected into the fourth ventricle where there was an increase of heart rate and no effect on blood pressure.[4,5] Additionally, Roerig and colleagues[6] observed that whereas neither intrethecal nor ICV administration of agmatine had an impact on morphine–clonidine antinociceptive synergy, subcutaneous administration of agmatine reduced that interaction to additivity. These observations serve as strong examples of the importance of considering the route of administration of agmatine when interpreting data from in vivo discoveries.

In addition, the species of the experimental subject must be considered when analyzing data. The apparent differences in the cardiovascular effects of agmatine across species is illustrated by comparing the observations in rats[4,5] with the results in an experiment conducted by Head,[7] in which agmatine injected into the fourth ventricle of rabbits decreased heart rate, but had no effect on blood pressure. Furthermore, Head and colleagues[7] showed that agmatine potentiated the bradycardia produced by clonidine and moxonidine but did not alter the hypotensive effects of these agents. Therefore, this study shows the importance of considering both the route of administration and the species of the experimental subject when proposing the broader implications of the experimental results of any particular study.

TABLES 1 through 7 summarize the in vivo studies of agmatine to date with attention to species, dose, route of administration, and dependent measure of agmatine effects. We have also included a column listing the mechanism the authors propose for their observed effects. In some cases, the proposed mechanisms are based on pharmacologic evidence; in other cases, the proposed mechanisms are speculations. The results of these studies are described in the following section.

DELIVERY OF AGMATINE

Agmatine has been delivered by intravenous,[3,7–14] subcutaneous,[15,16] intraperitoneal,[17–40] intracerebroventricular (ICV),[4,5,7,17,34,41–46] intrathecal,[47–50] oral,[35,51,52] and intrarenal[42] routes. The doses, species, dependent measures, and outcomes from more than 50 in vivo studies are shown in TABLES 1 through 7. The effective systemic doses for which positive outcomes have been noted for agmatine range from 10 to 400 mg/kg with one outlying value of 3000 mg/kg. The most commonly reported effective systemic dose is 100 mg/kg.

The polar character of agmatine reduces its ability to cross the blood–brain barrier. Although the existence of an agmatinergic transporter has been suggested, there are no apparent data indicating the presence of such a transporter at this time. In support of the transporter concept, there are now many reports in which systemically administered agmatine has affected phenomena mediated by central processing. These effects are summarized in TABLES 1 through 7.

TABLE 1. Subcutaneous administration of agmatine

Citations	Species	Agmatine Dose (Source)	Frequency of Delivery	Dependent Measure	Outcome	Proposed Mechanisms of Actin
Kolesniko (1996)[16]	Male CD-1 mice	0.1, 1, 10 mg/kg agmatine (Sigma)	Once daily for 5 days with opioid ligand	Opioid analgesia and opioid tolerance. Tail flick assay	Dose-dependent enhancement of opioid analgesia and prevention of opioid tolerance	Analgesic potentiation: imidazoline receptors; Tolerance prevention: NMDA receptor/NOS cascade
Roerig (2003)[6]	Male ICR mice	10 mg/kg agmatine sulfate, (Sigma)	Once	Enhancement of antinociception induced by morphine and clonidine	Decreased intrathecal morphine/clonidine antinociceptive synergism to an additive interaction	Brain: α_2AR and imidazoline receptors; Spinal cord: imidazoline receptors and, perhaps, NMDA receptors

TABLE 2. Intraperitoneal administration of agmatine

Citations	Species	Agmatine Dose (Source)	Frequency of Delivery	Dependent Measure	Outcome	Proposed Mechanisms
Aricioglu-Kartal (1997)[20]	Male Wistar rats	20, 30, 40 mg/kg agmatine SO$_4$ (Sigma)	Once (72 hours after morphine implantation) 45 minutes before tests	Attenuation of behavioral signs or morphine abstinence syndrome	Dose-dependent prevention of all signs of naloxone-precipitated abstinence syndrome in morphine-dependent rats	Imidazoline receptor or central inhibition of NOS
Arteni (2002)[30]	Male Wistar rats	0.1, 1, 10, 20 mg/kg agmatine	Once daily (1 hour pretreatment or immediately post-training)	Memory of an inhibitory avoidance task	Post-test treatment with agmatine showed facilitation of memory, pretest treatment had no effect	Imidazoline receptors
Bence (2003)[35]	Male Sprague Dawley rats and albino mice	30, 60, 120 mg/kg (rat) 30, 100, 300 mg/kg (mice) agmatine SO$_4$ (Sigma)	Once	Antiseizure activity: maximal electroshock seizure (MES) test; Acute neurotoxicity: Rats: positional sense and gait tests; Mice: rotarod test	MES: Mouse: not effective; Rat: minimal effect; no neurotoxic effects	

TABLE 2. Intraperitoneal administration/continued.

Citations	Species	Agmatine Dose (Source)	Frequency of Delivery	Dependent Measure	Outcome	Proposed Mechanisms
Feng (2002)[31]	M/F Sprague Dawley rat pups (7–22 days old)	50, 100, 150 mg/kg, i.p. agmatine SO_4 (Sigma)	Once daily for 3 days	Inhibition of hypoxic-ischemic (HI) brain injury (evaluated by weight deficit 22 days post-treatment)	150-mg/kg dose reduced brain weight deficits; 100-mg/kg dose inhibited the formation of brain NO metabolites following HI injury	Suppression of NO production after hypoxia through inhibition of NOS
Gilad (1996)[18]	Male Wistar rats, male Mongolian gerbils	10, 50, 100 mg/kg agmatine	Once daily for 3 days	Motor deficits and neuronal cell death following forebrain or cerebral ischemia	Neuroprotection and significant reduction in motor function deficits	Unknown, synthesis of bioamines, modulation of neurotransmission; inhibition of NOS or action on NMDA, α_2AR, or imidazoline receptors
Gilad (2000)[22]	Male Wistar rats	100 mg/kg	Once daily for 4 days	Motor deficits following spinal cord ischemia	Significant recovery of motor deficits	Multiple, unknown
Glavin (1995)[17]	Male Sprague Dawley rats	0.1, 1, 10, and 20 mg/kg agmatine (Sigma)	Once (4 hours pretreatment)	Gastric secretions	Augmented basal gastric section by 40%; depleted mucus; increased stress injury; increased total secretion volume and pepsin and gastric acid output in pylorus-ligated rats	Action as an inverse agonist at central imidazoline receptors
Ishizuka (2000)[23]	Male Sprague Dawley rats	50 mg/kg agmatine, (Sigma)	Daily (up to 7 days)	Renal function in Anti-Thy-1 glomerulonephritis	Prevented reduction in glomerular filtration rate on day 1 and proteinuria on days 5–7	Inhibition of NOS, ornithine decarboxylase activity, and cell proliferation
Karadag (2003)[37]	Wistar rat (either sex)	10, 30, 100 mg/kg agmatine	Once	Attenuation of neuropathic pain models: spinal nerve ligation and streptozocin-induced diabetic neuropathy	100 mg/kg reduced mechanical allodynia	Action on central α_2-AR, agonist activity at imidazoline receptor, central inhibition of NOS or NMDA receptors

TABLE 2. Intraperitoneal administration/continued.

Citations	Species	Agmatine Dose (Source)	Frequency of Delivery	Dependent Measure	Outcome	Proposed Mechanisms
Li (1999)[53]	Mice	0.125, 2.5, 10 mg/kg	Once	Opioid-induced tolerance and withdrawal syndrome	Prevention of tolerance to morphine and naloxone-induced signs of withdrawal	Activation of imidazoline receptors
Li (1999)[12]	Mice	------	------	Opioid withdrawal	Agmatine inhibited naloxone-induced withdrawal jumps and prevented an increased in NOS in cerebellum, forebrain, and thalamus	Inhibition of NOS and activation of imidazoline receptors
Li (1999)[54]	Mice, rats	------	------	Analgesia (tail flick, acetic acid writhing, 4% saline [rat])	Tail flick test: no effect; Acetic acid writhing: reduction of responses; 4% saline: ablation of responses; potentiation of morphine and clonidine analgesia	Activation of imidazoline receptors
McKay (2002)[32]	Male and female Wistar rats	1, 5, 10 or 50 mg/kg agmatine	Once 20 minutes pretreatment or immediately after training	Behavioral inferences of specific types of learning and memory. Water maze	Dose-dependent impairment in acquisition of learned fear to contextual but not auditory stimuli; no effect on latencies for maze place learning	Selective action in the ventral hippocampus; action on NMDA receptor
McKay (2003)[38]	Male Wistar rats	4 mg/kg agmatine (Sigma)	Once immediately before conditioning	Additive impairment of contextual fear learning with agmatine and theta-burst stimulation patterned complex magnetic field treatments	Significant additive impairment measured by a decrease in freezing behavior	Antagonism of NMDA receptors
Onal (2001)[28]	Male albino mice	37.5–600 mg/kg agmatine (Sigma)	Once	Nociceptive responses; formalin test; tail flick; (radiant heat) rotarod	Decreased nociceptive behaviors in first and second phase of formalin test; Tail flick: no effect; Rotarod: slight motor decrement at 300 mg/kg; profound decrement at 600 mg/kg	α_2AR or imidazoline receptors; NMDA receptors

TABLE 2. Intraperitoneal administration/continued.

Citations	Species	Agmatine Dose (Source)	Frequency of Delivery	Dependent Measure	Outcome	Proposed Mechanisms
Onal (2003)[39]	Male Sprague Dawley rats	10–400 mg/kg agmatine	Once	Neuropathic pain (sciatic nerve ligation) Ugo Basile Analgesymeter	Agmatine increased pain threshold at high doses (300–400 mg/kg) and decreased nitrate and MHPG levels in brainstem and cerebellum	Alterations in NO and noradrenergic activity
Prasad (1996)[19]	Male Sprague Dawley rats	0.5, 1, 5, 10 mg/kg agmatine (Sigma)	Once daily for 3 days	Caloric intake in satiated rats	Agmatine increases caloric intake in satiated rats (10 mg/kg)	α_2AR agonism or increased norepinephrine availability
Stewart (2000)[24]	Male Wistar rats	1, 5, 10 mg/kg agmatine	Once before conditioning (all doses) or after conditioning (10-mg/kg dose only)	Pretreatment: acquisition of contextual fear (defensive freezing); Posttreatment: consolidation of memory formation	Pretreatment impaired the acquisition of contextual fear; Post-treatment impaired consolidation of contextual stimuli at 30 minutes and at 2 hours	NMDA receptor antagonism in the hippocampus
Utkan (2000)[25]	Wistar rats (either sex)	0.5, 1, 10, 50 mg/kg agmatine	Once (10 minutes before intragastric ethanol)	Increase in ethanol-induced gastric mucosal injury	1 mg/kg significantly increased ethanol-induced gastric mucosal injury	Ulcergenic effect mediated by both α_2AR and imidazoline receptors
Uzbay (2000)[26]	Male Wistar rats	20, 40, 80, 160 mg/kg agmatine SO$_4$ (Sigma)	30 minutes pre- and 6 hours post-ethanol withdrawal	Ethanol withdrawal syndrome	Dose-dependent inhibition of withdrawal behaviors with no impairment of motor coordination or function	Clonidine-like effect on α_2AR; agonist activity at imidazoline receptor; central inhibition of NOS; or through inhibition of NMDA receptors
Uzbay (2002)[33]	Male Long-Evans hooded rats	20, 40, 60 mg/kg, 5 mL/kg agmatine SO$_4$	Once daily (10 minutes pretreatment)	Effect of NOS inhibition on pentylene-tetrazol (PTZ) discriminative stimulus (anxiety model)	No effect	PTZ discriminative stimulus may not be related to NO-mediated central mechanisms

TABLE 2. Intraperitoneal administration/continued.

Citations	Species	Agmatine Dose (Source)	Frequency of Delivery	Dependent Measure	Outcome	Proposed Mechanisms
Yesilyurt (2001)[29]	Male albino Swiss Webster mice	10, 20, 40 mg/kg agmatine SO_4 (Sigma)	Once (15 minutes before morphine)	Opioid analgesia; radiant heat; tail flick test	Potentiation of morphine-induced analgesia during (reversed by yohimbine)	Clonidine-like effect on α_2AR
Yu (2000)[27]	Female Sprague Dawley rats	100 mg/kg agmatine, (Sigma)	Once daily for 42 days	Locomotor function and tissue damage following spinal cord injury	Mean BBB locomotor scale rating scores were increased significantly more following bilateral hindlimb paralysis; 30% less mean tissue damage in treated group	Antagonism of NMDA receptors and inhibition of NOS
Yu (2003)[40]	Rats	100 mg/kg/day agmatine (Sigma)	Once daily for 14 days, 30 minutes after quisqualate (QUIS) injection	Prevention and treatment of excessive grooming behavior	Final area of skin targeted for excessive grooming reduced; onset time of spontaneous grooming increased; severity of grooming behavior lower than in QUIS or saline groups	Agmatine selectively blocks the NMDA receptor and also inhibits NOS
Zomkowski (2002)[34]	Swiss mice (either sex)	0.01–50 mg/kg, agmatine (Sigma)	Once (30 minutes pretreatment)	Anti-depressant–like effects in forced swim test (FST) and tail suspension test (TST), measured by duration of immobility	Decreased the duration of immobility in FST (10 mg/kg) and TST (0.1 mg/kg) comparable to imipramine (15 mg/kg), without impairing motor function	Antagonism of NMDA receptors and inhibition of NOS; possible involvement of α_2ARs

TABLE 3. Intravenous administration of agmatine

Citations	Species	Agmatine Dose (Source)	Frequency of Delivery	Dependent Measure	Outcome	Proposed Mechanism
Bradley (1997)[11]	Male Wistar rats	25–200 mg/kg agmatine (Sigma)	Dose doubled every 6 minutes up to cumulative 200 mg/kg (repeated after 60 minutes)	Spinal nociceptive reflexes: noxious pinch potentiation of fentanyl antinociception	Spinally intact animals with non-inflamed paws: 200 mg/kg reduced reflex responses; doses > 25 mg/kg decreased mean blood pressure; no effect on fentanyl antinociception	Not through $\alpha_2 AR$; possibly cardiovascular and peripheral toxicity
Gao (1995)[8]	Sprague Dawley rats (either sex)	1–10 mg bolus agmatine SO_4 (Sigma)	Once	Hemodynamics, vasodilatory effects	Dose-dependently decreased systemic arterial pressure	Unknown
Häuser (1995)[9]	Male SHRs	10–5000 μg/kg/minute	—	Effects on catecholamine release	5000 μg/kg/minute resulted in an increase in epinephrine release at highest dose, with no change in norepinephrine overflow	Action on imidazoline receptors on the adrenal medulla but not on presynaptic $\alpha_2 AR$
Li (1999)[21]	Rats	10 mg/kg	—	Cellular mechanisms of hemodynamic effects	Decreased heart rate, mean arterial pressure, left ventricular pressure, cardiac index, and total peripheral resistance index	Mediated by vasodilatory effects of agmatine and its action on imidazoline receptors and $\alpha_2 AR$
Li (2001)[65]	Rats	0.01, 0.05, 1 mg/kg	—	Effects on femoral, renal, and mesenteric vascular beds	Dose-dependently increased perfusion pressure in femoral vascular beds (blocked by idazoxan and yohimbine) and renal vascular beds (blocked by idazoxan); decreased perfusion pressure in mesenteric vascular beds (blocked by idazoxan)	Differential action on vascular beds and interactions with imidazoline and $\alpha_2 AR$

TABLE 3. Intravenous administration/continued.

Citations	Species	Agmatine Dose (Source)	Frequency of Delivery	Dependent Measure	Outcome	Proposed Mechanism
Li (2001)[13]	Dahl salt-sensitive (DS) hypertensive and Dahl salt-resistant rats	1, 10, 20 mg/kg	----	Hemodynamic effects	Dose-dependently decreased heart rate, mean arterial pressure, left ventricular pressure, CI, and TPRI (completely blocked by efaroxan, and partially blocked by yohimbine and idazoxan)	Action on I1-imidazoline receptor, with some participation of I2-imidazoline receptor and $\alpha_2 AR$
Morgan (2002)[14]	Male Wistar rats	10, 30, 60 mg/kg agmatine SO_4 (Sigma)	Twice daily or three times daily for 6–30 days	Escalation of intravenous cocaine and fentanyl self-administration	Agmatine pretreatment significantly decreased the escalation of administration of fentanyl, but not cocaine	Antagonism of NMDA receptors or inhibition of NOS
Raasch (2002)[5]	Male SHRs	0.01–100 mg/kg agmatine (Sigma)	Bolus-given 1 minute before clonidine bolus	Antagonism of clonidine-mediated blood pressure reaction	Reduced blood pressure and heart rate in anaesthetized rat, reduced norepinephrine when α_2ARs are blocked with rauwolscine	Central action for decreasing blood pressure and heart rate; action on I1-imidazoline receptor for norepinephrine release
Raasch (2003)[68]	Male SHRs	6, 33, 60 mg/kg agmatine	----	Influence of agmatine on noradrenaline overflow	Agmatine reduced noradrenaline overflow	I1-binding sites in ganglia might be involved
Schäfer (1999)[4]	Male SHRs	0.01–100 mg/kg	Once	Cardiovascular effects	33–100 mg/kg decreased blood pressure and heart rate	Inhibition of sympathetic ganglionic transmission, and differing central mechanisms
Smyth (1995)[10]	Male Sprague Dawley rats	3, 30 nmol/kg/minute infusion agmatine, (Sigma)	----	Natriuresis	No change on blood pressure, heart rate; increased urine flow rate at 30 nmol/kg/minute infusion; increased osmolar clearance at 3 nmol/kg/minute infusion	Involvement of I1-imidazoline receptor with the kidney
Sun (1995)[3]	Male Sprague Dawley rats	60, 400 μmoles bolus infusion	----	Arterial pressure and sympathetic nerve activity	60 μmoles: decreased arterial blood pressure; 400 μmoles: no effect	Inhibition of sympathetic ganglionic transmission and direct dilation of smooth muscle

TABLE 4. Intrathecal administration of agmantine

Citations	Species	Agmantine Dose (Source)	Frequency of Delivery	Dependent Measure	Outcome	Proposed Mechanism
Fairbanks (1997)[47]	Male Institute of Cancer Research mice	0.2, 0.6, 2, 8, 20, 30, 100 nmol agmantine SO_4 (Sigma)	Once before test	Tail flick (warm water immersion); spinal morphine tolerance	Agmatine alone had no effect on tail flick; agmatine did not potentiate morphine antinociception but did prevent induction of acute spinal morphine tolerance	Antagonism of NMDA receptor or NOS inhibition
Fairbanks (2000)[49]	Male ICR mice and Sprague Dawley rats	0.3, 1, 5, 10, 60 nmol agmantine SO_4 (Sigma)	Once after confirmation of hyperalgesia	Allodynia, hyperalgesia and autotomy-like responses	Antiallodynic and antihyperalgesic	Antagonism of NMDA receptor, inhibition of NOS
Horvath (1999)[48]	Male Wistar rats	1, 10, 50, 100 μg agmantine, (Sigma)	Once	Carrageenan-induced thermal hyperalgesia (paw withdrawal to radiant heat stimulus)	Dose-dependent 35%–76% attenuation of thermal hyperalgesia when given pretreatment; lesser effect when given post-treatment; potentiation of antihyperalgesic effect of morphine	Actions at imidazoline receptor and inhibition of inducible and/or constitutive NOS
Hou (2003)[50]	Wistar rats (either sex)	20, 40, 100, 200 nmol agmantine (Sigma)	Once	Extracellular single-unit recordings of noxiously evoked discharges of parafiscular (PF) neurons of the medial thalamus	No effect on spontaneous PF discharges, dose-dependently suppressed nociceptive discharges (blocked by idazoxan but not yohimbine)	Activation of imidazoline receptors at the spinal level
Roerig (2003)[6]	Male ICR mice	10 nmoles agmantine SO_4 (Sigma)	Once	Potentiation of spinal morphine-induced anti-nociception	Potentiated intrathecal morphine analgesia; attenuated intrathecal clonidine-induced analgesia	Action at imidazoline receptors in the spinal cord

TABLE 5. Brain area administration of agmatine

Citations	Species	Agmatine Dose (Source)	Frequency of Delivery	Dependent Measure	Outcome	Proposed Mechanism
Glavin (1995)[17]	Male Sprague Dawley rats	0.5–2.5 µg ICV-lateral cerebral ventricle	Once	Gastric secretion	Significantly augmented basal gastric section by 33% (1 µg), 44% (2.5 µg)	Action as an inverse agonist at central ICV receptors
Head (1997)[7]	Rabbits (either sex)	0.01–100 µg/kg fourth ventricle	Every 15 minutes (x 5 doses)	Cardiovascular actions of agmatine	No effect on mean arterial pressure; dose-dependent bradycardia when given alone (reversed by efaroxan and idazoxan); potentiation of clonidine and moxonidine-induced bradycardia	Action on α2AR
Penner (1996)[42]	Male Sprague Dawley rats	0, 10, 100, 300, or 1,000 nmol agmatine ICV (Sigma)	Once	Alteration of sodium excretion (natriuresis)	Increased sodium excretion and osmolar clearance; decreased free water clearance	Agmatine functions as a physiologic agonist resulting in alterations in sodium excretion
Pineda (1996)[43]	Male Sprague Dawley rats	1–10 mM agmatine SO_4 intracerebroventricularly-fourth ventricle (Sigma)	3–10 nL x 1–10 mM	Activity of agmatine at α2ARs which modulate locus coeruleus neuron firing rate	Application of agmatine to the locus coeruleus showed a slight but significant increase in cell firing rate	I2-IBS, sodium channels, or other proteins
Raasch (2002)[5]	Male SHRs	10–1,000 nmol ICV-fourth ventricle	—————	Cardiovascular responses	ICV agmatine caused a significant dose-dependent increase in blood pressure and an increase in heart rate	
Roerig (2003)[6]	Male ICR mice	1 nmol, 4 µL agmatine SO_4 ICV (Sigma)	Once	Morphine-enhancing activity	ICV agmatine potentiated spinal morphine antinociception; co-adminstration ICV of α2 and imidazoline antagonists attenuated the action of ICV agmatine	Action at both α2AR and imidazoline receptors in the brain

TABLE 5. Brain administration/continued.

Citations	Species	Agmatine Dose (Source)	Frequency of Delivery	Dependent Measure	Outcome	Proposed Mechanism
Ruiz-Durantez (2002)[46]	Male Sprague Dawley rats	10, 20, 40 μg agmatine SO_4 ICV-left lateral ventricle (Sigma)	Once	Locus coeruleus neuron firing rate	Dose-dependently increased firing rate (blocked by L-NAME)	Through NOS mechanisms in the locus coeruleus
Sanchez-Blazquez (2000)[44]	Male albino mice (CD-1)	10 μg agmatine sulphate, ICV- right lateral ventricle (Sigma)	Once (30 minutes before ICV morphine)	Activation of I2-imidazoline receptor; enhancement of morphine analgesia; tail flick test: 52°C warm water immersion	Agmatine increased antinoceptive morphine to opioids	Functional interaction between I2-imidazoline and opioid receptors; involvement of Gi-Go transducer proteins
Schäfer (1999)[4]	Male SHRs	10–1,000 nmol/5μL agmatine, ICV-fourth ventricle	Once	Cardiovascular effects (blood pressure and heart rate)	Increased blood pressure; no effect on heart rate	Mechanism is unclear
Sugawara (2001)[45]	Male Holtzman rats	80 nmol agmatine ICV-third cerebral ventricle (Sigma)	Single pulse	Suppression of water intake in 24-hour water-deprived rats	No effect	Selective, non-imidazoline α_2-AR activation suppresses water intake
Sun (1995)[3]	Male Sprague-Dawley rats	40–400 nmol intracisternal agmatine	-----	Aterial pressure and sympathetic nerve activity	Increased aterial pressure; increased sympathetic nerve activity; blocked baroreflex transmissionic nerve activity	Central inhibition of baroreflexes
Sun et al. (1995)[3]	Male Sprague-Dawley rats	0.2 M (10 nmol/50 ml/site; 10s) agmatine rostral ventrolateral medulla	-----	Baroreceptor activity	No effect	Blockade within nucleus of the solitary tract or in an interposed neuron in baroreceptor reflex

TABLE 6. Oral administration of agmatine

Citations	Species	Agmatine Dose (Source)	Frequency of Delivery	Dependent Measure	Outcome	Proposed Mechanism
Bence (2003)[35]	Male Sprague Dawley rats	30, 60, 120 mg/kg 480 mg/kg (neurotoxicity) agmatine sulfate (Sigma)	Once	Antiseizure activity: maximal electroshock seizure (MES) test; acute neurotoxicity: positional sense and gait tests	Protection in less than 20% of rats at 15, 30 minutes, 1 hour, 2 hours, and 6 hours; protection in 50% of rats at 4 hours after injection; no neurotoxic effects	Action at α_2AR and other CNS sites, or regulation of polyamines
Marx (1995)[51]	Diabetic db/db mice	50 mg/kg agmatine	Once daily	Collagen accumulation in diabetic kidney	Reduced collagen accumulation (lower kidney OH-proline content and carboxymethyllysine concentrations, and higher acid solubility in treated group)	Nucleophilic structure of agmatine blocks reactive carbonyls (inhibits glucose carbonyl-mediated cross linking)
Moore (2001)[52]	C57/BL6 infant mice	0.16 mg (~32 mg/kg) Agmatine	Twice daily on days 5–12 of age	Inhibition of *Crytosporidium parvum* infection	Treated mice were significantly less infected with *C. parvum* than untreated	Alters polyamine matabolism of *C. parvum*

TABLE 7. Intrarenal administration of agmatine

Citation	Species	Agmatine Dose (Source)	Frequency of Delivery	Dependent Measure	Outcome	Proposed Mechanism
Penner (1996)[42]	Male Sprague Dawley rats	0, 3, 10, 30, 100, 300, nmol/kg/minute	3.4 µL/minute	Alteration of sodium excretion (natriuresis)	Increased creatine clearance at lowest and highest doses, dose-related inc in urine flow rate, inc in sodium excretion and osmolar clearance	AG functions as a physiologic agonist resulting in alterations in sodium excretion

IN VIVO OBSERVATIONS OF AGMATINERGIC FUNCTION

One of the early reports of agmatine's action on an in vivo phenomenon revealed that subcutaneously administered agmatine (10 mg/kg) delivered concomitantly with toleragenic doses of morphine prevented the development of chronically induced morphine tolerance.[16] Since then, others have shown that intraperitoneally administered agmatine also inhibits manifestations of morphine[20,53,54] and ethanol[26] withdrawal. Consistent with those observations, Morgan and colleagues[14] reported that intravenously administered agmatine decreased the escalation of fentanyl (but not cocaine) self-administration. Clearly, systemically administered agmatine affects the opioidergic systems of tolerance and dependence, which are demonstrably CNS processes.

Systemically administered agmatine has also been shown to prevent other manifestations of neuronal plasticity, including brain and spinal cord injury and seizures. Gilad and colleagues[18] observed that agmatine-treated Mongolian gerbils subjected to cerebral ischemia showed reduced neurotoxicity relative to saline-treated controls. This same group observed similar agmatine-mediated neuroprotection in a model of rat spinal cord injury.[22] Consistent with those observations, Yezierski and colleagues[27,40,49] have observed significant anatomic and functional recovery in rats intraperitoneally injected with agmatine following chemical lesions or weight-drop injuries to the spinal cord of rats. Bence and colleagues[35] observed that orally administered agmatine prevented seizures in rats. That agmatine is able to protect against these events of neuronal dysfunction clearly illustrates the ability of systemically administered agmatine to act within the CNS.

Further evidence that systemically administered agmatine acts centrally is presented in the studies that have evaluated the ability of agmatine to modulate hypersensitivity of rodents to noxious stimuli, which represent models of various pain states. Agmatine has been evaluated in three distinct phenomena that are related to the pain and analgesia systems. The distinctions among these areas are important. The first screen of the effects of any new compound is identifying the effect of the compound in a standard antinociceptive (analgesic) assay. The investigator attempts to determine whether the new compound can interrupt the pain conduction pathway and relieve perceived pain, as morphine does. The second area that may be assessed in studies of pain is whether the new compound can enhance the analgesic properties of a known or standard analgesic, such as morphine or clonidine. In this case, the new compound may or may not have analgesic properties of its own. Some studies have shown that agmatine does not seem to have analgesic properties when delivered alone but does seem to enhance the analgesic properties of morphine and clonidine (see Roerig, Ref. 6). The third area that is assessed is the ability of the new compound to reverse hypersensitivity to non-noxious (allodynic) or noxious (hyperalgesic) stimuli that develops following an injury to the organism and is caused by a reorganization of the CNS. Various novel compounds may not themselves be analgesic (i.e., do not relieve pain in the normal condition) but rather show antiallodynic or antihyperalgesic efficacy (i.e., return to normal sensitivity an organism previously made hypersensitive to non-noxious or noxious stimuli). For example, the relatively recently discovered endogenous cannabinnoid agonist anandamide was classified in this category.[55] The observation that agmatine does not seem to be analgesic but reverses mechanical and thermal hypersensitivity following inflammation and neuropathic lesions suggests that agmatine may also fall into this category. In our report[49] on the antihyperalgesic effects of agmatine in models of neuropathic and inflammatory pain, we intended to make it clear that we do not believe spinally administered agmatine is, in and of itself, antinociceptive or analgesic. We realize, however, that those not well versed in the pain and analgesia literature may not understand the subtleties of these categories and may misunderstand our interpretation of the data. Consequently, we are sometimes cited inaccurately as having reported that agmatine induces analgesia mediated through α_2 adrenergic receptors (α_2ARs) or imidazoline receptors, whereas our observations actually indicated that spinally administered agmatine is antiallodynic/antihyperalgesic and that these effects are most likely mediated by the NMDA receptor/nitric oxide synthase pathway.

Yezierski and colleagues[49] have shown that intraperitoneally administered agmatine reduced manifestations of spontaneous pain-related grooming behavior that arises following chemical lesioning of the spinal cord by quisqualate. In this study agmatine delayed both the onset and severity of the grooming when given before treatment and reversed the grooming when delivered after treatment. In a different model of pain, Onal and Soykan[28] tested intraperitoneally administered agmatine for modulation in both the first and second phases of the formalin model of tonic pain. In this model, formalin is injected into the hindpaw, causing a biting and flinching behavior that persists for 1 to 5 minutes (first phase) followed by a 20-minute quiescent period and a second phase of an hour or more. This model has been previously demonstrated to be inhibited by opioids,[56,57] α_2AR agonists,[56,57] NSAIDS,[58] NMDA receptor antagonists,[59] and NOS inhibitors.[60,61] Onal and Soykan[28] observed that intraperitoneal agmatine inhibited both the first and second phases of the formalin model of tonic pain. In this case, the second phase was inhibited in a yohimbine-sensitive manner. Yesilyurt and Uzbay[29] also observed that intraperitoneal agmatine potentiated the effects of morphine in a yohimbine-sensitive manner. These observations suggest the participation of α_2ARs in the effect of agmatine in the formalin model. Bradley and Headley,[11] however, reported that intravenously delivered agmatine inhibited spinal reflexes in an electrophysiologic preparation only at doses high enough (200 mg/kg) to cause cardiotoxicity. Their results support the concept that, although agmatine may reverse manifestations of mechanical and thermal hypersensitivity, it is not likely to be an analgesic agent in and by itself; rather it acts as an antihyperalgesic agent, like anandamide. In support of that idea, Karadag and colleagues[37] have shown that acute intraperitoneal administration of agmatine reduces expression of mechanical allodynia (hypersensitivity to normally non-noxious tactile stimuli) following spinal nerve ligation (Chung model) or streptozocin-induced diabetes. The same group, however, also observed that agmatine had no effect on responses of normal subjects to tactile stimulation.

One neurochemical mechanism that chronic neuropathic pain, spinal cord injury, opioid-induced tolerance, and opioid dependence and self-administration share is activation of the NMDA-receptor–NOS system. Agmatine has been shown to antagonize NMDA receptors[49,62] and to inhibit NOS.[63,64] In fact, for many of the studies listed in TABLES 1 through 7, the action of agmatine on these entities has been proposed as a mechanism for its effects. If that were the case, one might expect that systemically administered agmatine could affect the performance of rodents subjected to models of learning and memory. In fact, several studies have addressed this question. McKay and colleagues[32] observed that systemic pretreatment with intraperitoneal agmatine dose-dependently impaired the magnitude of learned fear to contextual (but not auditory or mace place) learning. In contrast, Arteni and colleagues[30] observed that administration of agmatine after training facilitated memory. The effect of agmatine on the memory of the subject is an extremely important consideration, particularly for studies that use systemic routes to deliver agmatine; once agmatine crosses the blood–brain barrier, brain regions that govern learning and memory formation are affected. More studies are needed to determine the types of learning and memory processes that agmatine effects.

Because systemically administered agmatine seems to affect centrally mediated processes such as opioid tolerance and dependence, spinal cord injury, and chronic pain, and possibly learning and memory, it is not surprising that it would have effects on other centrally mediated systems. Agmatine was originally discovered during the search for the clonidine-displacing substance; therefore the impact of agmatine on centrally mediated cardiovascular responses was assessed. Intravenously administered agmatine has reportedly dose-dependently evoked bradycardia[3–5,7,65] and potentiated bradycardia invoked by moxonidine and clonidine.[7] Intravenous agmatine also decreases blood pressure and is accompanied by vasodilatation.[8] As are learning and memory, these cardiovascular effects are critical considerations when evaluating the effect of systemically administered agmatine on other phenomena, such as opioid and nerve injury effects.

EVIDENCE BASED ON HIGH-PRESSURE LIQUID CHROMATOGRAPHY

The best evidence for agmatine transport to the central nervous system following systemic administration is data representing HPLC-mediated detection of agmatine in CNS regions following systemic administration of agmatine. We and others have conducted some limited studies along these lines. In one study, we injected the median effective dose (ED_{50}) of agmatine sulfate (100 mg/kg) or saline in ICR-CD1 mice (25–30 g). At 1 minute and 30 minutes after injection, the mice were killed, trunk blood was collected, and spinal cords were extracted by hydraulic extrusion and then were frozen in liquid nitrogen. Serum and spinal cords were prepared for HPLC analysis 49. As shown in TABLE 8, we detected 20 ± 6.1 pmoles/mg (n = 3) in spinal cords of mice killed 1 minute after intraperitoneal injection of 100 mg/kg agmatine; we also detected 40 ± 0.39 pmoles/μL (n = 3) in serum at the same time point (TABLE 9). At 30 minutes after injection, we detected 0.54 ± 0.12 pmoles/mg (n = 3) in spinal cord and 6.7 ± 2.4 pmoles/μL (n = 3) in serum (TABLE 8 and TABLE 9, respectively). The marked decrease in agmatine levels in the serum was also found by Raasch and colleagues,[5] who saw substantial decreases in serum agmatine after 35 minutes. For comparison we conducted the same experiment with subjects implanted with Alzet minipumps (Durect Corp., Cupertino, CA) infusing 100 mg/kg/12 μL/day for 13 days. We were unable to detect appreciable levels of agmatine in either the spinal cord (0.27 ± 0.11 pmoles/mg) (n = 6) or serum (0.024 ± 0.016 pmoles/μL) (n = 6) of these subjects. Therefore, it would seem that the volume of delivery and/or rate of infusion contributes to the ability of the compound to enter the CNS. Investigators considering the use of continuous infusion using minipump technology should confirm central levels of agmatine before planning large-scale experiments or interpreting data.

TABLE 8. Agmatine in homogenized spinal cord: systemic delivery by bolus injection (100 mg/kg) versus continuous infusion by Alzet minipump (100 mg/kg/day)

	IP Q20pmol/mg[a]		Pump pmol/mg[a]
Agmatine 1 minute (n = 3)	20 ± 6.1	Agmatine infusion (n = 6)	0.27 ± 0.11
Saline 1 minute (n = 3)	0.118 ± 0.047	Saline infusion (n = 6)	−0.008 ± 0.0005
Agmatine 30 minutes (n = 3)	0.54 ± 0.12	—	—
Saline 30 minutes (n = 3)	−0.018 ± 0.005	—	—
Naïve (n = 4)	−0.017 ± 0.001	Naïve (n = 4)	−0.008 ± 0.002

[a] Mg measured in wet weight.

CENTRAL ADMINISTRATION

The initial studies of central delivery of agmatine focused in large part on the cardiovascular effects of centrally administered agmatine. Sun and colleagues[3] observed that intracisternally administered agmatine (100, 400 nmoles) dose-dependently increased arterial pressure and sympathetic nerve activity in Sprague Dawley rats. These actions were confirmed to be central because the same doses given systemically did not elicit those responses. Similarly, in rabbit, Szabo and colleagues[41] showed that blood pressure, renal sympathetic neve activity, and plasma concentrations of noradrenaline and adrenaline were increased following intracisternal administration of 30, 100, and 300 μg/kg agmatine. Head and colleagues[7] observed that cumulative doses of agmatine (0.01–10 μg/kg) into the fourth ventricle of rabbits did not alter resting mean arterial pressure but caused a reduction in heart rate. A higher dose of agmatine (100 μg/kg) caused both agitation and an increase in blood pressure accompanied by a reversal of the bradycardia. In contrast, Schafer and colleagues[4] showed that in anesthetized SHRs agmatine (ED_{50} value: 55 nmole) delivered to the fourth ventricle increased the heart rate and had no effect on blood pressure. Shafer and colleagues,[4] however, also showed that, in these same rats, ICV agmatine (ED_{50} value: 130 nmole) increased blood pressure and failed to affect heart rate. Raasch and colleagues[5] microinjected agmatine directedly into the central lateral ventricle

TABLE 9. Agmatine in serum: systemic delivery by bolus injection (100 mg/kg) versus continuous infusion by Alzet minipump (100 mg/kg/day)

	IP pmol/μL		Pump pmol/μL
Agmatine 1 minute (n = 3)	40 ± .39	Agmatine infusion (n = 6)	0.024 ± 0.016
Saline 1 minute (n = 3)	−0.014 ± 1.8	Saline infusion (n = 6)	−0.014 ± 0.013
Agmatine 30 minutes (n = 3)	6.7 ± 2.4	—	—
Saline 30 minute (n = 3)	0.002 ± 0.016	—	—
Naïve (n = 4)	0.014 ± 1.4	Naïve (n = 4)	−0.006 ± 0.008

of SHRs and observed that agmatine (ED_{50} value: 201 nmol) increased diastolic blood pressure with no effect on heart rate. Similar to the results of Shafer and colleagues[4], injection of agmatine (ED_{50} value: 53 nmole) into the fourth cerebral ventricle of SHRs increased heart rate with no effect on blood pressure. These studies of the effects of centrally administered agmatine on cardiovascular responses clearly illustrate the importance of considering drug transport and distribution to the CNS as well as to the site of action when interpreting data obtained from experiments using systemic delivery.

We provided the first evidence that spinally delivered agmatine affects established centrally mediated phenomena in vivo.[47] In that study, we demonstrated that spinally administered agmatine (4 nmoles/5 µL) delivered concomitantly with toleragenic doses of morphine prevented the development of acutely induced morphine tolerance. We then assessed how spinally delivered agmatine affected paw-withdrawal responses of mice following inflammation-induced and neuropathy-induced hyperalgesia. We noted that spinally delivered agmatine successfully reduced tactile hyperalgesia induced by the inflammatory agent, carrageenan, in a dose-dependent fashion. (Dosages ranged from 0.3 to 60 nmoles.) The most effective dose (60 nmoles) completely inhibited tactile hyperalgesia at 15 minutes after injection; however, the tactile hyperalgesia returned by 60 minutes after injection. Horvath and colleagues[48] had previously observed similar results in rats where intrathecal pretreatment with agmatine attenuated both the development and the maintenance of the carrageenan-evoked thermal hyperalgesia.

We also gave a single injection of agmatine following induction of tactile hyperalgesia by either a chemical insult (high-dose dynorphin) or spinal nerve injury. This single injection of agmatine 1 day after the injury reversed the tactile allodynia or hyperalgesia in both models of neuropathic pain. This reversal seemed permanent because we tested the animals out to 28 days after that one injection. The most effective dose in this experiment was the lower dose (0.3 nmoles); higher doses were ineffective in producing this reversal. Our study differs from that of Karadag and colleagues[37] who showed that tactile hyperalgesia induced by spinal nerve ligation was reduced for 2 hours following a single administration of intraperitoneal agmatine. This group did not report testing at later time points.

We also showed in this study that spinally delivered agmatine dose-dependently inhibited NMDA-evoked scratching and biting behavior as well as NMDA-evoked thermal hyperalgesia. Interestingly, the ED_{50} value of spinal agmatine inhibition of NMDA-evoked scratching and biting behavior is 30 nmoles (similar to the ED_{50} of agmatine against inflammation). In addition, the ED_{50} value of spinal agmatine's inhibition of NMDA-evoked thermal hyperalgesia is 0.3 nmoles, the same as the ED_{50} value for agmatine's ability to reverse manifestations of neuropathic pain. Kitto *et al*.[69] (1992) proposed that activation of the NMDA receptor is sufficient to govern the NMDA-evoked scratching and biting behavior, whereas activation of both the NMDA receptor and NOS enzyme is required for induction of the NMDA-evoked thermal hyperalgesia. We speculate that the action of agmatine on carrageenan-evoked hyperalgesia may require action only at the NMDA receptor, whereas the action of agmatine on the neuropathic pain–evoked hyperalgesia is mediated by agmatine's action on both the NMDA receptor and the NOS enzyme.

Others have now shown that, whereas intrathecal, ICV, or subcutaneous agmatine does not demonstrate analgesic activity in and of itself, agmatine delivered by these routes does significantly increase the potency of spinal morphine to produce analgesia.[6] These observations are consistent with several reports showing that agmatine when given intracerebroventricularly[44] or systemically[16,29,54] potentiates opioid-evoked analgesia. In contrast, Roerig and colleagues[6] also observed that spinally administered agmatine decreased the potency of clonidine-evoked analgesia by approximately 4.5-fold. Interestingly, agmatine had no effect on intrathecally delivered norepinephrine-induced analgesia, the potency of which was decreased by the selective α_2AR antagonists yohimbine and SK&F 86466. Taken together, these data support the concept that agmatine's effect on clonidine-induced analgesia might be non–α_2AR-mediated and perhaps implicate the participation of imidazoline receptors.

REASONS FOR CENTRAL DELIVERY

At least two rationales should be considered in an investigator's decision to incorporate central administration in experimental designs using agmatine. First, as illustrated in this review, for many indications, agmatine is thought to have a central site of action coupled with limited or varied access from blood to brain. To define better agmatine's mechanism of action in the CNS and its potential as a therapeutic agent, central administration can reduce dosage and intersubject variability, simplifying analysis and interpretation of results. Second, because almost all studies (shown in TABLES 1–7) report that effective systemic doses of agmatine are 100 mg/kg or greater, it is likely that the therapeutic index of agmatine administered systemically will prove to be low. Third, our early-stage pharmacokinetic studies suggest that the tissue levels of agmatine attained in CNS after central bolus administration are higher and of longer duration than levels after systemic administration of thousand-fold higher amounts. Although the mechanism of this apparent distinction is unknown, the implication is that understanding the central actions of agmatine will require carefully controlled central kinetics. Understanding the action of these drugs in distinct regions of the CNS will also contribute to the investigators' attempt to understand and interpret the effect of the systemically administered drug.

CONCLUSION

In vivo administration of agmatine in animal models of a variety of disease states and conditions has provided proof-of-concept for the therapeutic potential of agmatine and future agmatine analogues and have demonstrated that agmatine probably has multiple mechanisms, regions, and sites of action in the CNS .

Our understanding of the physiologic role of endogenous agmatine and the utility of exogenously administered agmatine remains in the earliest stages. There has been a recent report of the cloning of the degradative enzyme (agmatinase)[66,67] and a report of the cloning of the synthetic enzyme is, presumably, close to disclosure. A full characterization of those enzymes will contribute substantially to our understanding of the nature of endogenous agmatinergic systems. Identification of the location and roles of these and other (e.g., transport) proteins and the development of techniques to manipulate the levels of endogenous agmatine by manipulating these proteins will provide the knowledge needed to define the roles of endogenous agmatine in the

CNS. Our understanding of the implications of central delivery with respect to distribution, site of action, and effects on systems has also expanded dramatically during the last 30 years. In addition, techniques to conduct central drug delivery in animal models (both rat and mouse) have become more sophisticated and precise. Therefore, it should be possible to pinpoint the regions of the CNS where agmatine (both exogenous and endogenous) acts to understand better its putative role as a neuromodulator or neurotransmitter. That information will provide a gateway to the development of agmatine or an agmatinergic drug and will enable efficient and safe translation of these basic research observations to therapeutic usefulness.

ACKNOWLEDGMENTS

We would like to extend our great appreciation to those who have contributed significantly to our agmatine studies over the years: Drs. Laura S. Stone, George L. Wilcox, and Robert Yezierski, Donald Shoeman, Hoang Yen X. Nguyen, Brent M. Grocholski, John C. Roberts, and Kelley F. Kitto. We would like to also thank Drs. Sandra Roerig, Soundar Regunathan, and John Piletz for many valuable conversations on agmatine during the years. These studies have been supported by NIDA DA-00509 and DA-15387-01 awarded to C.A.F. In addition, T32DA007097 supports A.D.M.

REFERENCES

1. ROERIG, S.C. & J.M. FUJIMOTO. 1989. Multiplicative interaction between intrathecally and intracerebroventricularly administered mu opioid agonists but limited interactions between delta and kappa agonists for antinociception in mice. J. Pharmacol. Exp. Ther. **249:** 762–768.
2. BILSKY, E.J., *et al.* 1994. Selective inhibition of [D-Ala2, Glu4]deltorphin antinociception by supraspinal, but not spinal, administration of an antisense oligodeoxynucleotide to an opioid delta receptor. Life Sci. **55:** PL37–PL43.
3. SUN, M.K., S. REGUNATHAN & D.J. REIS. 1995. Cardiovascular responses to agmatine, a clonidine-displacing substance, in anesthetized rat. Clin. Exp. Hypertens. **17:** 115–128.
4. SCHAFER, U., *et al.* 1999. Effects of agmatine on the cardiovascular system of spontaneously hypertensive rats. Ann. N.Y. Acad. Sci. **881:** 97–101.
5. RAASCH, W., *et al.* 2002. Agmatine, an endogenous ligand at imidazoline binding sites, does not antagonize the clonidine-mediated blood pressure reaction. Br. J. Pharmacol. **135:** 663–672.
6. ROERIG, S.C. 2003. Spinal and supraspinal agmatine activate different receptors to enhance spinal morphine antinociception. Ann. N.Y. Acad. Sci. This volume.
7. HEAD, G.A., C.K.S. CHAN & S.J. GODWIN. 1997. Central cardiovascular actions of agmatine, a putative clonidine-displacing substance in conscious rabbits. Neurochem. Int. **30:** 37–45.
8. GAO, Y., *et al.* 1995. Agmatine: a novel endogenous vasodilator substance. Life Sci. **57:** L83–L86.
9. HAUSER, W., *et al.* 1995. Influence of imidazolines on catecholamine release in pithed spontaneously hypertensive rats. Ann. N.Y. Acad. Sci. **763:** 573–579.
10. SMYTH, D.D. & S.B. PENNER. 1995. Renal I1-imidazoline receptor-selective compounds mediate natriuresis in the rat. J. Cardiovasc. Pharmacol. **26:** S63–S67.
11. BRADLEY, K.J. & P.M. HEADLEY. 1997. Effect of agmatine on spinal nociceptive reflexes–lack of interaction with alpha(2)-adrenoceptor or mu-opioid receptor mechanisms. Eur. J. Pharmacol. **331:** 133–138.

12. LI, J., et al. 1999. Correlation between inhibitions of morphine withdrawal and nitric-oxide synthase by agmatine. Zhongguo Yao Li Xue Bao/Acta Pharmacologica Sinica **20:** 375–380.
13. LI, Q. & R.R. HE. 2001. Hemodynamic effects of agmatine in Dahl salt-sensitive hypertensive and Dahl salt-resistant rats. Sheng Li Hsueh Pao - Acta Physiologica Sinica **53:** 355–360.
14. MORGAN, A.D., et al. 2002. Effects of agmatine on the escalation of i.v. cocaine and fentanyl self-administration in rats. Pharmacol. Biochem. Behav. **72:** 873–880.
15. OYANAGUI, Y. 1984. Anti-inflammatory effects of polyamines in serotonin and carrageenan paw edemata–possible mechanism to increase vascular permeability inhibitory protein level which is regulated by glucocorticoids and superoxide radical. Agents Actions **14:** 228–237.
16. KOLESNIKOV, Y., S. JAIN & G.W. PASTERNAK. 1996. Modulation of opioid analgesia by agmatine. Eur. J. Pharmacol. **296:** 17–22.
17. GLAVIN, G.B., M.A. CARLISLE & D.D. SMYTH. 1995. Agmatine, an endogenous imidazoline receptor agonist, increases gastric secretion and worsens experimental gastric mucosal injury in rats. J. Pharmacol. Exp. Ther. **274:** 741–744.
18. GILAD, G.M., et al. 1996. Metabolism of agmatine into urea but not into nitric oxide in rat brain. Neuroreport **7:** 1730–1732.
19. PRASAD, A. & C. PRASAD. 1996. Agmatine enhances caloric intake and dietary carbohydrate preference in satiated rats. Physiol. Behav. **60:** 1187–1189.
20. ARICIOGLU-KARTAL, F. & I.T. UZBAY. 1997. Inhibitory effect of agmatine on naloxone-precipitated abstinence syndrome in morphine dependent rats. Life Sci. **61:** 1775–1781.
21. LI, X.T. & R.R. HE. 1999. Hemodynamic effects of agmatine and its cellular mechanism in anesthetized rats. Sheng Li Hsueh Pao - Acta Physiologica Sinica **51:** 229–233.
22. GILAD, G.M. & V.H. GILAD. 2000. Accelerated functional recovery and neuroprotection by agmatine after spinal cord ischemia in rats. Neurosci. Lett. **296:** 97–100.
23. ISHIZUKA, S., et al. 2000. Agmatine inhibits cell proliferation and improves renal function in anti-thy-1 glomerulonephritis. J. Am. Soc. Nephrol. **11:** 2256–2264.
24. STEWART, L.S. & B.E. MCKAY. 2000. Acquisition deficit and time-dependent retrograde amnesia for contextual fear conditioning in agmatine-treated rats. Behav. Pharmacol. **11:** 93–97.
25. UTKAN, T., et al. 2000. Investigation on the mechanism involved in the effects of agmatine on ethanol-induced gastric mucosal injury in rats. Life Sci. **66:** 1705–1711.
26. UZBAY, I.T., et al. 2000. Effects of agmatine on ethanol withdrawal syndrome in rats. Behav. Brain Res. **107:** 153–159.
27. YU, C.G., et al. 2000. Agmatine improves locomotor function and reduces tissue damage following spinal cord injury. Neuroreport **11:** 959–965.
28. ONAL, A. & N. SOYKAN. 2001. Agmatine produces antinociception in tonic pain in mice. Pharmacol. Biochem. Behav. **69:** 93–97.
29. YESILYURT, O. & I.T. UZBAY. 2001. Agmatine potentiates the analgesic effect of morphine by an alpha(2)-adrenoceptor-mediated mechanism in mice. Neuropsychopharmacology **25:** 98–103.
30. ARTENI, N.S., et al. 2002. Agmatine facilitates memory of an inhibitory avoidance task in adult rats. Neurobiol. Learn. Mem. **78:** 465–469.
31. FENG, Y., J.E. PILETZ & M.H. LEBLANC. 2002. Agmatine suppresses nitric oxide production and attenuates hypoxic-ischemic brain injury in neonatal rats. Pediatr. Res. **52:** 606–611.
32. MCKAY, B.E., et al. 2002. Learning and memory in agmatine-treated rats. Pharmacol. Biochem. Behav. **72:** 551–557.
33. UZBAY, I.T. & H. LAL. 2002. Effects of NG-nitro-L-arginine methyl ester, 7-nitro indazole, and agmatine on pentylenetetrazol-induced discriminative stimulus in Long-Evans rats. Prog. Neuropsychopharmacol. Biol. Psychiatry **26:** 567–573.
34. ZOMKOWSKI, A.D., et al. 2002. Agmatine produces antidepressant-like effects in two models of depression in mice. Neuroreport **13:** 387–391.
35. BENCE, A.K., et al. 2003. An in vivo evaluation of the antiseizure activity and acute neurotoxicity of agmatine. Pharmacol. Biochem. Behav. **74:** 771–775.

36. DUDKOWSKA, M., et al. 2003. Agmatine modulates the in vivo biosynthesis and interconversion of polyamines and cell proliferation. Biochim. Biophys. Acta **1619:** 159–166.
37. KARADAG, H.C., et al. 2003. Systemic agmatine attenuates tactile allodynia in two experimental neuropathic pain models in rats. Neurosci. Lett. **339:** 88–90.
38. MCKAY, B.E. & M.A. PERSINGER. 2003. Combined effects of complex magnetic fields and agmatine for contextual fear learning deficits in rats. Life Sci. **72:** 2489–2498.
39. ONAL, A., et al. 2003. Agmatine attenuates neuropathic pain in rats: possible mediation of nitric oxide and noradrenergic activity in the brainstem and cerebellum. Life Sci. **73:** 413–428.
40. YU, C.G., et al. 2003. Effects of agmatine, interleukin-10, and cyclosporin on spontaneous pain behavior after excitotoxic spinal cord injury in rats. J. Pain **4:** 129–140.
41. SZABO, B., et al. 1995. Cardiovascular effects of agmatine, a "clonidine-displacing substance", in conscious rabbits. Naunyn-Schmiedebergs Arch. Pharmacol. **351:** 268–273.
42. PENNER, S.B. & D.D. SMYTH. 1996. Natriuresis following central and peripheral administration of agmatine in the rat. Pharmacology **53:** 160–169.
43. PINEDA, J., et al. 1996. Agmatine does not have activity at alpha 2-adrenoceptors which modulate the firing rate of locus coeruleus neurones: an electrophysiological study in rat. Neurosci. Lett. **219:** 103–106.
44. SANCHEZ-BLAZQUEZ, P., et al. 2000. Activation of I(2)-imidazoline receptors enhances supraspinal morphine analgesia in mice: a model to detect agonist and antagonist activities at these receptors. Br. J. Pharmacol. **130:** 146–152.
45. SUGAWARA, A.M., et al. 2001. Effects of central imidazolinergic and alpha2-adrenergic activation on water intake. Brazilian Journal of Medical and Biological Research **34:** 1185–1190.
46. RUIZ-DURANTEZ, E., et al. 2002. Effect of agmatine on locus coeruleus neuron activity: possible involvement of nitric oxide. Br. J. Pharmacol. **135:** 1152–1158.
47. FAIRBANKS, C.A. & G.L. WILCOX. 1997. Acute tolerance to spinally administered morphine compares mechanistically with chronically induced morphine tolerance. J. Pharmacol. Exp. Ther. **282:** 1408–1417.
48. HORVATH, G., et al. 1999. Effect of intrathecal agmatine on inflammation-induced thermal hyperalgesia in rats. Eur. J. Pharmacol. **368:** 197–204.
49. FAIRBANKS, C.A., et al. 2000. Agmatine reverses pain induced by inflammation, neuropathy, and spinal cord injury. Proc. Natl. Acad. Sci. U. S. A. **97:** 10584–10589
50. HOU, S.W., et al. 2003. Spinal antinociceptive effect of agmatine and tentative analysis of involved receptors: study in an electrophysiological model of rats. Brain Res. **968:** 277–280.
51. MARX, M., et al. 1995. Agmatine and spermidine reduce collagen accumulation in kidneys of diabetic db/db mice. Nephron. **69:** 155–158.
52. MOORE, D., et al. 2001. Treatment with agmatine inhibits Cryptosporidium parvum infection in infant mice. J. Parasitol. **87:** 211–213.
53. LI, J., et al. 1999. Effects of agmatine on tolerance to and substance dependence on morphine in mice. Chung-Kuo Yao Li Hsueh Pao - Acta Pharmacologica Sinica **20:** 232–238.
54. LI, J., et al. 1999. Analgesic effect of agmatine and its enhancement on morphine analgesia in mice and rats. Zhongguo Yao Li Xue Bao/Acta Pharmacologica Sinica **20:** 81–5.
55. RICHARDSON, J.D., L. AANONSEN & K.M. HARGREAVES. 1998. Antihyperalgesic effects of spinal cannabinoids. Eur. J. Pharmacol. **345:** 145–153.
56. MALMBERG, A.B. & T.L. YAKSH. 1993. Pharmacology of the spinal action of ketotrolac, morphine, ST-91, U-50488 and L-PIA on the formalin test and an isobolographic analysis of the NSAID interaction. Anesthesiology **79:** 1276–1279.
57. SAWAMURA, S., et al. 1999. Opioidergic and adrenergic modulation of formalin-evoked spinal c-fos mRNA expression and nocifensive behavior in the rat. Eur. J. Pharmacol. **379:** 141–149.
58. MALMBERG, A.B. & T.L. YAKSH. 1992. Antinociceptive actions of spinal nonsteroidal anti-inflammatory agents on the formalin test in the rat. J. Pharmacol. Exp. Ther. **263:** 136–146.

59. CHAPLAN, S.R., A.B. MALMBERG & T.L. YAKSH. 1997. Efficacy of spinal NMDA receptor antagonism in formalin hyperalgesia and nerve injury evoked allodynia in the rat. J. Pharmacol. Exp. Ther. **280:** 829–838.
60. MOORE, P.K., *et al*. 1993. Characterization of the novel nitric oxide synthase inhibitor 7-nitro indazole and related indazoles: antinociceptive cardiovascular effects. Br. J. Pharmacol. **110:** 219–224.
61. SAKURADA, T., *et al*. 1996. Effect of spinal nitric oxide inhibition on capsaicin-induced nociceptive response. Life Sci. **59:** 921–930.
62. YANG, X.C. & D.L. REIS. 1999. Agmatine selectively blocks the N-methyl-D-aspartate subclass of glutamate receptor channels in rat hippocampal neurons. J. Pharmacol. Exp. Ther. **288:** 544–549.
63. AUGUET, M., *et al*. 1995. Selective inhibition of inducible nitric oxide synthase by agmatine. Jpn. J. Pharmacol. **69:** 285–287.
64. GALEA, E., *et al*. 1996. Inhibition of mammalian nitric oxide synthases by agmatine, an endogenous polyamine formed by decarboxylation of arginine. Biochem. J. **316:** 247–249.
65. LI, Q., *et al*. 2001. Differential responses of regional vascular beds to local injection of agmatine in rats. Sheng Li Hsueh Pao - Acta Physiologica Sinica **53:** 451–455.
66. IYER, R.K., *et al*. 2002. Cloning and characterization of human agmatinase. Mol. Genet. Metab. **75:** 209–218.
67. MISTRY, S.K., *et al*. 2002. Cloning of human agmatinase. An alternate path for polyamine synthesis induced in liver by hepatitis B virus. Am. J. Physiol. Gastrointest. Liver Physiol. **282:** G375–G381.
68. RAASCH, W., *et al*. 2003. Modification of noradrenaline release in pithed spontaneously hypertensive rats by I1-binding sites in addition to alpha2-adrenoceptors. J. Pharmacol. Exp. Ther. **304:** 1063–1071.
69. KITTO, K.F., J.E. HALEY & G.L. WILCOX. 1992. Involvement of nitric oxide in spinally mediated hyperalgesia in the mouse. Neurosci. Lett. **148:** 1–5.

Effect of Agmatine on Acute and Mononeuropathic Pain

FEYZA ARICIOGLU,[a] EYLEM KORCEGEZ,[a] AYHAN BOZKURT,[b] AND SULEYMAN OZYALCIN[c]

[a]*Department of Pharmacology, Faculty of Pharmacy, Marmara University, Haydarpasa, Istanbul, Turkey*

[b]*Department of Physiology, Faculty of Medicine, Marmara University, Haydarpasa, Istanbul, Turkey*

[c]*Department of Algology, Istanbul Medical Faculty, Istanbul University, Çapa, Istanbul, Turkey*

ABSTRACT: Agmatine is a polycationic amine synthesized from L-arginine by arginine decarboxylase in brain and several tissues. It binds to N-methyl-D-aspartate (NMDA) subtype of glutamatergic, α_2-adrenergic and imidazoline (I) receptors. The present study was designed to investigate effect of agmatine on acute and mononeuropathic pain after chronic constriction injury (CCI). CCI was created by four loose ligations around the right sciatic nerve. The analgesic threshold in rats was evaluated by using thermal hyperalgesia/allodynia (THA) at 4°C. The evaluations were made preoperatively, on postoperative day 15, and after drug administration. Agmatine (10, 20, 40, 80, and 100 mg/kg) was administered intraperitoneally for 5 days beginning on postoperative day 15. Agmatine significantly reduced the hyperalgesia in all doses applied. When agmatine was injected intraperitoneally (10, 20, 40, 80, and 100 mg/kg), it increased the nociceptive threshold in the tail-immersion test in a dose-dependent manner, but it had no effect in the hot-plate test. This effect of agmatine in the tail-immersion test was blocked by both yohimbine (1 mg/kg) and idazoxan (0.5 mg/kg). When agmatine was administered intracerebroventricularly (25–200 μg/10 μL), it increased the nociceptive threshold in the hot-plate but not in the tail-immersion test. We conclude that agmatine, an endogenous substance derived from arginine, can modulate both acute and chronic pain.

KEYWORDS: agmatine; imidazoline; alpha$_2$-adrenoceptors; nitric oxide; tail-immersion test; hot-plate test; allodynia

INTRODUCTION

It is well established from radioligand studies that imidazoline receptors are discrete entities. Two different subtypes of imidazoline sites have already been described based on ligand selectivity and regional distributions.[1–4] Sites that show high affinity for clonidine have been classed as imidazoline I$_1$ receptors, whereas those

Address for correspondence: Feyza Aricioglu, Ph.D., Department of Pharmacology, Faculty of Pharmacy, Marmara University, 81010 Tibbiye Cad. No: 49, Haydarpasa, Istanbul, Turkey. Voice: 0216 418 95 73; fax: 0216 345 29 52.
  e-mail: feyzak@turk.net

showing high affinity for idazoxan have been termed imidazoline I_2 receptors.[1-4] Imidazoline receptors are widely distributed both centrally and peripherally. Imidazoline I_1 receptors have a limited distribution in brain, especially in the brain stem. In contrast, imidazoline I_2 receptors are widely distributed in the central nervous system,[1-4] but their functional role is still not fully established.

Agmatine, a guanidinium analogue, is an endogenous imidazoline receptor ligand that interacts with both subtypes of imidazoline receptors (I_1 and I_2) as well as with α_2-adrenoceptors. Agmatine is synthesized in brain from L-arginine and is biologically active in a number of neuronally related and endocrine tissues. It dose-dependently releases catecholamines from adrenal chromaffin cells, releases insulin from pancreatic islet cells exposed to glucose, and enhances gastric secretion.[5] There is inferential evidence that agmatine may modulate the action of L-glutamate. In addition, agmatine has properties of an endogenous neurotransmitter. It is locally synthesized in brain by a specific enzyme, arginine decarboxylase, is stored in a large number of neurons, is released from synaptosomes in a Ca^{2+}-dependent manner, and can be enzymatically degraded by agmatinase.[5] It has been shown that agmatine potentiates morphine analgesia,[6] attenuates all the behavioral signs of the morphine abstinence syndrome in rats[7] and mice,[8] and attenuates many signs of ethanol withdrawal syndrome in ethanol-dependent rats.[9]

Agmatine blocks the ligand-gated N-methyl-D-aspartate (NMDA) receptor channel and competitively inhibits the activity of all isoforms of nitric oxide synthase (NOS).[10,11] Most of the NMDA receptor blockers[12,13] and NOS inhibitors are known to be analgesic.[14-16] The drugs that have selective agonistic activity on imidazoline/α_2-adrenoceptors, such as clonidine and moxonidine, produce an antinociceptive effect.[17-19] Therefore the present study is designed to investigate the effect of agmatine on the nociceptive threshold in acute and mononeuropathic pain.

MATERIALS AND METHODS

Animals

Male (200–250 g) Wistar albino rats were used for neuropathic pain experiments, and Balb/c mice (20–30 g) were used only for acute pain models. Rats and mice were housed at 22°C ± 2°C under a 12-hour light/dark cycle with access to water and food ad libitum. The experiments were reviewed and approved by the Institutional Animal Care and Use Committee. All experiments were performed at the same time in the light period of the day. Each animal served as its own control, the latency-to-response ratio being measured before and after drug administration. Animals were divided into several groups as shown in TABLE 1.

Drugs

Agmatine sulfate, idazoxan HCl, and yohimbine HCl (Sigma, St. Louis, MO, USA) were dissolved in distilled water. Fresh solution of drugs was prepared each day and was administered once daily for acute pain experiments or twice daily for 5 days for mononeuropathic pain experiments. Agmatine sulfate was administered in dosages of either 25 to 200 µg/10 µL intracerebroventricularly (i.c.v.) or 10, 20, 40, 80, and 100 mg/kg intraperitoneally (i.p.) in a volume of 0.1 mL/100 g.

TABLE 1. Groups and injection protocols for acute experiments

Group	Treatment
1	Saline i.p. (n = 10 mice)
2	Agmatine 10 mg/kg i.p (n = 10 mice)
3	Agmatine 20 mg/kg i.p (n = 10 mice)
4	Agmatine 40 mg/kg i.p (n = 10 mice)
5	Agmatine 80 mg/kg i.p (n = 10 mice)
6	Agmatine 100 mg/kg i.p (n = 10 mice)
7	Saline + saline i.p. (n = 8 mice)
8	Yohimbine 1 mg/kg (n = 8 mice)
9	Idazoxan 0.5 mg/kg (n = 8 mice)
10	Yohimbine 1 mg/kg + agmatine 40 mg/kg i.p (n = 8 mice)
11	Idazoxan 0.5 mg/kg + agmatine 40 mg/kg i.p (n = 8 mice)
12	Saline 10 µl i.c.v. (n = 6 rats)
13	Agmatine 25 µg/10 µl i.c.v. (n = 6 rats)
14	Agmatine 50 µg/10 µl i.c.v. (n = 6 rats)
15	Agmatine 100 µg/10 µl i.c.v. (n = 6 rats)
16	Agmatine 200 µg/10 µl i.c.v. (n = 6 rats)

Locomotor Activity

The activity cage was a wooden box with a floor 35 × 50 cm and clear plastic walls 21 cm high. The cage was divided into 12 equal areas, and there were 12 equally spaced holes in the center of each area, 3 cm diameter and 1 cm deep. Rats or mice were placed in a corner, and locomotor activity was measured by counting the number of lines between squares crossed in 5 minutes.

Hot-Plate Test

The hot-plate test was based on that described by Eddy and Leimbach.[20] A cylinder (25 cm in diameter, 40 cm high) was used to keep the mouse on heated surface of the plate, which was kept at a temperature of 56°C ± 1°C. The latency period until the mouse jumped or licked its hind paw was registered using a stopwatch (cut-off time, 60 seconds).

Tail-Flick Test

The responsiveness was determined using the warm water (56°C ± 1°C) immersion tail-flick test.[21] The latency to the rapid tail-flick represented the behavior endpoint (cut-off time, 15 seconds). Baseline measurements of tail-flick latencies were collected for all mice before testing. Animals received either idazoxan (0.5 mg/kg i.p.) or yohimbine (1 mg/kg i.p.) 30 minutes before agmatine administration.

Neuropathic Pain Model

Peripheral mononeuropathy was described by Bennett and Xie.[22] Procedures were carried out under halothane anesthesia. A chronic constructive injury (CCI) was created on the right sciatic nerve. The CCI was performed by four loose ligations around the right sciatic nerve. Each of four chromic gut sutures was tied loosely with a square knot around the sciatic nerve. A brief twitch in the muscle surrounding the exposure served as an indicator of the desired degree of constriction. The left sciatic nerve was only mobilized. Incisions were closed layer-to-layer with silk sutures, and the rats were allowed to recover from anesthesia. After surgery, the animals were individually maintained in clear plastic cages with solid floors covered with sawdust. All animals postoperatively displayed normal feeding and drinking behavior. Rats were then placed in a clear plastic cage ($18 \times 28 \times 13$ cm) with a metal floor (1/8-inch aluminum) that was chilled or warmed by an underlying water bath. With counterbalanced stimulus order, the animals were exposed for 20 minutes on successive days to a floor that was chilled by cold water or warmed by a 30°C bath. A thermometer placed on the floor indicated surface temperatures of 4°C and 30°C, respectively. Recordings were made of the animal's behavior and the time during which either hind paw was held above the floor while the animal was sitting or standing. The observation period was 20 minutes.

Cannulation for I.C.V. Administration

A group of rats was prepared for i.c.v. treatment by stereotaxically implanting stainless-steel guide cannulas into a brain lateral ventricle (Paxinos and Watson), under ketamine plus xylazine anesthesia, and by fixing the cannulas to the skull with a plastic cap and dental acrylic. The guide cannula was kept in place until drug injection. Correct placement was verified at the end of the experiment by injecting 5 µL of toluidine blue dye through an internal cannula, followed by decapitation under ethyl ether anesthesia and dissection of the brain.

Statistical Analysis

The groups were compared before surgery (pre-op), on day 15 (post-op), and day 21 (post-treatment) by ANOVA with the Tukey multiple comparison test. Results are expressed as means ± SD, and differences were considered statistically significant if $P < 0.05$.

RESULTS

In initial experiments, the effect of agmatine on locomotor activity was measured. Thirty minutes after injection of 10, 20, 40, 80, or 100 mg/kg of agmatine i.p. or i.c.v. (25–200 µg/10 µL), animals were observed for 5 minutes. The control group received the same volume of saline. Agmatine alone did not produce any significant change in locomotor activities of rats or mice compared with saline ($P > 0.05$) (data not shown).

When agmatine was injected i.p. (10, 20, 40, 80, or 100 mg/kg), it increased the nociceptive threshold in the tail-immersion test (FIG. 1A) in a dose-dependent manner,

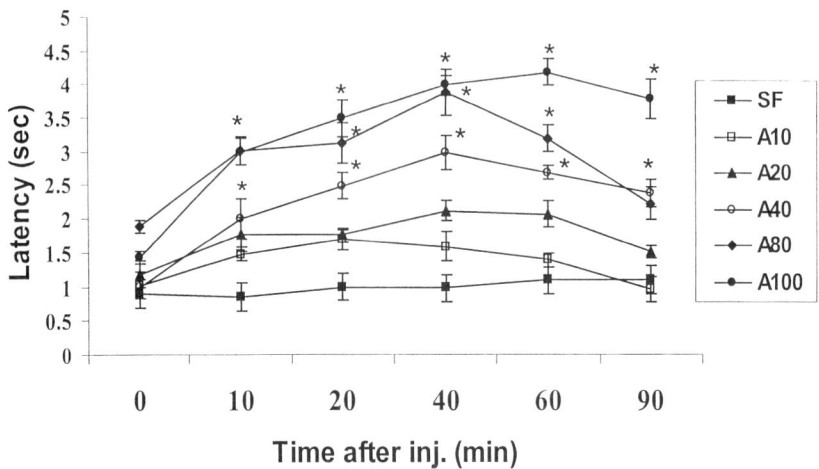
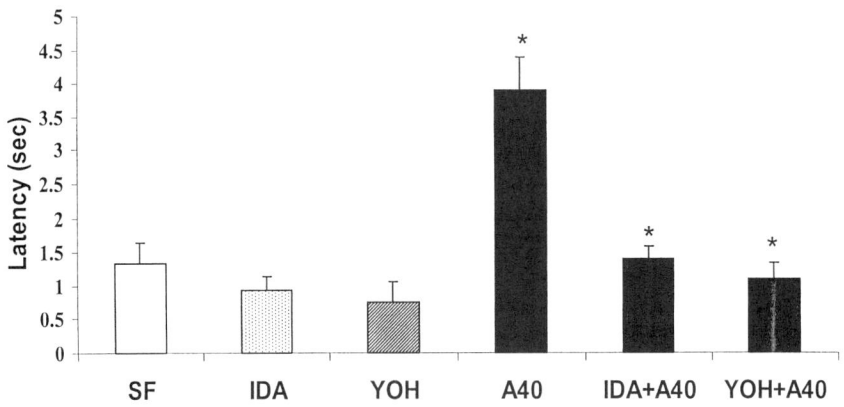

FIGURE 1. Effect of agmatine on nociceptive threshold in tail-immersion test. (**A**) Agmatine (10, 20, 40, 80, or 100 mg/kg) or saline. (**B**) Saline, agmatine, idazoxan, and yohimbine administered alone or in combination. * $P < 0.05$. A, agmatine; IDA, idazoxan; YOH, yohimbine.

but it had no effect in the hot-plate test (data not shown). This effect of agmatine in tail-immersion test was blocked by both yohimbine (1 mg/kg) and idazoxan (0.5 mg/kg) (FIG. 1B). When agmatine was administered i.c.v., it increased the nociceptive threshold in the hot-plate test (FIG. 2) but not in the tail-immersion test (data not shown).

Allodynia was detected by recording the cumulative time and the number of hind paw withdrawals in 20 minutes. CCI significantly decreased the threshold 15 days after the nerve injury (saline group, TABLE 1) whereas the sham-operated group showed no changes (data not shown). The response to 4°C induced on day 15 was

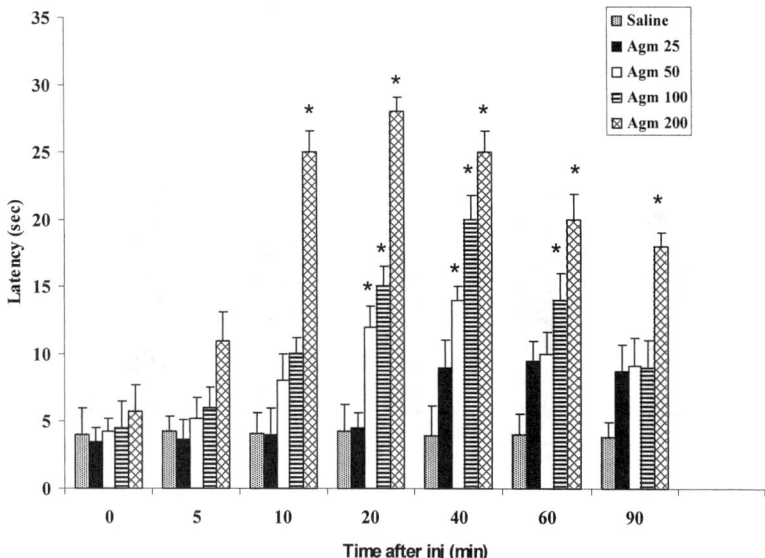

FIGURE 2. Effect of i.c.v. agmatine (25, 50, 100, or 200 μg/10 μL) on nociceptive threshold in hot-plate test. * $P < 0.05$. Agm, agmatine.

reduced after agmatine treatment for 5 days (FIG. 3 A,B); agmatine had no effect on sham-operated animals (data not shown). The effect of agmatine on the number of hind paw withdrawals was statistically significant in a dose-dependent manner, $F_{5,54} = 21.29$ ($P < 0.05$) (FIG. 3B). The effect of harman on the cumulative time of hind paw withdrawal was also found significant for all doses when compared with the postoperated value of the same group, $F_{5,54} = 28.32$ ($P < 0.05$) (FIG. 3A). None of the animals withdrew paws from the 30°C surface, and no difference was observed between control and sham-operated rats in any of the tests applied (data not shown).

DISCUSSION

This study clearly demonstrated that (1) agmatine dose-dependently increased the nociceptive threshold in the tail-immersion when administered i.p. but not i.c.v.; (2) agmatine dose-dependently increased latency in the hot-plate test when administered i.c.v. but not i.p.; and (3) agmatine decreased both the number of hind paw withdrawals and the cumulative duration of paw withdrawals after 5 days of treatment in mononeuropathic pain model. The dose range in our study was 10 to 100 mg/kg. Recently it has been shown that the effect of agmatine on neuropathic pain may result from the reduction of nitric oxide (NO) levels and noradrenergic activity in the brain.[23] The doses in the study were extremely high (i.e., 300 and 400 mg/kg). Systemic doses of agmatine of 200 mg/kg cause cardiovascular disturbances.[24] Therefore the mechanism by which agmatine produces an anti-allodynic effect is still unclear.

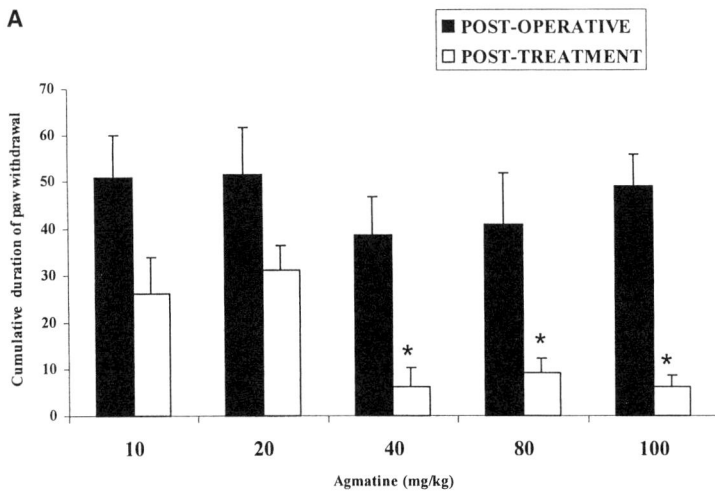

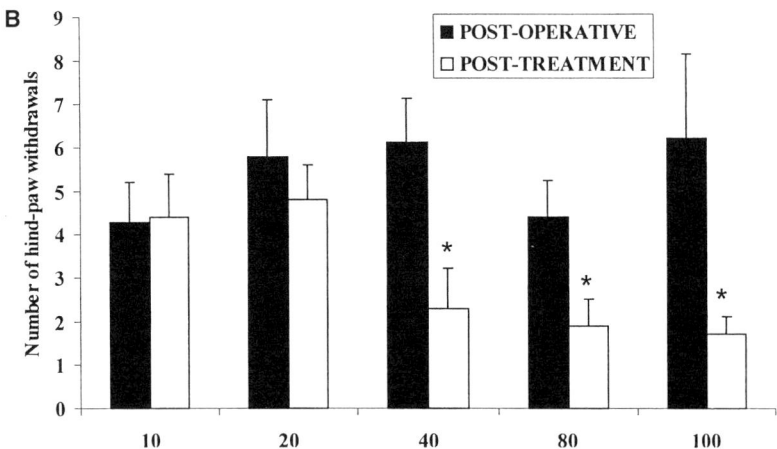

FIGURE 3. Effect of agmatine on (**A**) cumulative duration of paw withdrawals and (**B**) number of paw withdrawals on 4°C floor for 20 minutes. Experiments were conducted on day 15 after sciatic nerve ligation (POST-OP) which are untreated groups, and on day 21 after 5 days of treatment with agmatine (10, 20, 40, 80, or 100 mg/kg) or saline (POST-TREATMENT). Data presented as mean ± SD; n = 10 rats in each group. Post-op and post-treatment groups were compared; * $P < 0.05$.

The localization of agmatine and its synthetic and degradative enzymes in mammalian brain established a potentially novel neurotransmitter/neuromodulatory agent.[5] The characterization of its dual-activity profile (NMDA receptor antagonism with NOS inhibition) may have impact in several areas of neuroscience relating to glutamatergic neurotransmission and synaptic plasticity. There is inferential evidence that agmatine may modulate the action of L-glutamate. Agmatine displaces binding to MK-801, an open-channel blocker of NMDA receptor channels.[25] It has been shown that agmatine is a selective blocker of the NMDA subclass of glutamate receptor channels. The blocking effect of agmatine is mediated by interaction between the guanidine group of agmatine and the pore of the NMDA receptor channel.[10] NMDA involvement in altered spinal neuron activity following peripheral nerve injury has been investigated in a rat model of chronic constriction injury of the sciatic nerve.[26,27] Blockage of NMDA receptors decreases nociceptive transmission in the thalamus and can modulate hyperalgesia.[12] It has been shown that the neuropathic pain is mediated by low-threshold mechanoreceptors, is sympathetically dependent, and is sensitive to both α_2-adrenoceptor agonists and NMDA antagonists.[13]

Agmatine has been detected biochemically[28,29] and immunocytochemically in neurons in various brain regions.[30–32] One important site of agmatine in brain is the hippocampus, where immunoreactive agmatine is stored in perikarya, processes, and axon terminals of the pyramidal cells.[31] In ultrastructural studies, it has been observed that immunoreactive agmatine is associated with vesicles in axons that make asymmetric (excitatory) synapses on pyramidal neurons.[31] Because these axons innervating pyramidal cells are glutamatergic, and pyramidal cells express the NMDA subclass of glutamate receptors, it has been proposed that agmatine may be co-stored and released with glutamate as a counterregulatory molecule. In fact, electrophysiologic studies in cultured hippocampal neurons have supported this contention, because agmatine selectively inhibited NMDA channels.[10]

Although previous studies revealed a possible regulatory role for agmatine in normal glutamatergic neurotransmission, it is speculated that agmatine may also play a role in pathologic conditions involving increased activation of NMDA receptors. Thus, agmatine is protective against ischemic injury, spinal cord injury, and neuropathic pain, conditions that arise from higher NMDA receptor activation and are reversed by NMDA receptor antagonists.[18,19,33] The amount of endogenous agmatine in specific regions of brain ranges from 100 to 700 ng/g,[29] comparable to the levels of other neurotransmitters. It should be emphasized that agmatine is an endogenous molecule, locally synthesized and stored in neurons and glia, and, therefore, the concentration at the synaptic region could reach much higher levels especially during increased synthesis, as in ischemia.[34] Therefore, it is conceivable that agmatine, co-released with glutamate, may act to inhibit the activation of NMDA receptors during conditions leading to higher glutamate release. Further in vivo studies, measuring the release of agmatine along with glutamate are required to verify this hypothesis.

It has been shown that agmatine potentiates morphine analgesia.[6] Agmatine joins a number of agents that act on the NMDA receptor/NOS cascade in the modulation of opioid tolerance.[35,36] Like NMDA receptor antagonists and NOS inhibitors, agmatine blocks opioid tolerance in mice.[6] In the present study agmatine was found to be a potent antinociceptive agent in mononeuropathic pain. CCI is associated with a local inflammatory reaction mediated at least in part by iNOS. Local activation of the iNOS-NO system may play an important role in the pathogenesis of peripheral nerve injury and neuropathic pain. Much evidence indicates that NO plays an important role in the development of thermal hyperalgesia after nerve injury.[37] Agmatine has been shown to reduce the induction of iNOS in astrocytes and macrophages after inflammatory stimuli.[38] There is also considerable evidence that NO plays a role in synaptic transmission in both the central and the peripheral nervous systems. In the rat model of neuropathic pain it has been found that intrathecal administration of either L-NAME or methylene blue, but not the inactive enantiomer D-NAME, reversed the persistent thermal hyperalgesia.[39]

In conclusion, we have provided evidence that agmatine has beneficial effects against mononeuropathic pain by increasing the nociceptive threshold, probably acting as an inhibitor of NMDA receptor or NOS. Because agmatine is synthesized from arginine by ADC[5,40] and is degraded by agmatinase[41,42] in mammalian brain, increasing endogenous agmatine by increasing ADC or by blocking agmatinase may provide a novel approach in the treatment of mononeuropathic pain and related conditions.

REFERENCES

1. LEHMANN, J., E. KOENIG-BERARD & P. VITOU. 1989. The imidazoline-preferring receptor. Life Sci. **45:** 1609–1615.
2. MICHEL, M.C. & P. ERNSBERGER. 1992. Keeping an eye on the I site: imidazoline-preferring receptors. Trends Pharmacol. Sci. **13:** 369–370.
3. PABLO, V.E., et al. 1998. Pharmacological characterization of imidazoline receptor proteins identified by immunological techniques and other methods. Ann. N. Y. Acad. Sci. **881:** 8–25.
4. OLMOS, G., et al. 1998. Pharmacological and molecular discrimination of I2 imidazoline receptor subtypes. Ann. N. Y. Acad. Sci. **881:** 144–160.
5. REIS, D.J. & S. REGUNATHAN. 2000. Is agmatine a novel neurotransmitter in brain? Trends Pharmacol. Sci. **247:** 187–193.
6. KOLESNIKOV, Y., S. JAIN & G.W. PASTERNAK. 1996. Modulation of opioid analgesia by agmatine. Eur. J. Pharmacol. **296:** 17–22.
7. ARICIOGLU-KARTAL, F. & T. UZBAY. 1997. Inhibitory effect of agmatine on naloxone-precipitated abstinence syndrome in morphine dependent rats. Life Sci. **61:** 1775–1781.
8. ARICIOGLU, F., I.A. PAUL & S. REGUNATHAN. Agmatine reduces only peripheral-related behavioral signs, not the central signs, of morphine withdrawal in nNOS deficient transgenic mice. Neurosci. Lett. In press.
9. UZBAY, I.T., et al. 2000. Effects of agmatine on ethanol withdrawal syndrome in rats. Behav. Brain Res. **107:** 153–159.
10. YANG, X.C. & D.J. REIS. 1999. Agmatine selectively blocks the N-methyl-D-aspartate subclass of glutamate receptor channels in rat hippocampal neurons. J. Pharmacol. Exp. Ther. **288:** 544–549.
11. GALEA, E., et al. 1996. Inhibition of mammalian nitric oxide synthases by agmatine, an endogenous polyamine formed by decarboxylation of arginine. Biochem. J. **316:** 247–249.
12. BORDI, F. & M. QUARTAROLI. 2000. Modulation of nociceptive transmission by NMDA/glycine site receptor in the ventroposterolateral nucleus of the thalamus. Pain **84:** 213–224.
13. LEE, Y.W. & T.L. YAKSH. 1995. Analysis of drug interaction between intrathecal clonidine and MK-801 in peripheral neuropathic pain rat model. Anesthesiology **82:** 741–748.
14. FERREIRA, J., A.R. SANTOS & J.B. CALIXTO. 1999. The role of systemic, spinal and supraspinal L-arginine-nitric oxide-cGMP pathway in thermal hyperalgesia caused by intrathecal injection of glutamate in mice. Neuropharmacology **38:** 835–842.
15. BUDZINSKI, M., et al. 2000. Inhibition of inducible nitric oxide synthase in persistent pain. Life Sci. **66:** 301–305.
16. RODELLA, L., et al. 2000. Nitric oxide involvement in the trigeminal hyperalgesia in diabetic rats. Brain Res. **865:** 112–115.
17. EISENACH, J.C., et al. 1995. Epidural clonidine analgesia for intractable cancer pain. The epidural clonidine study group. Pain **61:** 391–399.
18. FAIRBANKS, C.A., et al. 2000. Moxonidine, a selective imidazoline/alpha(2) adrenergic receptor agonist, synergizes with morphine and deltorphin II to inhibit substance P-induced behavior in mice. Pain **84:** 13–20.

19. FAIRBANKS, C.A. & G.L. WILCOX. 1999. Moxonidine, a selective alpha2-adrenergic and imidazoline receptor agonist, produces spinal antinociceptive in mice. J. Pharmacol. Exp. Ther. **290:** 403–412.
20. EDDY, N.B. & D. LEIMBACH. 1953. Synthetic analgesics. II. Dithienylbutenyl- and dithienylbutylamines. J. Pharmacol. Exp. Ther. **107:** 385–393.
21. SEWELL, R.D. & P.S. SPENCER. 1976. Antinociceptive activity of narcotic agonist and partial agonist analgesics and other agents in the tail-immersion test in mice and rats. Neuropharmacology **15:** 683–688.
22. BENNETT, G.J. & Y.K. XIE. 1988. A peripheral mononeuropathy in rat that produces disorders of pain sensation like those seen in man. Pain **33:** 87–107.
23. ONAL, A., et al. 2003. Agmatine attenuates neuropathic pain in rats: possible mediation of nitric oxide and noradrenergic activity in the brainstem and cerebellum. Life Sci. **73:** 413–428.
24. BRADLEY, K.J. & P.M. HEADLEY. 1997. Effect of agmatine on spinal nociceptive reflexes: lack of interaction with alpha 2-adrenoceptor or µ-opioid receptor mechanisms. Eur. J. Pharmacol. **331:** 133–138.
25. ANIS, N., et al. 1990. Structure-activity relationship of philanthotoxin analogs and polyamines on N-methyl-D-aspartate and nicotinic acetylcholine receptors. J. Pharmacol. Exp. Ther. **254:** 764–773.
26. SOTGIU, M.L. & G. BIELLA. 2000. Contribution of central sensitization of the pain-related abnormal activity in neuropathic rats. Somatosens. Mot. Res. **17:** 32–38.
27. SOTGIU, M.L. & G. BIELLA. 2000. Differential effects of MK-801, a N-methyl-D-aspartate non-competitive antagonist, on the dorsal horn neuron hyperactivity and hyperexcitability in neuropathic rats. Neurosci. Lett. **283:** 153–156.
28. LI, G., et al. 1994. Agmatine: an endogenous clonidine-displacing substance in the brain. Science **263:** 966–969.
29. FENG, Y., A.E. HALARIS & J.E. PILETZ. 1997. Determination of agmatine in brain and plasma using high-performance liquid chromatography with fluorescence detection. J. Chromotgr. **691:** 277–286.
30. OTAKE, K., et al. 1998. Regional localization of agmatine in the rat brain: an immunocytochemical study. Brain Res. **787:** 1–14.
31. REIS, D.J., X.C. YANG & T.A. MILNER. 1998. Agmatine containing axon terminals in rat hippocampus from synapses on pyramidal cells. Neurosci. Lett. **250:** 185–188.
32. GORBATYUK, O.S., et al. 2002. Localization of agmatine in vasopressin and oxytocin neurons of the rat hypothalamic paraventricular and supraoptic nuclei. Exp. Neurol. **171:** 235–245.
33. FAIRBANKS, C.A., et al. 2000. Agmatine reverses pain induced by inflammation, neuropathy, and spinal cord injury. Proc. Natl. Acad. Sci. U. S. A. **97:** 10584–10589.
34. FENG, Y., J.E. PILETZ & M.H. LEBLANC. 2002. Agmatine suppresses nitric oxide production and attenuates hypoxic-ischemic brain injury in neonatal rats. Pediatr. Res. **52:** 1–6.
35. TRUJILLO, K.A. & H. AKIL. 1991. Opiate tolerance and dependence: recent findings and synthesis. New Biol. **3:** 915–923.
36. TRUJILLO, K.A. & H. AKIL. 1991. The NMDA receptor antagonist MK-801 increases morphine catalepsy and lethality. Pharmacol. Biochem. Behav. **38:** 673–675.
37. KHALIL, Z. & B. KHODR. 2001. A role for free radicals and nitric oxide in delayed recovery in aged rats with chronic constriction nerve injury. Free Radic. Biol. Med. **31:** 430–439.
38. REGUNATHAN, S., D.L. FEINSTEIN & J. REIS. 1999. Anti-proliferative and anti-inflammatory actions of imidazoline agents. Ann. N. Y. Acad. Sci. **881:** 410–419.
39. MELLER, S.T., C. DYKSTRA & G.F. GEBHART. 1992. Production of endogenous nitric oxide and activation of soluble guanylyl cyclase are required for N-methyl-D-aspartate-produced facilitation of the nociceptive tail-flick reflex. Eur. J. Pharmacol. **214:** 93–96.
40. REGUNATHAN, S., et al. 1995. Agmatine, the decarboxylated arginine is localized and synthesized in glial cells. Neuroreport **6:** 1897–1900.
41. SASTRE, M., S. REGUNATHAN & D.J. REIS. 1996. Agmatinase activity in rat brain: a metabolic pathway for the degradation of agmatine. J. Neurochem. **67:** 1761–1765.
42. IYER, R.K., et al. 2002. Cloning and characterization of human agmatinase. Mol. Gen. Metab. **75:** 209–218.

Spinal and Supraspinal Agmatine Activate Different Receptors to Enhance Spinal Morphine Antinociception

SANDRA C. ROERIG

Department of Pharmacology and Therapeutics, LSU Health Sciences Center, Shreveport, Louisiana 71130, USA

ABSTRACT: The endogenous clonidine-displacing substance, agmatine, enhances morphine-induced antinociception and inhibits development of tolerance to morphine. Because agmatine binds with relatively high affinity to both α_2 adrenergic and imidazoline (I) receptors, the following studies were designed to determine which receptor type is involved in the morphine-enhancing activity. Mice were injected by various routes with agmatine, clonidine or norepinephrine as well as selective antagonists, and tail flick antinociception was measured. Agmatine administered subcutaneously (s.c.), intracerebroventricularly (i.c.v.), or intrathecally (i.t.) had no antinociceptive activity, but enhanced the antinociception produced by i.t. morphine. The morphine-enhancing activity of i.c.v. agmatine (and clonidine) was attenuated by coadministered yohimbine, idazoxan and SK&F 86466 (α_2 antagonists). When given i.t., agmatine, yohimbine and SK&F 86466 attenuated the antinociception produced by coadministered i.t. clonidine. In contrast, i.t. yohimbine and SK&F 86466, but not agmatine, attenuated antinociception produced by i.t. norepinephrine. These results suggested that agmatine actions were different at brain and spinal sites. Thus, agmatine may act at both α_2 and I receptors in the brain and I receptors in the spinal cord.

KEYWORDS: agmatine; clonidine; antinociception; morphine

INTRODUCTION

The endogenous clonidine-displacing substance, agmatine (decarboxylated arginine), is synthesized in brain and, like clonidine, binds with relatively high affinity to both α_2 adrenergic and imidazoline (I_1 and I_2) receptors.[1,2] However, the physiologic consequences of agmatine binding to these receptors are not identical to clonidine-induced effects. For example, clonidine inhibits the firing rate of locus coeruleus neurons, but agmatine is not an agonist or antagonist for this α_2 receptor mediated event.[3] When administered into the fourth cerebral ventricle of rabbits, agmatine does not produce the same cardiovascular effects as do clonidine and the I_1/α_2 receptor agonist moxonidine.[4] Agmatine appears to display unique biologic

---

Address for correspondence: Sandra C. Roerig, Department of Pharmacology and Therapeutics, LSU Health Sciences Center, 1501 Kings Highway, Shreveport, LA 71130, USA. Voice: 318-675-7877; fax: 318-675-4343.
 e-mail: sroeri@lsuhse.edu

activity different from that of clonidine (and moxonidine), even though these agents bind to the same receptors.

Although endogenous agmatine is widely expressed and may possess multiple roles, one possible role in the central nervous system is the regulation of opioid-induced analgesia. Agmatine, like clonidine, enhances morphine-induced antinociception in the tail flick test of acute thermal nociception[5] when given systemically. However, unlike clonidine, agmatine alone has no antinociceptive activity when tested in the tail flick test.[5–7] The thermal antinociceptive effects of clonidine are blocked by a number of α_2 adrenergic receptor antagonists,[8] most of which are also antagonists of I receptors.[9] Thus, it is not clear which receptors, α_2 or I, are responsible for clonidine-induced antinociception. Results from antinociceptive tests and binding studies with [^{3}H]clonidine suggest that spinal clonidine-induced antinociception is mediated by α_2, rather than by I receptors.[10] Also, recent studies in mutant mice deficient in the α_{2A} receptor suggest that spinally administered clonidine produces antinociception entirely through the α_{2A} receptor subtype.[11] Because agmatine has no antinociceptive activity the tail flick test, it has been difficult to characterize the receptors through which it may affect nociception. An indirect indication of receptor involvement comes from studies by Kolesnikov et al.,[12] who showed that idazoxan, an antagonist at both α_2 and I receptors, reverses agmatine-induced enhancement of s.c. morphine antinociception. However, the identity of the receptor (α_2 or I) responsible for this activity is not clear. The following studies utilized the ability of agmatine to enhance i.t. morphine-induced antinociception in an attempt to determine whether the enhancing effects are due to activity at α_2 adrenergic receptors or I receptors.

METHODS

Male, ICR mice (Harlan Sprague Dawley, Indianapolis, IN) weighing 25 to 35 g were used in all studies. They were housed five per cage with food and water continuously available and exposed to 12 hours/12 hours light/dark cycles. Each animal was used only one time for drug testing.

Drugs for s.c. administration were dissolved in sterile saline (0.9% NaCl) in a volume of 0.1 mL/10 g body weight. For central administration, drugs were dissolved in artificial cerebrospinal fluid (aCSF) and administered intracerebroventricularly (i.c.v.), 4 µL, under halothane anesthesia,[13] or intrathecally (i.t., spinal intrathecal space), 5 µL.[14] Agents used were: morphine sulfate (National Institutes on Drug Abuse); clonidine HCl, agmatine sulfate, yohimbine HCl, idazoxan HCl, norepinephrine HCl (Sigma Chemical Co., St. Louis, MO). SK&F 86466 was a generous gift from Dr. Paul Heibel at SmithKline Beecham Pharmaceuticals (King of Prussia, PA).

Antinociception was measured using the radiant heat tail flick test with a cut-off time of 10 seconds as previously described.[15] The per cent maximum possible effect (%MPE) was calculated according to the formula: (Drug Time – Control Time/ 10 – Control Time) × 100. The %MPE values were used to construct dose response curves with at least four drug doses per curve and eight animals per dose.

For experiments with s.c. agmatine and i.t. morphine or clonidine, the agmatine was administered 15 minutes before the i.t. drug, then the tail flick test was performed 10 minutes later. For the experiments with i.c.v. plus i.t. drug, the i.c.v. drug was administered first, then 5 minutes later the i.t. drug was given and 10 minutes later the tail flick test was performed. When two drugs were administered i.t., the drugs were coadministered and antinociception was measured after 10 minutes.

Antinociceptive median effective dose (ED_{50}) values were computed from %MPE values in the dose response curves using the Graded Dose Response method of Tallarida and Murray.[16]

RESULTS

To establish the agmatine effect on i.t. morphine-induced antinociception, agmatine was given s.c. (15 minutes before morphine), i.c.v. (10 minutes before morphine), or i.t. (coadministered with morphine), and tail flick responses were measured 10 minutes after the i.t. morphine administration. None of the doses of agmatine tested by any route altered tail flick latency times (data not shown). As shown in FIGURE 1A, all the agmatine treatments shifted the i.t. morphine dose response curve to the left, to about the same extent. The morphine ED_{50} values calculated from these curves (TABLE 1) show that agmatine decreased these values two- to three-fold. Both i.t. doses of agmatine tested (1 nmol and 10 nmol) were effective in enhancing the morphine effect.

Because i.t. clonidine is synergistic with i.t. morphine, the effects of i.t. agmatine on i.t. morphine were directly compared with clonidine. The ED_{50} value for clonidine-induced antinociception was 0.46 nmol (TABLE 2); thus, clonidine and morphine were given together in a 1:4 (morphine:clonidine) equi-effect constant dose ratio. As shown in FIGURE 1B, clonidine shifted the morphine dose response curve to the left and the morphine ED_{50} value decreased four-fold (TABLE 1). Agmatine was given as a single constant dose since by itself it did not affect the tail flick latency. The 10 nmol dose agmatine also shifted the morphine dose response curve to the left, but to a lesser extent than did clonidine. Thus, both clonidine, which has antinociceptive activity, and agmatine, which has no antinociceptive activity, enhanced morphine-induced antinociception.

The next experiments were designed to determine whether agmatine was acting at the same spinal receptors as clonidine, and whether these were α_2 adrenergic receptors. Agmatine, and the non-imidazoline α_2 antagonists yohimbine and SK&F 86466 were given i.t. along with clonidine or norepinephrine. None of these agents had any effect on tail flick latency times at the doses used (doses shown on TABLE 2) (data not shown). Dose response curves for clonidine and norepinephrine in the presence and absence of the other agents are shown in FIGURE 2. The 1 nmol dose agmatine had no effect on the clonidine ED_{50} value (TABLE 2). Agmatine (10 nmol dose), yohimbine and SK&F 86466 all shifted the clonidine dose response curve to the right (FIG. 2A) and increased the clonidine ED_{50} value three- to four-fold (TABLE 2). On the other hand, while both yohimbine and SK&F 86466 also shifted the norepinephrine dose curve to the right and increased the norepinephrine ED_{50} value, agmatine (10 nmol) had no effect on antinociception produced by norepinephrine (FIG. 1B, TABLE 1). Thus, agmatine had differential effects on clonidine (α_2 and I agonist) and norepinephrine (α_2 agonist). These results suggested that agmatine did not interact with the same spinal receptor as norepinephrine (α_2) to produce antinociception.

As described above, i.c.v. agmatine also enhanced i.t. morphine-induced antinociception. To determine which brain receptors agmatine activated to produce this

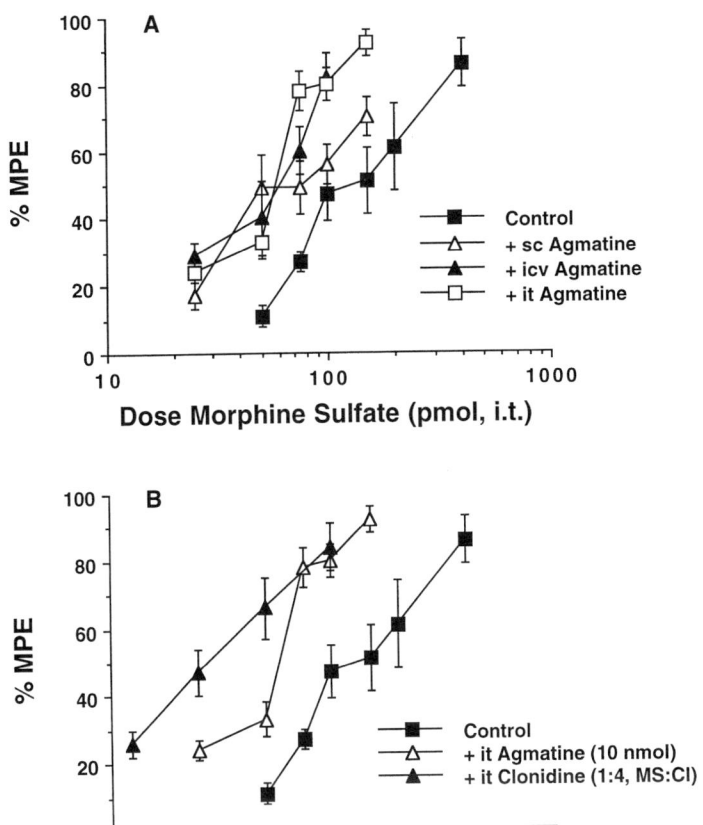

FIGURE 1. Dose response curves for intrathecal (i.t.) morphine in the presence of agmatine or clonidine. **(A)** Agmatine was given subcutaneously (s.c.; 10 mg/kg, 15 minutes prior), intracerebroventricularly (i.c.v.; 1 nmol, 5 minutes prior) or i.t. (1 nmol, concurrently) with i.t. morphine and tail flick response was measured after 10 minutes. **(B)** Agmatine (10 nmol) or clonidine (various doses in an equi-effect ratio) was given i.t. along with i.t. morphine and tail flick response was measured after 10 minutes.

effect, agmatine was given i.c.v. along with various antagonists, yohimbine, idazoxan and SK&F 86466, followed by morphine given i.t. Idazoxan, is an antagonist at both α_2 and I receptors, while yohimbine and SK&F 86466 are highly selective for α_2 receptors.[9,17] None of the antagonists given i.c.v. in the doses used altered tail flick latency times (data not shown). Results of these studies are shown in FIGURE 3A and ED_{50} values calculated from the morphine dose response curves are in TABLE 3. Agmatine administered i.c.v. shifted the i.t. morphine dose response curve to the left

TABLE 1. Effect of s.c, i.c.v. or i.t. agmatine or i.t. clonidine on i.t. morphine-induced antinociception

Treatment			Morphine ED_{50} (95% CI) (pmol, i.t.)
Drug	Route	Dose	
None			127 (103–157)
Agmatine	s.c.	10 mg/kg	73 (56–95)*
Agmatine	i.c.v.	1 nmol	51 (42–64)*
Agmatine	i.t.	1 nmol	77 (60–100)*
Agmatine	i.t.	10 nmol	52 (45–61)*
Clonidine	i.t.	4:1 ratio	29 (23–37)*

Agmatine in the indicated doses was administered to mice before (15 minutes for s.c., 5 minutes for i.c.v.) or concurrently (i.t.) with morphine and tail flick response was measured 10 minutes later. Various doses of clonidine were administered concurrently with various doses of i.t. morphine in a constant 4:1 ratio.
* Significantly different from no treatment, $P < 0.05$

(FIG 3A) and decreased the morphine ED_{50} value twofold. This enhancing effect of agmatine was reversed by yohimbine, idazoxan and SK&F 86466 (FIG. 3A, TABLE 3).

For comparison to agmatine, i.c.v. clonidine was given in the same experimental protocol and results are shown in FIGURE 3B and TABLE 3. The dose of clonidine used in these studies was 500 pmol, a dose that produces a 24% MPE when administered alone. Clonidine administered i.c.v. also shifted the i.t. morphine dose response curve to the left and decreased the morphine ED_{50} value to a similar extent

TABLE 2. Effect of i.t. agmatine, yohimbine or SK&F 86466 on i.t. clonidine or norepinephrine-induced antinociception

Agonist	"Antagonist" (Dose)	Agonist ED_{50} (95% CI) (nmol, i.t.)
Clonidine	—	0.46 (0.31–0.69)
Clonidine	Agmatine (1 nmol)	0.69 (0.48–0.97)
Clonidine	Agmatine (10 nmol)	2.08 (1.80–2.40)*
Clonidine	Yohimbine (10 nmol)	2.41 (2.09–2.79)*
Clonidine	SK&F 86466 (1 nmol)	1.77 (1.53–2.04)*
Norepinephrine	—	1.98 (1.67–2.36)
Norepinephrine	Agmatine (10 nmol)	1.85 (1.49–2.30)
Norepinephrine	Yohimbine (10 nmol)	3.16 (2.54–3.93)*
Norepinephrine	SK&F 86466 (1 nmol)	3.43 (2.55–4.61)*

Indicated doses of "antagonists" were coadministered i.t. with indicated agonists and tail flick antinociception was measured.
* Significantly different from agonist alone, $P < 0.05$.

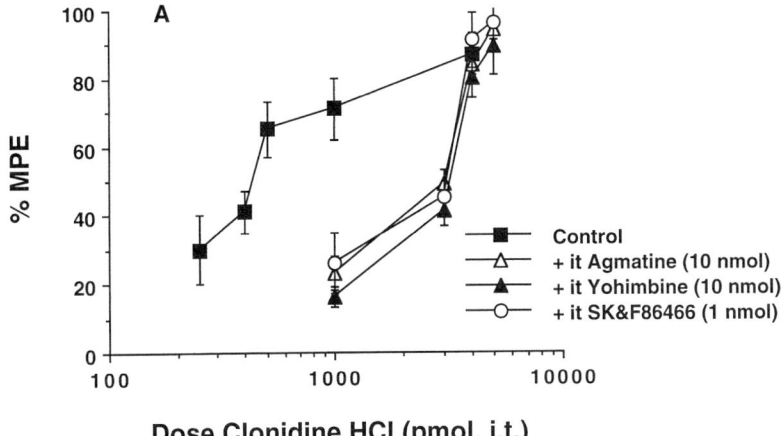

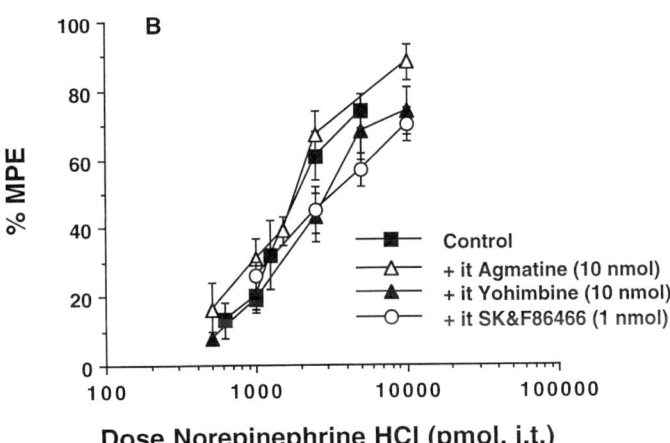

FIGURE 2. Dose response curves for i.t. clonidine and norepinephrine in the presence of "antagonists." **(A)** Clonidine was coadministered with the indicated doses of agmatine, yohimbine, or SK&F 86466 and tail flick response was measured as in Figure 1. **(B)** Norepinephrine was given in the same protocol.

as did agmatine. This effect of clonidine was also reversed by yohimbine, idazoxan and SK&F 86466. Thus, in the brain, agmatine and clonidine appeared to activate the same receptors to enhance the spinal morphine effect. Because the non-imidazoline antagonists yohimbine and SK&F 86466 blocked both clonidine and agmatine-induced enhancement, α_2 receptors are likely involved in this effect. The involvement of I receptors is also possible since idazoxan reversed the effects of both clonidine and agmatine, but since selective I antagonists were not tested, the involvement of the I receptor remains speculative.

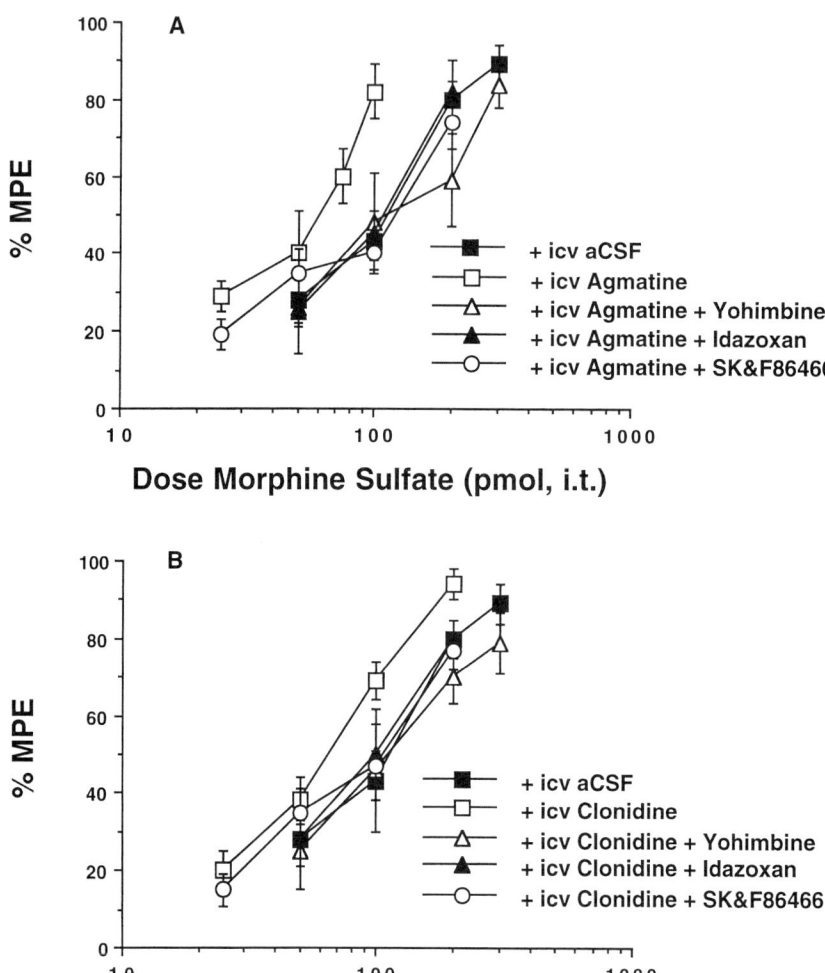

FIGURE 3. Dose response curves for i.t. morphine after pretreatment with i.c.v. agents. **(A)** aCSF, agmatine (1 nmol), agmatine (1 nmol) + yohimbine (5 nmol), agmatine (1 nmol) + idazoxan (5 nmol) or agmatine (1 nmol) + SK&F 86466 (5 nmol) was given i.c.v. 5 minutes prior to i.t. morphine. **(B)** Clonidine (500 pmol) was used instead of agmatine in the same protocol.

In additional studies, the effects of norepinephrine given i.c.v. on i.t. morphine-induced antinociception was determined. The ED_{50} value for i.c.v. norepinephrine was 1.46 (1.10 to 1.94) nmol (dose response curve not shown). For these studies, a 500 pmol dose of norepinephrine was used, which produces a 29% MPE when given alone. Results shown in TABLE 3 show that i.c.v. norepinephrine, similar to agmatine

TABLE 3. Effect of i.c.v. agmatine, clonidine or norepinephrine on i.t. morphine-induced antinociception

i.c.v. Pretreatment[a]		Morphine ED$_{50}$ (95% CI) (pmol, i.t.)
aCSF		100 (85–117)
Agonist	Antagonist	
Agmatine	—	54 (49–62)*
Agmatine	Yohimbine	114 (91–141)
Agmatine	Idazoxan	104 (87–124)
Agmatine	SK&F 86466	98 (75–127)
Clonidine	—	61 (54–70)*
Clonidine	Yohimbine	104 (79–137)
Clonidine	Idazoxan	96 (84–109)
Clonidine	SK&F 86466	89 (74–107)
Norepinephrine	—	65 (53–78)*

Indicated drugs were administered i.c.v. 5 minutes before i.t. administration of morphine. Tail flick antinociception was measured 10 minutes later. i.c.v. drugs were given 10 minutes before i.t. morphine.

[a] i.c.v. doses: agmatine, 1 nmol; clonidine, 500 pmol; norepinephrine, 500 pmol; yohimbine, 5 nmol; idazoxan, 5 nmol; SK&F 86466, 5 nmol.

* Significantly different from aCSF, $P < 0.05$.

and clonidine, enhanced the i.t. morphine effect. These results support the involvement of α_2 receptor activation in the agmatine and clonidine effects. Because the ED$_{50}$ values (for i.t. morphine) obtained in the presence of the antagonists were not different from the ED$_{50}$ value after aCSF treatment, it appeared that the antagonists blocked only the effects of the applied agmatine and clonidine. There was no apparent involvement of endogenous agmatine or norepinephrine.

Because the earlier studies showed that i.t. agmatine attenuated i.t. clonidine-induced antinociception (TABLE 2), similar experiments were performed to determine whether i.c.v. agmatine also affects i.c.v. clonidine action. Clonidine was given i.c.v. alone or along with 1 nmol agmatine, the dose that enhanced i.t. morphine antinociception. Results shown in TABLE 4 show that agmatine at this dose did not alter the clonidine ED$_{50}$ value. The antinociception produced by i.t. clonidine was also not changed by either s.c. agmatine or i.c.v. agmatine (TABLE 4), there was no change in the clonidine ED$_{50}$ values.

DISCUSSION

A confounding factor in determining which receptors in pain pathways are affected by agmatine has been the universal finding that agmatine, unlike clonidine, has no antinociceptive activity in the tail flick test[5–7] (and present studies). Thus, studies

TABLE 4. Effect of agmatine on clonidine-induced antinociception

Route Clonidine	Route (Dose) Agmatine	Clonidine ED_{50} (95% CI) (nmol, i.t.)
i.c.v.	—	1.18 (1.21–2.44)
i.c.v.	i.c.v. (1 nmol)	1.95 (1.54–2.48)
i.t.	—	0.46 (0.31–0.69)
i.t.	s.c. (10 mg/kg)	0.51 (0.32–0.81)
i.t.	i.c.v. (1 nmol)	0.67 (0.49–0.97)

Agmatine was administered concurrently (i.c.v.) with i.c.v. clonidine or prior to (15 minutes, s.c. or 5 minutes i.c.v.) i.t. clonidine, and tail flick response was measured after 10 minutes.

utilizing receptor-selective antagonists to block agmatine-induced antinociception cannot be used to determine the receptor targets of agmatine. The current studies used indirect measurements, agmatine-induced enhancement of morphine antinociception and agmatine-induced effect on antinociception produced by clonidine and norepinephrine, in attempts to determine whether agmatine interacts with α_2 or I receptors in nociceptive pathways.

Initial studies showed that agmatine administered by s.c., i.c.v. and i.t. routes enhanced the antinociception produced by i.t. morphine to similar extents. Thus, agmatine administered s.c. likely accesses the central nervous system (CNS) to interact with receptors at both brain and spinal sites. Although others have shown using a similar test (hot water tail flick) that 4 nmol i.t. agmatine does not alter i.t. morphine antinociception,[6] the present results show that both 1 and 10 nmol agmatine decreased the i.t. morphine ED_{50} value. It is possible that this difference in results arises from the difference in sensitivity between tests since the morphine ED_{50} value in the previous study was in the nmol range, while the morphine ED_{50} value in the present study was tenfold lower (127 pmol). Subsequent studies were directed toward determining whether the actions of agmatine at both sites resulted from interaction with the same receptor(s), α_2 and/or I.

Results from these studies suggest that the actions of agmatine are mediated through different receptors in the brain than in the spinal cord. When administered i.c.v., the ability of agmatine to enhance i.t. morphine-induced antinociception was attenuated by both α_2 adrenergic receptor-selective (yohimbine, SK&F 86466) and mixed α_2/I antagonists (idazoxan). Similar results were found for i.c.v. clonidine. These results, along with the finding that i.c.v. administered norepinephrine (α_2 receptor agonist) also enhanced i.t. morphine-induced antinociception suggest that the morphine-enhancing effects of these drugs involves at least α_2 receptors. However, these studies could not rule out the possibility of a role for brain I receptors in the morphine-enhancing effect.

When administered i.t., agmatine attenuated clonidine-induced antinociception (an α_2/I receptor effect) but not norepinephrine-induced antinociception (an α_2 receptor effect). These results suggest that agmatine may act as an antagonist at I receptors, but not α_2 receptors, in spinal thermal sensory pathways. On the other hand, Horvath et al.[18] recently reported that i.t. agmatine attenuates carrageenan-induced thermal hyperalgesia, suggesting an agonist action in the spinal cord. Also, recent electrophysiological studies in rats suggests that spinal agmatine activates I receptors, but not α_2 receptors, to inhibit transmission of mechanical nociception.[19] Thus, spinal agmatine appears to have both agonist and antagonist properties in spinal sensory pathways, likely through I receptors.

In summary, the current studies suggest that agmatine acted at both spinal and supraspinal sites to enhance morphine-induced analgesia and that the mechanisms involved at the separate sites are not the same. The multiple actions of agmatine on different signaling systems may contribute differently at brain versus spinal sites to the overall observed effects.

ACKNOWLEDGMENTS

This work was supported by National Institutes of Health Grant DA07972. A preliminary report of this work was presented at the Experimental Biology meeting, April 1999. The expert technical assistance of Timothy Busch is gratefully acknowledged. The helpful discussions with Carolyn Fairbanks, Ph.D., and George Wilcox, Ph.D., are much appreciated.

REFERENCES

1. LI, G., S. REGUNATHAN, C.J. BARROW, *et al.* 1994. Agmatine: an endogenous clonidine-displacing substance in the brain. Science **263:** 966–969.
2. PILETZ, J.E., D.N. CHIKKALA & P. ERNSBERGER. 1995. Comparison of the properties of agmatine and endogenous clonidine-displacing substance at imidazline and alpha-2 adrenergic receptors. J. Pharmacol. Exp. Ther. **272:** 581–587.
3. PINEDA, J., J.A. RUIZ-ORTEGA, R. MARTIN-RUIZ, *et al.* 1996. Agmatine does not have activity at α_2-adrenoceptors which modulate the firing rate of locus coeruleus neurones: an electrophysiological study in rat. Neurosci. Lett. **219:** 103–106.
4. HEAD, G.A., C.K. CHAN & S.J. GODWIN. 1997. Central cardiovascular actions of agmatine, a putative clonidine-displacing substance, in conscious rabbits. Neurochem. Int. **30:** 37–45.
5. KOLESNIKOW, Y., S. JAIN & G.W. PASTERNAK. 1996. Modulation of opioid analgesia by agmatine. Eur. J. Pharmacol. **296:** 17–22.
6. FAIRBANKS, C.A. & G.L. WILCOX. 1997. Acute tolerance to spinally administered morphine compares mechanistically with chronically induced morphine tolerance. J. Pharmacol. Exp. Ther. **282:** 1408–1417.
7. ONAL, A. & N. SOYKAN. 2001. Agmatine produces antinociception in tonic pain in mice. Pharm. Biochem. Behav. **69:** 93–97.
8. TAKANO, Y. & T.L. YAKSH. 1992. Characterization of the pharmacology of intrathecally administered alpha$_2$ agonists and antagonists in rats. J. Pharmacol. Exp. Ther. **261:** 764–772.
9. HIEBLE, J.P. & R.R. RUFFOLO. 1995. Possible structural and functional relationships between imidazoline receptors and α_2-adrenoceptors. Ann. N.Y. Acad. Sci. **763:** 8–21.
10. MONROE, P.J., D.L. SMITH, H.R. KIRK, *et al.* 1995. Spinal nonadrenergic imidazoline receptors do not mediate the antinociceptive action of intrathecal clonidine in the rat. J. Pharmacol. Exp. Ther. **273:** 1057–1062.
11. FAIRBANKS, C.A. & G.L. WILCOX. 1999. Moxonidine, a selective α_2-adrenergic and imidazoline receptor agonist, produces spinal antinociception in mice. J. Pharmacol. Exp. Ther. **290:** 403–412.
12. KOLESNIKOV, Y.A., C.G. PICK, G. CISZEWSKA, *et al.* 1993. Blockade of tolerance to morphine but not to k opioids by a nitric oxide synthase inhibitor. Proc. Natl. Acad. Sci. U.S.A. **90:** 5162–5166.

13. HALEY, T.J. & W.G. MCCORMICK. 1957. Pharmacological effects produced by intracerebral injections of drugs in the conscious mouse. Br. J. Pharmacol. **12:** 12–15.
14. HYLDEN, J.L.K. & G.L. WILCOX. 1980. Intrathecal morphine in mice: A new technique. Eur. J. Pharmacol. **67:** 313–316.
15. ROERIG, S.C. 1995. Decreased spinal morphine/clonidine antinociceptive synergism in morphine-tolerant mice. Life Sci. **56:** PL115–PL122.
16. TALLARIDA, R.J. & R.B. MURRAY. 1987. Graded dose-response. *In* Manual of Pharmacologic Calculations.: 26–31. Springer-Verlag. New York, NY.
17. MIRALLES, A., G. OLMOS, M. SASTRE, *et al.* 1993. Discrimination and pharmacological characterization of I_2-imidazoline sites with [^{3}H]idazoxan and alpha-2 adrenoceptors with [^{3}H]RX821002 (2-methoxy idazoxan) in the human and rat brains. J. Pharmacol. Exp. Ther. **264:** 1187–1197.
18. HORVATH, G., G. KEKESI, I. DOBOS, *et al.* 1999. Effect of intrathecal agmatine on inflammation-induced thermal hyperalgesia in rats. Eur. J. Pharmacol. **368:** 197–204.
19. HOU, S.-W., J.-S. QI, Y. ZHANG, *et al.* 2003. Spinal antinociceptive effect of agmatine and tentative analysis of involved receptors: study in an electrophysiological model of rats. Brain Res. **968:** 277–280.

Is Agmatine an Endogenous Factor Against Stress?

FEYZA ARICIOGLU,[a,b] SOUNDAR REGUNATHAN,[b] AND JOHN E. PILETZ[b]

[a]*Department of Pharmacology, Faculty of Pharmacy, Marmara University, Haydarpasa, Istanbul, Turkey*

[b]*Department of Psychiatry and Human Behavior, Division of Neurobiology and Behavior Research, University of Mississippi Medical Center, Jackson, Mississippi 39216, USA*

ABSTRACT: Agmatine is an endogenous amine synthesized from the decarboxylation of arginine. A proposed intracellular role of agmatine is to balance the production of polyamines (a promitotic process) and nitric oxide (an inflammatory process). Agmatine is also released from neurons upon depolarization. We previously reported that agmatine concentrations are increased in rat pups' brains shortly after hypoxic-ischemia and in the plasma of depressed patients. Herein, male rats (270–290 g) were divided into four groups receiving different degrees of known stress: 2-hour restraint at 21°C, 4-hour restraint at 21°C, 4-hour restraint at 4°C, and control rats only handled at 21°C. Cortex, cerebellum, medulla, hippocampus, hypothalamus, and blood plasma samples were collected for determination of endogenous agmatine levels. No changes in agmatine levels were detected after 2-hour and 4-hour restraint at room temperature, but concentrations of agmatine were increased in all brain regions except cerebellum after 4-hour restraint in the cold. Plasma agmatine levels (ng/mL) were 6.8 ± 0.6 in controls versus 58.1 ± 12.8 in the 4-hour restraint-plus-cold group. Cortical agmatine levels (ng/g wet tissue) were 15.3 ± 2.4 in controls versus 57.4 ± 19.6 in the 4-hour restraint-plus-cold group. Therefore, endogenous agmatine was increased in response to cold-restraint stress, possibly as a neuroprotective agent.

KEYWORDS: agmatine; stress; cold restraint; imidazoline; NMDA; nitric oxide

INTRODUCTION

Stress is defined as that which causes functional adaptation of an organism to cope with a new circumstance. Accordingly, a stressor is envisioned as any physiologic, psychologic, or environmental stimulus capable of altering homeostasis. The biologic substrate of the human stress response is thought to be a complex interaction between limbic structures of the central nervous system (CNS), the hypothalamus-pituitary-adrenal axis, and components of the visceral system. Cortical neural networks are also known to regulate the activity of stress-response systems. The ability to cope with a stressor is a crucial determinant of health and disease.

Address for correspondence: Feyza Aricioglu, Ph.D., Department of Pharmacology, Faculty of Pharmacy, Marmara University, 81010 Tibbiye Cad. No: 49, Haydarpasa, Istanbul, Turkey. Voice: 0216 418 95 73; fax: 0216 345 29 52.
e-mail: feyzak@turk.net

Agmatine (1-amino-4-guanidinobutane) is an endogenous amine synthesized from the decarboxylation of arginine. Agmatine has been quantified in nearly all organs of the rat including brain and plasma.[1] The concentration of agmatine is higher in brain than in plasma but is approximately 20-fold less than in small intestine and threefold less than in the adrenal gland.[1] Agmatine exerts a wide range of biologic activities on several organ systems, including the CNS, where it has been proposed to act as a neurotransmitter.[2] Agmatine interacts with imidazoline receptors, α_2-adrenoceptors, nicotinic-cholinergic receptors, and 5-HT$_3$ receptors.[2] Agmatine selectively modulates the NMDA class of glutamate receptors in rat hippocampal neurons through an interaction between the guanidino group of agmatine and the NMDA channel pore.[3] Intracellularly, agmatine is reported to modulate the production of polyamines (involved in promitotic processes) and nitric oxide (involved in inflammatory processes).[4–6] Other studies have shown that agmatine is stored in synaptic vesicles, accumulated by active uptake, released by depolarization, and inactivated by agmatinase.[2,7,13]

It has been suggested that agmatine may modulate memory and other behavioral functions,[8] because it produces an amnesic effect when administered before fear conditioning,[9] In addition, the post-training injection of agmatine facilitated memory consolidation in an inhibitory avoidance task.[9] It was also reported that agmatine attenuates the withdrawal syndrome in morphine- and ethanol-dependent rats.[10,11] Other studies have indicated that agmatine exerts significant neuroprotective effects in models of neurotoxicity and brain ischemia.[7] Agmatine also causes antidepressant-like effects in tests of forced swimming and tail suppression in mice.[12] We have also previously reported agmatine levels to be increased in plasma of depressed patients.[8] The present study was designed to evaluate the effect of acute stress on endogenous agmatine.

MATERIALS AND METHODS

Animals

All procedures were conducted in accordance with the Guide for the Care and Use of Laboratory Animals as adopted by the National Institutes of Health (USA) and the declaration of Helsinki. Adult male Sprague-Dawley rats (270–290 g) were housed in a quiet room with controlled temperature (20°C ± 2°C) and humidity (60% ± 3%) and a 12-hour light-dark cycle (light 7:00–19:00 hours). The rats were fed standard lab chow, with tap water ad libitum. All the experiments were carried out during the light period of the day (9:50–15:00 hours).

Animals were divided into four groups receiving different degrees of known stressors: (1) 2-hour restraint at 21°C (n = 4), (2) 4-hour restraint at 21°C (n = 4), (3) 4-hour restraint at 4°C (n = 8), and (4) control rats only handled at 21°C (n = 6). To create restraint stress, the rats were firmly fit into a clean transparent plastic cylinder and remained in this position for 2 or 4 hours in a lit, quiet room. For restraint stress plus cold, the rats were restrained in the same cylinder and remained in this position for 4 hours at 4°C in a lit, quiet, cold room. Rats exposed to these stressors were decapitated immediately afterwards. Blood samples were collected during decapitation, and brain regions (hypothalamus, hippocampus, frontal cortex, cerebellum, and medulla) were collected for determination of endogenous agmatine. Brains were excised quickly on an ice-cold Petri dish. Dissection of brain regions was performed as previously described.[14]

Statistical Analysis

Comparisons between the three stressor groups and the control group were carried out using ANOVA followed by Tukey test. The statistical significance was set at $P < 0.05$. The data are expressed as mean ± SD.

RESULTS

No change in agmatine concentrations was detected in the 2-hour and 4-hour restraint groups in comparison either with each other or with the control group (TABLE 1). In the control group, agmatine concentrations in the cortex, hypothalamus, medulla, cerebellum, andhippocampus were found to be 5.3 ± 2.4, 23.9 ± 3.8, 23.5 ± 0.9, 37.0 ± 10.3, and 33.1 ± 4.4 ng/g wet tissue, respectively. Agmatine concentrations were not changed significantly in any of these brain regions after 2-hour or 4-hour of restraint stress at 21°C (TABLE 1). Finally, the combined stressor test (4-hour restraint-plus-cold) led to an increase in agmatine concentrations in most tissues (FIG. 1). Among the brain regions studied, only cortical agmatine levels were found to be statistically higher than control values after 4-hour restraint-plus-cold. Cortical agmatine concentrations (ng/g wet tissue) were 57.4 ± 19.6 in the 4-hour restraint-plus-cold group versus 15.3 ± 2.4 in controls ($P < 0.05$). Agmatine concentrations in the other brain regions from the 4-hour restraint-plus-cold group were 33.7 ± 7.7, 37.1 ± 7.8, 44.5 ± 9.2, and 46.2 ± 8.9 ng/g wet tissue, in hypothalamus, medulla, cerebellum, and hippocampus, respectively. Plasma agmatine concentrations (ng/mL) were also elevated by 4-hour restraint-plus-cold: 58.1 ± 12.8 ng/mL in the 4-hour restraint-plus-cold group versus 6.18 ± 0.6 ng/mL in controls ($P < 0.05$).

TABLE 1. Effect of restraint at room temperature on agmatine concentrations in brain regions (ng/g wet weight) and plasma (ng/mL)

Tissue	Controls	Res-2H	Res-4H
Plasma	6.18 ± 0.6	7.1 ± 1.4	6.5 ± 0.7
Cortex	15.3 ± 2.4	16.6 ± 0.9	14.9 ± 0.7
Hypothalamus	23.9 ± 3.8	19.5 ± 2.7	22.6 ± 2.7
Medulla	23.5 ± 0.9	22.2 ± 1.5	25.9 ± 0.5
Cerebellum	37.0 ± 10.3	20.6 ± 1.4	24.8 ± 1.5
Hippocampus	33.1 ± 4.4	23.6 ± 1.4	24.5 ± 1.2

Values were compared to control rats, which were only handled. Data are presented as mean ± SD. There were no significant differences among the groups. Res-2H, restraint for 2 hours; Res-4H, restraint for 4 hours.

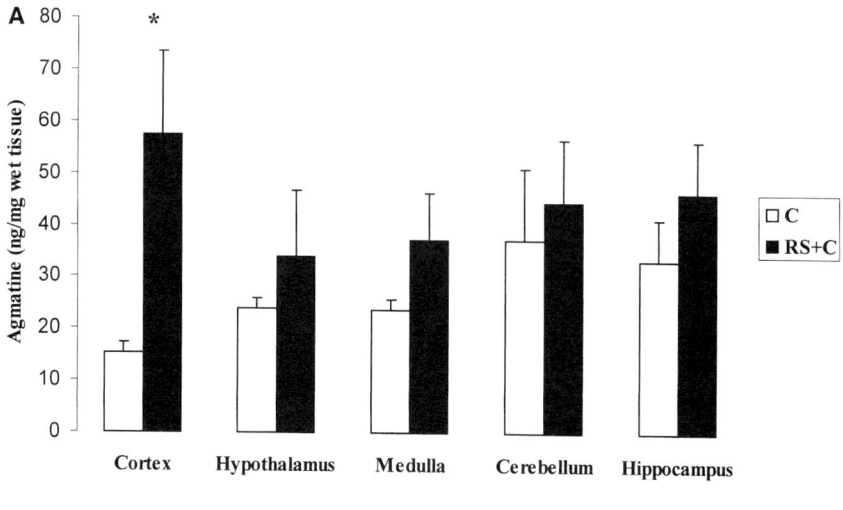
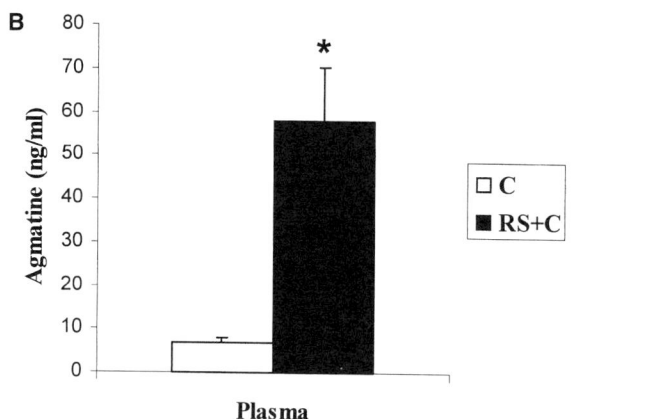

FIGURE 1. Effect of restraint stress in the cold for 4 hours on agmatine concentrations in brain regions (**A**) and plasma (**B**). Values were compared to control rats, which were only handled. Data are presented as mean ± SD. * $P < 0.05$. C, control rats; RS+C, restraint stress plus cold.

DISCUSSION

Agmatine immunoreactivity has previously been reported[15] to be enriched in frontal cortex, several nuclei of the hypothalamus, nucleus accumbens, ventral tegmental area, and locus coeruleus. It has also been shown that arginine decarboxylase exhibits relatively high activity in some of the same brain regions (Neurosci. Abstr. **33:** 449-8). Collectively, these brain regions suggest that agmatine might be involved in functions of emotional behavior, neuroendocrine responses, or pain regulation. In fact, several studies in rats and mice have reported that exogenously administrated agmatine has beneficial effects in fear conditioning, drug abuse, learning/memory, pain threshold, and models of depression.[6,9–12] Whether the endogenous synthesis of agmatine regulates these functions is not known.

Our present study indicates that agmatine concentrations are significantly increased in the frontal cortex of rats during restraint-plus-cold stress. Little is known about what mechanisms may underlie this increase. Arginine decarboxylase is known to be regulated under certain conditions, such as inflammation and morphine exposure[16,17]; however the restraint-plus-cold stress for 4 hours may not allow sufficient time to induce this enzyme. The large increase in agmatine concentration in plasma suggests that agmatine is released into the circulation during restraint-plus-cold stress. Although the source of agmatine is not known in plasma, we can predict that the hypothalamus, pituitary, adrenals, and sympathetic nerve terminals may all contribute. For example, the hypothalamus and posterior pituitary normally have high levels of agmatine as measured by high-pressure liquid chromatography (HPLC) or immunohistochemistry[15,18] that could be released into circulation. A possible release of agmatine from the hypothalamus into the circulation might explain why agmatine levels in the hypothalamus were not increased during restraint-plus-cold stress. Stress hormones such as adrenocorticotrophic hormone (ACTH) and corticotrophin-releasing factor (CRF) follow a similar pattern in which acute stress leads to higher circulating levels without increasing (or even with decreasing) tissue hormone levels. Additional chronic stress studies are planned to address these issues.

In conclusion, this study has for the first time demonstrated that an acute stressor can increase endogenous agmatine concentrations in the plasma and some brain regions. We suggest that this effect might be related to stress-response systems. The suggestion is that agmatine might be increased in response to certain stressors as a neuroprotective agent.[7] Additional studies of acute and chronic stressors are needed to define better the role of agmatine in the stress response.

REFERENCES

1. RAASCH, W., et al. 1995. Agmatine, the bacterial amine, is widely distributed in mammalian tissues. Life Sci. **56:** 2319–2330.
2. REIS, D.J. & S. REGUNATHAN. 2000. Is agmatine a novel neurotransmitter in brain? Trends Pharmacol. Sci. **21:** 187–193.
3. YANG, X.-C. & D.J. REIS. 1999. Agmatine selectively blocks the NMDA subclass of glutamate receptor channels in cultured mouse hippocampal neurons. J. Pharmacol. Exp. Ther. **288:** 544–549.
4. GALEA, E., et al. 1996. Inhibition of mammalian nitric oxide synthases by agmatine, an endogenous polyamine formed by decarboxylation of arginine. Biochem. J. **316:** 247–249.
5. DEMADY, D.R., et al. 2001. Agmatine enhances the NADPH oxidase activity of neuronal NO synthase and leads to oxidative inactivation of the enzyme. Mol. Pharmacol. **59:** 24–29.
6. FAIRBANKS, C.A., et al. 2000. Agmatine reverses pain induced by inflammation, neuropathy, and spinal cord injury. Proc. Natl. Acad. Sci. U. S. A. **97:** 10584–10589.
7. GILAD, G.M. & V.H. GILAD. 2000. Accelerated functional recovery and neuroprotection by agmatine after spinal cord ischemia in rats. Neurosci. Lett. **296:** 97–100.
8. HALARIS, A., et al. 1999. Plasma agmatine and platelet imidazoline receptors in depression. Ann. N. Y. Acad. Sci. **881:** 445–451.

9. MCKAY, B.E., *et al*. 2002. Learning and memory in agmatine treatment. Pharmacol. Biochem. Behav. **72:** 551–557.
10. ARICIOGLU-KARTAL, F. & I.T. UZBAY. 1997. Inhibitory effect of agmatine on naloxone-precipitated abstinence syndrome. Life Sci. **61:** 1775–1781.
11. UZBAY, I.T., *et al*. 2000. Effects of agmatine on ethanol withdrawal syndrome in rats. Behav. Brain Res. **107:** 153–159.
12. ZOMKOWSKI, A.D.E., *et al*. 2002. Agmatine produces antidepressant-like effects in two models of depression in mice. Neuroreport **13:** 387–391.
13. SASTRE, M., S. REGUNATHAN & D.J. REIS. 1996. Agmatinase activity in rat brain: a metabolic pathway for the degradation of agmatine. J. Neurochem. **67:** 1761–1765.
14. PALKOVITS, M. & M.J. BROWNSTEIN. 1998. Maps and Guide to Microdissection of the Rat Brain. Elsevier. New York, NY.
15. OTAKE, K., *et al*. 1998. Regional localization of agmatine in the rat brain: an immunocytochemical study. Brain Res. **787:** 1–14.
16. SASTRE, M., *et al*. 1998. Metabolism of agmatine in macrophages: modulation by lipopolysaccharide and inhibitory cytokines. Biochem. J. **330:** 1405–1409.
17. ARICIOGLU-KARTAL, F. & S. REGUNATHAN. 2002. Effect of chronic morphine treatment of the biosynthesis of agmatine in rat brain and other tissues. Life Sci. **71:** 1695–1701.
18. FENG, Y., A.E. HALARIS & J.E. PILETZ. 1997. Determination of agmatine in brain and plasma using high performance liquid chromatography with fluorescence detection. J. Chromatogr. **691:** 277–286.

Agmatine-Morphine Interaction on Nociception in Mice

EDUARDO RUIZ-DURÁNTEZ, JAVIER LLORENTE, ISABEL ULIBARRI, JOSEBA PINEDA, AND LUISA UGEDO

Department of Pharmacology, Faculty of Medicine, University of the Basque Country, Leioa, Vizcaya, Spain

> ABSTRACT: The aim of this study was to investigate the possible participation of nitric oxide in the agmatine-mediated potentiation of morphine-induced analgesia in mice. Agmatine and L-NAME (a nitric oxide synthesis inhibitor) enhanced morphine-induced analgesia in the tail flick test, but not in the hot plate test. L-NAME did not block the agmatine-induced potentiation of morphine effect. Our results indicate that agmatine potentiates morphine-induced spinal but not supraspinal analgesia, and that this effect is not mediated by a nitric oxide-dependent mechanism.
>
> KEYWORDS: agmatine; nitric oxide; spinal analgesia; supraspinal analgesia

Interactions between agmatine and the opioid system have been reported in recent years. Thus, it has been shown that agmatine potentiates opioid analgesia and blocks the development of opiate tolerance in mice.[1–3] Using electrophysiological techniques, we previously reported that agmatine increases the neuronal activity of the locus coeruleus by a nitric oxide-dependent mechanism, and that an interaction between agmatine and morphine was not involved.[4] The aim of this study was to investigate whether nitric oxide was also involved in the effect of agmatine on morphine-induced analgesia in mice by using the hot plate (supraspinal analgesia quantification) and tail flick (spinal analgesia quantification) tests.

Nociceptive effects were assessed using the hot plate and the tail flick tests, with cut-off times of 600 seconds and 10 seconds respectively, to minimize the risk of tissue damage. Agmatine or saline was injected 10 minutes after L-NAME or saline and 10 minutes before morphine or saline, and the analgesic responses were assessed 30 minutes after the morphine or saline injections. The degree of analgesia was calculated as the latency of jump response to the hot plate stimulus or, in the case of the tail flick test, as the percentage of the maximum possible effect (MPE) according to the following formula: % MPE = $100 \times$ (test latency – baseline latency) $\times$ (cut-off time – baseline latency)$^{-1}$. Statistical comparisons were evaluated using one-way ANOVA followed by the Newman-Keuls test. The level of significance was chosen as $P = 0.05$.

In the hot plate test, morphine (1 to 6 mg/kg) administration induced a significant and dose-dependent increase in jump response latency, as expected. In an initial

---

Address for correspondence: Luisa Ugedo, Department of Pharmacology, Faculty of Medicine, University of the Basque Country, E-48940 Leioa, Vizcaya, Spain. Voice: (+34) 94-601-5574; fax: (+34) 94-480-0128.

e-mail: kfpugurl@lg.ehu.es

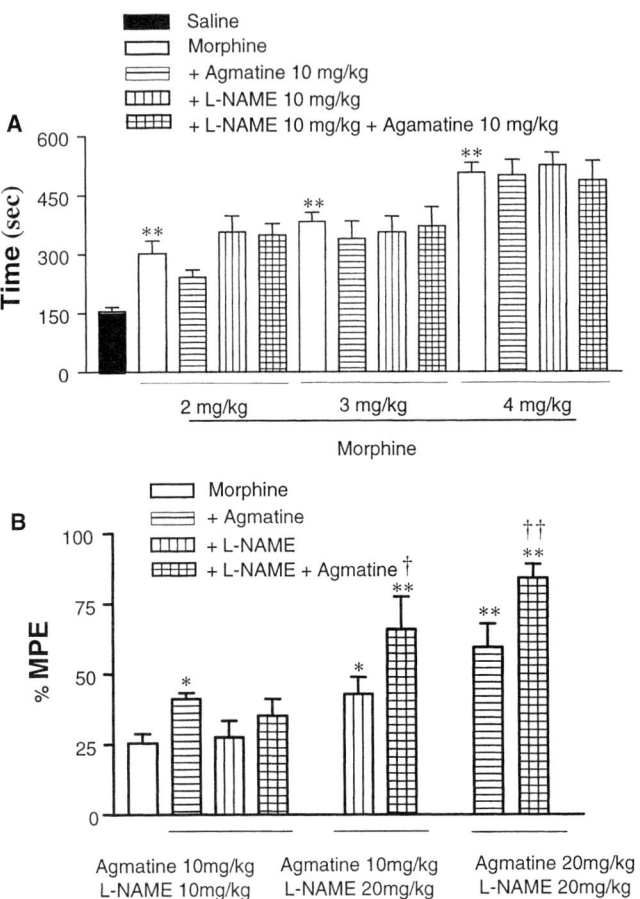

FIGURE 1. (**A**) Effect of the administration of agmatine, L-NAME or both on the increase in latency induced by morphine in the hot plate test. Bar histograms show the analgesic effect of morphine i.e., increase in latency (** $P < 0.001$ one-way ANOVA followed by Newman-Keuls) and the lack of effect of agmatine, L-NAME or both on the morphine-induced supraspinal analgesic effects. Bars represent means ± s.e.m. (**B**) Effect of the administration of agmatine or L-NAME or both, on the analgesic effect induced by morphine in the tail flick test. Bar histograms show the potentiation of the morphine analgesic effect by agmatine (10 and 20 mg/kg i.p.; * $P < 0.01$; ** $P < 0.001$, respectively). L-NAME (20 mg/kg i.p.) also increased the analgesic effect of morphine (* $P < 0.01$), but it failed to block the agmatine-induced potentiation of the analgesic effect of morphine († $P < 0.01$; †† $P < 0.001$ compared with the corresponding "+agmatine" groups; one-way ANOVA followed by Newman-Keuls). Bars represent means ± s.e.m. for the percentage of the maximal possible effect (MPE) in this spinal analgesic paradigm.

series of experiments, it was found that latency values after agmatine (10 mg/kg i.p.; 182 ± 11, n = 12), L-NAME (10 mg/kg i.p.; 184 ± 19, n = 9) or both agmatine and L-NAME (10 mg/kg each, i.p.; 145 ± 19, n = 6) were not different to those of the control group (saline; 155 ± 11, n = 20). Prior administration of agmatine (10 mg/kg i.p.) or L-NAME (10 mg/kg i.p.), or both agmatine and L-NAME, did not modify latency values after morphine administration (2, 3, and 4 mg/kg s.c.) (FIG. 1A).

In the tail flick test, the MPE obtained after agmatine (10 mg/kg i.p.; 8 ± 3%, n = 14) or L-NAME (10 mg/kg i.p.; 10 ± 3%, n = 11), or both agmatine and L-NAME (14 ± 3%, n = 11) did not differ statistically from that measured for the control group (6 ± 2%, n = 18). However, as shown in Figure 1B, pretreatment with agmatine (10 and 20 mg/kg i.p.) enhanced morphine-induced (6 mg/kg s.c.) analgesia by 52% and 122%, respectively. L-NAME, administered at 20 mg/kg i.p., but not at lower doses, enhanced morphine-induced analgesia by 59%. Unexpectedly, L-NAME pretreatment did not block the agmatine-induced potentiation of the morphine effect in either case. Thus, when both L-NAME and agmatine were administered, the potentiation of the morphine effect was larger than when each drug was administered separately, suggesting that an addition of both drug effects occurred.

In conclusion, our results indicate that agmatine potentiates morphine-induced spinal (tail flick test) but not supraspinal (hot plate) analgesia and that this effect is not mediated by a nitric oxide-dependent mechanism. It has been suggested that agmatine potentiates the analgesic effect of morphine by an α_2-adrenoceptor-mediated mechanism[2] and that agmatine antinociceptive effects are due to the activation of α_2-adrenoceptors.[5] However no interaction between α_2-adrenoceptors and opioid receptors has been found in the locus coeruleus.[4] Further studies will be required to determine the precise mechanism of action involved in this interaction.

ACKNOWLEDGMENTS

This work was supported by the Spanish CICYT (SAF 99/0046) and the UPV/EHU (00026.327-13590/2001). Eduardo Ruiz-Durántez was supported by a fellowship from the Basque Government.

REFERENCES

1. KOLESNIKOV, Y., S. JAIN & G.W. PASTERNAK. 1996. Modulation of opioid analgesia by agmatine. Eur. J. Pharmacol. **296:** 17–22.
2. YESILYURT, O. & I.T. UZBAY. 2001. Agmatine potentiates the analgesic effect of morphine by an alpha (2)-adrenoceptor-mediated mechanism in mice. Neuropsychopharmacology **25:** 98–103.
3. SÁNCHEZ-BLÁZQUEZ, P., M.A. BORONAT, G. OLMOS, et al. 2000. Activation of I(2)-imidazoline receptors enhances supraspinal morphine analgesia in mice: a model to detect agonist and antagonist activities at these receptors. Br. J. Pharmacol. **130:** 146–152.
4. RUIZ-DURÁNTEZ, E., J.A. RUIZ-ORTEGA, J. PINEDA, et al. 2002. Effect of agmatine on locus coeruleus neuron activity: possible involvement of nitric oxide. Br. J. Pharmacol. **135:** 1152–1158.
5. HOU, S.W., J.S. QI, Y. ZHANG, et al. 2003. Spinal antinociceptive effect of agmatine and tentative analysis of involved receptors: study in an electrophysiological model of rats. Brain Res. **968:** 277–280.

Is Agmatine an Endogenous Anxiolytic/Antidepressant Agent?

FEYZA ARICIOGLU AND HALE ALTUNBAS

Department of Pharmacology, Faculty of Pharmacy, Marmara University, Haydarpasa, Istanbul, Turkey

ABSTRACT: Agmatine, an endogenous cationic amine, exerts a wide range of biologic effects, but its physiologic role is still to be determined. The aim of the present experiments was to investigate the role of agmatine in anxiety and depression. The forced swim test (FST) and the elevated plus maze (EPM) were used to determine the antidepressant and anxiolytic effects of agmatine in comparison with imipramine (30 mg/kg i.p.). Agmatine (10, 20, 40, 80, or 100 mg/kg, i.p.), saline, or imipramine was given 30 minutes before the tests. Agmatine decreased immobility time in the FST and increased the time spent in the open arms in the EPM, as compared with the saline group. As an endogenous substance, agmatine have modulatory effect on anxiety and depression.

KEYWORDS: agmatine; forced swim test; elevated plus maze; imidazoline; NMDA; nitric oxide

INTRODUCTION

Agmatine, 4-aminobutyl guanidine, has recently been found in various mammalian organs and is thought to act as a neurotransmitter or neuromodulatory agent.[1] It stimulates the release of catecholamines from adrenal chromaffin cells,[2] and increases the release of luteinizing hormone-releasing hormone from hypothalamus.[3] The physiologic roles of agmatine in the central nervous system (CNS) are not well established. When exogenously administered to rodents, agmatine enhances morphine analgesia,[4] blocks tolerance to opioids,[4] and attenuates withdrawal syndrome both in morphine-,[5] and ethanol-dependent[6] rats. Agmatine blocks spinal nociceptive reflexes when administered systemically,[7] and reverses chronic pain induced by inflammation, neuropathy, and spinal cord injury.[8,9] Agmatine is also released from neurons and has neuroprotective properties.[10,11]

Agmatine binds to α_2-adrenergic and imidazoline receptors with high affinity.[12] In addition, agmatine can evoke a noncompetitive voltage- and concentration-dependent block of the N-methyl-D-aspartate (NMDA) ionophore[13] and inhibits all isoforms of nitric oxide (NO) synthase. Both NMDA antagonists and NO synthase inhibitors are known to have anti-depressant-like effects in animal models.[15,16]

The present study was designed to investigate the potential antidepressant and anxiolytic effects of agmatine by using the elevated plus maze (EPM) and forced swim tests (FST) in rats.

Address for correspondence: Feyza Aricioglu, Ph.D., Department of Pharmacology, Faculty of Pharmacy, Marmara University, 81010 Tibbiye Cad. No: 49, Haydarpasa, Istanbul, Turkey. Voice: 0216 418 95 73; fax: 0216 345 29 52.
e-mail: feyzak@turk.net

MATERIALS AND METHODS

Animals

The experiments performed in this study have been carried out according to the rules in the Guide for the Care and Use of Laboratory Animals adopted by the National Institute of Health (USA) and Declaration of Helsinki. Male adult Sprague-Dawley rats (180–200 g) were used. Animals maintained on a 12-hour light/dark cycle and given ad libitum access to food and water.

Drugs

Agmatine sulfate and imipramine was purchased from Sigma Chemical (St. Louis, MO, USA) and dissolved in saline. The drugs or saline were injected intraperitoneally (i.p.) at a volume of 0.1 mL/100 g.

Elevated Plus Maze

The EPM was made of wood and consisted of two opposite open arms, 50×10 cm^2, and two opposite arms of equal size enclosed by walls 40 cm in height. The arms were connected by a central 10×10 cm^2 square, and thus the maze had the shape of a plus sign. The maze was elevated 50 cm from the floor and lit by dim light. Rats were placed individually in the center of the maze facing a closed arm and allowed 5 minutes of free exploration.[17] The maze was cleaned thoroughly after each test. Thirty minutes before the test, the rats received agmatine at doses of 20, 40, 80, and 100 mg/kg i.p.

Forced Swim Test

Rats were taken from the cage and transported to a separate treatment room. They were immediately placed in a cylinder (45 cm high, 20 cm in diameter) filled with 30 cm of water that was meticulously maintained at $25°C \pm 1°C$. Rats were forced to swim for 15 minutes. The rats initially struggled to escape from the water, but eventually they adopted a posture of immobility in which they made only the movements necessary to keep their heads above water.[18] After 15 minutes the rats were removed from the water, dried, and placed in a warmed enclosure for 30 minutes. The cylinders were emptied and cleaned between tests. Twenty-four hours after the first session, the rats received 10, 20, 40, 80, and 100 mg/kg agmatine. The 15-minute FST was repeated 30 minutes after the administration of agmatine, and again the immobilization time was recorded. All tests were conducted between 10:00 a.m. and 4:00 p.m.

Statistical Analysis

Data obtained are expressed as mean ± SE. Differences between groups were analyzed by ANOVA. Duncan's post hoc comparisons, when appropriate, were carried out if significant overall $F-$ values were obtained ($P < 0.05$).

RESULTS AND DISCUSSION

Agmatine significantly decreased the duration of immobility in the FST ($P < 0.05$) (FIG. 1). When the efficacy of agmatine (10, 20, 40, 80, or 100 mg/kg i.p.) was

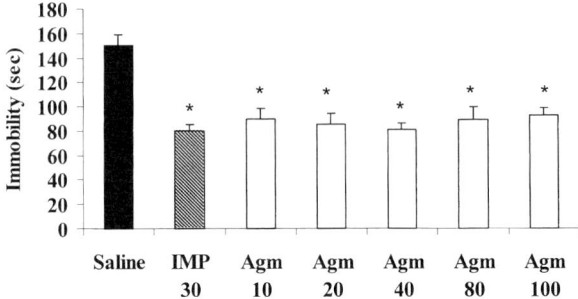

FIGURE 1. Effect of agmatine on forced swimming test in rats. Agmatine (10, 20, 40, 80, or 100 mg/kg i.p.) or imipramine (30 mg/kg i.p.) was administered 30 minutes before the test. Values are expressed as mean ± SD; n = 10 in each group. *$P < 0.05$ versus saline group. Agm, agmatine; IMP, imipramine.

compared with the saline group, agmatine (40 and 80 mg/kg) was found as effective as imipramine (30 mg/kg i.p.). In the EPM, agmatine significantly increased the total time spent in the arms ($P < 0.05$) (FIG. 2). Agmatine (40 and 80 mg/kg i.p.) increased the time spent in the open arms of the EPM in comparison with the saline group. Doses lower or higher than 40 to 80 mg/kg of agmatine did not differ significantly from controls (FIGS. 1 & 2); therefore the effect of agmatine was not found to be dose-dependent.

This study used the FST, a model of depression, and the EPM, a model of anxiety. Both methods are accepted models and are widely used to screen new antidepressant and anxiolytic drugs. The results presented here show that agmatine is a antidepressant and anxiolytic compound. The effect of agmatine was compared with imipramine in both tests. Agmatine significantly but not dose-dependently increased the

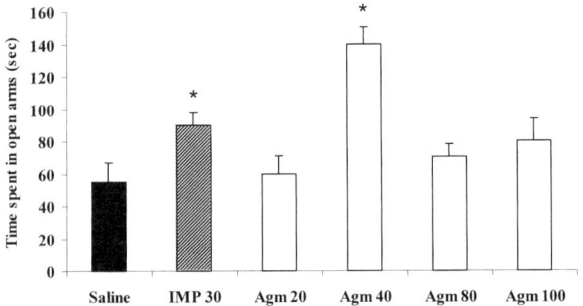

FIGURE 2. Effect of agmatine on elevated plus maze test in rats. Agmatine (20, 40, 80, or 100 i.p.) or imipramine (30 mg/kg i.p.) was administered 30 minutes before the test. Data are presented as time spent in open arms. Values are expressed as mean ± SD; n = 10 in each group. *$P < 0.05$ versus saline group. Agm, agmatine; IMP, imipramine.

duration of immobility in the FST. It was also dose-dependently effective in increasing the time spent in open arms in the EPM.

Because agmatine interacts with several receptors, this effect of agmatine may be caused by multiple mechanisms.

Clonidine is an adrenergic agonist with high affinity for α_2-adrenoceptors and also has affinity for I_1 imidazoline receptors. Clonidine has previously been shown to reduce immobility in the FST.[19] Both I_1 and I_2 imidazoline receptors are altered in depressed patients. The I_2 sites have been shown to be decreased in platelet internal membranes of depressed patients.[20] When compounds with selective affinity for I_2 receptors were tested in the FST, they were found to be inactive.[19] Like clonidine, agmatine is an endogenous imidazoline receptor ligand that interacts with both I_1 and I_2 subtypes as well as with α_2-adrenoceptors. The effect of agmatine might result from its action at α_2-adrenoceptors.

Chronic antidepressant treatment reduces the function of the glutamate/NMDA receptor complex in rodent brain. It is well known that NMDA receptors are involved in depression and that NMDA receptor antagonists possess antidepressant-like effects in animal models. Noncompetitive NMDA receptor antagonists such as amantadine, memantine, and neramexane have antidepressant-like effects in the FST.[21] As an NMDA receptor blocker, a part of agmatine's action may result from blockade of NMDA receptors.

The L-arginine-NO pathway is important in the modulation of depression. The NO precursor L-arginine abolishes the anxiolytic effect of diazepam in the EPM test in rats. S-nitroso-N-acetylpenicillamine (SNAP), a NO donor, blocks the anxiolytic effect of ethanol. NOS inhibitors NG-nitro-L-arginine-methyl-ester (L-NAME) and NG-nitro-L-arginine induced an anxiolytic effect in the plus maze test[22,23] and 7-nitroindazole (7-NI) enhanced anxiolytic efficacy without tolerance in rats.[24] Thus it is possible that the NO pathway may underline anxiety. NG-nitro-L-arginine has also been shown to reduce open-arm activity in the EPM test. It has been also shown that NG-nitro-L-arginine and L-NAME have antidepressant properties in the FST.[25] Agmatine is an endogenous inhibitor for all isoforms of NOS; therefore, the antidepressant and anxiolytic properties of agmatine may also result from NOS inhibition.

In summary, the results of the present study demonstrate that agmatine modulates anxiety and depression in rat models. Because agmatine is an endogenous substance, it probably has a modulatory or protective role against anxiety and depression. Further studies are necessary to understand the mechanism of action of agmatine in anxiety and depression.

REFERENCES

1. REIS, D.J. & S. REGUNATHAN. 2000. Is agmatine a novel neurotransmitter in brain? Trends Pharmacol. Sci. **21:** 187–193.
2. LI, G., et al. 1994. Agmatine: an endogenous clonidine-displacing substance in the brain. Science **263:** 966–969.
3. KALRA, S.P., et al. 1995. Agmatine, a novel hypothalamic amine, stimulates pituitary luteinizing hormone release in vivo and hypothalamic luteinizing hormone-releasing hormone release in vitro. Neurosci. Lett. **194:** 165–168.
4. KOLESNIKOV, Y., S. JAIN & G.W. PASTERNAK. 1996. Modulation of opioid analgesia by agmatine. Eur. J. Pharmacol. **296:** 17–22.
5. ARICIOGLU-KARTAL, F. & I.T. UZBAY. 1997. Inhibitory effect of agmatine on naloxane-precipitated abstinence syndrome. Life Sci. **61:** 1775–1881

6. UZBAY, I.T., et al. 2000. Effects of agmatine on ethanol withdrawal syndrome in rats. Behav. Brain Res. **107:** 153–159.
7. BRADLEY, K.J. & P.M. HEADLEY. 1997. Effect of agmatine on spinal nociceptive reflexes: lack of interaction with alpha2-adrenoceptor or mu-opioid receptor mechanisms. Eur. J. Pharmacol. **331:** 133–138.
8. FAIRBANKS, C.A., et al. 2000. Agmatine reverses pain induced by inflammation, neuropathy, and spinal cord injury. Proc. Natl. Acad. Sci. U. S. A. **97:** 10584–10589
9. FAIRBANKS, C.A. & G.L. WILCOX. 1997. Acute tolerance to spinally administered morphine compares mechanistically with chronically induced morphine tolerance. J. Pharmacol. Exp. Ther. **282:** 1408–1417
10. GILAD, G.M. & V.H. GILAD. 2000. Accelerated functional recovery and neuroprotection by agmatine after spinal cord ischemia in rats. Neurosci. Lett. **296:** 97–100.
11. FENG, Y., J.E. PILETZ & M.H. LEBLANC. 2002. Agmatine suppresses nitric oxide production and attenuates hypoxic-ischemic brain injury in neonatal rats. Pediatr. Res. **52:** 1–6
12. PILETZ, J.E., D.N. CHIKKALA & P. ERNSBERGER. 1995. Comparison of the properties of agmatine and endogenous clonidine-displacing substance at imidazoline and alpha-2 adrenergic receptors. J. Pharmacol. Exp. Ther. **272:** 581–587.
13. YANG, X.-C. & D.J. REIS. 1999. Agmatine selectively blocks the NMDA subclass of glutamate receptor channels in cultured mouse hippocampal neurons. J. Pharmacol. Exp. Ther. **288:** 544–549.
14. GALEA, E., et al. 1996. Inhibition of mammalian nitric oxide synthases by agmatine, an endogenous polyamine formed by decarboxylation of arginine. Biochem. J. **316:** 247–249.
15. YILDIZ, F., et al. 2000. Antidepressant-like effect of 7-nitroindazole in the forced swimming test in rats. Psychopharmacology **149:** 41–44.
16. DA SILVA G.D., et al. 2000. Evidence for dual effects of nitric oxide in the forced swimming test and in the tail suspension test in mice. Neuroreport **11:** 3699–3702.
17. PELLOW, S., et al. 1985. Validation of open:closed arm entries in an elevated plus-maze as a measure of anxiety in the rat. J. Neurosci. Methods **14:** 149–167.
18. PORSOLT, R.D., A. BERTIN & M. JALFRE. 1977. Behavioral despair in mice: a primary screening test for antidepressants. Arch. Int. Pharmacodyn. Ther. **229:** 327–336.
19. O'NEILL, M.F., et al. 2001. Selective imidazoline I2 ligands do not show antidepressant-like activity in the forced swim test in mice. Psychopharmacology **15:** 18–22.
20. HALARIS, A., et al. 1999. Plasma agmatine and platelet imidazoline receptors in depression. Ann. N. Y. Acad. Sci. **881:** 445–452.
21. ROGOZ, Z., et al. 2002. Synergistic effect of uncompetitive NMDA receptor antagonists and antidepressant drugs in the forced swimming test in rats. Neuropharmacology **42:** 1024–1030.
22. FARIA, M.S., et al. 1997. Acute inhibition of nitric oxide synthesis induced anxiolysis in the plus-maze test. Eur. J. Pharmacol. **323:** 37–43.
23. CATON, P.W., S.A. TOUSMAN & R.M. QUOCK. 1994. Involvement of nitric oxide anxiolysis in the elevated plus maze. Pharmacol. Biochem. Behav. **48:** 689–692.
24. DUNN, R.W., et al. 1998. The nitric oxide synthase inhibitor 7-nitroindazole displays enhanced anxiolytic efficacy without tolerance in rats following subchronic administration. Neuropharmacology **37:** 899–904.
25. HARKIN, A.J., et al. 1999. Nitric oxide synthase inhibitors have antidepressant-like properties in mice. 1. Acute treatments are active in the forced swim test. Eur. J. Pharmacol. **372:** 207–213.

Effect of Agmatine on Electrically and Chemically Induced Seizures in Mice

FEYZA ARICIOGLU,[a] BILGE KAN,[a] OKAN YILLAR,[b] EYLEM KORCEGEZ,[a] AND KEMAL BERKMAN[c]

[a]*Department of Pharmacology, Faculty of Pharmacy, Marmara University, Haydarpasa, Istanbul, Turkey*

[b]*Department of Pharmacology, Faculty of Medicine, Istanbul University, Cerrahpasa, Turkey*

[c]*Department of Pharmacology, Faculty of Medicine, Marmara University, Istanbul University, Haydarpasa, Istanbul, Turkey*

ABSTRACT: Agmatine, an amine and organic cation, is formed by the decarboxylation of L-arginine by arginine decarboxylase. It binds to α_2-adrenergic and imidazoline receptors. It blocks N-methyl-D-aspartate (NMDA) subtype of glutamate receptors and inhibits nitric oxide (NO) synthase. Because the importance of NMDA receptors and the NO system are well known in seizure activity, this study was designed to investigate the effect of agmatine on electrically and chemically induced seizures by using maximal electroshock (MES) and pentilentetrazole (PTZ) models in mice. Initial studies established convulsive current 50 (CC_{50}) for MES and effective dose 50 (ED_{50}) for PTZ to produce seizures. Agmatine (20, 40, 80, and 100 mg/kg intraperitoneally) increased the threshold of seizures in MES dose dependently. In PTZ-induced convulsions, the highest dose of agmatine (100 mg/kg) increased the seizure onset time and decreased percent survival. The percentage of grade V seizures was found to be increased by agmatine doses greater than 20 mg/kg.

KEYWORDS: agmatine; maximal electroshock; pentilentetrazole; imidazoline; adrenoceptors; NMDA; nitric oxide

INTRODUCTION

Agmatine (1-amino-4-guanidobutane) is a polycationic amine synthesized from L-arginine by the enzyme arginine decarboxylase (ADC). Long recognized as a product of bacteria, plants, and some invertebrates, agmatine and ADC have recently been identified in a number of mammalian tissues including stomach, intestine, aorta, and brain.[1] In the periphery, agmatine modulates insulin release from islet cells exposed to glucose, has insulin-like properties on isolated adipocytes, and releases adrenaline and noradrenaline from chromaffin cells. In kidney, agmatine is natriuretic, increasing the excretion of Na^+ independently of action on blood flow. Furthermore, agmatine blocks

Address for correspondence: Feyza Aricioglu, Ph.D., Department of Pharmacology, Faculty of Pharmacy, Marmara University, 81010 Tibbiye Cad. No: 49, Haydarpasa, Istanbul, Turkey. Voice: 0126 418 95 73; fax: 0216 345 29 52.
  e-mail: feyzak@turk.net

the stimulated proliferation of vascular smooth muscle cells.[2,3] Agmatine interacts with imidazoline receptors and α_2-adrenoceptors, but it is not known whether it activates or inhibits these receptors. Agmatine blocks N-methyl-D-aspartate (NMDA) and nicotinic, cholinergic, and serotoninergic (5-HT3) receptors and inhibits all isoforms of nitric oxide synthase (NOS).[2,3] In the central nervous system, agmatine enhances morphine analgesia, prevents morphine tolerance, and attenuates all of the behavioral signs of the morphine abstinence syndrome in rats.[4,5] There is inferential evidence that agmatine may modulate the action of L-glutamate. The association between agmatine and NMDA receptor function has been confirmed, in that agmatine selectively modulates the NMDA subclass of glutamate receptors in the hippocampal neurons.[6] Because the importance of NMDA receptors and nitric oxide (NO) system are well known in seizure activity, this study was designed to investigate the effect of agmatine on electrically and chemically induced seizures by using maximal electroshock (MES) and pentylenetetrazol (PTZ) models in mice.

MATERIAL AND METHODS

Animals

Male and female Swiss albino mice weighing 20 to 30 g were housed in colony cages, under standard laboratory conditions, with free access to food and tap water. All mice were maintained at 20°C and on a natural light/dark cycle. Each mouse was used only once.

Drugs

Agmatine HCl and pentylenetetrazol were purchased from Sigma Chemicals (St. Louis, MO, USA) and dissolved in saline. The drugs, or saline, were injected intraperitoneally (i.p) at a volume of 0.1 mL/10 g.

MES Model

Electrodes were attached to each animal's ears, and the animals were positioned on their backs with their tails fixed so that tonic and clonic convulsions were clearly observed. Electroshocks were evoked through a current transmitter producing 60 Hz square waves (Ugo Basile Biological Research Apparatus, ECT unit). The shock was applied between 2:00 and 5:00 p.m. Flow duration of the current and the duration of each square wave were fixed at 0.2 seconds and at 0.4 milliseconds, respectively. Maximal electroshock seizures were defined by a latency period (lasting 1.6 seconds) followed by a short initial flexion period, then 13.2 seconds of tonic hindlimb extension and 7.6 seconds of terminal clonus.[8] Total duration of the seizure averaged 22.3 seconds. At the beginning of the study, the convulsive current 50 (CC_{50}) value for mice and its 95% fiducial limits were calculated by the method of Litchfield and Wilcoxon.[7]

PTZ Model

The procedure for the PTZ model has been reported in detail elsewhere.[8,9] Animals were given agmatine (20, 40, 80, or 100 mg/kg) 30 minutes before convulsive stimuli (80 mg/kg PTZ). Following each PTZ injection, mice were placed individually in acrylic observation chambers for 30 minutes, and behavioral seizures were rated according to the following scale: 0, no change in behavior; I, myoclonic jerks (MKJ); II, minimum seizures, with convulsive wave through the body; III, fully developed minimal seizures, clonus of the head muscles and forelimbs, righting reflex present; IV, major seizures (generalized without the tonic phase); V, generalized tonic-clonic seizures beginning with running, followed by the loss of righting ability, then a short tonic phase (flexion or extension of fore and hind limbs) progressing to clonus of all four limbs that sometimes led to the death of the animal. The time between the injection of the PTZ and the MKJ is defined as the seizure-onset time.

Statistical Analysis

The group pretreated with agmatine was compared with the PTZ group. Data (seizure-onset time, the percentage of grade V seizures, and the survival percentage) were analyzed with ANOVA. If appropriate, this analysis was followed by a Tukey multiple comparison test. Data are presented as percentage response or mean ± SD; $P < 0.05$.

RESULTS AND DISCUSSION

The value of CC_{50} is 47 mA (53.5 mA upper limit and 41.2 mA lower limit). We stimulated the mice 45 minutes after i.p. administration of 20, 40, 80, or 100 mg/kg agmatine. Pretreatment with agmatine at all doses decreased the threshold of MES (TABLE 1). These groups were compared with a control group treated with saline only; all results in the MES model were statistically significant. None of the animals in the MES group died, as shown in TABLE 1.

Single injection of PTZ in a dose of 80 mg/kg i.p. produced MKJ at 93.29 ± 25.39 seconds after PTZ administration. FIGURE 1 shows the effect of agmatine on PTZ-induced convulsions in terms of seizure-onset time (FIG. 1A), grade V tonic-clonic convulsions (FIG. 1B), and survival percentage 30 minutes after PTZ injection

TABLE 1. Effect of agmatine on maximal electroshock seizures in mice

Treatment	Number of Animals		
	Total	Seizure	Died
Saline	50	25	5
Agmatine (20 mg/kg i.p.)	25	10*	2
Agmatine (40 mg/kg i.p.)	25	5*	1*
Agmatine (80 mg/kg i.p.)	25	1*	0*
Agmatine (100 mg/kg i.p.)	25	0*	0*

Agmatine or saline was administered i.p. 45 minutes before MES. Data show the total number of mice in each group, the number of seizures (end point of the measurement of hind limb tonic extension), and the number of deaths (observed immediately after seizure).

* $P < 0.05$ compared with saline group.

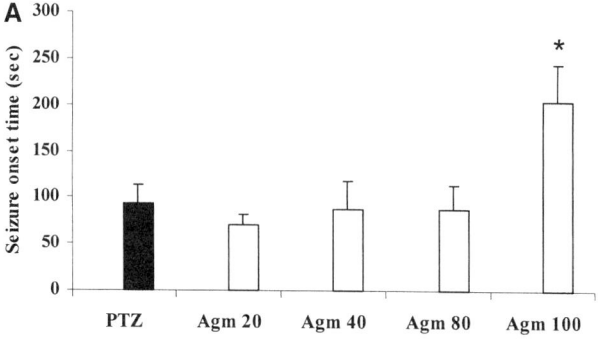
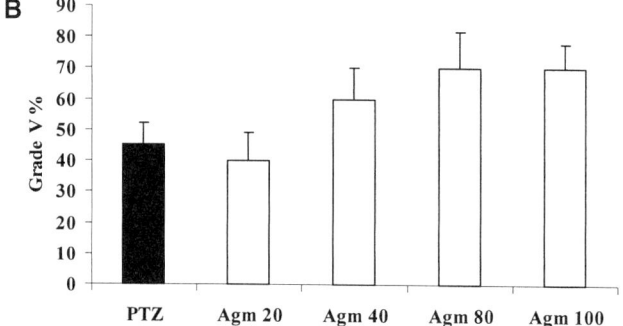
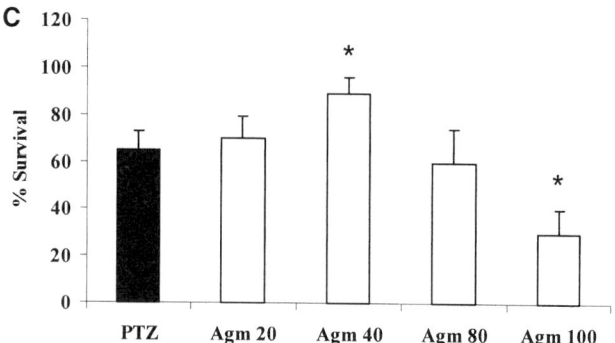

FIGURE 1. Effect of agmatine on PTZ-induced convulsions. Agmatine (Agm) (20, 40, 80, and 100 mg/kg i.p.) was administered 30 minutes before PTZ (80 mg/kg). Measurements were (**A**) seizure onset time; (**B**) tonic-clonic convulsions (grade V); (**C**) survival percentage. Data are presented as mean ± SD; n = 12 in each group). * $P < 0.05$ compared with the PTZ group.

(FIG. 1C). Agmatine (20, 40, 80, or 100 mg/kg) produced MKJ at 70.43 ± 13.29 seconds; 87.80 ± 31.94 seconds; 88.50 ± 27.05 seconds; and 204.9 ± 26.32 seconds after PTZ administration, respectively. In comparison with the PTZ-only group, high-dose agmatine (100 mg/kg) significantly ($P < 0.05$) increased the seizure-onset time. In PTZ-induced convulsions, the percentage of grade V seizures was found to be increased by doses greater than 20 mg/kg ($P < 0.05$). The survival percentage was decreased only in highest dose (100 mg/kg) of agmatine ($P < 0.05$).

Results of this study show that agmatine increased the threshold of MES but not in a dose-dependent manner. In PTZ-induced convulsions, agmatine had a different pattern of action: it increased onset time of seizures but also increased tonic-clonic convulsions. This effect of agmatine may be related to different mechanisms, because it interacts with NMDA and α_2-adrenergic and imidazoline receptors and inhibits NOS. First, it is evident that excitatory amino acids are involved in the generation of seizure activity through inotropic or metabotropic receptors.[8,9] The excitatory amino acid receptor agonist NMDA is known to be a potent convulsant in rodents and primates. Antagonists of NMDA receptors were found to be anticonvulsant in animal models. Interestingly NMDA antagonists such as MK-801 and CPPene reduce the ED_{50} values in MES. MK-801 has been found to be proconvulsant in some other animal models.[10,11]

Second, it has been shown that the NO system is involved in modulation of convulsive threshold. NOS inhibitors such as NG-nitro-L-arginine methyl ester (L-NAME), an unspecific NOS inhibitor, is able to reduce the protective activity of some conventional antiepileptics.[12,13] It has been reported that both N-omega-nitro-L-arginine methyl ester and NG-nitro-L-arginine increased the tonic CD_{50} of pentylenetetrazol in mice and that NG-nitro-L-arginine (NNA) did not affect the susceptibility of mice to pentylenetetrazol and electroconvulsions.[14] Despite a rapidly accumulating body of literature, the effect of NMDA receptor blockers and NOS inhibitors on convulsions are not clear.[15–19]

Third, it has been shown that α_2-adrenergic receptors may be important in mediating anticonvulsant activity.[20] Agents such as tizanidine, which binds to both α_1- and α2-adrenergic receptors, have anticonvulsant effect. Antagonists of α_2-adrenergic receptors reverse the anticonvulsant effect of α_2-adrenergic receptors agonists like tizanidine.[20] It is known that agmatine binds to α_2-adrenergic receptors as well as to imidazoline receptors, but it is still not clear if agmatine is an agonist or antagonist of these receptors.

Agmatine is an endogenous neuropharmacologically active agent. Our results indicate that agmatine can influence epileptic activity both in MES and PTZ models in mice. This endogenous substance may have a role in modulating the convulsive threshold, and its study may lead to new understandings of the mechanism of epilepsy.

REFERENCES

1. RAASCH, W., et al. 1995. Agmatine is widely and unequally distributed in rat organs. Ann. N.Y. Acad. Sci. **763:** 330–334.
2. REIS, D.J. & S. REGUNATHAN. 1998. Agmatine: a novel neurotransmitter? Adv. Pharmacol. **42:** 645–649.
3. REIS, D.J. & S. REGUNATHAN. 2000. Is agmatine a novel neurotransmitter in brain? Trends Pharmacol. Sci. **21:** 187–193.

4. KOLESNIKOV, Y., S. JAIN & G.W. PASTERNAK. 1996. Modulation of opioid analgesia by agmatine. Eur. J. Pharmacol. **296:** 17–22.
5. ARICIOGLU-KARTAL, F. & I.T. UZBAY. 1997. Inhibitory effect of agmatine on naloxone-precipitated abstinence syndrome. Life Sci. **61:** 1775–1781.
6. YANG, X.C. & D.J. REIS. 1999. Agmatine selectively blocks the N-methyl-D-aspartate subclass of glutamate receptor channels in rat hippocampal neurons. J. Pharmacol. Exp. Ther. **288:** 544–549.
7. LITCHFIELD, J.T. & F. WILCOX. 1949. A simplified method of evaluating dose-effect experiments. J. Pharmacol. Exp. Ther. **96:** 99–113.
8. RACINE, R.J. 1972. Modification of seizure activity by electrical stimulation. II. Motor seizure. Electroencephalogr. Clin. Neurophysiol. **32:** 281–294.
9. RACINE, R.J. 1972. Modification of seizure activity by electrical stimulation. I. After-discharge threshold. Electroencephalogr. Clin. Neurophysiol. **32:** 269–279.
10. SWINYARD, E.A., et al. 1963. Some neurophysiological and neuropharmacological characteristics of audiogenic-seizure-susceptible mice. J. Pharmacol. Exp. Ther. **106:** 319–330.
11. URBANSKA, E.M., et al. 1999. AMPA/kainate-related mechanisms contribute to convulsant and proconvulsant effects of 3-nitropropionic acid. Eur. J. Pharmacol. **370:** 251–256.
12. STARR, M.S. & B.S. STARR. 1993. Paradoxical facilitation of pilocarpine-induced seizures in the mouse by MK-801 and the nitric oxide synthesis inhibitor L-NAME. Pharmacol. Biochem. Behav. **45:** 321–325.
13. CZUCZWAR, S.J., et al. 1995. Influence of combined treatment with NMDA and non-NMDA receptor antagonists on electroconvulsions in mice. Eur. J. Pharmacol. **281:** 327–333.
14. MULSCH, A., et al. 1994. Nitric oxide promotes seizure activity in kainate-treated rats. Neuroreport **5:** 2325–2328.
15. MOLLACE, V., G. BAGETTA & G. NISTICO. 1991. Evidence that L-arginine possesses proconvulsant effects mediated through nitric oxide. Neuroreport **2:** 269–272.
16. DEL-BEL, E.A., et al. 1997. Anticonvulsant and proconvulsant roles of nitric oxide in experimental epilepsy models. Braz. J. Med. Biol. Res. **30:** 971–979.
17. WANG, Q., et al. 1994. Nitric oxide (NO) is an endogenous anticonvulsant but not a mediator of the increase in cerebral blood flow accompanying bicuculline-induced seizures in rats. Brain Res. **658:** 192–198
18. ALEXANDER, C.B., et al. 1998. Further studies on anti- and proconvulsant effects of inhibitors of nitric oxide synthase in rodents. Eur. J. Pharmacol. **344:** 15–25
19. KIRKBY, R.D., et al. 1996. Factors determining proconvulsant and anticonvulsant effects of inhibitors of nitric oxide synthase in rodents. Epilepsy Res. **24:** 91–100.
20. DENIZBASI, A., et al. 1999. The effect of tizanidine on maximal electroshock seizures (MES) in mice. Gen. Pharmacol. **32:** 513 516.

Agmatine Inhibits Naloxone-Induced Contractions in Morphine-Dependent Guinea Pig Ileum

FEYZA ARICIOGLU, ESER ERCIL, AND GUL DULGER

Department of Pharmacology, Faculty of Pharmacy, Marmara University, Istanbul, Turkey

ABSTRACT: This study investigates the effects of agmatine on naloxone-precipitated withdrawal syndrome in morphine-dependent guinea pig ileum. Male guinea pigs that were starved for 24 hours were decapitated after cervical dislocation, and terminal portions of the ilea were removed. Segments were fixed at a resting tension of 1 g in an organ bath containing 1×10^{-6} M morphine in Tyrode solution at 37°C, which was bubbled with 95% O_2 and 5% CO_2. Tissues were incubated in morphine containing Tyrode solution for 4 hours before agmatine was added. Naloxone and agmatine had no effect on naïve ilea. Naloxone (1×10^{-6} M) contracted morphine-dependent ilea. Agmatine significantly inhibited the contractile response to naloxone in a dose-dependent manner (1×10^{-7} M, 44%; 1×10^{-6} M, 80%; 1×10^{-5} M, 95%). This effect of agmatine was partly abolished by pretreatment with yohimbine and was almost completely abolished by idazoxan.

KEYWORDS: agmatine; morphine; imidazoline; α_2-adrenergic; NMDA; nitric oxide; ileum

INTRODUCTION

The chronic use of opioids is often accompanied by the development of tolerance to or dependence on these agents. The mechanisms involved with these phenomena are not entirely clear. Although all the mechanisms by which tolerance to and dependence on morphine have yet to be determined, a growing body of evidence suggests the participation of a nitric oxide (NO) system.[1–6] In addition, the involvement of the nitridergic system in the naloxone-precipitated withdrawal signs in animal models has been reported[7]. NOS inhibitors are known to block the development of morphine dependence.[1,7,8]

Agmatine is synthesized in brain from L-arginine by arginine decarboxylase and is biologically active in a number of neuronal and endocrine tissues. Agmatine, a guanidinium amine, is an endogenous ligand/modulator of imidazoline receptors and α_2-adrenoceptors as well as N-methyl-D-aspartate (NMDA) receptor channels.[8–10] In addition, agmatine is an endogenous inhibitor of nitric oxide synthase (NOS).[11]

Address for correspondence: Feyza Aricioglu, Ph.D., Department of Pharmacology, Faculty of Pharmacy, Marmara University, 81010 Tibbiye Cad. No: 49, Haydarpasa, Istanbul, Turkey. Voice: 0216 418 95 73; fax: 0216 345 29 52.
e-mail: feyzak@turk.net

Ann. N.Y. Acad. Sci. 1009: 147–151 (2003). © 2003 New York Academy of Sciences.
doi: 10.1196/annals.1304.016

Based on functional studies, it has been suggested that agmatine has neuromodulatory properties.[9] Recently it has been shown that agmatine attenuates the escalation of fentanyl self-administration.[12] It has been also shown that agmatine potentiates morphine analgesia[13] and attenuates all the behavioral signs of the morphine abstinence syndrome in rats.[14]

Because the inhibitory effect of agmatine on morphine dependence has been demonstrated in vivo,[14] and because of the importance of above-mentioned systems in morphine dependence, the present study was designed to investigate the effect of agmatine on morphine-dependent guinea pig ileum.

MATERIALS AND METHODS

Animals

All procedures were performed in accordance with the Guide for the Care and Use of Laboratory Animals as adopted by the National Institutes of Health (USA) and the declaration of Helsinki.

Adult male guinea pigs (300–400 g) were used in the study. They were housed in a quiet, temperature-controlled (20°C ± 2°C) and humidity-controlled (60% ± 3%) room in which a 12-hour light/dark cycle was maintained (light, 07:00–19:00). The rats were fed standard lab chow and tap water ad libitum during the study.

Drugs

Naloxone HCl and agmatine sulfate were purchased from Sigma Chemical (St. Louis, MO, USA). Morphine sulfate was purchased from the Solid Products Office from Ministry of Agriculture of Turkey. All drugs were dissolved in deionized water.

Male guinea pigs (300–400 g) were starved for 24 hours and decapitated after cervical dislocation. Terminal portions of the ilea were removed, placed in Tyrode solution (NaCl 8.0 g, KCl 0.2 g, $CaCl_2$ 0.2 g, $NaHCO_3$ 1 g, NaH_2PO_4 0.05 g, and glucose 2.0 g), and thoroughly washed by flushing Tyrode solution through the lumen. Consequently, they were cut into 5-cm segments, and these segments were mounted in 20-mL organ chambers for isometric tension measurement. The organ chambers contained Tyrode solution with 10^{-6} M morphine. The solution was gassed with 95% O_2 and 5% CO_2 during study, and the temperature was maintained at 37°C by a thermoregulatory water circuit. Each tissue was connected to a force-displacement transducer for the measurement of isometric force, which was continuously displayed. After mounting, each tissue was allowed to equilibrate with a basal tension of 1 g for 4 hours; during this time morphine containing Tyrode solution was replaced every 15 minutes with fresh solution. After the equilibration period, naloxone was added to the medium either alone or following preincubation with various concentrations of agmatine for 15 minutes. In another series of experiments, yohimbine or idazoxan was added to the tissue bath, and after 25 minutes the same protocol was repeated. One agonist or antagonist was tested in each preparation. The effects of agonists or antagonists on naloxone-induced contraction were evaluated by comparing the response before and after the addition of agonists or antagonists in the same preparation.

Statistical Analysis

Contractions were compared by ANOVA followed by paired t-test. Inhibitions (%) were compared by the Mann-Whitney U test. $P < 0.05$ was considered statistically significant.

RESULTS AND DISCUSSION

None of these agents had a contractile response on naive ilea. In the present study naloxone (10^{-6} M) had no effect on naive ilea, whereas it contracted the ilea made morphine-dependent by preincubation with morphine (10^{-6} M) for 4 hours. Agmatine also had no effect on naive ilea, but it significantly inhibited the contractile response to naloxone in a concentration-dependent manner (1×10^{-7} M, 44%; 1×10^{-6} M, 80%; 1×10^{-5} M, 95%) in morphine-dependent ilea (FIG. 1). This effect of agmatine was partly abolished by pretreatment with yohimbine, an α_2-adrenoceptor antagonist, and was abolished almost completely by idazoxan, an imidazoline and α_2-adrenoceptor antagonist (FIG. 2).

The present study demonstrates that agmatine, an arginine metabolite, has prominent inhibitory effects on naloxone-induced contractions. This inhibitory effect of agmatine on morphine dependence may be related to several mechanisms including α_2-adrenoceptors and NMDA receptors.

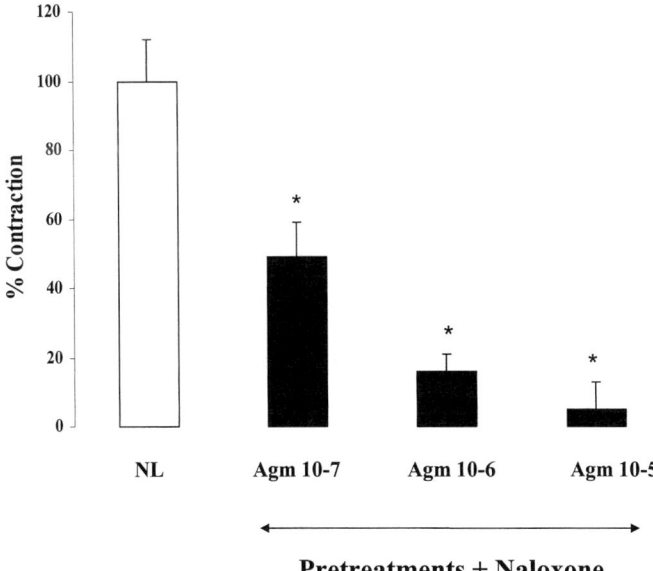

FIGURE 1. Effect of agmatine (1×10^{-7}, 1×10^{-6}, 1×10^{-5} M) on naloxone (1×10^{-6} M)-induced contractions in morphine-dependent guinea pig ileum. Data are presented as percentage of contractions (n = 8 in each group). *$P < 0.05$ compared with naloxone group. Agm, agmstine; NL, naloxone.

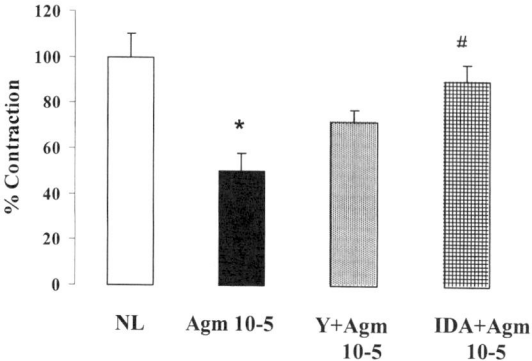

FIGURE 2. Effect of pretreatment with idaxozane (1×10^{-6} M) or yohimbine (1×10^{-6} M) on agmatine (1×10^{-5} M) response in morphine-dependent guinea pig ileum. Data are presented as percentage of contractions (n = 8 in each group). *$P < 0.05$ compared with naloxone group; #$P < 0.05$ compared with agmatine group. Agm, agmatine; IDA, idaxozane; NL, naloxone; Y, yohimbine.

Agmatine is an α_2-adrenoceptor ligand. Ligands such as clonidine that bind to these receptors also have prominent inhibitory effects on the morphine withdrawal syndrome.[15] In addition, clonidine has been reported to possess an antinociceptive action that is reversed by yohimbine and to reduce significantly the force of contractures induced by naloxone in the isolated ileum taken from morphine-dependent guinea pig.[15,16] Tizanidine, an α_2-adrenoceptor/imidazoline ligand, attenuates the intensity of naloxone-precipitated abstinence syndrome in vivo and in vitro.[17,18] Because the effect of agmatine is partly blocked by yohimbine, α_2-adrenoceptors are involved, at least in part, in the inhibitory effect of agmatine on morphine dependence in guinea pig ileum.

Another explanation of this inhibitory effect may be NOS inhibition of agmatine caused by NMDA receptor antagonism. Activation of excitatory amino acid receptors, particularly the NMDA subtype, causes an influx of calcium into neurons, leading to calmodulin-dependent activation of NOS. Thus, activation of NMDA receptors may be accompanied by formation of NO. Several studies indicate that peripheral administration of a variety of NOS inhibitors that are arginine derivatives can inhibit the development of physical dependence on morphine and attenuate symptoms of antagonist-induced withdrawal in morphine-dependent mice and rats.[18,19] Agmatine has been shown to inhibit NOS in various tissues.[11] In our previous study agmatine decreased the severity of all signs of morphine abstinence in vivo.[13,14] The existence of the NMDA in the mesenteric plexus of the guinea pig has long been known. The role of NMDA receptors and excitatory amino acid stimulation in the development of physical dependence on morphine is also well known.[20,21] The activation of NMDA receptors and enhanced sensitivity to glutamate are important components of naloxone-precipitated contractions of the guinea pig ileum after incubation with morphine.[22] Competitive and noncompetitive antagonists of NMDA inhibit naloxone-induced contractions.[23]

In conclusion, agmatine can inhibit naloxone-induced contractions in morphine-dependent ilea. This inhibitory effect of agmatine was partly abolished by pretreatment with an α_2-adrenoceptor antagonist and was almost completely abolished by an imidazoline and α_2-adrenoceptor antagonist. We believe that agmatine as an endogenous substance may have an important role in compensatory mechanisms that take place during morphine dependence.

REFERENCES

1. ADAMS, M.L., et al. 1993. Inhibition of morphine withdrawal syndrome by a nitric oxide synthase inhibitor, NG-nitro-L-arginine methyl ester. Life Sci. **52:** 245–249.
2. KOLESNIKOV, Y.A., C.G. PICK & G.W. PASTERNAK. 1992. NG-nitro-L-arginine prevents morphine tolerance. Eur. J. Pharmacol. **221:** 399–400.
3. KOLESNIKOV, Y.A., et al. 1993. Blockade of tolerance to morphine but not to κ-opioids by a nitric oxide synthase inhibitor. Proc. Natl. Acad. Sci. U. S. A. **90:** 5162–5166.
4. BHARGAVA, H.N. 1994. Nitric oxide synthase inhibition blocks tolerance to the analgesic action of kappa-opioid receptor agonist in the rat. Pharmacology **48:** 234–241.
5. BHARGAVA, H.N. 1995. Attenuation of tolerance to, and physical dependence on, morphine in the rat by inhibition of nitric oxide synthase. Gen. Pharmacol. **26:** 1049–1053.
6. BHARGAVA, H.N. & J.T. BIAN. 1998. Effects of acute administration of L-arginine on morphine antinociception and morphine distribution in central and peripheral tissues in mice. Pharmacol. Biochem. Behav. **61:** 29–33.
7. DEHPOUR, A.R., N. AKBARLOO & P. GHARFORIFAR. 1998. Endogenous nitric oxide modulates naloxone-precipitated withdrawal signs in a mouse model with acute cholestasis. Behav. Pharmacol. **9:** 77–80.
8. LI, G., et al. 1994. Agmatine: an endogenous clonidine-displacing substance in the brain. Science **263:** 966–969.
9. REIS, D.J. & S. REGUNATHAN. 2000. Is agmatine a novel neurotransmitter in brain? Trends Pharmacol. Sci. **21:** 187–193.
10. YANG, X.-C. & D.J. REIS. 1999. Agmatine selectively blocks the NMDA subclass of glutamate receptor channels in cultured mouse hippocampal neurons. J. Pharmacol. Exp. Ther. **288:** 544–549.
11. GALEA, E., et al. 1996. Inhibition of mammalian nitric oxide synthases by agmatine, an endogenous polyamine formed by decarboxylation of arginine. Biochem. J. **316:** 247–249.
12. KOLESNIKOV, Y., S. JAIN & G.W. PASTERNAK. 1996. Modulation of opioid analgesia by agmatine. Eur. J. Pharmacol. **296:** 17–22.
13. ARICIOGLU-KARTAL, F. & I.T. UZBAY. 1997. Inhibitory effect of agmatine on naloxane-precipitated abstinence syndrome. Life Sci. **61:** 1775–1781.
14. MORGAN, A.D., et al. 2002. Effects of agmatine on the escalation of intravenous cocaine and fentanyl self-administration in rats. Pharmacol. Biochem. Behav. **72:** 873–880.
15. GEORGES, F. & G. ASTON-JONES. 2003. Prolonged activation of mesolimbic dopaminergic neurons by morphine withdrawal following clonidine: participation of imidazoline and norepinephrine receptors. Neuropsychopharmacology **28:** 1140–1149.
16. JUNGNICKEL, S. & L.A. CHAHL. 2002. The effect of the naltrexone-induced withdrawal response in morphine-treated guinea-pigs. J. Pharm. Pharmacol. **54:** 127–132.
17. KOYUNCUOGLU H., et al. 1992. Effects of tizanidine on morphine physical dependence: attenuation and intensification. Pharmacol. Biochem. Behav. **42:** 693–698.
18. CUELLAR, B., et al. 2000. Up-regulation of neuronal NO synthase immunoreactivity in opiate dependence and withdrawal. Psychopharmacology **148:** 66–73.
19. THORAT, S.N., et al. 1994. Comparative effects of NG-monomethyl-L-arginine and MK-801 on the abstinence syndrome in morphine-dependent mice. Brain Res. **642:** 153–159.
20. TRUJILLO, K.A. & H. AKIL. 1994. Inhibition of opiate tolerance by non-competitive N-methyl-D-aspartate receptor antagonists. Brain Res. **633:** 178–188.
21. TRUJILLO, K.A. & H. AKIL. 1991. Inhibition of morphine tolerance and dependence by the NMDA receptor antagonist MK-801. Science **251:** 85–87.
22. KOYUNCUOGLU H., et al. 1992. Morphine and naloxone act similarly on glutamate-caused guinea pig ileum contraction. Pharmacol. Biochem. Behav. **43:** 479–482.
23. KOYUNCUOGLU, H. & F. ARICIOGLU. 1991. Previous blockade of NMDA receptors intensifies morphine dependence in rats. Pharmacol. Biochem. Behav. **39:** 575–579.

Effect of Agmatine on the Time Course of Brain Inflammatory Cytokines After Injury in Rat Pups

YANGZHENG FENG AND MICHAEL H. LeBLANC

Department of Pediatrics, University of Mississippi Medical Center, Jackson, Mississippi 39216, USA

ABSTRACT: Pro-inflammatory cytokines play an important role in brain injury. Agmatine reduces brain injury. Does agmatine act by reducing cytokines? Seven-day-old rat pups had the right carotid artery ligated and then were subjected to 2.5 hours of 8% oxygen. Agmatine (100 mg/kg) or vehicle was administered at 5 minutes after reoxygenation. Cytokines were measured in the cortex by enzyme-linked immunosorbent assay. Interleukin (IL)-6, IL-1β, and tumor necrosis factor-alpha (TNF-α) were significantly increased after reoxygenation. Agmatine had no effect.

KEYWORDS: newborn; ischemia; hypoxia; imidazoline agonist

INTRODUCTION

Inflammatory mediators play an important role in brain damage after injury. Placental infections in premature neonates correlates with the degree brain injury.[1] The pro-inflammatory cytokines interleukin-1β (IL-1β), tumor necrosis factor-α (TNF-α) and interleukin-6 (IL-6) are increased in the cerebral spinal fluid of human newborns after birth asphyxia,[2] and their concentration correlates with the degree of injury. In the newborn rat hypoxic ischemia model, leukocytes infiltrate the brain after injury and eliminating the white cells reduces the severity of injury.[3] Blocking interleukin converting enzyme, which produces IL-1β, reduces injury in adult and newborn animal stroke model.[4–6] In an adult rat focal ischemia model, blocking TNF-α will reduce brain injury while adding exogenous TNF-α will increase injury.[7] TNF-α and IL-1β both stimulate inflammation through membrane receptors that activate nuclear factor-κB[8] (NF-κB). NF-κB stimulates production of inducible nitric oxide synthase and other compounds.[9,10] We have shown that agmatine, the endogenous neurotransmitter of the imidazoline receptors,[11] given after reoxygenation prevents hypoxic-ischemic brain injury in the newborn rat model and eliminates the inducible nitric oxide synthase-related peak in nitric oxide production that occurs 3 to 6 hours after reoxygenation.[12] Since treatment with blockers of nitric oxide synthase are ineffectual when given after reoxygenation in the newborn rat,[13] how then does agmatine protect against brain damage? Blocking inducible nitric oxide synthase activity prior

Address for correspondence: Michael H. LeBlanc, M.D., University of Mississippi Medical Center, 2500 North State Street, Jackson, MS 39216, USA. Voice: 601-984-5260; fax: 601-815-3666.
e-mail: mleblanc@ped.umsmed.edu

to injury in newborn rats,[14] or after injury in adult rats[15] is neuroprotective. Perhaps increases in IL-1β, IL-6 and TNF-α both stimulate nitric oxide production and increase the severity of brain injury by different mechanisms. Does agmatine reduce these pro-inflammatory cytokines? In order to better understand the role of IL-1β and IL-6, and TNF-α in hypoxic-ischemic brain injury in the newborn rat model, we measured the time course of changes in TNF-α, IL-1β, and IL-6 after hypoxia-ischemia brain injury using the well-described Rice model.[16]

METHODS

Animal Protocol

Seven-day-old Sprague-Dawley (Harlan Sprague Dawley, Indianapolis, IN) rat pups of either sex, weighing between 12 and 17 g, were anesthetized with isoflurane (4% induction, 2% maintenance). The right common carotid artery was exposed, isolated and doubly ligated. After surgery, the rat pups were returned to their dams for 2- to 3-hour recovery. Pups were then placed in sealed jars in a 37°C water bath and subjected to a warmed, humidified mix of 8% oxygen and 92% nitrogen delivered at 4 L/minutes for 2.5 hours. After this hypoxic exposure, pups were returned to their dams and allowed to recover.

Pups from each litter were randomly assigned to a vehicle group or for treatment with agmatine sulfate salt (Sigma Chemical Company, St. Louis, MO). Agmatine in doses of 100 mg/kg was dissolved in 0.9% saline and administered by intraperitoneal injection (i.p.) at 5 minutes after hypoxia exposure. The vehicle group was given a similar volume of 0.9% saline alone. These doses were chosen as most effective from our previous experiments.[13]

Measurement of Cytokine

Pups were randomly assigned to an untreated sham group ($n = 11$), a vehicle group treatment with saline and subjected to hypoxia and ischemia ($n = 38$), or treatment with agmatine at a dose of 100 mg/kg ($n = 26$) at 5 minutes after hypoxia, and sampled at 0.5, 3, 4.5, 6, and 12 hours after hypoxia. At each time point, the pups were decapitated, brains were removed, and each side of the cerebral cortex was dissected on ice and frozen at −80°C. Brain samples were later homogenized in ice cold buffer as described by Tha et al.[16] Total protein was mechanically dissociated from tissue using an ultrasonic cell disrupter. The sonicated samples were immediately centrifuged at 20,000× g for 30 minutes at 4°C and supernatants were removed and stored at −80°C until an enzyme-linked immunosorbent assay (ELISA) was performed.[17] Samples were normalized for protein concentration. The ELISAs for rat IL-1β, IL-6, and TNF-α were performed using antibodies and other materials from R&D Systems (Minneapolis, MN, USA).

Statistics

All data are presented as mean ± SEM and the statistical significance of differences between groups were determined using multivariant analysis and only where there was overall statistical significance seen were individual values compared.

Dunnett's test was used to compare other time points to shams and the Student *t*-test was used to compare left (no carotid ligation) and right hemispheres (carotid ligation). Differences were considered significant at $P < 0.05$.

RESULTS AND DISCUSSION

There were no significant group differences between the agmatine and the vehicle groups for IL-1β, IL-6, or TNF-α. Differences with time were highly significant,

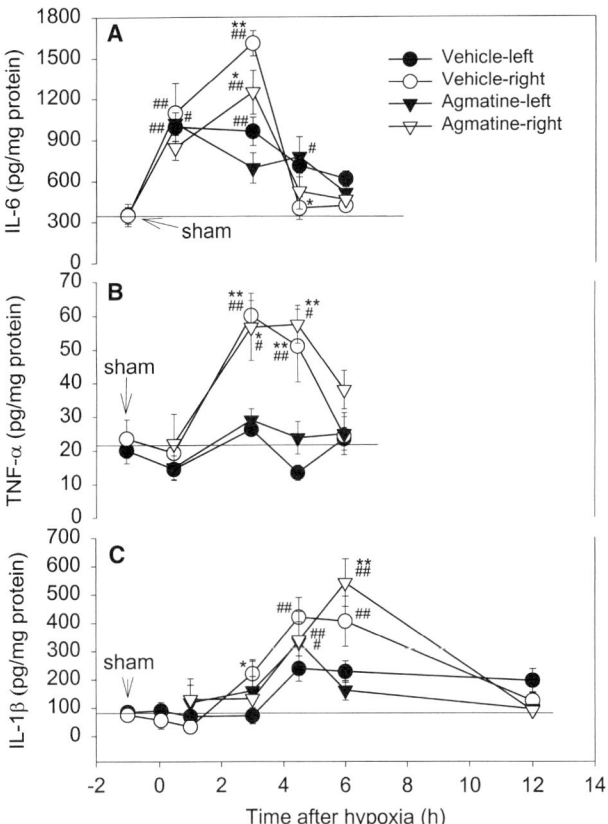

FIGURE 1. Changes in interleukin (IL)-6 (**A**), tumor necrosis factor-alpha (TNF-α; **B**), and IL-1β (**C**) caused by hypoxic ischemic brain injury (right side, open symbols) or hypoxia alone (left side, filled symbols). Pups were treatment with 100 mg/kg of agmatine (triangles), or vehicle (circles) i.p. 5 minutes after reoxygenation. Data are presented as mean ± SEM. Agmatine had no significant effect on the time coarse of the brain levels of the three proinflammatory cytokines. IL-6 was elevated first, followed TNF-α, with IL-1β the most delayed. The return to baseline followed the same order. Hypoxia alone without ischemia significantly increased IL-6, but not IL-1β, or TNF-α. Hypoxia alone does not cause brain injury.[16] # $P < 0.05$ vs. sham, ## $P < 0.01$ vs. sham, * $P < 0.05$ vs. left side, ** $P < 0.01$ vs. left side.

$P < 0.0001$, for all three cytokines. Differences between hemisphere were also significant (IL-1β, $P < 0.0025$; IL-6, $P < 0.01$; and TNF-α, $P < 0.0002$; FIG. 1).

Agmatine has no effect on brain levels of IL-1β, IL-6, or TNF-α. Therefore, the neuroprotective effect of agmatine is not related to changes in these three cytokines. Szaflarski et al.[18] measured mRNA for IL-1β and TNF-α in the Rice model and found elevated levels at 4 hours after reoxygenation but not at 0 or 8 hours. Hagberg et al.[5] found an increase in IL-1 and IL-6 by bioassay at 6 hours after hypoxia. IL-1 was elevated from 3 to 48 hours while IL-6 was significantly elevated only at 6 hours. There are reports of dissociation between transcription and translation for IL-1β[19] and TNF-α.[20] Our findings are similar to those previously reported, but the more accurate ELISA technique allows the sequential rise and fall of the three cytokines, IL-6 followed by TNF-α, followed by IL-1β to be seen. Is this a cascade with each cytokine stimulating the production or release of the subsequent members? Both IL-1β and TNF-α are thought to simulate production of IL-6 rather than the other way around.[21] TNF-α can stimulate production of IL-1β.[21]

TNF-α levels were significantly elevated in the brain from 3- to 5-hours postinjury, IL-1β between 4.5 and 6 hours after injury, and IL-6 levels from 0.5 to 3 hours after injury. There is a peak in nitric oxide production 3 to 6 hours after reoxygenation, that is thought to be from NF-κB activation.[9] This peak is suppressible by inhibitors of inducible nitric oxide syntheses[22] or inhibitors of sphingomylinase.[23] Imidazoline receptors are present on astrocytes.[24] Agmatine can inhibit inducible nitric oxide synthase in cultured astrocytes stimulated with TNF-α, and IL-1β.[24]

The elevation of the inflammatory mediators is occurring at approximately the same time as the early mediators of the apoptotic system are being activated, at least in thalamus in this model.[25] Since TNF-α can activate the caspase system through caspase-8, which activates caspase-3, this association may not coincidental.

Hypoxic ischemic injury in the newborn rat causes a brief elevation in inflammatory cytokines that begins 0.5 hour after injury and has returned to normal by 12 hours. Agmatine does not affect this process.

REFERENCES

1. MURPHY, D.J., et al. 1995. Case control study of antenatal and intrapartum risk factors for cerebral palsy in very preterm singleton babies. Lancet **346:** 1449–1454.
2. SAVMAN, K., et al. 1998. Cytokine response in cerebrospinal fluid after birth asphyxia. Pediatr. Res. **43:** 746–751.
3. HUDOME, S., et al. 1997. The role of neutrophils in the production of hypoxic-ischemic brain injury in the newborn rat. Pediatr. Res. **41:** 607–616.
4. FREIDLANDER, R.M., et al. 1997. Expression of dominant negative mutant of ICE in transgenic mice prevents neuronal death induced by trophic factor withdrawal and ischemic brain injury. J. Exp. Med. **185:** 933–940.
5. MARTIN, D., N. CHINOOKOSWONG & G. MILLER. 1994. The interleukin-1 receptor antagonist (rhIL-1ra) protects against cerebral infarction in a rat model of hypoxia-ischemia. Exp. Neurol. **130:** 362–367.
6. HAGBERG, H., et al. 1996. Enhanced expression of interleukin (IL)-1 and IL-6 messenger RNA and bioactive protein after hypoxia-ischemia in neonatal rats. Pediatr. Res. **40:** 603–609.
7. BARONE, F.C., et al. 1997. Tumor necrosis factor-α: A mediator of focal ischemic brain injury. Stroke **28:** 1233–1244.
8. ALLAN, S.M. & N.J. ROTHWELL. 2001. Cytokines and acute neurodegeneration. Nature Rev. Neurosci. **2:** 734–744.

9. GRISCAVAGE, J.M., S. WILKS & L.J. IGNARRO. 1995. Serine and cysteine proteinase inhibitors prevent nitric oxide production by activated macrophages by interfering with signal transcription of the inducible NO synthase gene. Biochem. Biophys. Res. Com. **215:** 721–729.
10. RUETTEN, H. & C. THIEMERMANN. 1997. Effect of calpain inhibitor 1, an inhibitor of the proteolysis of IκB, on the circulatory failure and multiple organ dysfunction caused by endotoxin in the rat. Br. J. Pharmacol. **121:** 695–704.
11. FENG, Y.Z., J.E. PILETZ & M.H. LEBLANC. 2002. Agmatine suppresses nitric oxide production and attenuates hypoxic-ischemic brain injury in neonatal rats. Pediatr. Res. **52:** 606–611.
12. XIAO, F., et al. 1998. Post-treatment with NOS inhibitors and hypoxic-ischemic brain injury in newborn rats [abstract]. Soc. Neurosci. **24:** 1234.
13. TSUJI, M., et al. 2000. Protective effect of aminoguanidine on hypoxic-ischemic brain damage and temporal profile of brain nitric oxide in neonatal rat. Pediatr. Res. **47:** 79–83.
14. ZHANG, F., et al. 1996. Aminoguanidine ameoliorates and L-arginine worsens brain damage from intraluminal middle cerebral artery occlusion. Stroke **27:** 317–323.
15. RICE, J.E., R.C. VANNUCCI & J.B. BRIERLEY. 1981. The influence of immaturity on hypoxic-ischemic brain damage in the rat. Anal. Neurol. **9:** 131–141.
16. THA, K.K., et al. 2000. Changes in expressions of proinflammatory cytokines IL-1β, TNF-α, and IL-6 in the brain of senescence accelerated mouse (SAM) P8. Brain Res. **885:** 25–31.
17. BRADFORD, M.M. 1976. A rapid and sensitive method for quantitation of microgram quantities of protein utilizing the principle of protein dye binding. Anal. Biochem. **72:** 248–254.
18. SZAFLARSKI, J., D. BURTRUM & F.S. SILVERSTEIN. 1995. Cerebral hypoxia ischemia stimulates cytokine gene expression in perinatal rats. Stroke **26:** 1093–1100.
19. SCHINDLER, R., B.D. CLARK & C.A. DINARELLO. 1990. Dissociation between interleukin-1β mRNA and protein synthesis in human peripheral blood mononuclear cells. J. Biol. Chem. **265:** 10232–10237.
20. SCHINDLER, R., J.A. GELFAND & C.A. DINARELLO. 1990. Recombinant C5a stimulates transcription rather than translation of IL-1 and TNF; cytokine synthesis by LPS, IL-1 or PMA. Blood **76:** 1631–1638.
21. ST. PIERRE, B.A., J.E. MERRILL & J.M. DOPP. 1996. Effects of cytokines on CNS cells: Glia. In Cytokines and the CNS. R.M. Ransohoff & E.N. Benveniste, Eds.: 151–168. CRC Press. New York, NY.
22. HIGUCI, Y., et al. 1998. Increase in nitric oxide in the hypoxic-ischemic neonatal rat brain a suppression by 7-nitroindazole and aminoguanidine. Eur. J. Pharmacol. **342:** 47–49.
23. LEBLANC, M.H., Y.Z. FENG & J.D. FRATKIN. 2000. TPCK pretreatment reduces hypoxic ischemic brain injury in the newborn rat. Eur. J. Pharmacol. **390:** 249–256.
24. REGUNATHAN, S., D.L. FEINSTEIN & D.J. REISS. 1999. Imidazolin receptors and their endogenous ligands: Current concepts and therapeutic potential. Ann. N. Y. Acad. Sci. **881:** 410–419.
25. NORTHINGTON, F.J., D.M. FERRIERO & L.J. MARTIN. 2001. Neurodegeneration in the thalmus following neonatal hypoxia-ischemia is programmed cell death. Dev. Neurosci. **23:** 186–191.

Endogenous β-Carbolines as Clonidine-Displacing Substances

E.S.J. ROBINSON,[a] N.J. ANDERSON,[a] J. CROSBY,[b] D.J. NUTT,[a] AND A.L. HUDSON[a]

[a]*Psychopharmacology Unit, School of Medical Sciences, University Walk, Bristol BS8 1TD, UK*

[b]*School of Chemistry, School of Medical Sciences, Bristol BS8 1TD, UK*

ABSTRACT: Endogenous β-carbolines, such as harmane, are known to occur in mammalian species including humans. Radioligand binding studies have revealed that certain β-carbolines display high affinity for both I_1 and I_2 imidazoline-binding sites (IBS). Functional studies have shown that the β-carboline harmane elicits many characteristics expected of an endogenous ligand IBS. This article discusses the evidence relating to β-carbolines as endogenous ligands and presents a case for harmane and related compounds as endogenous ligands for IBS.

KEYWORDS: β-carboline; clonidine-displacing substance (CDS); harmane

INTRODUCTION

In 1999, Hudson and coworkers[1] reported that certain β-carbolines display high affinity for imidazoline-binding sites (IBS). In a subsequent publication, Husbands *et al.*[2] also reported that a number of β-carbolines display high affinity for I_1- and I_2-binding sites. It was particularly interesting that some of the β-carbolines that were shown to have high affinity also occur endogenously in mammalian tissue,[3] raising the possibility that harmane, norharmane, and tetrahydro-norharmane (THN) may represent endogenous ligands for IBS.

Since the discovery of the IBS, a number of candidates have been put forward as endogenous clonidine-displacing substances (CDS). The first studies of CDS described an impure extract isolated from calf brain.[4] The fact that this extract was able to displace [^{3}H]clonidine fully from rat brain membranes suggested the extract contained an endogenous ligand for IBS.[4] Since then, a number of different candidates have been put forward as CDSs. The first substance identified as a CDS was agmatine, which was extracted using a modified CDS-extraction procedure.[5] Agmatine, however, does not meet many of the criteria for classical CDS and is unlikely to represent the active component of the original extract. Further studies have since identified imidazoleacetic acid-ribotide as a CDS, but, again, this substance is not believed to represent the active component of classical CDS.[6] Research in our laboratory has

Address for correspondence: A.L. Hudson, Psychopharmacology Unit, School of Medical Sciences, University Walk, Bristol BS8 ITD, UK. Voice: (+44) 117 928 8608; fax: (+44) 117 928 9700.
e-mail: a.l.hudson@bristol.ac.uk

recently identified β-carbolines within the active fraction of bovine lung CDS (J. Crosby. 2003. Harmane and harmalan are active constituents of bovine lung CDS [unpublished report]). This paper discusses recent findings in relation to identification of the active component of classical CDS and the evidence supporting the β-carbolines as endogenous ligands at IBS.

CLASSICAL CDS

Atlas and Burnstein[4,7] undertook the first experiments to ascertain whether there was an endogenous compound that had clonidine-like activity. A methanolic extraction of rat[7] and bovine[4] brain, followed by reverse-phase high performance liquid chromatography (RP-HPLC) purification yielded a partially purified extract exhibiting such activity. This substance, termed classical CDS, was divided into the crude and the RP-HPLC–pure forms.

Research in our laboratory has been aimed at identifying the structure of the active component of classical CDS. Using the method described by Singh and coworkers,[8] a crude methanolic extract from bovine lung was prepared, and, when the preparation was run on a reverse-phase C_{18} column with a methanolic gradient, a three-peak profile as described by Atlas and Burnstein was demonstrated.[4] Using radioligand binding studies, the elution time of the active fraction was ascertained, and electrospray mass spectroscopy was used to determine mass fragmentation patterns and structural properties. Using this technique, tryptophan was identified as an inactive contaminant of CDS.[9] Subsequent studies also identified an inactive β-carboline, 1-carboxyl tetrahydro-β-carboline. These substances made it difficult to detect and identify other molecules that were eluting in the active fraction but at significantly lower levels. A number of potential candidates were run on HPLC, and a β-carboline, harmalan was shown to elute within the active fraction. The extraction procedure was subsequently revised and optimized for the detection of β-carbolines. Both harmane and harmalan were shown to be present in bovine lung.

ENDOGENOUS β-CARBOLINES

The nomenclature used for β-carbolines can be confusing. The original chemical names, originating from 9H-pyrido [3,4-b] indoles, have been replaced by the β-carboline terminology. In this report the harmalan nomenclature and numbering of carbon and nitrogen atoms is used as illustrated in FIGURE 1.

There is no doubt that the beta-carbolines, harmane, harmalan, tetrahydroharmane (THN), and norharmane, display high affinity for IBS, but the question still remains as to whether they are truly endogenous substances. Furthermore, there would need to be some level of regulation present if these substances were involved in a neuromodulatory or hormonal role. Detailed studies quantifying endogenous β-carbolines have shown regional differences in their distribution as well as changes in their levels under different circumstances. Their endogenous formation, however, has been a subject for debate.

The first endogenous β-carboline, pinoline, (6-methoxy-tetrahydro-β-carboline), was identified from pineal gland tissue by McIsaac in 1961.[10] Since its discovery

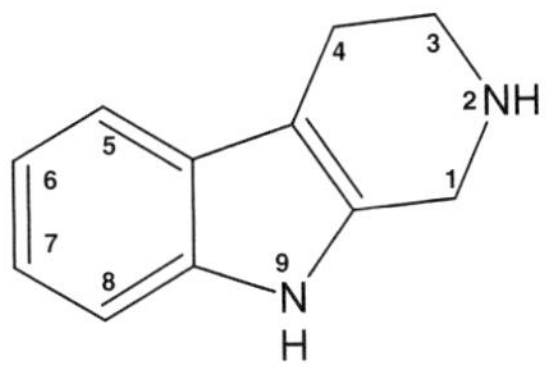

FIGURE 1. Structure of norharmane (β-carboline) and standard numbering of carbon and nitrogen atoms. Harmane has a methyl substitution at the 1 position, which is known to increase binding to MAO-A, whereas substitutions at the 5, 6, and 7 position are associated with I_2 binding.

various extraction, detection, and quantification methods have been used to characterize these substances in biological samples (TABLE 1). Unfortunately, the study of β-carbolines has been complicated because they can be readily formed artifactually. Bosin and coworkers[20] found that a significant amount of artifact β-carboline, 6-methoxy-tetrahydroharmane, could be formed from the condensation of endogenous serotonin (5-HT) with exogenous formaldehyde in the dichloromethane organic solvent. Bosin also showed that many research groups were not using aldehyde-trapping reagents, such as semicarbazide, or ensuring that the organic solvents used were aldehyde-free.[20] This demonstration prompted a review of the procedures to minimize artifactual β-carboline formation and demonstrate that the compounds identified were truly endogenous substances and not artifacts of the extraction procedure. To date, endogenous levels of harmane, harmalan, norharmane, and several tetra-hydroβ-carbolines have been quantified in mammalian tissues (TABLE 1).

TABLE 1. Identification of endogenous β-carbolines in mammalian tissue

β-Carboline	Tissue	Detection Method	Ref.
Harmane	Rat arcuate nucleus	Spectral studies and TLC	11
	Human platelets	TLC, UV, fluorimetry, GC-MS	12
		C18 RP-HPLC and fluorometric detection	13
Norharmane	Human plasma	HPLC with fluorometric detection	14
	Rat plasma, brain, liver, kidney, spleen, heart and lung		15
THN	Rat forebrain	TLC and GC-MS	16
	Rat brain	GC-MS	17
	Human platelets	GC-MS	3
6-MeO-THN	Rat arcuate nucleus	Spectral studies and TLC	18
	Rat brain	GC-MS	17
	Rat adrenal gland		
	Pineal Gland	GC-MS	19

Abbreviations: TLC, thin-layer chromatography; GC-MS, gas chromatography-mass spectroscopy; HPLC, high-performance liquid chromatography; RP, reverse phase; UV, ultraviolet.

IN VIVO SYNTHESIS OF β-CARBOLINES

Evidence from in vitro studies has shown that β-carbolines are formed spontaneously through the Pictet-Spengler cyclization of indolamines with carbonyl-containing compounds such as formaldehyde.[21] Therefore, stimulation of pathways in vivo that lead to the formation of formaldehyde and acetaldehyde could result in increased synthesis of β-carbolines.[22] An alternative route for synthesis, using glyoxylic acid, results in the rapid formation of β-carbolines from tryptamine.[3] Pyruvic acid is closely related to glyoxylic acid and occurs in mammalian tissues. In the presence of a monoamine oxidase inhibitor, [^{3}H]typtamine and pyruvic acid were shown to form β-carbolines in vivo (FIG. 2). This process seemed to be enzymatic, because it did not occur in vitro under pseudophysiologic conditions.[23,24] Taken together, these data showed that some of the β-carbolines of high affinity for IBS exist endogenously in mammalian tissues. Formation of these substances may be enzymatic, although the mechanisms have yet to be elucidated.

BINDING AND SIGNALLING

The pharmacology of β-carbolines is complex because they are known to bind to many different sites within mammalian tissue (TABLE 2). Studies investigating the existence of an endogenous ligand for the benzodiazepine site identified β-carboline 3-carboxylic acid ethyl ester (β-CCE), a substance later shown to be an artifact of

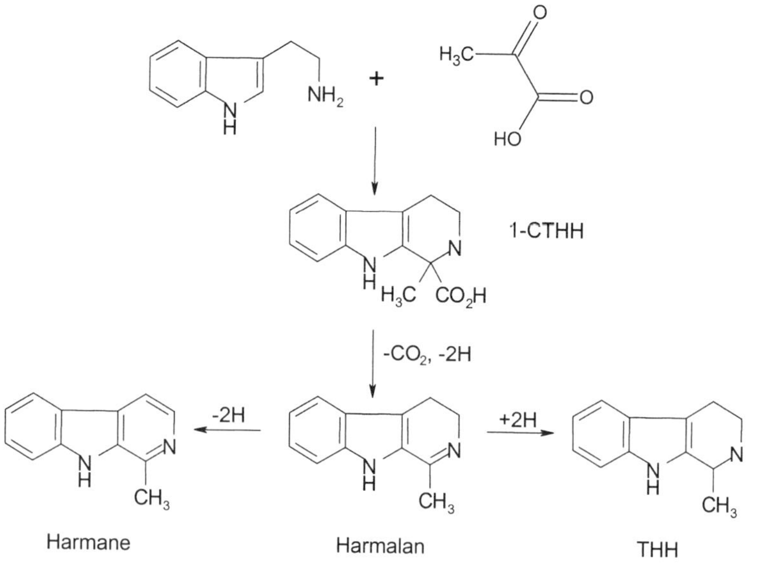

FIGURE 2. Proposed synthetic pathway for endogenous β-carbolines from tryptamine and pyruvic acid through the intermediate products 1-carboxyl-tetrahydroharmane (1-CTHH) and harmalan.

TABLE 2. Examples of endogenous β-carboline binding sites

Binding Site	Compound and Affinity	Ref.
Benzodiazepine site	Harmane and norharmane (MA)	25, 26
MAO-A	Harmane (HA), norharmane (MA)	27
MAO-B	Norharmane (HA), harmane (MA)	27
Monoamine re-uptake sites	THN (MA), Pinoline (MA)	28, 29
G-proteins	Harmane, norharmane and THN (MA)	30, 31
Cytochrome P-450	Norharmane (HA)	32
DNA intercalation	Harmol>harmine>harmaline>harmane>norharmane	33
Unknown	Norharmane (HA)	34

Abbreviations: HA, high affinity (<100 nM); MA, moderate affinity (100 nM–100 μM).

the extraction procedure. The endogenous β-carbolines have moderate affinity at the benzodiazepine site, but they show interaction with aspects of monoamine neurotransmission. Harmane and other β-carbolines with a methyl substitution in the 1 position are inhibitors of monoamine oxidase (MAO) A.[27] In addition, affinity for the 5-HT reuptake site has been reported for THN and pinoline.[28,29] It is unlikely that concentrations of endogenous β-carbolines are high enough for these targets to represent their primary sites of action. Furthermore, radioligand-binding studies have suggested that harmane and norharmane bind to an unknown high-affinity site in the brain[34] and adrenal glands.[27] In 1997, Lichtenberg-Kraag and coworkers[30] showed that harmane and norharmane could activate small G-proteins in a human neuroblastoma cell line and that this effect was dose-dependent with a bell-shaped dose-response curve. The SHSY5Y cell expressed a high-affinity [^{3}H]norharmane site, and it has been concluded that activation of this β-carboline receptor facilitates phosphoinositide-specific phospholipase C activation by the muscarinic agonist carbachol.[30] In a different study, norharmane and harmane were shown to activate G-proteins in a receptor-independent manner with EC_{50} values of 60 μM and 300 μM, respectively.[31] Unfortunately, no further studies into the signaling mechanisms of endogenous β-carbolines have been reported.

FUNCTIONAL CHARACTERISTICS OF IBS AND ENDOGENOUS β-CARBOLINES

The β-carbolines have been shown to induce a diverse range of functional effects often attributed to the inhibition of MAO-A. The β-carbolines are selective inhibitors of MAO-A and, with the exception of norharmane, are only weak inhibitors of MAO-B.[27] As a consequence of their interactions with the MAOs, many of the functional properties associated with endogenous β-carbolines can be attributed to modulation of noradrenaline, dopamine, and 5-HT. Many of the β-carbolines found in plants are also potent monoamine receptor ligands.[35] Their binding to 5-HT$_{2A}$ receptors is associated with hallucinations.[35] Among the brain β-carbolines, only pinoline is believed to be hallucinogenic, perhaps because of its high affinity for the 5-HT re-uptake site.[30]

TABLE 3. Summary of functional data for endogenous β-carbolines and IBS

	Ref.
Harmane, norharmane, 1-methyl harmane and tetrahydro-β-carboline displace [^{3}H]2-BFI and/or [^{3}H]clonidine with low nanomolar affinity.	1
IBS ligand, 2-BFI and harmane interact in vivo to modulate body temperature.	Fig. 3
Harmane induces a hypotensive response when injected into the rostrolateral ventrolateral medulla of rats, an effect which is antagonized by the mixed I_1–$α_2$AR antagonist efaroxan.	36
Harmane, norharmane, and harmaline substitute for 2-BFI in the rat drug discrimination paradigm.	37
Harmane and imidazoline ligands modulate monoamine levels in specific brain areas.	38, 39
Norharmane and the selective IBS ligand, BU224, reduce parameters associated with morphine withdrawal syndrome.	39, 40
Harmane is found in high density in the arcuate nucleus, a region of the hypothalamus associated with IBS.	11, 41
Harmane and norharmane bind to a high (nanomolar)-affinity site in the brain, which is not MAO.	34
Harmane and atypical 'I_3' ligands modulate insulin secretion.	44
Harmane and THN modulate food intake.	45, 46

Several studies have investigated the possibility that harmane is an endogenous ligand for IBS, and many aspects of harmane, norharmane, and THN pharmacology overlap with that describing IBS ligands (TABLE 3). Harmane has been shown to induce a hypotensive effect in spontaneously hypertensive rats following central administration.[36] This hypotensive effect was fully reversed by the mixed I_1/$α_2$-adrenoceptor antagonist, efaroxan. In this study harmane was equipotent with the positive control clonidine but lacked the tachycardiac effects seen with the mixed I_1-/$α_2$-adrenoceptor agonist.[36] Previous studies have shown that certain β-carbolines effect cardiovascular parameters,[42] but this study was the first demonstration of direct antagonism of a β-carboline–mediated effect by an imidazoline ligand.

Studies in our laboratory have investigated the ability of an I_2-selective ligand, 2-BFI, to antagonize the hypothermic response induced by harmane (FIG. 3). Previous studies had shown that harmane induces a hypothermic response, which is not mediated by inhibition of MAO.[38] Results from our laboratory have shown that 2-BFI pretreatment can significantly attenuate the hypothermic response induced by harmane (10 mg kg^{-1}). At present, the mechanisms underlying this response are not clear but may relate to an interaction with monoaminergic systems. Studies using other I_2-selective ligands and a number of different β-carbolines have shown that both classes of compounds can modulate monoamine levels in vivo.[38,39]

Other functional effects mediated by IBS include modulation of food intake and regulation of insulin secretion.[43] The I_3 site is associated with potentiation of insulin secretion, and harmane has been shown to induce insulin secretion.[44] Furthermore,

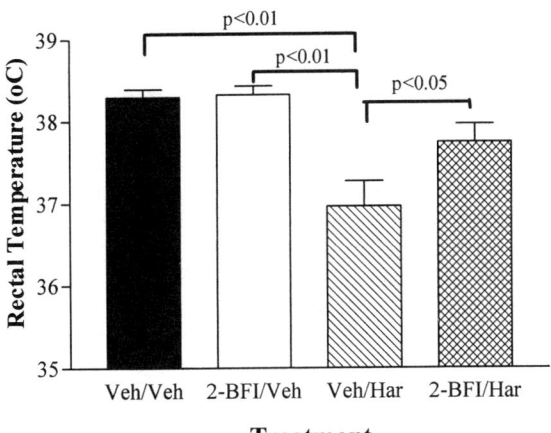

FIGURE 3. Effect of 2-BFI (10mg kg^{-1}) pretreatment on harmane- (10mg kg^{-1})–induced hypothermia, 15 minutes after Harmane administration. Data shown as mean ± SE mean for 9–10 animals per group; statistical comparison made using a one-way ANOVA with Tukey's test post hoc.

when given to rats, harmane and THN inhibit food intake in a dose-dependent manner.[45,46] These results suggest a role for endogenous β-carbolines in regulating food intake and energy homeostasis.

The β-carbolines have also been extensively studied in relation to their mutagenesis and toxicity.[47,48] Mutagenic and comutagenic properties have been reported for harmane and norharmane. The mutagenic and comutagenic properties of harmane, norharmane, and related compounds are associated with their interaction with DNA and enzymatic systems such as cytochrome P-450.[48] The β-carbolines are also likely to modify and increase genotoxic and toxic consequences of other compounds.[48] In relation to neurotoxicity, the β-carbolinium cations formed enzymatically from harmane and norharmane are of particular interest. β-carboline N-methyltransferase is found in mammalian brain and catalyses the 2N-methylation of simple β-carbolines. The resulting products, 2N-methylated β-carbolinium cations, are structural and functional analogues of the neurotoxic agent MPP$^+$. As such, these compounds have been investigated as factors involved in the etiology of Parkinson's disease.[47] In a recent study, significant increases in β-carboline 9N-methyltransferase activity were observed in postmortem examinations of the frontal cortex of Parkinson's disease patients.[49] The mechanism by which these neurotoxic agents are associated with the pathogenesis of Parkinson's disease is not known, but interaction between N-methylated β-carbolines and specific cellular proteins has been reported.[50] Further investigations will determine the significance of these findings.

DISCUSSION

Two endogenous β-carbolines, harmane and harmalan, are active constituents of bovine lung CDS and probably represent the active component of classical CDS described by Atlas and Burnstein.[4] The procedure for preparing classical CDS involved the heating of tissue and was likely to result in the further production of β-carbolines by spontaneous formation. Therefore the original extraction protocols may have resulted in high levels of artifactual β-carbolines. Future studies of CDS should strive to use extraction protocols that prevent artifactual formation of β-carbolines. Several different research groups have shown that a number of different β-carbolines can be extracted from mammalian tissues and that these β-carbolines represent endogenous molecules. Furthermore, mechanisms for their endogenous synthesis, source, and site of action have been hypothesized. Taken together, these substances and the IBS represent a novel neuroendocrine system. Future studies of β-carbolines and IBS in combination should provide greater insight into the existence and importance of this proposed system.

ACKNOWLEDGMENTS

This work was funded by the Wellcome Trust and Roche Biosciences, Palo Alto, CA, USA.

REFERENCES

1. HUDSON, A.L., *et al*. 1999. Harmane, norharmane and tetrahydro-β-carboline have high affinity for rat imidazoline binding sites. Br. J. Pharmacol. **126:** 2P.
2. HUSBANDS, S.M. 2001. β-Carboline binding to imidazoline receptors. Drug Alcohol Depend. **64:** 203–208.
3. AIRAKSINEN, M.M. & I. KARI. 1981. β-Carbolines, psychoactive compounds in the mammalian body. Part I: occurrence, origin and metabolism. Med. Biol. **59:** 21–34.
4. ATLAS, D. & Y. BURNSTEIN. 1984. Isolation and partial purification of clonidine-displacing endogenous brain substance. Eur. J. Biochem. **144:** 287–293.
5. LI, G., *et al*. 1994. Agmatine: an endogenous clonidine-displacing substance in the brain. Science **263:** 966–969.
6. PRELL, G.D., *et al*. 2003. Imidazoleacetic acid-ribotide is an endogenous imidazoline receptor (IR) ligand. Presented at the Fourth International Symposium on Agmatine and Imidazoline Systems, San Diego, April 2003.
7. ATLAS, D. & Y. BURNSTEIN. 1984. Isolation of an endogenous clonidine-displacing substance from rat brain. FEBS Lett. **170:** 387–390.
8. SINGH, G., *et al*. 1995. Evidence for the presence of a non-catecholamine, clonidine-displacing substance in crude, methanolic extracts of bovine brain and lung. Naunyn-Schmiedberg's Arch. Pharmacol. **351:** 17–26.
9. PARKER, C.A., *et al*. 1999. Tryptophan: a distinct but biologically inactive component of clonidine-displacing substance. Br. J. Pharmacol. **127:** 72P.
10. MC ISSAC, W.M. 1961. Formation of 1-methyl-6-methoxy-1,2,3,4-tetrahydro-2-carboline under physiological conditions. Biochem. Biophys. Acta **52:** 607–609.
11. SHOEMAKER, D.W., *et al*. 1980. Identification of harmane in the rat arcuate nucleus. Naunyn-Schmiedeberg's Arch. Pharmacol. **310:** 227–230.
12. BIDDER, T.G., *et al*. 1980. Harmane in human platelets. Life Sci. **25:** 157–164.
13. ZHENG, W., *et al*. 2000. Determination of harmane and harmine in human blood using reversed-phased high performance liquid chromatography and fluorescence detection. Anal. Biochem. **279:** 125–129.
14. FEKKES, D. & W.T. BODE. 1993. Occurrence and partition of the β-carboline norharmane in rat organs. Life Sci. **52:** 2045–2054.
15. FEKKES, D., *et al*. 1992. Norharmane, a normal body constituent. Lancet **339:** 506.
16. HONECKER, H. & H. ROMMELSPACHER. 1978. Tetrahydroharmane (tetrahydro-β-carboline), a physiologically occurring compound of indole metabolism. Naunyn Schmiedeberg's Arch. Pharmacol. **305:** 135–141.

17. BARKER, S.A., et al. 1979. Identification and quantification of 1,2,3,4-tetrahydro-β-carboline, 2-methyl-1,2,3,4-tetrahydro-β-carboline, and 6-methoxy-1,2,3,4-tetrahydro-β-carboline as *in vivo* constituents of rat brain and adrenal gland. Biochem. Pharmacol. **30:** 9–17.
18. SHOEMAKER, D.W., J.T. CUMMINS & T.G. BIDDER. 1978. β-carbolines in rat arcuate nucleus. Neurosci. **3:** 233–239.
19. KARI, I., et al. 1983. Mass spectrometric identification of 6-methoxy-1,2,3,4-tetrahydro-β-carboline in pineal gland. In Recent Developments in Biochemistry, Medicine and Environmental Research. Vol 8: 19–24. Elsevier. Amsterdam, The Netherlands.
20. BOSIN, T.R., et al. 1983. Presence of formaldehyde in biological media and organic solvents: artifactual formation of tetra-hydro-β-carbolines. Analyt. Biochem. **128:** 287–293.
21. BROSSI, A. 1993. Mammalian alkaloids II. In The Alkaloids. G.A. Cordell, Ed.: 119–183. Academic Press. New York, NY.
22. ROMMELSPACHER, H., et al. 1976. On the mode of formation of tetrahydro-β-carbolines. Life Sci. **18:** 81–88.
23. SUSILO, R. & H. ROMMELSPACHER. 1987. Formation of a β-carboline (1,2,3,4-tetrahydro-1-methyl-β-carboline-1-carboxylic acid) following intracerebro-ventricular injection of tryptamine and pyruvic acid. Naunyn-Schmiedeberg's Arch. Pharmacol. **335:** 70–76.
24. SUSILO, R. & H. ROMMELSPACHER. 1988. Formation of 1-methyl-β-carbolines in rats from their possible carboxylica acid precursor. Naunyn-Schmiedeberg's Arch. Pharmacol. **335:** 566–571.
25. ROMMELSPACHER, H., et al. 1980. 1-Methyl-β-carboline (harmane) a potent inhibitor of bezodiadepine receptor binding. Naunyn Schmiedeberg's Arch. Pharmacol. **314:** 97–100.
26. MORIN, A.M., I.A. TANKAA & C.G. WASTERLAIN. 1981. Norharmane inhibition of [^{3}H]-diazepam binding in mouse brain. Life Sci. **28:** 2257–2263.
27. MAY, T., et al. 1994. Comparison of the *in vitro* binding characteristics of the β-carbolines harmane and norharmane in rat brain and liver and bovine adrenal medulla. Naunyn Schmiedeberg's Arch. Pharmacol. **349:** 308–317.
28. KELLER, K.J., et al. 1976. Tryptoline inhibition of serotonin uptake in rat forebrain homogenates. J. Pharmacol. Exp. Ther. **198:** 619–625.
29. FAIVRE, V., et al. 2000. Ligand interaction with the purified serotonin transporter in solution and at the air/water interface. FEBS Lett. **471:** 56–60.
30. LICHTENBERG-KRAAG, B., et al. 1997. The natural β-carbolines facilitate inositol phosphate accumulation by activating small G-proteins in human neuroblastoma cells (SHSY5Y). Neuropharmacology **36:** 1771–1778.
31. KLINKER, J.F., et al. 1997. Activation by β-carbolines of G-proteins in HL-60 membranes and the bovine retinal G-protein transducin in a receptor independent manner. Biochem. Pharmacol. **53:** 1621–1626.
32. STOWOWY, P., R. BONNET & H. ROMMELSPACHER. 1999. The high-affinity binding of [^{3}H]norharmane ([^{3}H]β-carboline) to the ethanol-inducible cytochrome P450 2E1 in rat liver. Biochem. Pharmacol. **57:** 511–20.
33. TIARA, Z., et al. 1997. Intercalationof six β-carboline derivatives into DNA. Jap. J. Toxicol. Environ. Health **43:** 83–91.
34. PAWLIK, M. & H. ROMMELSPACHER. 1988. Demonstration of a distinct class of high-affinity binding sites for [^{3}H]norharmane ([^{3}H]β-carboline) binding sites in the rat brain. Eur. J. Pharmacol. **147:** 163–171.
35. GLENNON, R.A., et al. 2000. Binding of β-carbolines and related serotonin (5–HT2 and 5-HT 1A) dopamine (D2) benzodiazepine receptors. Drug Alcohol Depend. **60:** 121–132.
36. MUSGRAVE, I.F. & E. BADOER. 2000. Harmane produces hypotension following microinjection into the RVLM: possible role of I_1-imidazoline receptors. Br. J. Pharmacol. **129:** 1057–1059.
37. MACKINNES, N. & S.L. HANDLEY. 2002. Characterization of the discriminable stimulus produced by 2-BFI: effects of imidazoline I2-site ligands, MAOIs, beta-carbolines, agmatine and ibogaine. Br. J. Pharmacol. **135:** 1227–1234.

38. ADELL, A., et al. 1996. Action of harmane (1-methyl-β-carboline) on the brain: body temperature and in vivo efflux of 5-HT from hippocampus of the rat. Neuropharmacology **8:** 1101–1107.
39. HUDSON, A.L., et al. 1999b. Novel selective compounds for the investigation of imidazoline receptors. Annals. N. Y. Acad. Sci. **881:** 81–91.
40. CAPPENDIKJ, S.L.T., D. FEKKES & M.R. DZOLJIC. 1994. The inhibitory effect of norharmane on morphine withdrawal syndrome in rats: comparison with ibogaine. Behav. Brain Res. **65:** 117–119.
41. LIONE, L.A., D.J. NUTT & A.L. HUDSON. 1998. Characterisation and localisation of [^{3}H]2-(2-benzofuranyl)-2-imidazoline binding in rat brain: a selective ligand for imidazoline I_2 receptors. Eur. J. Pharmacol. **353:** 123–135.
42. WIBLE, J.H., et al. 1996. Cardiovascular effects of β-carbolines in conscious rats. Hypertens. Res. **19:** 161–170.
43. JACKSON, H.C. & D.J. NUTT. 1996. Imidazoline receptors and ingestion. In Drug Receptor Subtypes and Ingestive Behaviour. Cooper, S.J. & P.G. Clifton, Eds.: 267–83. Academic Press. London.
44. MORGAN, N.G., et al. 2003. Comparative effects of efaroxan and β-carbolines on the secretory activity of rodent and human β cells. Ann. N. Y. Acad. Sci. This volume.
45. EDWARDS, M.M. 2003. Imidazoline ligands and feeding behaviour: the role of imidazoline binding sites. Ph.D. thesis, University of Bristol, Bristol, UK.
46. ROMMELSPACHER, H., et al. 1977. Pharmacological properties of tetrahydronorharmane (tryptoline). Naunyn-Schmiederberg's Arch. Pharmacol. **298:** 83–91.
47. COLLINS, M.A. 2002. Alkaloids, alcohol and Parkinson's disease. Parkinsonism Relat. Disord. **8:** 417–422.
48. DE MEESTER, C. 1995. Genotoxic potential of β-carbolines: a review. Mutation Res. Rev. Gen. Toxicol. **7. 339:** 139–153.
49. GEARHART, D.A., et al. 2000. Increased β-carboline 9N-methyltransferase activity in the frontal cortex in Parkinson's disease. Neurobiol. Dis. **7:** 201–211.
50. GEARHART, D.A., P.F. TOOLE & J.W. BEEACH. 2002. Identification of brain proteins that interact with 2-methylnorharman. An analog of the Parkinsonian-inducing toxin, MPP+. Neurosci. Res. **44:** 255–265.

Comparative Effects of Efaroxan and β-Carbolines on the Secretory Activity of Rodent and Human β Cells

NOEL G. MORGAN,[a,b] E. JANE COOPER,[b] PAUL E. SQUIRES,[c] CLAIRE E. HILLS,[c] CHRISTINE A. PARKER,[d] AND ALAN L. HUDSON[d]

[a]*Institute of Biomedical and Clinical Science, Peninsula Medical School, Plymouth, Devon PL6 8BX, UK*

[b]*School of Life Sciences, Keele University, Keele ST5 5BG, UK*

[c]*Biomedical Research Institute, University of Warwick, Coventry CV4 7AL, UK*

[d]*Psychopharmacology Unit, University of Bristol, Bristol BS8 1TS, UK*

ABSTRACT: The pancreatic β-cell expresses an imidazoline-binding site that is involved in the regulation of insulin secretion. This site is pharmacologically atypical in comparison with the I_1 and I_2 sites described in other tissues, and it has been classified as I_3. The structural requirements for binding of ligands to the I_3 site have not been fully defined, although a range of synthetic I_3 ligands have been characterized in functional terms. Evidence has been presented that an endogenous I_3 ligand may exist, because extracts of brain contain an active principle that stimulates insulin secretion in a manner consistent with the involvement of I_3 sites. The active component has not been identified but has been equated with the long-sought clonidine displacing substance (CDS) that is proposed as the endogenous ligand for imidazoline-binding sites. Recent evidence has indicated that one active component of CDS may be a β-carboline, but it is not known whether β-carbolines can stimulate insulin secretion. Thus, we have studied the effects of β-carbolines on insulin secretion and cytosolic Ca^{2+} levels in rodent and human islet cells. The results reveal that harmane, pinoline, and norharmane cause a dose- and glucose-dependent increase in insulin secretion but show that this response differs in a number of ways from that elicited by the well-characterized I_3-agonist, efaroxan. Thus, β-carbolines represent a new class of insulin secretagogues, although it remains unclear whether their action is mediated solely by I_3 sites in the β cell.

KEYWORDS: efaroxan; harmane; I_3-binding sites; β-cell; insulin secretion; islets of Langerhans

INTRODUCTION

It is well established that a variety of imidazoline compounds stimulate insulin secretion,[1–4] and this stimulation seems to be mediated by two mechanisms that can

Address for correspondence: Prof. N.G. Morgan, Room N32, ITTC Building, Peninsula Medical School, Tamar Science Park, Plymouth, Devon PL6 8BX, UK. Voice: (+44) 1752-764274; fax: (+44) 1752-764234.
e-mail: noel.morgan@pms.ac.uk

operate either independently or in concert. For example, some imidazoline reagents interact directly with the pore-forming component (Kir6.2) of the ATP-sensitive potassium (K_{ATP}) channel to promote channel closure, membrane depolarization, Ca^{2+} influx, and insulin secretion.[5,6] By contrast, others seem to activate a mechanism that operates downstream of the K_{ATP} channel and that has the ability to promote exocytosis directly, even when membrane depolarization is precluded.[7–9] This latter mechanism may be the more important for stimulation of insulin secretion, because the latest generation of imidazoline secretagogues activate this response but have no effect on the K_{ATP} channel.[9–11]

On the basis of this evidence, it may be concluded that pancreatic β cells express at least two distinct imidazoline-binding proteins that can each play a role in the control of insulin release. One of these (Kir6.2) occupies a proximal position within the pathway of stimulus–secretion coupling, whereas the second is more distally located. The identity of this second imidazoline-binding site (the putative I_3-site) has not yet been disclosed, and its characterization remains an important priority. Candidate molecules are beginning to emerge; among them the low molecular weight GTP-binding protein Rhes seems to be a strong contender.[12]

Another unresolved issue concerns the possibility that an endogenous ligand may exist that has functional activity at the imidazoline-binding proteins expressed in β cells.[13,14] This endogenous ligand might be expected to have higher potency than the synthetic compounds and might thereby form an appropriate prototype for the development of a new class of antidiabetic agents.

Evidence of the existence of an endogenous ligand having activity in the endocrine pancreas has been provided by the demonstration that extracts of rat brain contain an active principle that potently increases insulin release[13,14] (and inhibits glucagon secretion[15]) in a manner consistent with the involvement of imidazoline-binding sites. This compound, known as clonidine-displacing substance (CDS), has so far eluded firm characterization, but recent evidence indicates that it could possess a β-carboline structure rather than an imidazoline moiety.[16,17]

To our knowledge, there have been no previous studies examining the secretory effects of β-carbolines in islets of Langerhans. To this end, we have now investigated whether the β-carboline harmane, and its structural analogues norharmane and pinoline, can induce insulin secretion. We have compared their effects with that of efaroxan, an imidazoline drug whose ability to stimulate insulin secretion has been extensively characterized in previous publications.[18]

METHODS

Male Wistar rats (180–220 g) were allowed free access to food and water. Islets were isolated by collagenase digestion of the pancreata. The isolation medium was a bicarbonate-buffered physiologic saline solution containing 4 mM glucose and 1 mM $CaCl_2$. This medium was also used for islet incubations, supplemented with bovine serum albumin (1 mg/mL). In some experiments, islets were used within 2 hours of isolation (freshly isolated islets), whereas others were cultured in RPMI-1640 medium containing 10% fetal bovine serum at 37°C for 18 hours before use in individual experiments (cultured islets).

Human islets were isolated from heart-beating cadaver organ donors at the Diabetes UK Core Islet Transplant Laboratory, Leicester, UK and were transported to the laboratory in CMRL-1066 medium containing 20% fetal bovine serum. On arrival, they were washed and resuspended in RPMI-1640 medium containing 10% fetal bovine serum. The islets were used within 1 to 4 days.

MIN6 β cells (passage 38-44) were cultured in DMEM medium supplemented with 15% bovine fetal serum and were plated onto 3-aminopropyltriethoxysilane (APES)-coated slides for microfluorimetry. Cells were loaded with Fura-2/AM, and changes in fluorescence intensity were monitored with a CoolSnap HQ CCD camera (Roper Scientific, Marlow, Bucks, UK).

For insulin secretion studies, islets were incubated in groups of three for 1 hour, and the incubation medium was sampled for measurement of insulin by radioimmunoassay.

RESULTS

Initial experiments revealed that, like efaroxan, harmane and pinoline caused a marked increase in insulin secretion from isolated human islets incubated in the presence of 6 mM glucose (TABLE 1). These effects were dose-dependent (FIG. 1) and, in common with efaroxan, both harmane and pinoline antagonized the inhibition of glucose-induced insulin secretion caused by diazoxide in human islets (TABLE 2).

The effects of harmane were glucose-dependent (FIG. 2) in that the β-carboline failed to increase insulin secretion at sub-threshold glucose concentrations (0–4 mM) but potentiated the secretory response when the glucose concentration was raised to 6 mM (FIG. 2). Harmane also increased the extent of insulin secretion when human islets were incubated with 20 mM glucose (FIG. 2). This result contrasts with the secretory response to the I_3-imidazoline agonist, efaroxan (which is ineffective when islets are incubated in the presence of 20 mM glucose[2,18]), suggesting there may be some differences between the mechanisms by which harmane and efaroxan stimulate insulin secretion from islet cells. This conclusion was further strengthened when the secretory responses to these two agents were compared in isolated rat islets (FIG. 3). Surpris-

TABLE 1. Effects of β-carbolines and efaroxan on insulin secretion from isolated human islets

Incubation Conditions	Insulin Secretion (% control)
Control	100 ± 15
Harmane (100 μM)	270 ± 32*
Norharmane (100 μM)	235 ± 25*
Pinoline (100 μM)	220 ± 20*
Efaroxan (100 μM)	230 ± 20*

Isolated human islets were exposed to test reagents in the presence of 6 mM glucose for 1 hour. Insulin secretion was measured after this time. The rate of secretion obtained in the presence of 6 mM glucose alone (control) was defined as 100%, and the effects of test reagents were expressed relative to this value. Each value represents the mean ± SEM obtained from three separate islet preparations.

* $P < 0.01$ relative to control.

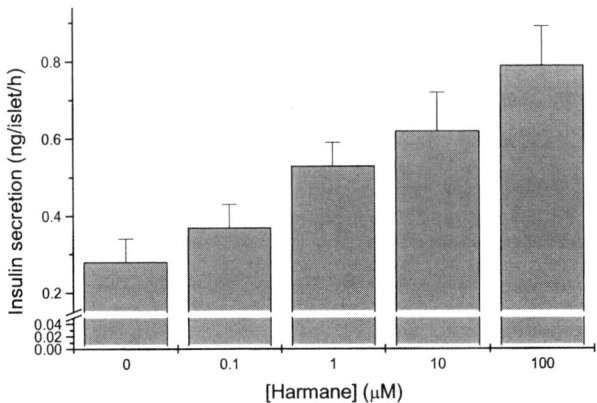

FIGURE 1. Dose–response relationship for stimulation of insulin secretion by harmane. Isolated human islets were incubated with 6 mM glucose and increasing concentrations of harmane for 1 hour. The medium was sampled for measurement of insulin secretion by radioimmunoassay. Data are presented as mean values ± SEM from six replicates.

ingly, treatment of freshly isolated rat islets with harmane failed to promote an increase in insulin secretion, whereas, as expected, efaroxan induced a marked increase. One important distinction between the protocols with rat and human islets was that the latter were in tissue culture medium for a prolonged period during transport to the laboratory, whereas rat islets were used immediately after isolation. Thus, we examined whether harmane would stimulate insulin secretion from rat islets that had been cultured for 18 hours before exposure to the β-carboline. Under these conditions, harmane induced a significant increase in insulin secretion (FIG. 3), whereas the secretory response to efar-

TABLE 2. Effects of β-carbolines and efaroxan on inhibition of glucose-induced insulin secretion mediated by diazoxide

Incubation Conditions	Insulin Secretion (% control)
Glucose + diazoxide	100 ± 12
Glucose + diazoxide + harmane (100 μM)	275 ± 25*
Glucose + diazoxide + pinoline (100 μM)	195 ± 20*
Glucose + diazoxide + efaroxan (100 μM)	220 ± 25*

Isolated human islets were exposed to test reagents in the presence of 20 mM glucose plus 200 μM diazoxide for 1 hour. Insulin secretion was measured after this time. The rate of secretion obtained in the presence of 20 mM glucose plus diazoxide was defined as 100% and the effects of test reagents were expressed relative to this value. Each value represents the mean ± SEM obtained from three separate islet preparations.

* $P < 0.01$ relative to control.

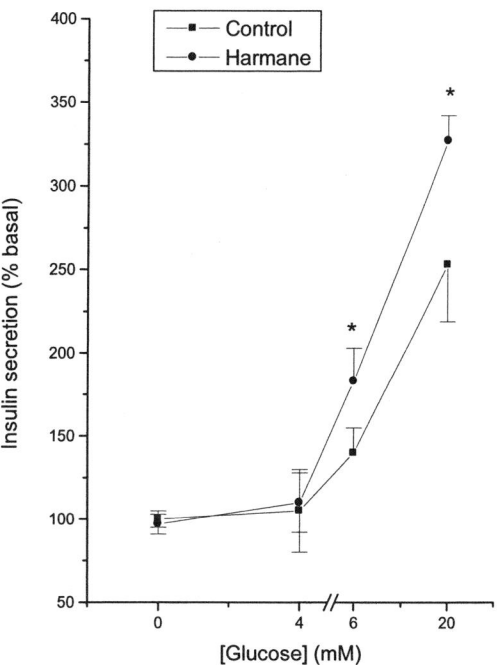

FIGURE 2. Glucose dependency of the stimulatory effects of harmane in human islets. Isolated human islets were incubated with increasing concentrations of glucose in the absence (*squares*) or presence (*circles*) of 100 µM harmane for 1 hour. The medium was then sampled for measurement of insulin secretion by radioimmunoassay. The rate of secretion measured in the absence of glucose was set at 100%, and all other values were expressed relative to this. Data are presented as mean values ± SEM from three islet preparations.

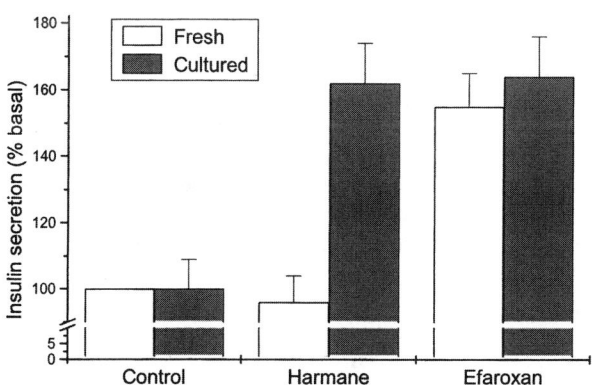

FIGURE 3. Comparison of the effects of harmane on insulin secretion from freshly isolated and cultured rat islets. Isolated rat islets were either used within 2 hours of isolation (*fresh*) or were cultured for 18 hours before the experiment (*cultured*). They were then incubated in the presence of 6 mM glucose and either 100 µM harmane or 100 µM efaroxan, as shown. The rate of insulin secretion was measured and expressed relative to the control rate measured in the presence of 6 mM glucose alone (100%). Results represent mean values ± SEM from three separate islet preparations in each case.

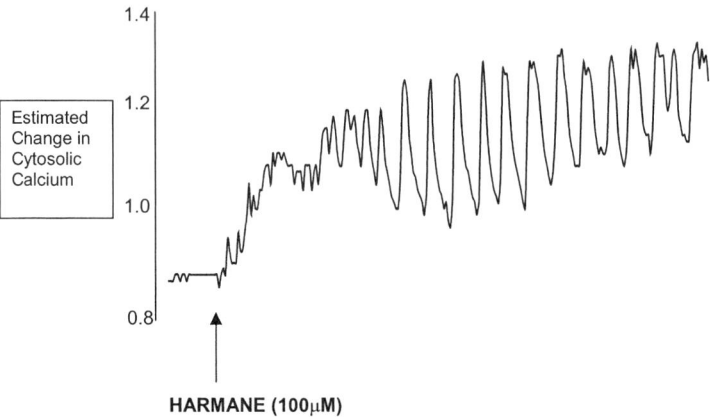

FIGURE 4. Effects of harmane on the cytosolic Ca^{2+} concentration in clonal MIN6 β cells. MIN6 cells were loaded with Fura-2 (Sigma, Dorset, UK) then exposed to harmane as shown. The cytosolic free Ca^{2+} concentration was monitored according to the fluorescence ratio of the dye. The trace shown is representative of that seen in 23 cells in three separate experiments.

oxan was unaffected (still robust) by culture of the islets. These results confirmed that the two agents must exert differential effects in the β cell.

The possibility was also examined that the failure of harmane to increase insulin secretion from freshly isolated rat islets may have resulted from an enhancement of prostaglandin E_2 (PGE_2) production, leading to inhibition of insulin secretion, as reported previously for the imidazoline RX871024.[19] Incubation of freshly isolated rat islets with the cyclooxygenase inhibitors flurbiprofen or indomethacin failed to reveal any stimulatory effects of harmane in freshly isolated rat islets, however (not shown).

In another set of experiments, clonal β cells were employed to investigate whether harmane caused any change in cytosolic Ca^{2+} concentrations. The results revealed that exposure of β cells to harmane was associated with initiation of trains of regular Ca^{2+} oscillations (FIG. 4). The first of these oscillations was preserved when extracellular Ca^{2+} was removed, although subsequent oscillations were abolished (not presented). This result suggested that the oscillations might have been generated by a process of Ca^{2+}-induced Ca^{2+} release in harmane-treated cells.

DISCUSSION

Harmane and other β-carbolines have attracted attention following the suggestion that a member of this class of molecules may represent one of the active components in preparations of CDS.[16,17] Because crude extracts of rat brain CDS have been shown to stimulate insulin secretion,[13] we have studied the effects of harmane on insulin secretion from isolated rat and human islets.

It has been discovered that three structurally related β-carbolines (harmane, norharmane, and pinoline) cause a marked increase in insulin secretion from isolated human islets (see TABLE 1). This effect is similar in magnitude to that elicited by the putative I_3-agonist efaroxan and, like efaroxan, the β-carbolines also antagonized the inhibition of insulin secretion caused by the ATP-sensitive channel agonist diazoxide. The secretory response to harmane was glucose dependent, but during the course of these experiments it became clear that there were some differences in the mechanisms of action of harmane and efaroxan.

Harmane was able to enhance insulin secretion beyond that elicited by a maximal glucose concentration (20 mM) alone. By contrast, efaroxan did not increase insulin secretion from islets exposed to 20 mM glucose.[2,18] Furthermore, the ability of efaroxan to stimulate insulin secretion from freshly isolated rat islets has been well documented[1,2,8,18] and was reproduced in the present studies. Despite its potent activity in human islets, harmane was entirely ineffective in freshly isolated rat islets. This lack of effect was reproduced in a large number of experiments and points to a marked difference between the actions of harmane and efaroxan. Indeed, our results indicate that these agents cannot act by a common mechanism.

We considered the possibility that differences in experimental protocol might underlie such marked differences in the secretory responses between rat and human islets treated with harmane. Of necessity, the human islets had to be placed in culture before their transport to the laboratory, whereas rat islets were used immediately after isolation. Therefore, rat islets were next placed in tissue culture before exposure to harmane. Surprisingly, following this longer culture period, harmane provoked a marked increase in insulin secretion from rat islets. Hence, it seems that either the islet isolation method leads directly to loss of responsiveness (perhaps by removal of a critical cell surface molecule during collagenase digestion) or that the culture period induces a change in the β cells so that they develop the capacity to respond to harmane. A similar dichotomy has been observed when freshly isolated or cultured rat islets were exposed to the imidazoline RX871024.[19] In that case, the agent was inhibitory in freshly isolated islets but stimulatory in cultured islets. The reversal was attributed to the differential production of PGE_2 under the two conditions, and blockade of PGE_2 generation prevented the inhibitory response.[19] In view of these results, we then treated freshly isolated rat islets with each of two structurally dissimilar cyclooxygenase inhibitors in the presence or absence of harmane, to examine whether a stimulatory response could be revealed. No response was seen. Thus, increased PGE_2 production does not seem to account for the differential effects of harmane in freshly isolated versus cultured islets.

Overall, we can conclude that certain β-carbolines are potent, glucose-dependent potentiators of insulin secretion. Although this response shares certain features in common with that of the I_3-agonist, efaroxan, there are also differences. Thus, it is suggested that harmane stimulates insulin secretion by mechanisms different from those used by efaroxan. Studies of intracellular Ca^{2+} handling in β cells exposed to harmane revealed that the agent promotes the development of regular Ca^{2+} oscillations (FIG. 4). These oscillations could underlie its ability to promote insulin secretion, although further studies are required to discover the extent to which the secretory response correlates with the generation of Ca^{2+} oscillations. Preliminary evidence indicates that the oscillations may be mediated by a process of Ca^{2+}-induced Ca^{2+} release. If so, these results suggest that harmane may gain access to an intracellular pool of Ca^{2+} that can be mobilized in the presence of the drug. Therefore, the β-carboline structure should be investigated further as a potential means to generate novel insulin secretagogues.

ACKNOWLEDGMENTS

We thank Diabetes UK and Roche Biosciences for financial support of this work. Thanks are also owed to Drs. Roger James and Sue Swift (University of Leicester) for provision of human islets.

REFERENCES

1. EGLEN, R.M., A.L. HUDSON, D.A. KENDALL, *et al.* 1998. "Seeing through a glass darkly": casting light on imidazoline "I" sites. Trends Pharmacol. Sci. **19:** 381–390.
2. MORGAN, N.G. & S.L.F. CHAN. 2001. Imidazoline binding sites in the endocrine pancreas: can they fulfill their potential as targets for the development of new insulin secretagogues? Curr. Pharm. Des. **7:** 1413–1431.
3. RUSTENBECK, I., M. KOPP, P. RATZKA, *et al.* 1999. Imidazolines and the pancreatic B-cell. Actions and binding sites. Ann. N. Y. Acad. Sci. **881:** 229–240.
4. EFENDIC, S., A.M. EFANOV, P.-O. BERGGREN, *et al.* 2002. Two generations of insulinotropic imidazoline compounds. Diabetes **51**(Suppl 3): S448–S454.
5. PROKS, P. & F.M. ASHCROFT. 1997. Phentolamine block of K_{ATP} channels is mediated by Kir6.2. Proc. Natl. Acad. Sci. U. S. A. **94:** 11716–11720.
6. MONKS, L.K., K.E. COSGROVE, M.J. DUNNE, *et al.* 1999. Affinity isolation of imidazoline binding proteins from rat brain using 5-amino-efaroxan as ligand. FEBS Lett. **447:** 61–64.
7. ZAITSEV, S.V., A.M. EFANOV, I.B. EFANOVA, *et al.* 1996. Imidazoline compounds stimulate insulin release by inhibition of K(ATP) channels and interaction with the exocytotic machinery. Diabetes **45:** 1610–1618.
8. CHAN, S.L.F., M. MOURTADA & N.G. MORGAN. 2001. Characterization of a K_{ATP} channel-independent pathway involved in potentiation of insulin secretion by efaroxan. Diabetes **50:** 340–347.
9. EFANOV, A.M., S.V. ZAITSEV, H.-J. MEST, *et al.* 2001. The novel imidazoline compound BL11282 potentiates glucose-induced insulin secretion in pancreatic beta-cells in the absence of modulation of K(ATP) channel activity. Diabetes **50:** 797–802.
10. JAKOBSEN, P., P. MADSEN & H. ANDERSEN. 2003. Imidazolines as efficacious glucose-dependent stimulators of insulin secretion. Eur. J. Med. Chem. **38:** 357–362.
11. HOY, M., H.L. OLSEN, H.S. ANDERSEN, *et al.* 2003. Imidazoline NNC77–0074 stimulates insulin secretion and inhibits glucagon release by control of Ca^{2+}-dependent exocytosis in pancreatic α- and β-cells. Eur. J. Pharmacol. **466:** 213–221.
12. CHAN, S.L.F., L.K. MONKS, H. GAO, *et al.* 2002. Identification of the monomeric G-protein, Rhes, as an efaroxan-regulated protein in the pancreatic β-cell. Br. J. Pharmacol. **137:** 31–36.
13. CHAN, S.L.F., D. ATLAS, R.F.L. JAMES, *et al.* 1997. The effect of the putative endogenous imidazoline receptor ligand, clonidine-displacing substance, on insulin secretion from rat and human islets of Langerhans. Br. J. Pharmacol. **120:** 926–932.
14. CHAN, S.L.F. 1998. Clonidine-displacing substance and its putative role in control of insulin secretion: a minireview. Gen. Pharmacol. **31:** 525–529.
15. HOY, M., S.L.F. CHAN, X.J. WENG, *et al.* 2001. Clonidine displacing substance reduces glucagon secretion from mouse pancreatic α-cells by K_{ATP}-independent inhibition of exocytosis. Biochem. Biophys. Res. Commun. **288:** 309–312.
16. HUSBANDS, S.M., R.A. GLENNON, S. GORGERAT, *et al.* 2001. Beta-carboline binding to imidazoline receptors. Drug Alcohol Depend. **64:** 203–208.
17. MUSGRAVE, I.F. & E. BADOER. 2000. Harmane produces hypotension following microinjection into the RVLM: possible role of I(1)-imidazoline receptors. Br. J. Pharmacol. **129:** 1057–1059.
18. CHAN, S.L.F. & N.G. MORGAN. 1990. Stimulation of insulin secretion by efaroxan may involve interaction with potassium channels. Eur. J. Pharmacol. **176:** 97–101.
19. MOURTADA, M., S.L.F. CHAN, S.A. SMITH, *et al.* 1999. Multiple effector pathways regulate the insulin secretory response to the imidazoline RX871024 in isolated rat pancreatic islets. Br. J. Pharmacol. **127:** 1279–1287.

Characterization of [^{3}H]Harmane Binding to Rat Whole Brain Membranes

N.J. ANDERSON,[a] E.S.J. ROBINSON,[a] S.M. HUSBANDS,[b] P. DELAGRANGE,[c] D.J. NUTT,[a] A.L. HUDSON[a]

[a]*Psychopharmacology Unit, School of Medical Sciences, University of Bristol, Bristol BS8 1TD, UK*

[b]*School of Pharmacy and Pharmacology, University of Bath, Bath BA2 7AY, UK*

[c]*IRIS, 92415 Courbevoie Cedex, France*

ABSTRACT: This study investigates the binding of [^{3}H]harmane to rat whole brain homogenates. Saturation studies revealed [^{3}H]harmane labels a single, saturable, high-capacity population with high affinity. All the test compounds displaced [^{3}H]harmane completely and in an apparently monophasic manner. The displacement profile of the test ligands indicated labeling of MAO-A. Given the high level of MAO-A binding, it is unlikely that a low-capacity I_2 site would be distinguishable from the total [^{3}H]harmane population.

KEYWORDS: β-carboline; harmane; imidazoline$_2$ binding site; monoamine oxidase A; radioligand binding

INTRODUCTION

There are currently three candidates for the endogenous ligand for the imidazoline-binding sites (IBS). Previously, an extract of bovine lung and brain was shown to displace [^{3}H]clonidine potently from α_2-adrenoceptors[1,2] and nonadrenergic binding sites[3] in the bovine brainstem. This extract, termed clonidine-displacing substance (CDS) was therefore proposed to contain the endogenous ligand for the imidazoline binding sites. Agmatine, decarboxylated arginine, has been proposed as a candidate[4]; however subsequent binding experiments have demonstrated a low affinity for the IBS.[5,6] Another compound, imidazoleacetic acid-ribotide, has also been shown to exhibit many of the properties expected for an endogenous ligand for the IBS.[7]

Radioligand binding studies have indicated that the β-carbolines harmane and harmalan demonstrate high affinity for the IBS,[8] and this finding has been confirmed by an extensive structure–activity study.[9] Subsequently, β-carboline precursor compounds were identified in the active methanolic extracts used to study CDS, and harmane and harmalan were shown to be endogenous components of bovine lung.[10] These data highlighted the potential of harmane and harmalan as endogenous modulators of the IBS. As with many I_2 compounds, harmane was also shown to be a

---

Address for correspondence: Dr. Alan L. Hudson, Head of Preclinical Science, Psychopharmacology Unit, School of Medical Sciences, University of Bristol, Bristol BS8 1TD, UK. Voice: (+44) 0 117 928 8608; fax: (+44) 0 117 928 9700.

e-mail: a.l.hudson@bristol.ac.uk

potent inhibitor of the A isoform of monoamine oxidase (MAO),[11] an enzyme known to possess an I_2 site.[12]

The present study has investigated the binding profile of the tritiated form of harmane using both saturation and competition assays to compare the [^{3}H]harmane binding site to what is currently known about MAO and I_2 binding.

METHODS

[^{3}H]harmane Synthesis

Di-bromo harmane was synthesized by Stephen Husbands, University of Bath, and tritiated by catalytic halogen-tritium exchange at Tocris-Cookson, Bristol, UK.

Radioligand-binding Experiments

Radioligand binding experiments were carried out according to the method of Lione et al[6] with the following modifications. For saturation assays, membrane aliquots were incubated with 0.03 to 100 nM of either [^{3}H]harmane (30 mins) or [^{3}H]Ro41-1049 for 60 minutes, with specific binding defined by either 10 μM harmane or 10 μM 2BFI for both radioligands. In the competition assays, membrane aliquots were incubated with 4 nM [^{3}H]harmane to equilibrium (30 minutes) in the presence of the displacing drugs (0.01 nM–10 μM). Specific binding was defined as described in TABLE 1.

RESULTS

Saturation experiments indicated that [^{3}H]harmane labeled a single, saturable population of sites in the rat brain with high affinity (K_D 15.1 ± 2.0 nM) (FIG. 1). When nonspecific binding was defined by 10 μM harmane, a maximal binding den-

TABLE 1. Summary of K_i values for [^{3}H]harmane displacement studies

		K_i (nM) ± SD
I_1 compounds	Clonidine	>10 000
	Efaroxan	>10 000
I_2 compounds	2BFI	1651.8 ± 409.0*
	BU224	482.73 ± 86.23
β-carbolines	Harmane	18.91 ± 1.10*
	Norharmane	188.63 ± 38.37
MAOIs	Clorgyline	1.06 ± 0.18
	R(-)-deprenyl	884.50 ± 153.42
	Pargyline	687.47 ± 94.14

Specific binding is defined by 100 μM norharmane, except where * denotes 10 μM harmane was used.

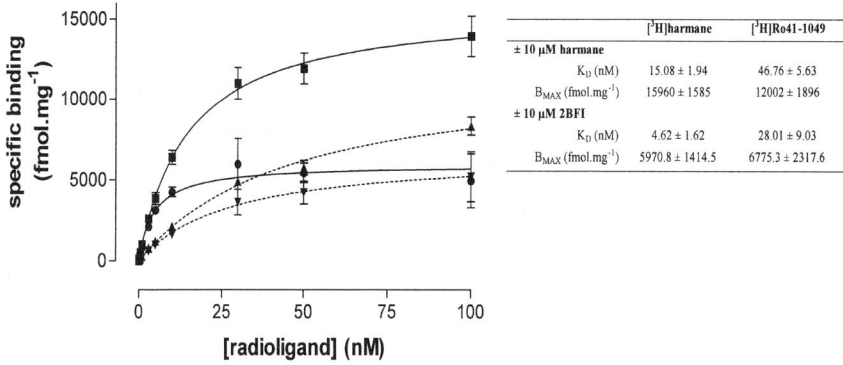

FIGURE 1. Specific binding of 0.03 to 100 nM [³H]harmane (*solid lines*) and [³H]Ro41-1049 (*dashed lines*) to rat whole brain membranes. Specific binding is defined by 10 μM harmane (■, ▲) or 10 μM 2BFI (●,▼). All data points and values represent the mean of three of four experiments ± SD. Analyses of the saturation data by nonlinear regression using GraphPad Prism version 3.03 (GraphPad Software, Inc., San Diego, CA) resolved a single high-affinity binding site for both radioligands.

sity (B_{MAX}) of 15960 ± 1585 fmol.mg^{-1} was measured. Using [³H]Ro41-1049 to label MAO-A selectively, saturation studies in the presence of 10 μM harmane suggest approximately 75% of the [³H]harmane sites are recognized by [³H]Ro41-1049. The number of sites recognized by 10 μM 2BFI was similar for both the [³H]harmane- and [³H]Ro41-1049–labeled populations (5970.8 ± 1414.5 fmol.mg^{-1} and 6775.3 ± 2317.6 fmol.mg^{-1}, respectively) (FIG. 1).

To profile the [³H]harmane binding site in rat brain, a series of competition assays were performed using four classes of compounds: I_1 ligands, I_2 ligands, endogenous β-carbolines, and MAO inhibitors (TABLE 1). Compounds previously shown to exhibit high affinity for MAO-A also displaced [³H]harmane with high affinity. The irreversible MAO-A inhibitor clorgyline and harmane itself demonstrated the highest affinities (1.1 ± 0.2 nM and 18.9 ± 1.1 nM, respectively). The MAO-B–selective drug deprenyl demonstrated only moderate affinity. The I_2 ligands 2BFI and BU224 also showed moderate affinity, whereas the classical I_1 ligands clonidine and efaroxan were of low affinity. Statistically, all curves were found to fit better the more simple, one-site model, indicating displacement from a single binding site/affinity state.

DISCUSSION

It has been previously documented that [³H]harmane[13] and [³H]Ro41-1049[14] both label MAO-A. This study aimed to investigate the binding of I_1 and I_2 ligands to the [³H]harmane site in an attempt to identify a non–MAO-A component. However, the apparent monophasic nature of the binding curves in this study indicates labeling of a single site. It has previously been shown that the I_2 site, as labeled by [³H]2BFI, is of low capacity (144 ± 4.8 fmol.mg^{-1}),[6] and that harmane has high affinity for and displaces completely from this population.[8,9] Furthermore, there is growing evidence that this I_2 site is distinct from MAO.[15] Although in this assay [^{3}H]Ro41-1049 seems to saturate to only approximately 75% of the capacity of the [^{3}H]harmane population, the monophasic displacement does not indicate the presence of any distinct subpopulations labeled by 4 nM [^{3}H]harmane. In a previous study using [^{3}H]harmane to label a purified mitochondrial preparation, the same rank order of K_i values was obtained (clorgyline > harmane > norharmane > pargyline > deprenyl).[16] In addition, the rank order of K_i values observed here is very similar to the corresponding values for the inhibition of rat brain MAO-A (clorgyline >> deprenyl > BU224 > 2BFI >> clonidine > efaroxan).[17] These data suggest that, under the conditions described herein, [^{3}H]harmane labeled predominantly MAO-A. As with the saturation experiments, given its small capacity, the I_2 site is unlikely to be resolved against the high-density [^{3}H]harmane population. Defining specific binding with 10 µM 2BFI yielded similar B_{MAX} values with both [^{3}H]harmane and [^{3}H]Ro41-1049, again suggesting that the same population of sites is labeled by both radioligands. These are smaller-capacity sites than those defined by 10 µM harmane, but the underlying reason is as yet unclear.

This study has demonstrated that [^{3}H]harmane labels a large population of sites in rat brain. The monophasic nature of the binding and the displacement profile of the test ligands indicate that [^{3}H]harmane labels predominantly MAO-A. The possibility that [^{3}H]harmane also labels a lower-capacity (by ~100-fold smaller) I_2 site is not excluded by these findings. Further work to investigate the regional binding of [^{3}H]harmane in brain using autoradiography may identify these sites.

ACKNOWLEDGMENTS

We would like to thank Dr. Borroni at Hoffmann La Roche for the kind gift of [^{3}H]Ro41-1049 and the Wellcome Trust for financial support. Neil Anderson is a doctoral student funded by the MRC.

REFERENCES

1. ATLAS, D. & Y. BURSTEIN. 1984. Isolation and partial purification of a clonidine-displacing endogenous brain substance. Eur. J. Biochem. **144:** 287–293.
2. ATLAS, D. & Y. BURSTEIN. 1984. Isolation of an endogenous clonidine-displacing substance from rat brain. FEBS Lett. **170:** 387–390.
3. ERNSBERGER, P., M.P. MEELEY & D.J. REIS. 1988. An endogenous substance with clonidine-like properties: selective binding to imidazole sites in the ventrolateral medulla. Brain Res. **441:** 309–318.
4. LI, G., et al. 1994. Agmatine: an endogenous clonidine-displacing substance in the brain. Science **263:** 966–969.
5. LIONE, L.A., D.J. NUTT & A.L. HUDSON. 1996. [^{3}H]2-(2-benzofuranyl)-2-imidazoline: a new selective high affinity radioligand for the study of rabbit brain imidazoline I_2 receptors. Eur. J. Pharmacol. **304:** 221–229.
6. LIONE, L.A., D.J. NUTT & A.L. HUDSON. 1998. Characterisation and localisation of [^{3}H]2-(2-benzofuranyl)-2-imidazoline binding in rat brain: a selective ligand for imidazoline I2 receptors. Eur. J. Pharmacol. **353:** 123–135.
7. PRELL, G.D., et al. 2003. Imidazoleacetic acid-ribotide is an endogenous imidazoline receptor (IR) ligand. Ann. N. Y. Acad. Sci. Presented at the Fourth International Symposium on Agmatine and Imidazoline Systems, San Diego, April 2003.

8. HUDSON, A.L., et al. 1999. Harmane, Norharmane and tetrahydro β-carboline have high affinity for rat imidazoline binding sites. Br. J. Pharmacol. **126:** 2P.
9. HUSBANDS, S.M., et al. 2001. Beta-carboline binding to imidazoline receptors. Drug Alcohol Depend. **64:** 203–208.
10. ROBINSON, E.S.J., et al. 2003. Identification of harman and harmalan in bovine lung CDS. Ann. N. Y. Acad. Sci. Presented at the Fourth International Symposium on Agmatine and Imidazoline Systems, San Diego, April 2003.
11. ROMMELSPACHER, H., T. MAY & B. SALEWSKI. 1994. Harman (1-methyl-beta-carboline) is a natural inhibitor of monoamine oxidase type A in rats. Eur. J. Pharmacol. **252:** 51–59.
12. PARINI, A., et al. 1996. The elusive family of imidazoline binding sites. Trends Pharmacol. Sci. **17:** 13–16.
13. MAY, T., S. STRAUSS & H. ROMMELSPACHER. 1990. [^{3}H]Harman labels selectively and with high affinity the active site of monoamine oxidase (EC 1.4.3.4) subtype A (MAO-A) in rat, marmoset, and pig. J. Neural Transm. Suppl. **32:** 93–102.
14. SAURA, J., et al. 1992. Quantitative enzyme radioautography with [^{3}H]-Ro 41–1049 and [^{3}H]-Ro 19–6327 in vitro: localization and abundance of MAO-A and MAO-B in rat CNS, peripheral organs, and human brain. J. Neurosci. **12:** 1977–1999.
15. EGLEN, R.M., et al. 1998. "Seeing through a glass darkly": casting light on imidazoline "I" sites. Trends Pharmacol. Sci. **19:** 381–390.
16. MAY, T., H. ROMMELSPACHER & M. PAWLIK. 1991. [^{3}H]harman binding experiments. I: A reversible and selective radioligand for monoamine oxidase subtype A in the CNS of the rat. J. Neurochem. **56:** 490–499.
17. LALIES, M.D., et al. 1999. Inhibition of central monoamine oxidase by imidazoline2 site-selective ligands. Ann. N. Y. Acad. Sci. **881:** 114–117.

Effect of Harmane on Mononeuropathic Pain in Rats

FEYZA ARICIOGLU,[a] EYLEM KORCEGEZ,[a] AND SULEYMAN OZYALCIN[b]

[a]*Department of Pharmacology, Faculty of Pharmacy, Marmara University, Haydarpasa, Istanbul, Turkey*

[b]*Department of Algology, Istanbul Medical Faculty, Istanbul University, Çapa, Istanbul, Turkey*

> ABSTRACT: This study was designed to investigate the effect of the endogenous β-carboline, harmane, on neuropathic pain produced by chronic constriction injury (CCI) of the sciatic nerve. Thermal allodynia evaluations were made preoperatively, postoperatively on the fifteenth day, and after harmane administration. Harmane (1, 2.5, 5, 10, or 20 mg/kg) was administered intraperitoneally for 5 days beginning from postoperative day 15. Treatment with harmane had a profound anti-allodynic effect in a dose-dependent manner. In conclusion, harmane might provide a new approach to treatment of neuropathic pain.
>
> KEYWORDS: harmane; chronic constriction injury; imidazoline; allodynia

INTRODUCTION

Harmane (1-methyl-β-carboline) and related alkaloids have a wide spectrum of neuropharmacologic actions, including convulsive and anticonvulsive actions, tremorogenesis, and psychotropic effects.[1–3] Harmala alkaloids have been found endogenously in mammalian tissues, including the central nervous system, liver, platelets, plasma, and urine.[4] Harmane has long been known to bind to several receptors in the brain, including those for 5-hydroxytryptamine, dopamine, and the benzodiazepines.[5,6] Nanomolar concentrations of harmane also inhibit monoamine oxidase A in vitro.[7] More recently, harmane has been shown to have nanomolar affinity for imidazoline receptors.[8] Although imidazoline binding sites have been discovered only recently, and their pharmacologic role is still being elucidated, there is growing evidence to suggest that they could be important therapeutic targets for a number of conditions.

The present study was designed to investigate the effect of harmane on the nociceptive threshold for neuropathic pain in rats.

Address for correspondence: Feyza Aricioglu, Ph.D., Department of Pharmacology, Faculty of Pharmacy, Marmara University, 81010 Tibbiye Cad. No: 49, Haydarpasa, Istanbul, Turkey. Voice: 0216 418 95 73; fax: 0216 345 29 52.

e-mail: feyzak@turk.net

MATERIALS AND METHODS

Animals

Adult (200–250 g) Wistar albino rats were used in the neuropathic pain model. Postoperatively the animals were housed in groups of two or three in clear plastic cages with a solid floor covered with soft bedding. The rats were housed at 22°C ± 2°C under a 12-hour light/dark cycle with access to water and food ad libitum. The animals were inspected every 1 or 2 days during the first 14 postoperative days. All procedures were in accordance with the Guide for the Care and Use of Laboratory Animals as adopted by the National Institutes of Health (USA) and the Declaration of Helsinki. Ethical approval was granted by the Marmara University Ethics Committee. All experiments were performed at the same time during the light period every day.

Drugs

Harmane HCl was purchased from Sigma Chemical (St. Louis, MO, USA) and dissolved in saline. Harmane or saline was injected intraperitoneally (i.p.), at a volume of 0.1 mL/100 g. Fresh solutions were prepared daily, 30 minutes before the test.

Mononeuropathic Pain Model

Peripheral mononeuropathy has been described by Bennett and Xie.[9] Procedures were carried out under halothane anesthesia. A chronic constrictive injury (CCI) was created by four ligations made with chromatic gut sutures that were tied loosely with square knots around the right sciatic nerve. A brief twitch in the muscle surrounding the exposure served as an indicator of the desired degree of constriction. The left sciatic nerve was only mobilized. Incisions were closed layer-to-layer with silk sutures, and the rats were allowed to recover from anesthesia. After surgery, the animals were individually maintained in clear plastic cages with solid floors covered with sawdust. All animals postoperatively displayed normal feeding and drinking behavior.

Animals were divided into the sham-operated group (with the same surgery, but without nerve constriction) and the CCI group (n = 10 per group). With counterbalanced stimulus order, the animals were exposed for 20 minutes on successive days to a metal floor that was either chilled by cold water (4°C) or warmed by a 30°C bath. The rat was placed in a clear plastic cage (18 × 28 × 13 cm) with a 1/8-inch aluminum floor. For a 20-minute session, the time was recorded during which the animal held either hind paw above the floor while animal sitting or standing. Animals in the operated group were observed at baseline, 15 days after surgery, and then again following 5 days' i.p. administration of harmane beginning on postoperative day 15.

Statistical Analysis

The two groups were compared by ANOVA with the Tukey multiple comparison test before surgery (pre-op), on day 15 (post-op), and day 21 (post-treatment). Results are expressed as means ± SD, and differences were considered statistically significant if $P < 0.05$.

TABLE 1. Effect of harmane on number of hind paw withdrawals on 4°C-floor over 20 minutes

Dosage (mg/kg i.p.)	Number of Paw Withdrawals	
	Post-op	Post-treatment
Saline	11.72 ± 3.4	12.01 ± 2.15
Harmane 1	8.83 ± 2.13	8.16 ± 2.10
Harmane 2.5	9.50 ± 1.64	5.33 ± 1.03*
Harmane 5	10.17 ± 2.63	4.0 ± 0.63*
Harmane 10	8.80 ± 2.10	3.16 ± 0.75*
Harmane 20	10.1 ± 2.48	1.50 ± 0.83*

Measurements were first made on day 15 day after sciatic nerve ligation (Post-op). Subsequent measurements were made on day 21 after 5 more days of saline or harmane treatments at doses shown (Post-treatment). Data are presented as mean ± SD (n = 10 rats/group). Post-op and post-treatment groups were compared.
*$P < 0.05$.

RESULTS AND DISCUSSION

We tested nerve-operated (CCI) and sham-operated rats for cold allodynia (4°C). Allodynia was quantified by means of cumulative time and number of hind paw withdrawals in 20 minutes. CCI significantly decreased the allodynia threshold 15 days after the nerve injury (saline group, TABLES 1 and 2), whereas the sham-operated group showed no changes from naive controls (data not shown). The response to 4°C induced on day 15 was reduced after the harmane treatment for 5 days (TABLE 1).

TABLE 2. Effect of harmane on cumulative duration of paw withdrawals on 4°C-floor over 20 minutes

Harmane (mg/kg i.p.)	Cumulative Duration of Paw Withdrawals (seconds)	
	Post-op	Post-treatment
Saline	52.34 ± 9.41	50.87 ± 8.25
1	46.68 ± 8.90	45.95 ± 9.67
2.5	48.25 ± 8.07	33.17 ± 6.21*
5	50.02 ± 8.17	24.11 ± 4.20*
10	50.17 ± 8.64	16.32 ± 2.91*
20	49.85 ± 10.07	8.84 ± 4.57*

Measurements were made on the fifteenth day after sciatic nerve ligation (Post-op). Subsequent measurements were made on the 21st day after 5 more days of saline or harmane treatments at doses shown (Post-treatment). Data are presented as mean ± SD (10 rats/group). Post-op and post-treatment groups were compared.
*$P < 0.05$.

Harmane had no effect on sham-operated animals (data not shown). The effect of harmane on numbers of hind paw withdrawals was statistically significant in a dose-dependent manner: $F_{5,54} = 21.29$ ($P < 0.05$) (TABLE 1). The effect of harmane on cumulative time of hind paw withdrawals was also found significant for all doses when compared with the postoperative value of the same group: $F_{5,54} = 28.32$ ($P < 0.05$) (TABLE 2). None of the animals withdrew hind paws from the 30°C surface, and no difference was observed between control and sham-operated rats in any of the tests applied (data not shown).

Because harmane is known to interact with many receptors, its anti-allodynic effects may be caused by several mechanisms. It is known that drugs that have selective agonistic activity on imidazoline receptors such as tizanidine, moxonidine, and clonidine produce antinociceptive effects in rodents.[10,11] Some recent studies have also indicated a modulatory effect of imidazoline receptor ligands on analgesia in mice and rats.[12,13] Our results with harmane are also similar to those obtained with agmatine, another endogenous ligand for imidazoline receptors that is ameliorative of persistent pain and neuronal injury.[14] It has also been reported that systemic imidazoline ligands such as agmatine may exert anti-allodynic effects in spinal nerve–ligated rats and also in streptozosine-induced diabetic rats.[15] Therefore, the action of harmane and agmatine might be similarly mediated.

In conclusion, the exogenous administration of harmane has been shown to modulate neuropathic pain by preventing allodynia in a dose-dependent manner. This property of harmane may be advantageous for treatment of neuropathic pain.

REFERENCES

1. TSE, S.Y.H., I.T. MAK & B.F. DICKENS. 1991. Antioxidative properties of harmane and β-carboline alkaloids. Biochem. Pharmacol. **42:** 459–464.
2. LUTES, J., et al. 1988. Tolerance to the tremorogenic effects of harmaline: evidence for altered olivo-cerebellar function. Neuropharmacology **27:** 849–855.
3. AIRAKSINEN, M.M. & I. KARI. 1981. β-carbolines, psychoactive compounds in the mammalian body: part I. Occurrence, origin and metabolism. Med. Biol. **59:** 21–34.
4. BECK, O. & K.F. FAULL. 1986. Concentrations of the enantiomers of 5-hydoxymethtryptoline in mammalian urine: implications for in vivo biosynthesis. Biochem. Pharmacol. **35:** 2636–2639.
5. LOEW, G.H., et al. 1985. Theoretical structure-activity studies of β-carboline analogs. Requirements for benzodiazepine receptor affinity and antagonist activity. Mol. Pharmacol. **28:** 17–31.
6. MULLER, W.E., et al. 1981. On the neuropharmacology of harman and other β-carbolines. Pharmacol. Biochem. Behav. **14:** 693–699.
7. ROMMELSPACHER, H., T. MAY & B. SALWSKI. 1994. Harman (1-methyl-β-carboline) is a natural inhibitor of monoamine oxidase type A in rats. Eur. J. Pharmacol. **252:** 51–59.
8. HUSBANDS, S.M., et al. 2001. Beta-carboline binding to imidazoline receptors. Drug Alcohol Depend. **64:** 203–208.
9. BENNETT, G.J. & Y.K. XIE. 1988. A peripheral mononeuropathy in rat that produces disorders of pain sensation like those seen in man. Pain **33:** 87–107.
10. FAIRBANKS, C.A. & G.L. WILCOX. 1999. Moxonidine, a selective alpha2-adrenergic and imidazoline receptor agonist, produces spinal antinociceptive in mice. J. Pharmacol. Exp. Ther. **290:** 403–412.
11. KHAN, Z.P.A., C.N. FERGUSON & R.M. JONES. 1999. Alpha-2 and imidazoline receptor agonists. Anaesthesia **54:** 146–165.

12. LEE, Y.W. & T.L. YAKSH. 1995. Analysis of drug interaction between intrathecal clonidine and MK-801 in peripheral neuropathic pain rat model. Anesthesiology **82:** 741–748.
13. FAIRBANKS, C.A., *et al.* 2000. Moxonidine, a selective imidazoline and alpha2-adrenergic receptor agonist, produces spinal synergistic antihyperalgesia with morphine in nerve-injured mice. Anesthesiology **93:** 765–773.
14. FAIRBANKS, C.A., *et al.* 2000. Agmatine reverses pain induced by inflammation, neuropathy, and spinal cord injury. Proc. Natl. Acad. Sci. U. S. A. **97:** 10584–10589.
15. KARADAG, H.C., *et al.* 2003. Systemic agmatine attenuates tactile allodynia in two experimental neuropathic pain models in rats. Neurosci. Lett. **39:** 88–90.

Inhibitory Effect of Harmane on Morphine-Dependent Guinea Pig Ileum

FEYZA ARICIOGLU[a] AND TIJEN UTKAN[b]

[a]*Department of Pharmacology, Faculty of Pharmacy, Marmara University, Haydarpasa, Istanbul, Turkey*

[b]*Department of Pharmacology, Kocaeli Medical Faculty, Kocaeli, Turkey*

ABSTRACT: Studies on the occurrence and properties of β-carbolines structurally related to harmala alkaloids have gained attention since it was hypothesized that some of these compounds play a role in processes of substance abuse and dependence. This study investigates the effects of harmane on naloxone-precipitated withdrawal syndrome in morphine-dependent guinea pig ileum. Segments of ilea from starved male guinea pigs were obtained and fixed at a resting tension of 1 g in an organ bath containing 10^{-6} M morphine in Tyrode solution at 37°C, which was bubbled with 95% O_2 and 5% CO_2. Tissues were incubated in 10^{-6} M morphine containing Tyrode solution for 4 hours before harmane was added. Naloxone and harmane had no effect on naive ilea. Naloxone (10^{-6} M) contracted morphine-dependent ilea. Harmane significantly inhibited the contractile response to naloxone in a dose-dependent manner (10^{-7} M = 24%; 10^{-6} M = 49.3%; 10^{-5} M = 70%). These results suggest that harmane may have beneficial effects on morphine withdrawal syndrome.

KEYWORDS: Harmane; imidazoline; morphine dependence; ileum

INTRODUCTION

Harmane (1-methyl-β-carboline) and related alkaloids are distributed widely in medicinal plants.[1] β-Carbolines structurally related to harmala alkaloids have also been found endogenously in mammalian tissues, including the central nervous system, liver, platelets, plasma, and urine.[2,3] These alkaloids have a wide spectrum of pharmacologic actions, including monoamine oxidase inhibition,[4] binding to benzodiazepine receptors,[5] convulsive and anticonvulsive actions,[6] tremorogenesis,[7] and behavioral effects.[8] Harmane has nanomolar affinity for imidazoline receptors[9] and is considered an endogenous ligand of imidazoline receptors.[10]

In recent years there has been increasing interest in the antiaddictive properties of β-carboline indole alkaloids. Chronic infusion of harmane induces voluntary ethanol intake in rats.[11] Blood levels of harmane are elevated in alcoholics[12] and heroin addicts.[13,14] It has been shown that norharmane, harmane, and harmine have prominent inhibitory effects on naloxone-precipitated withdrawal syndrome in morphine-

---

Address for correspondence: Feyza Aricioglu, Ph.D., Department of Pharmacology, Faculty of Pharmacy, Marmara University, 81010 Tibbiye Cad. No: 49, Haydarpasa, Istanbul, Turkey. Voice: 0216 418 95 73; fax: 0216 345 29 52.

e-mail: feyzak@turk.net

dependent rats.[15,16] These findings suggest a role for some of the β-carbolines in alcoholism and drug dependence.

Literature investigating the effects of harmala alkaloids such as harmane on morphine dependence and withdrawal is limited. The present study was designed to investigate the effects of harmane on morphine-dependent guinea pig ileum.

MATERIALS AND METHODS

Animals

All procedures were in accordance with the Guide for the Care and Use of Laboratory Animals as adopted by the National Institutes of Health (USA) and the declaration of Helsinki. Ethical approval was granted by the Kocaeli University Ethics Committee.

Adult male guinea pigs (300–400 g) were housed in a quiet, temperature controlled (20°C ± 2°C) and humidity controlled (60% ± 3%) room in which a 12-hour light/dark cycle was maintained (07:00–19:00 light). The rats were fed standard lab chow and tap water ad libitum during the study.

Drugs

Naloxone-HCl, harmane-HCl, idazoxane-HCl, and yohimbine-HCl were purchased from Sigma Chemicals (St. Louis, MO, USA.). The morphine base was purchased from the Solid Products Office of the Ministry of Agriculture of Turkey.

Guinea pigs were decapitated after cervical dislocation. Terminal portions of their ilea were removed, placed in Tyrode solution, and thoroughly washed by flushing solution through the lumen. Subsequently, the ilea were cut into 5-cm segments, and the segments were mounted in 20-mL organ chambers for isometric tension measurements. The organ chambers contained Tyrode solution with 10^{-6} M morphine. The solution was gassed with 95% O_2 and 5% CO_2, and the temperature was maintained at 37°C by a thermoregulated water circuit. Each tissue was connected to a force-displacement transducer (FDT 10A May IOBS 99 COMMAT Iletisim, Ankara, Turkey) for measurement of isometric force, which was continuously displayed and recorded online by a four-channel transducer data acquisition system (MP 30 B-CE BIOPAC System Inc., Santa Barbara, CA, USA.) using software (BSL-PRO v 3.67, BIOPAC Systems, Inc.) to analyze the data. After mounting, each tissue was allowed to equilibrate with a basal tension of 1 g for 4 hours; during this time the morphine-containing Tyrode solution was replaced every 15 minutes with fresh solution. After the equilibration period, naloxone was added to the medium either alone or following preincubation for 15 minutes with various concentrations of harmane. In other experiments, the same protocol was repeated 25 minutes after either yohimbine (10^{-6} M) or idazoxan (10^{-6} M) was added to the tissue bath. The effects of these agents on naloxone-induced contractions were evaluated by comparing the responses before and after additions of agonists or antagonists in the same preparation.

Statistical Analysis

Contractions were compared by ANOVA followed by paired t-tests. The percentages of inhibitions were compared by the Mann-Whitney U test. $P < 0.05$ was considered statistically significant.

FIGURE 1. Effect of harmane (10^{-7}, 10^{-6}, or 10^{-5} M) on contractile response to naloxone (10^{-6} M) on morphine-dependent guinea pig ileum. Data are presented as percentage contraction (n = 8/group). * $P < 0.05$ compared with the naloxone group. NL, naloxone.

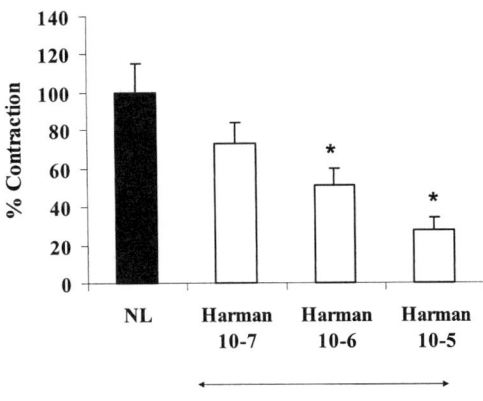

RESULTS AND DISCUSSION

Naloxone (10^{-6} M) had no effect on naive ilea, whereas it contracted the ilea made morphine-dependent by preincubation with morphine (10^{-6} M) for 4 hours. Likewise, harmane had no effect on naive ilea, but it significantly inhibited the contractile response to naloxone in a concentration-dependent manner in morphine-dependent ilea (FIG. 1). The effect of harmane was partly reversed by pretreatment with idazoxan, a mixed imidazoline receptor antagonist and α_2-adrenoceptor antagonist (FIG. 2). Yohimbine, a non-imidazoline α_2-adrenoceptor antagonist, had no such effect (FIG. 2).

The present study shows that harmane, a β-carboline, attenuates the intensity of naloxone-induced contractions in morphine-dependent ilea. This finding supports the hypothesis that harmala alkaloids have beneficial effects in morphine with-

FIGURE 2. Effect of pretreatment with idazoxan (10^{-6} M) or yohimbine (10^{-6} M) on harmane (10^{-5} M) response on morphine-dependent guinea pig ileum. Data are presented as percentage contraction (n = 8/group). * $P < 0.05$ compared with the naloxone group; # $P < 0.05$ compared with the harmane group. IDA, idazoxan; Y, yohimbine.

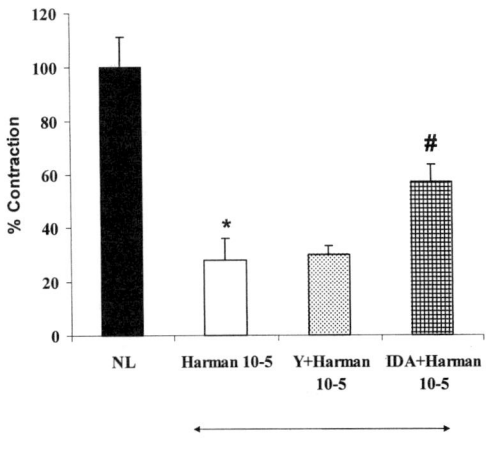

drawal, as first shown by Cappendijk and coworkers.[15] That group found that norharmane produced inhibitory effects on naloxone-precipitated withdrawal syndrome in morphine-dependent rats.

β-Carbolines such as harmane have been proposed to be endogenous ligands for imidazoline receptors.[14] Binding studies indicate that imidazoline receptors can be divided into at least two subtypes, I_1 and I_2 receptors. The functional role of these receptors is poorly understood. Some agents with affinity for imidazoline receptors, such as clonidine, agmatine, harmane, harmine, and norharmane, have been shown to produce beneficial effects on naloxone-precipitated signs of morphine withdrawal in rats.[15–19] In our study, the effect of harmane was diminished by pretreatment with idazoxan, an imidazoline receptor antagonist and α_2-adrenoceptor antagonist, but not by yohimbine, a selective α_2-adrenoceptor antagonist. Therefore, the inhibitory effect of harmane on morphine physical dependence in guinea pig ileum seems to be partly related to imidazoline receptors.

REFERENCES

1. TSE, S.Y.H., I.T. MAK & B.F. DICKENS. 1991. Antioxidative properties of harmane and β-carboline alkaloids. Biochem. Pharmacol. **42:** 459–464.
2. AIRAKSINEN, M.M. & I. KARI. 1981. β-carbolines, psychoactive compounds in the mammalian body: Part I. Occurrence, origin and metabolism. Med. Biol. **59:** 21–34.
3. BECK, O. & K.F. FAULL. 1986. Concentrations of the enantiomers of 5-hydroxymethtryptoline in mammalian urine: implications for in vivo biosynthesis. Biochem. Pharmacol. **35:** 2636–2639.
4. LOEW, G.H., et al. 1985. Theoretical structure-activity studies of β-carboline analogs. Requirements for benzodiazepine receptor affinity and antagonist activity. Mol. Pharmacol. **28:** 17–31.
5. MULLER, W.E., et al. 1981. On the neuropharmacology of harman and other β-carbolines. Pharmacol. Biochem. Behav. **14:** 693–699.
6. FULLER, R.W., C.J. WONG & S.K. HEMRICK-LUECKE. 1986. MD 240928 and harmaline: opposite selectivity in antagonism of the inactivation of types A and B monoamine oxidase by pargyline in mice. Life Sci. **8:** 409–412.
7. LUTES, J., et al. 1988. Tolerance to the tremorigenic effects of harmaline: evidence for altered olivo-cerebellar function. Neuropharmacology **27:** 849–855.
8. ROMMELSPACHER, H., T. MAY & B. SALWSKI. 1994. Harman (1-methyl-β-carboline) is a natural inhibitor of monoamine oxidase type A in rats. Eur. J. Pharmacol. **252:** 51–59.
9. HUSBANDS, S.M., et al. 2001. Beta-carboline binding to imidazoline receptors. Drug Alcohol Depend. **64:** 203–208.
10. RUIZ-DURANTEZ, E., et al. 2001. Stimulatory effect of harmane and other beta-carbolines on locus coeruleus neurons in anaesthetized rats. Neurosci. Lett. **308:** 197–200.
11. ADEL, A. & R.D. MYERS. 1994. Increased alcohol intake in low alcohol drinking rats after chronic infusion of the β-carboline harmane into the hippocampus. Pharmacol. Biochem. Behav. **49:** 949–953.
12. ROMMELSPACHER, H., L.G. SCHMIDITD & T. MAY. 1991. Plasma norharman (beta-carboline) levels are elevated in chronic alcoholics. Alcohol. Clin. Exp. Res. **15:** 553–559.
13. STOHLER, R., et al. 1993. Beta-carbolines (harman/norharman) are increased in heroin dependent patients. Ther. Umsch. **50:** 178–181.
14. STOHLER, R., H. ROMMELSPACHER & D. LADEWIG. 1995. The role of beta-carbolines (harman/norharman) in heroin addicts. Eur. Psychiatry **10:** 56–58.
15. CAPPENDIJK, S.L., D. FEKKES & M.R. DZOLJIC. 1994. The inhibitory effect of norharman on morphine withdrawal syndrome in rats: comparison with ibogaine. Behav. Brain Res. **65:** 117–119.

16. ARICIOGLU-KARTAL, F., H. KAYIR & I.T. UZBAY. 2003. Effect of harman and harmine on naloxone-precipitated withdrawal syndrome in morphine dependent rats. Life Sci. **73:** 2363–2371.
17. ARICIOGLU-KARTAL, F. & I.T. UZBAY. 1997. Inhibitory effect of agmatine on naloxone-precipitated abstinence syndrome in morphine dependent rats. Life Sci. **18:** 1775–1781.
18. DISTEFANO, P.S. & O.M. BROWN. 1985. Biochemical correlates of morphine withdrawal. 2. Effects of clonidine. J. Pharmacol. Exp. Ther. **233:** 339–344.
19. TAYLOR, J.R., *et al.* 1988. Clonidine infusions into the locus coeruleus attenuate behavioral and neurochemical changes associated with naloxone-precipitated withdrawal. Psychopharmacology **96:** 121–134.

Effect of Harmane on the Convulsive Threshold in Epilepsy Models in Mice

FEYZA ARICIOGLU,[a] OKAN YILLAR,[b] EYLEM KORCEGEZ,[a] AND KEMAL BERKMAN[c]

[a]*Department of Pharmacology, Faculty of Pharmacy, Marmara University, Haydarpasa, Istanbul, Turkey*

[b]*Department of Pharmacology, Faculty of Medicine, Istanbul University, Cerrahpasa, Turkey*

[c]*Department of Pharmacology, Faculty of Medicine, Marmara University, Haydarpasa, Istanbul, Turkey*

ABSTRACT: The study investigated the activity of harmane on maximal electroshock seizures (MES) and seizures induced by pentilentetrazole (PTZ) in mice. Initial studies established convulsive current 50 (CC_{50}) values or MES and effective dose 50 (ED_{50}) for PTZ to produce seizures. Harmane (2.5, 5.0, or 10 mg/kg intraperitoneally) increased the threshold of seizures in MES dose-dependently. The convulsions produced by PTZ were decreased by the low dose of harmane (2.5 mg/kg), but the high dose of harmane (10 mg/kg) resulted in worse grade V convulsions followed by more lethality compared with PTZ alone. Therefore, harmane seems to be protective against grand mal seizures in the MES model but not against a petit mal seizure model (PTZ) in mice.

KEYWORDS: harmane; maximal electroshock; pentylenetetrazol, imidazoline; benzodiazepine; monoamine oxidase

INTRODUCTION

Epilepsy is a cluster of disorders rather than a single disease, and it is the most common neurologic disorder worldwide. The understanding of the pathophysiology of the epilepsies is still incomplete.

Harmane and related alkaloids, such as harmine and harmaline, are agents with a β-carboline structure.[1] They form the basis of hallucinogenic preparations of South American and African tribes.[2] These compounds are also found endogenously in mammalian tissues, including central nervous system, liver, platelets, plasma, and urine.[3,4] These harmala alkaloids have some pharmacologic effects involved in convulsive or anticonvulsive actions,[5] tremorogenesis,[6] and psychopathology.[7]

Harmane and other related β-carbolines are putative endogenous ligands of the benzodiazepine receptor.[8] Harmane is a competitive inhibitor of benzodiazepine

Address for correspondence: Feyza Aricioglu, Ph.D., Department of Pharmacology, Faculty of Pharmacy, Marmara University, 81010 Tibbiye Cad. No: 49, Haydarpasa, Istanbul, Turkey. Voice: 0216 418 95 73; fax: 0216 345 29 52.

e-mail: feyzak@turk.net

receptor binding in vitro.[8] A variety of other biochemical properties have also been described for β-carbolines, including inhibition of monoamine oxidase A, competitive inhibition of serotonin uptake, general inhibition of sodium-dependent transport, binding to opiate receptors, and probable action on dopamine receptors.[9–11] Recently it has also been shown that harmane is an endogenous ligand of imidazoline receptors.[12]

The aim of the present study was to investigate the effects of harmane on electrically and chemically induced seizures by using maximal electroshock (MES) and pentylenetetrazol (PTZ) in mice.

MATERIALS AND METHODS

Animals

Male and female Swiss albino mice weighing 20 to 30 g were housed in colony cages, under standard laboratory conditions, with free access to food and tap water. All mice were maintained at 20°C and on a natural light/dark cycle. Each mouse was used only once.

Drugs

Harmane-HCl and pentilentetrazole were purchased from Sigma Chemicals (St. Louis, MO, USA) and dissolved in saline. The drugs, or saline, were injected intraperitoneally (i.p) at a volume of 0.1 mL/10 g.

MES Model

Electroshocks were evoked through a current transmitter producing 60 Hz square waves (Ugo Basile, ECT unit). The shock was applied in the afternoon between 2:00 and 5:00 p.m. Flow duration of the current and the duration of each square wave were fixed at 0.2 seconds and at 0.4 milliseconds, respectively. Electrodes were attached to each animal's ears, and the animals were positioned on their backs with their tails fixed. Thus, tonic and clonic convulsions were clearly observed. MES was defined by a latency period (lasting 1.6 seconds) followed by a short initial flexion period, then 13.2 seconds of tonic hind limb extension and 7.6 seconds of terminal clonus. Total duration of the seizure averaged 22.3 seconds. At the beginning of the study, the convulsive current 50 (CC_{50}) value for the animals and its 95% fiducial limits were calculated by the method of Litchfield and Wilcoxon.[13] Doses of 2.5, 5, or 10 mg/kg harmane were subsequently administered to groups consisting of 15 animals 45 minutes before MES.

PTZ Model

The procedure has been reported in detail elsewhere.[14,15] Animals were given harmane-HCl (2.5, 5, or 10 mg/kg) 30 minutes before convulsive stimulus (80 mg/kg PTZ). Following each PTZ injection, mice were placed individually in acrylic observation chambers for 30 minutes, and behavioral seizures were rated according to the following scale: 0, no change in behavior; I, myoclonic jerks; II, minimum seizures, with convulsive wave through the body; III, fully developed minimal seizures, clonus of the head muscles and forelimbs, with righting reflex present; IV, major seizures (generalized without the tonic phase); V, generalized tonic-clonic seizures that began with running, followed by the loss of righting ability, then a short tonic phase (flexion or extension of fore and hind limbs) progressing to clonus of all four limbs leading sometimes to the death of the animal. The time between the injection of PTZ and the onset of myoclonic jerks is defined as the seizure-onset time.

Statistical Analysis

Data (seizure-onset time, percentage of grade V seizures, and the survival percentage) were analyzed with ANOVA, followed by the Tukey multiple comparison test, if appropriate. Data are presented as the percentage of response or mean ± SD. The harmane pretreatment group was compared with PTZ group; $P < 0.05$ was considered statistically significant.

RESULTS AND DISCUSSION

In mice, the CC_{50} was found to be 47 mA, and its fiducial limits were 53.5 mA (upper limit) and 41.2 mA (lower limit). Pretreatment with harmane at all doses decreased the threshold of MES (TABLE 1). The frequencies of convulsions were 66% at 2.5 mg/kg, 46% at 5.0 mg/kg, and 20% at 10 mg/kg harmane. These groups were compared with a control group treated with saline only, and all results in the MES model were statistically significant. None of the animals in the MES group died in the MES group.

A single injection of PTZ in a dose of 80 mg/kg i.p. produced myoclonic jerks at 47.79 ± 6.87 seconds after PTZ administration. FIGURE 1 shows the effect of harmane on PTZ-induced convulsions in terms of seizure-onset time (FIG. 1A), grade V tonic-clonic convulsions (FIG. 1B), and survival percentage (FIG. 1C) for 30 minutes after PTZ injection. Harmane (2.5, 5, or 10 mg/kg) produced myoclonic jerks at 62.55 ± 6.5 seconds; 55.46 ± 5.49 seconds; 54.08 ± 7.32 seconds after PTZ administration, respectively. The difference in onset time of myoclonic jerks was not statistically different in any of the harmane groups when compared with the PTZ-only

TABLE 1. Effect of harmane on maximal electroshock seizure in mice

		Maximal Electroshock Seizure	
Dose (mg/kg)	Number of Animals	Numbers	%
Saline	50	25	50
Harmane (2.5)	15	10	66
Harmane (5)	15	7	46
Harmane (10)	15	3	20*

Harmane (2.5, 5, or 10 mg/kg i.p.) or saline administered 30 minutes before MES (60 Hz, 0.2 seconds).

* $P < 0.05$ compared with saline group.

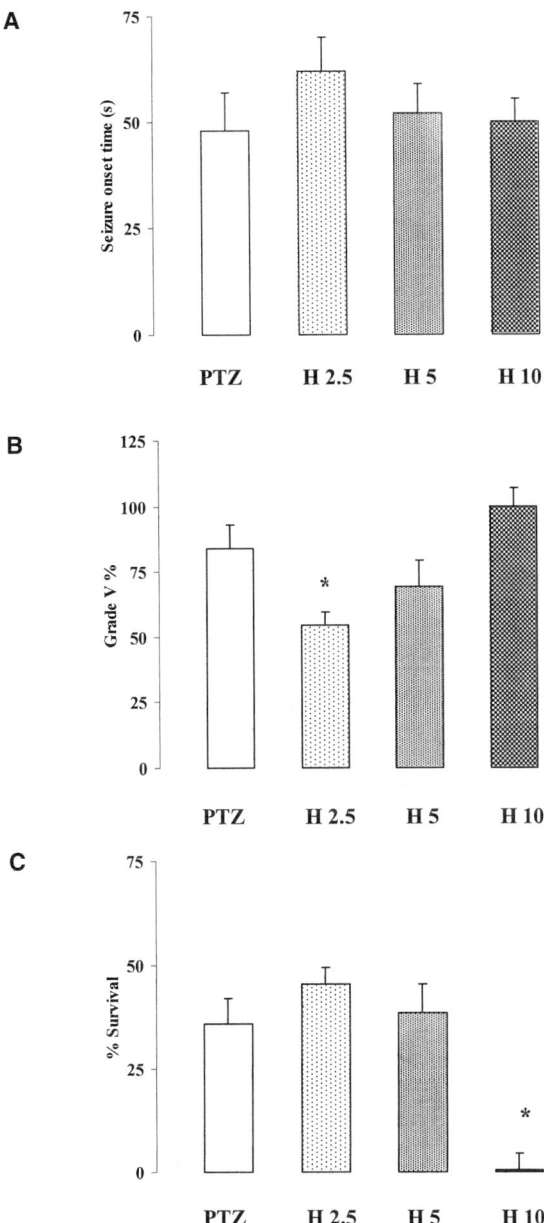

FIGURE 1. Effect of harmane on PTZ-induced convulsions. Harmane (2.5, 5, or 10 mg/kg i.p.) was administered 30 minutes before PTZ (80 mg/kg). Measurements were (**A**) seizure-onset time, (**B**) grade V tonic-clonic convulsions, (**C**) survival percentage. Data presented as mean ± SD; n = 15 in each group. H, harmane. * $P < 0.05$ compared with PTZ group.

group. In PTZ-induced convulsions, the percentage of grade V convulsions was found to be decreased by a low dose of harmane (2.5 mg/kg) ($P < 0.05$) but increased by a high dose (10 mg/kg) (results not statistically significant). The survival percentage was decreased with high-dose (10 mg/kg) ($P < 0.05$) and increased with low-dose (2.5 mg/kg) harmane (results not statistically significant).

The present study shows that harmane prevented MES-induced convulsions significantly and dose-dependently. PTZ-induced convulsions, however, were aggravated with high doses of harmane. This finding can be interpreted to mean that harmane is protective against a grand mal seizure model, but in the petit mal seizure model the dose of harmane is critical.

Harmane has been proposed to be an endogenous ligand for imidazoline receptors.[12] A possible interaction with imidazoline receptors may be responsible for the attenuating effects of harmane on the convulsive threshold. Noradrenaline acts as an inhibitory neurotransmitter within the brain, partly facilitating GABAergic transmission. In animals, the higher monoamine level produced by monoamine oxidase inhibitors protects them against seizure susceptibility.[16]

A second action known of harmane is stimulation of the benzodiazepine receptor in an inverse manner.[8] Harmane binds to the benzodiazepine receptor complex with an inhibition constant (Ki) value in the low micromolar range.[8] Reduction in benzodiazepine receptor density in the epileptogenic foci of patients with epilepsy has been reported.[17] In tonic-clonic generalized seizures, labeling of benzodiazepine receptors is enhanced in cerebellar nuclei and decreased in thalamus,[16] apparently because of corresponding modifications in receptor density.

A further explanation for the effects of harmane may involve changes in dopamine and serotonin levels. It has been shown that harmane increases extracellular dopamine and serotonin levels, probably by inhibition of monoamine oxidase A.[11] It has also been shown that high doses of harmane increase both homovanillic acid and 5-hydroxyindole acetic acid levels.[11,18] Inhibition of monoamine oxidase A elicits an increased efflux of both dopamine and serotonin. It is accepted that serotonin delays seizure generation, whereas a reduction in serotonin promotes the occurrence of seizures. Thus, serotonin depletion decreases the discharge threshold in rats pretreated with pentylenetetrazol, whereas administration of precursor serotonin increases it.[19]

Our study indicates that harmane can influence epileptic activity in the MES model in mice but not in PTZ-induced convulsions. As an endogenous substance, harmane may modulate the convulsive threshold and may provide a new understanding of the mechanism of epilepsy.

REFERENCES

1. TSE, S.Y.H., I.T. MAK & B.F. DICKENS. 1991. Antioxidative properties of harmane and β-carboline alkaloids. Biochem. Pharmacol. **42:** 459–464.
2. HOLMSTEDT, B. & J.E. LINDGREN. 1967. Chemical constituents and pharmacology of South American snuffs. *In* Ethnopharmacologic Search for Psychoactive Drugs. D.H. Efron, D. Holmstedt & N.D. Kline, Eds.: 339–373. Raven Press. New York, NY.
3. AIRAKSINEN, M.M. & I. KARI. 1981. β-carbolines, psychoactive compounds in the mammalian body: part I. Occurrence, origin and metabolism. Med. Biol. **59:** 21–34.
4. BECK, O. & K.F. FAULL. 1986. Concentrations of the enantiomers of 5-hydoxymethtryptoline in mammalian urine: implications for in vivo biosynthesis. Biochem. Pharmacol. **35:** 2636–2639.

5. MULLER, W.E., et al. 1981. On the neuropharmacology of harman and other β-carbolines. Pharmacol. Biochem. Behav. **14:** 693–699.
6. LUTES, J., et al. 1988. Tolerance to the tremorogenic effects of harmaline: evidence for altered olivo-cerebellar function. Neuropharmacology **27:** 849–855.
7. ROMMELSPACHER, H., P. DUFEU & L.G. SCHMIDT. 1996. Harman and norharman in alcoholism: correlation with psychopathology and long-term changes. Alcohol. Clin. Exp. Res. **20:** 3–8.
8. LOEW, G.H., et al. 1985. Theoretical structure-activity studies of β-carboline analogs. Requirements for benzodiazepine receptor affinity and antagonist activity. Mol. Pharmacol. **28:** 17–31.
9. ROMMELSPACHER, H., T. MAY & B. SALWSKI. 1994. Harman (1-methyl-β-carboline) is a natural inhibitor of monoamine oxidase type A in rats. Eur. J. Pharmacol. **252:** 51–59.
10. MAY, T., M. PAWLIK & H. ROMMELSPACHER. 1991. [3H]Harman binding experiments. II: regional and subcellular distribution of specific [3H]Harman binding and monoamine oxidase subtype A and B activity in marmoset and rat. J. Neurochem. **56:** 500–508.
11. ADEL, A. & R.D. MYERS. 1995. 5-HT, dopamine, norepinephrine and related metabolites in brain of low alcohol drinking (LAD) rats shift after chronic intra-hippocampal infusion of harmane. Neurochem. Res. **20:** 209–215.
12. HUSBANDS, S.M., et al. 2001. Beta-carboline binding to imidazoline receptors. Drug Alcohol Depend. **64:** 203–208.
13. LITCHFIELD, J.T. & F. WILCOX. 1949. A simplified method of evaluating dose-effect experiments. J. Pharmacol. Exp. Ther. **96:** 99–113.
14. RACINE, R.J. 1972. Modification of seizure activity by electrical stimulation. II. Motor seizure. Electroencephalogr. Clin. Neurophysiol. **32:** 281–294.
15. RACINE, R.J. 1972. Modification of seizure activity by electrical stimulation. I. Afterdischarge threshold. Electroencephalogr. Clin. Neurophysiol. **32:** 269–279.
16. MISHRA, P.K., et al. 1993. Anticonvulsant effects of intracerebroventricularly administered norepinephrine are potentiated in the presence of monoamine oxidase inhibition in severe seizure genetically epilepsy-prone rats (GEPR-9s). Life Sci. **52:** 1435–1441.
17. SAVIC, I., et al. 1994. In vivo demonstration of altered benzodiazepine receptor density in patients with generalized epilepsy. J. Neurosurg. Psychiatry **57:** 797–804.
18. BAUM, S.S., R. HILL & H. ROMMELSPACHER. 1996. Harmane-induced changes of extracellular concentrations of neurotransmitters in the nucleus accumbens of rats. Eur. J. Pharmacol. **314:** 75–82.
19. SGARAGLI, G., et al. 1981. Hypothermia induced in rabbits by intracerebroventricular taurine: specificity and relationships with central serotonin (5-HT) systems. J. Pharmacol. Exp. Ther. **219:** 778–785.

Harmane Induces Anxiolysis and Antidepressant-Like Effects in Rats

FEYZA ARICIOGLU AND HALE ALTUNBAS

Department of Pharmacology, Faculty of Pharmacy, Marmara University, Haydarpasa, Istanbul, Turkey

ABSTRACT: A forced swim test (FST) and an elevated plus maze (EPM) were used to determine antidepressant and anxiolytic effects of harmane in rats in comparison with a known antidepressant, imipramine (30 mg/kg i.p.). Harmane (2.5, 5.0, or 10 mg/kg, i.p.), saline, or imipramine were given 30 minutes before the tests. Administration of harmane decreased the time of immobility in the FST dose-dependently and increased the time spent in open arms in the EPM, as compared with the saline group. As an endogenous substance, harmane therefore has anti-anxiety and antidepressant effects.

KEYWORDS: harmane; forced swim test; elevated plus maze; imidazoline; benzodiazepine; monoamine oxidase

INTRODUCTION

The amine harmane (1-methyl-β-carboline) was originally identified in plants (*Peganum harmala*), and related alkaloids are found in medicinal plants.[1] β-Carboline alkaloids are also present in small concentrations in the food chain, in commonly eaten plant-derived foods (wheat, rice, corn, and barley), beverages (wine, beer, whisky, and sake),[2] and inhaled substances (tobacco).[3] Harmane occurs in blood, heart, kidney, liver, urine, and brain.[4] Many β-carboline alkaloids are highly lipophilic, and brain concentrations are as much as 55 times higher than those in plasma.[5] β-Carbolines have a wide spectrum of pharmacologic actions in Parkinson's disease,[14] cancer,[15] and addiction.[16] Previously it has been shown that a β-carboline infused acutely into the hypothalamus can induce an intense anxiety-like state as well as a strong preference for alcohol in rats.[17] There is evidence that harmane binds to imidazoline receptors and is considered an endogenous ligand of these receptors.[6] Furthermore, harmane is an endogenous ligand (inverse agonist) of the benzodiazepine receptors in vitro and in vivo.[7,8] Harmane also inhibits monoamine oxidase enzyme (MAO), particularly type A (MAO-A), and has been used as a short-acting MAO inhibitor.[9–13]

The present study was designed to investigate the potential antidepressant and/or anxiolytic effects of harmane by using the forced swim test (FST) and the elevated plus maze (EPM), respectively, in rats.

Address for correspondence: Feyza Aricioglu, Ph.D., Department of Pharmacology, Faculty of Pharmacy, Marmara University, 81010 Tibbiye Cad. No: 49, Haydarpasa, Istanbul, Turkey. Voice: 0216 418 95 73; fax: 0216 345 29 52.

e-mail: feyzak@turk.net

MATERIALS AND METHODS

Animals

Experiments performed in accordance with the Guide for the Care and Use of Laboratory Animals adopted by the National Institute of Health (USA) and Declaration of Helsinki. Male adult Sprague-Dawley rats (180–200 g) were used. Animals were maintained on a 12-hour light/dark cycle and given ad libitum access to food and water.

Drugs

Harmane-HCl and imipramine-HCl were purchased from Sigma Chemical Co. (St. Louis, MO, USA) and dissolved in saline. The drugs or saline were injected intraperitoneally (i.p.) at a volume of 0.1 mL/100 g body weight. Fresh solutions of drugs were prepared 30 minutes before the tests.

Elevated Plus Maze

The apparatus was made of wood and consisted of two opposite open arms, 50 cm × 10 cm, and two opposite arms of equal size enclosed by 40-cm–high walls. The arms were connected by a central 10 cm × 10 cm square, and thus the maze formed a "plus" shape. The maze was elevated 50 cm from the floor and lit by dim light. Rats were placed individually in the center of the maze facing a closed arm and allowed 5 minutes of free exploration. The maze was cleaned thoroughly after each test. Thirty minutes before the test, rats received harmane, i.p., at doses of 2.5, 5.0, or 10 mg/kg.

Forced Swim Test

Rats were placed in a glass cylinder (45 cm high, 20 cm in diameter) filled with water to a height of 30 cm that was meticulously maintained at 25°C ± 1°C. Rats were forced to swim for 15 minutes. After an initial struggle to escape from the water, the rats eventually adopted a posture of immobility in which they made only slight movements necessary to keep their heads above water. After 15 minutes of FST, the rats were removed from the water, dried, and placed in a warmed enclosure for 30 minutes. The cylinders were emptied and cleaned between uses. Twenty-four hours after the first session, rats received 2.5, 5.0, or 10 mg/kg harmane 30 minutes before the second FST. The 15-minute FST was repeated, and immobilization time was recorded. All tests were conducted between 10:00 am and 4:00 pm.

Statistical Analysis

Data obtained are expressed as mean ± SE. Differences between groups were analyzed by ANOVA. Duncan's post hoc comparisons, when appropriate, were carried out if significant overall $F-$ values were obtained ($P < 0.05$).

RESULTS AND DISCUSSION

Harmane decreased the duration of immobility in the FST in a dose-dependent manner (FIG. 1). Results with all doses of harmane (2.5, 5.0, or 10 mg/kg) were

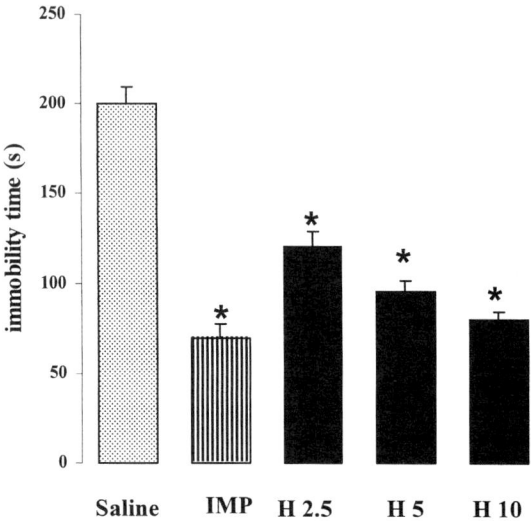

FIGURE 1. Effect of harmane (2.5, 5, or 10 mg/kg i.p.) on forced swim test in rats. Harmane or imipramine (30 mg/kg i.p.) was administered 30 minutes before the test. Values are expressed as mean ± SD (n = 10 in each group). * $P < 0.05$ versus saline group. H, harmane; IMP, imipramine.

significantly different from with saline controls, and the highest dose of harmane (10 mg/kg) was as effective as imipramine (30 mg/kg i.p.) in the FST (FIG. 1). Similarly, harmane (5.0 and 10 mg/kg i.p.) increased time spent in the open arms of the EPM, and the highest dose of harmane (10 mg/kg) was as effective as imipramine (30 mg/kg i.p.) (FIG. 2). Harmane also increased time spent in total arms of the EPM in a dose-dependent manner (data not shown). Rats receiving 2.5 mg/kg harmane did not significantly differ from controls in time spent in open arms of the EPM (FIG 2).

The FST and EPM are accepted models of depression and anxiety, respectively, and they are widely used to screen for new antidepressant and anxiolytic drugs. The effects of harmane have been compared with imipramine in both tests. Harmane significantly and dose-dependently increased the duration of immobility in the FST, as did imipramine (FIG. 1). Harmane was also effective in increasing the percentage of time spent in open arms of the EPM, as was imipramine (FIG. 2). These results indicate, for the first time, that harmane has both antidepressant-like and anxiolytic-like properties.

The effects of harmane in the FST and EPM may be caused by several mechanisms. Harmane binds to several receptors in the brain, including those for serotonin (5-HT2, IC50 = 6.75 µM), dopamine (D2, IC50 = 163 µM), and benzodiazepines (IC50 = 7 µM).[18] Because harmane is a potent endogenous ligand (inverse agonist) of the benzodiazepine receptor in vitro, the action of harmane could be caused by stimulation of benzodiazepine receptors in an inverse manner. Harmane also inhibits MAO-A in vitro by reversibly binding with high affinity (nM range) to the active site of the enzyme. Specific [^{3}H]-harmane binding is displaceable by substrates of the

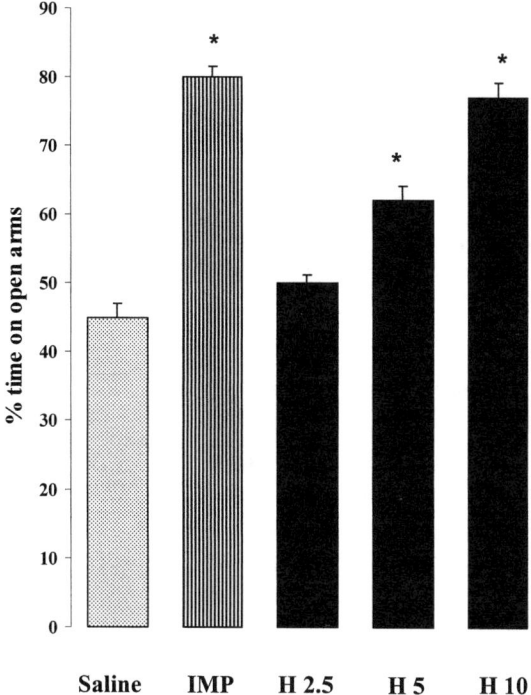

FIGURE 2. Effect of harmane (2.5, 5, or 10 mg/kg i.p.) on elevated plus maze test in rats. Harmane or imipramine (30 mg/kg i.p.) was administered 30 minutes before the test. Data are presented as percentage of time spent in open arms. Values are expressed as mean ± SD (n = 10 in each group), * $P < 0.05$ versus saline group. H, harmane; IMP, imipramine.

enzyme, such as serotonin and other biogenic amine neurotransmitters, as well as by potent and selective inhibitors of MAO-A; however harmane is not oxidized by MAO-A.[10,12,13] There are also ex vivo and in vivo experiments showing that harmane inhibits MAO-A specifically and reversibly.[9-13] It has also been shown that harmane operates as a natural inhibitor of MAO-A, but only a small percentage of the enzyme is inhibited under physiologic conditions.[9] The binding of harmane for imidazoline receptors may also play a role. I_2 sites are of interest to psychiatry because they are physically associated with MAO-A and B.[19]

A further explanation for the antidepressant and anxiolytic effects of harmane may involve dopamine and serotonin. It has been shown that harmane increases extracellular dopamine and serotonin levels, probably by inhibition of MAO-A.[9,11] It has also been shown that high doses of harmane increase their respective metabolites, homovanillic acid , and 5-hydroxyindole acetic acid levels.[9,11] It has also been shown that harmane infusion causes release of serotonin and norepinephrine in alcohol-drinking rats.[17]

In conclusion, exogenous administration of harmane attenuates behaviors associated with anxiety and depression in rat models in a dose-dependent manner. This action of harmane makes the compound a novel and potentially advantageous therapeutic agent for treatment of depression and anxiolysis. The existence of harmane in mammalian tissues raises speculation regarding its function as an endogenous antidepressant and anxiolytic.

REFERENCES

1. TSE, S.Y.H., I.T. MAK & B.F. DICKENS. 1991. Antioxidative properties of harmane and β-carboline alkaloids. Biochem. Pharmacol. **42:** 459–464.
2. ADACHI, J., et al. 1991. Determination of beta-carbolines in foodstuffs by high-performance liquid chromatography-mass spectrometry. J. Chromatogr. **538:** 331–339.
3. POINDEXTER, E.H. Jr. & R.D. CARPENTER. 1962. The isolation of harman and norharman from tobacco and cigarette smoke. Phytochemistry **1:** 215–221.
4. BECK, O. & K.F. FAULL. 1986. Concentrations of the enantiomers of 5-hydoxymethtryptoline in mammalian urine: implications for in vivo biosynthesis. Biochem. Pharmacol. **35:** 2636–2639.
5. SPIJKERMAN, R., et al. 2002. The impact of smoking and drinking on plasma levels of norharman. Eur. Neuropsycopharmacol. **12:** 61–71.
6. HUSBANDS, S.M., et al. 2001. Beta-carboline binding to imidazoline receptors. Drug Alcohol Depend. **64:** 203–208.
7. LOEW, G.H., et al. 1985. Theoretical structure-activity studies of β-carboline analogs. Requirements for benzodiazepine receptor affinity and antagonist activity. Mol. Pharmacol. **28:** 17–31.
8. CLOW A., et al. 1983. New endogenous benzodiazepine receptor ligand in human urine: identity with endogenous monoamine oxidase inhibitor? Life Sci. **33:** 735–741.
9. ROMMELSPACHER, H., T. MAY & B. SALWSKI. 1994. Harman (1-methyl-β-carboline) is a natural inhibitor of monoamine oxidase type A in rats. Eur. J. Pharmacol. **252:** 51–59.
10. MAY, T., M. PAWLIK & H. ROMMELSPACHER. 1991. [3H]Harman binding experiments. II: regional and subcellular distribution of specific [3H]Harman binding and monoamine oxidase subtype A and B activity in marmoset and rat. J. Neurochem. **56:** 500–508.
11. MAY, T. 1993. 1-methyl-4-phenylpridinium (MPP+) binds with high affinity to a β-carboline binding site located on monoamine oxidase type A in rat brain. Neurosci. Lett. **162:** 55–58.
12. MAY, T., S. STRAUSS & H. ROMMELSPACHER. 1991. [3H]Harman labels selectively and with high affinity the active site of monoamine oxidase (EC 1.4.3.4) subtype A (MAO-A) in rat, marmoset and pig. J. Neural Transm. **32:** 93–102.
13. MAY, T., H. ROMMELSPACHER & M. PAWLIK. 1991. [3H]Harman binding experiments. I: a reversible and selective radioligand for monoamine oxidase subtype A in the CNS of the rat. J. Neurochem. **56:** 490–499.
14. KUHN, W., et al. 1996. Elevated levels of harman and norharman in cerebrospinal fluid of parkinsonian patients. J. Neural Transm. **103:** 1435–1440.
15. WAKABAYASHI, K., et al. 1997. Human exposure to mutagenic/carcinogenic heterocyclic amines and comutagenic beta-carbolines. Mutat. Res. **376:** 253–259.
16. CAPPENDIJK, S.L., D. FEKKES & M.R. DZOLJIC. 1994. The inhibitory effect of norharmane on morphine withdrawal syndrome in rats: comparison with ibogaine. Behav. Brain Res. **65:** 117–119.
17. ROMMELSPACHER, H., C. BUCHAU & J. WEISS. 1987. Harman induces preference for ethanol in rats: is the effect specific for ethanol? Pharmacol. Biochem. Behav. **26:** 749–755.
18. BAUM, S.S., R. HILL & H. ROMMELSPACHER. 1996. Harman-induced changes of extracellular concentrations of neurotransmitters in the nucleus accumbens of rat. Eur. J. Pharmacol. **314:** 75–82.
19. LALIES, M.D., et al. 1999. Inhibition of central monoamine oxidase by imidazoline-2 site selective ligands. Ann. N. Y. Acad Sci. **881:** 114–118.

No Evidence for Activation of α_2-Adrenoceptors by Methanolic Extracts of Bovine Brain and Lung Containing Clonidine-Displacing Substance

D. PINTHONG,[a] D.A. KENDALL,[a] S.J. MacLENNAN,[b] R.M. EGLEN,[b] AND V.G. WILSON[a]

[a]*School of Biomedical Sciences, The Medical School, Queen's Medical Centre, Nottingham NG7 2UH, UK*

[b]*Center for Biological Research, Roche Bioscience, Palo Alto, California 94303, USA*

ABSTRACT: Methanolic extracts of bovine brain and lung are capable of displacing [^{3}H]-clonidine from α_2-adrenoceptor binding sites, indicating the presence of a clonidine-displacing substance (CDS). We have examined α_2-adrenergic responses and the extracts in three models: [^{3}H]-cyclic AMP accumulation in miniprisms of guinea pig cerebral cortex, isometric tension measurements of isolated segments of the rat vas deferens, and porcine palmar lateral vein. The selective α_2-adrenoceptor agonist, 5-bromo-6-2-imidazolin-2-ylamino]-quinoxaline bitartrate (UK-14304) inhibited forskolin-stimulated [^{3}H]-cyclic AMP accumulation in the cerebral cortex and elicited contractions of the porcine isolated palmar lateral vein. Clonidine (0.1–30 nM) inhibited neurogenic contractions of the rat vas deferens. Responses to both agonists were inhibited by the α_2-adrenoceptor antagonists, idazoxan or rauwolscine. Brain CDS (5 units/mL) reduced forskolin-stimulated [^{3}H]-cyclic AMP accumulation in the guinea pig cerebral cortex, whereas lung CDS (1 unit/mL) increased the accumulation of the cyclic nucleotide. Neither response to the extracts was inhibited by 1 µM idazoxan. Low concentrations of both extracts (0.05 unit/mL) reduced electrically evoked contractions of the rat vas deferens by approximately 20%, but higher concentrations enhanced neurogenic contractions by approximately 50%. Again, the effect of the brain extract was not altered by 1 µM idazoxan. Lung CDS (0.02–1 unit/mL) induced contractions of the porcine palmar lateral vein that were also insensitive to rauwolscine. The results suggest that brain and lung CDS do not activate either central or peripheral α_2-adrenoceptors.

KEYWORDS: α_2-adrenoceptors; rat vas deferens; guinea pig cerebral cortex; clonidine-displacing substance; harmane

INTRODUCTION

Atlas and Burstein[1] coined the term clonidine-displacing substance (CDS) to describe the ability of a noncatecholamine substance, contained in a partially purified

Address for correspondence: Vince Wilson, School of Biomedical Sciences, The Medical School, Queen's Medical Centre, Clifton Boulevard, Nottingham NG7 2UH, UK. Voice: 00 44 115 9709472; fax: 00 44 115 9709259.
  e-mail: Vince.wilson@nottingham.ac.uk

Ann. N.Y. Acad. Sci. 1009: 201–215 (2003). © 2003 New York Academy of Sciences.
doi: 10.1196/annals.1304.025

extract of rat and bovine brain, to displace [^{3}H]-clonidine from α_2-adrenoceptor binding sites on bovine cerebral cortex membranes. In subsequent experiments these workers[2] and others[3] reported that the extract was also able to recognize selectively nonadrenoceptor imidazoline binding sites labeled by either [^{3}H]-idazoxan or [^{3}H]-clonidine, sites latter classified as I_1 and I_2 imidazoline receptors (reviewed in Eglen et al.[4]). Agmatine[5] and, more recently, the β-carboline harmane[6] have been shown to be endogenous ligands for imidazoline receptors, but neither agent possesses appreciable affinity for α_2-adrenoceptors and cannot, therefore, account for the CDS activity originally described. Significantly, CDS has been shown to possess biologic activity commensurate with agonist properties at α_2-adrenoceptors. Atlas and coworkers[7,8] reported that CDS activates α_2-adrenoceptors on human platelets to produce a pro-aggregatory response and that CDS acts on pre-junctional α_2-adrenoceptors on the rat vas deferens to inhibit neurogenic contractions.

Because CDS is a candidate for an endogenous, noncatecholamine ligand for α_2-adrenoceptors,[4,9,10] it may account for two important aspects of α_2-adrenoceptor pharmacology. First, CDS could shed light on the differences between imidazoline derivatives and catecholamines in their structural requirements for receptor activation[11,12] and the characteristics of biologic responses (e.g., time course and calcium dependency) mediated by this receptor subtype.[13] Second, CDS, together with noradrenaline and adrenaline, could provide useful insights into the classification of α_2-adrenoceptors which currently is largely based on differences between receptor antagonists.[14,15]

Herein, three functional models are described to compare the effects of methanolic extracts containing CDS with known selective α_2-adrenoceptor agonists: (1) inhibition of [^{3}H]-cyclic AMP accumulation in the guinea pig isolated cerebral cortex, (2) inhibition of electrically evoked contractions of the rat isolated vas deferens,[16] and (3) contractile responses of the porcine isolated palmar lateral vein.[17] The vas deferens permits a direct comparison of the biologic properties of CDS extracted in our laboratory with those originally examined by Diamant and Atlas.[7] We have also compared the effects of brain and lung methanolic extracts of CDS with those of harmane to establish whether the β-carboline derivative could account for any of the non–α_2-adrenoceptor properties of the extracts.

MATERIALS AND METHODS

Preparation of Bovine Cerebral Cortex Membrane

Calf brains were obtained from a local abattoir immediately after the slaughter of the animals. The cerebral cortices were homogenized in 20 volumes of ice-cold Tris buffer (50 mM Tris HCl; pH 7.7 at 25°C) using an OMNI-GEN sealed macro-homogenizer (Camlab, Cambridge, UK; setting 5; 120 s) to minimize potential risks associated with aerosol formation. The homogenate was centrifuged at 20,000 rpm (40,000 gravity) for 10 minutes at 4°C (MSE Europa 24M; Berthold Hermle KG, Weisbaden, Germany). The supernatant was discarded, and the pellet resuspended in 20 volumes (w/v) of ice-cold 50 mM Tris buffer (pH 7.7 at 25°C) using an Ultra-turrax homogenizer (Northern Media Company, Humberside, UK) sited in a laminar airflow hood. The resuspended membranes were recentrifuged for a further 15 minutes, and the supernatant was discarded. The remaining pellets were weighed and resuspended in six volumes of ice-cold 50 mM Tris buffer and then aliquoted for direct use in binding assay or stored at $-20°C$.

Preparation of CDS from Bovine Brain and Lung

Bovine brain and lungs were obtained from a local abattoir immediately after slaughter of the animal. Half a bovine brain (110–160 g wet weight) was taken and the cerebellum and the pia mater removed before the brain was chopped into small pieces. The brain was homogenized in an OMNI-GEN sealed homogenizer (setting, 4.5 for 3×3 minutes) with 5 volumes (w/v) of distilled water. Lung (80 g wet weight) was finely chopped and placed in 10 volumes (w/v) of boiling distilled water. The extractions of both brain and lung were performed in the same manner with the addition of an earlier step of maceration of the chopped lung in 400 mL cold distilled water using a blender (3×1 minute at high speed, 1-minute intervals) before homogenization. Lung tissues were then homogenized using an OMNI-GEN sealed homogenizer (setting 4.5 for 3×3 minutes), and the resulting homogenates centrifuged at 65,000 gravity for 30 minutes at $4°C$ (MSE Superspeed 65). The supernatant was removed, boiled for approximately 40 to 60 minutes to precipitate soluble protein and to reduce the volume, and then allowed to cool to room temperature. The resulting solution was recentrifuged at 65,000 gravity for 15 minutes. The supernatant was removed from the pellets, divided into three or four equal portions, frozen at $-20°C$, and then freeze-dried. The freeze-dried materials were used for further extraction.

The lyophilized material (a yellowish brown, dry, fluffy residue) was extracted by sonication with 2×20 mL highly purified methanol (HPLC grade) at room temperature for 30 minutes. The methanolic extracts were combined and centrifuged at 3,000 rpm for 5 minutes (MSE Mistral 3000) to remove any particulate matter. These were evaporated to dryness in a rotary evaporator at low pressure. The residual material (a brown, viscous residue) was dissolved in 10 volumes (w/v) double-distilled water, frozen, and lyophilized again to remove all traces of the organic solvent. The final lyophilized material was redissolved in 10 volumes (w/v) double-distilled water and kept in 3-mL aliquots until required.

Determination of CDS Activity of the Extract

The CDS activity of the methanolic extracts was evaluated by determining the displacement of [^{3}H]-clonidine (1 nM) from α_2-adrenoceptor sites on bovine cerebral cortex membranes. The final assay volume was 0.5 mL, which contained 100 μL bovine cerebral cortex membranes, the radioligand (50 μL), and increasing amounts of the extract in 50 mM Tris buffer (pH 7.4 at room temperature). Nonspecific binding was determined in the presence of 100 μM noradrenaline. After an incubation period of 60 minutes at room temperature, bound radioactivity was separated from free by vacuum filtration over Whatman GF/B glass fiber (Siemat, Dorset, UK) using a Brandel cell harvester (Biomedical Research and Development Laboratories, Gaithersburg, MD, USA) followed by 2×3 mL washes with ice-cold assay buffers. The filters were then suspended in 4 mL of scintillation cocktail, and bound ligand was determined by scintillation spectrometry.

One unit of CDS activity is defined as the amount of the extract that produced 50% inhibition of [^{3}H]-clonidine (1 nM) binding to bovine cerebral cortex membranes. CDS activity was calculated in unit/g wet weight of tissue.

The Effect of CDS Extracts on Forskolin-Stimulated [^{3}H]-Cyclic AMP Accumulation

Male guinea pigs (250–300 g) were killed by cervical dislocation. The cerebral cortices were dissected out on ice and chopped into miniprisms (350 × 350 µm) using a McIlwain tissue chopper (Mickle Lab Engineering, Surrey, UK). The slices were dispersed into oxygenated modified Krebs-Henseleit (K-H) solution in a stoppered conical flask with several cycles of aspiration and re-addition of medium (one guinea pig cortex per 100 mL flask containing 30–40 mL medium). The cortex slices were pre-incubated for 60 minutes in modified K-H solution in a shaking water bath at 37°C, washed with K-H solution, and then labeled with 0.4 µM [^{3}H]-adenine (37 kBq/mL) for 45 minutes. After washing away the unincorporated [^{3}H]-adenine with three changes of K-H solution, the slices were allowed to settle. Aliquots of cortex slices (25 µL) were distributed into flat-bottomed vials containing K-H saline to maintain a final volume of 300 µL. Basal levels of [^{3}H]-cyclic AMP accumulation were assessed when slices were incubated in the K-H solution for 30 minutes. Forskolin-stimulated [^{3}H]-cyclic AMP accumulation was measured in slices maintained in K-H solution for 20 minutes and then exposed to 30 µM forskolin for 10 minutes. The effects of 5-bromo-6-2-imidazolin-2-ylamino-quinoxaline bitartrate (UK-14304), a selective α_2-adrenoceptor agonist, histamine (100 µM), and the methanolic extracts against basal or forskolin-stimulated [^{3}H]-cyclic AMP accumulation were determined by making additions 10 or 20 minutes, respectively, before the end of the exposure period. In some experiments the effects of these agents were examined against forskolin-stimulated [^{3}H]-cyclic AMP accumulation following addition of either idazoxan (1 µM) or a combination of 1 µM mepyramine or 100 µM cimetidine (added at the beginning of the 30-minute exposure period). Incubation tubes were re-sealed under an atmosphere of 95% O_2/5% CO_2 after each addition. At the end of the exposure period the incubations were terminated by the addition of 200 µL M HCl followed by 750 µL cold distilled water. All experiments were conducted in duplicate.

[^{3}H]-Cyclic AMP from the cerebral cortex miniprisms was isolated by sequential Dowex 50/alumina chromatography using [^{14}C]-cyclic AMP as a recovery marker. Aliquots of the supernatant (0.9 mL) were applied to Dowex 50 columns (Bio-Rad, filled with 1 mL resin). Distilled water (2 mL) was added to elute [^{3}H]-ATP and [^{3}H]-ADP to waste. [^{3}H]-cyclic AMP was desorbed from the Dowex resin by applying 4 mL water, which was allowed to drip directly onto alumina columns. [^{3}H]-Cyclic AMP was eluted from the alumina columns with 5 mL 0.1 M imidazole directly into scintillation vials. Scintillation cocktail (10 mL) was added to the effluent and mixed to form a gel before counting in a refrigerated liquid scintillation counter, using a dual channel [^{3}H]/[^{14}C] program. [^{3}H]-Cyclic AMP levels were corrected for recovery from Dowex/alumina chromatography and the total [^{3}H]-adenine taken into each individual tissue.

The Effect of CDS Extracts on Isolated Vas Deferens and Palmar Lateral Vein

Male Wistar rats (200–300 g) were killed by CO_2 asphyxiation. The prostatic end of the vas deferens was removed and placed in oxygenated, ice-cold modified K-H solution. The lower end of the vas deferens was secured to a plastic holder between parallel platinum wire electrodes. The upper end was attached by cotton to a Grass FT-03C isometric transducer connected to a Grass polygraph (Grass, Quincey, MA, USA). The holder was placed in an isolated organ bath containing 20 mL modified K-H solution with 1 µM propranolol (to block β-adrenoceptors) gassed with 95% O_2, 5% CO_2 and maintained at 37°C. After an equilibration period of 30 minutes, 1 g weight of tension was slowly applied, and the preparation allowed to relax to a final resting tension of 0.3 to 0.4 g weight over 60 minutes. Contractions of the tissue were elicited by (single-pulse) transmural stimulation by electrodes with a single supramaximal voltage (0.5 millisecond duration, 0.05 Hz, 70 volts) with an SRI stimulator (Scientific Research Instruments Ltd., Cambridge, UK). The effects of the methanolic CDS extracts were examined by cumulative addition (at 10-minute intervals) and compared with those produced by clonidine or harmane. Some preparations were also exposed, before the effect of clonidine was examined, to idazoxan (1 µM) for 30 minutes, a high concentration of the extract (1.7–4 units/mL), or 30 µM harmane.

Porcine fore-trotters were obtained from a local abattoir within 30 minutes of the death of the pig and transported to the laboratory on ice. The palmar lateral vein was dissected out, placed in oxygenated, ice-cold K-H solution containing 2% Ficoll, and stored overnight at 4°C. The following day the vein was allowed to equilibrate to room temperature (40 minutes), carefully cleaned of fat and connective tissue, and divided into 5-mm ring segments. Stainless steel wire supports (0.2 mm thick) were inserted into the lumen, and each segment was suspended in a 10-mL isolated organ bath containing K-H solution, maintained at 37°C, and gassed with 95% O_2 and 5% CO_2. No attempt was made to remove the endothelium. The lower support was fixed, and the upper support was connected to a Grass FT-03C transducer linked to a Grass polygraph. After 30 minutes equilibration in K-H solution, approximately 4 g weight of tension was slowly applied, and the tissue was allowed to relax to a final resting tension of 1.2 to 1.5 g weight of tension. After 60 minutes equilibration, each preparation was exposed to 60 mM KCl until a steady contraction was observed (usually 10 minutes) and then was washed with fresh K-H solution. The procedure was repeated until the magnitude of successive contractions to 60 mM KCl was within 10% of each other. Cumulative concentration-response curves to UK-14304 and the lung methanolic extract of CDS were determined in the absence or presence of either 0.1 µM prazosin, 0.1 µM rauwolscine, or 30 µM harmane (added 30 minutes before the agonists).

Analysis of Data

For the CDS extracts, the concentration of the extract (µL/mL) producing 50% inhibition of [^{3}H]-clonidine binding was calculated using a nonlinear least square method described by DeLean et al.[18] One unit of CDS was defined as the volume of extract required to produce 50% inhibition of 1 nM [^{3}H]-clonidine binding in bovine cerebral cortex membrane in a 1-mL assay volume. In guinea pig cerebral cortex slices, [^{3}H]-cyclic AMP accumulation was calculated as the percentage of conversion of [^{3}H]-adenine (mean of duplicate observations corrected for tissue variation and column recovery). Values are expressed as the mean ± SEM of four to eight experiments. Differences between mean responses in the presence and absence of antagonists were considered statistically significant if $P < 0.05$ (ANOVA followed by a Dunnett's test).

In the rat vas deferens and porcine isolated palmar lateral vein the effects were calculated as percentage of the electrically evoked contractions before the addition of the drugs or the response to 60 mM KCl, respectively, and were expressed as the mean ± SEM of five or six experiments. The negative logarithm of the agonist concentration producing 50% of the maximum response was calculated using a logistic equation.[18] Differences between mean responses in the presence and absence of antagonists were considered statistically significant if $P < 0.05$ using either Student's unpaired t-test or ANOVA followed by a Dunnett's test.

MATERIALS

The composition of modified K-H solution (in mM) was NaCl, 119; KCl, 4.7; $CaCl_2$, 2.5; $MgSO_4$, 1.2; $NaHCO_3$, 25; KH_2PO_4, 1.2; glucose, 11.1. Radiochemicals purchased from Amersham Biosciences (Amersham, Buckinghamshire, UK) were [^{3}H]-clonidine HCl (specific activity 30 Ci/mmol), [^{3}H]-adenine (specific activity 851 GBq/mmol), and [^{14}C]-cyclic AMP (specific activity 1.6 GBq/mmol). Scintillation cocktails (Emulsifier Scintillator 299; Packard Chemicals, Cambridge, UK) were purchased from Packard, UK. The following were purchased from Sigma Chemical Company (Poole, UK): clonidine hydrochloride; noradrenaline bitartrate; histamine; forskolin; Ficoll (80, 000 molecular weight); idazoxan (2-(2(1,4-benzodioxanyl)2-imidazoline hydrochloride); (–)–propranolol hydrochloride; harmane hydrochloride; and pyrilamine maleate (mepyramine). UK-14304 was a generous gift from Pfizer (Sandwich, UK). Cimetidine was purchased from Smith Kline Beecham Laboratories (Hertfordshire, UK). With the exception of forskolin (10 mM) and harmane (10 mM), which were dissolved in absolute alcohol, all drugs were dissolved in either K-H solution or distilled water. The maximum volume of the drugs added never exceeded 1% for the vas deferens and palmar lateral vein experiments or 3% for the [^{3}H]-cyclic AMP assay on the cerebral cortex slices. All other general chemicals were purchased from BDH (Poole, UK).

RESULTS

Effect of UK-14304 and CDS on Forskolin-Stimulated [^{3}H]-Cyclic AMP Accumulation in Guinea Pig Isolated Cerebral Cortex Slices

The basal level of [^{3}H]-cyclic AMP accumulation in guinea-pig cerebral cortex slices (0.26 ± 0.03% conversion of [^{3}H]-adenine, n = 4) was not affected by 1 µM UK-14304 (0.29 ± 0.04% conversion of [^{3}H]-adenine, n = 4). Forskolin (30 µM) caused a three- to fourfold increase in [^{3}H]-cyclic AMP accumulation which was inhibited by 1 µM UK-14304 (FIG. 1A). Idazoxan (1 µM) did not affect either basal or forskolin-stimulated [^{3}H]-cyclic AMP accumulation but abolished the inhibitory effect of UK-14304 (FIG.1A). These experiments show the presence of α_2-adrenoceptors on guinea pig cerebral cortex membranes that are negatively linked to cyclic AMP formation.

Brain methanolic CDS extract (1 unit/mL) did not affect conversion of [^{3}H]-adenine in the basal state (control, 0.24 ± 0.03% conversion, n = 8; plus extract, 0.29 ± 0.03%, n = 8). Brain methanolic CDS extract (1 unit/mL) also did not affect forskolin-stimulated [^{3}H]-cyclic AMP accumulation (FIG. 1B). Similarly, 5 units/mL brain

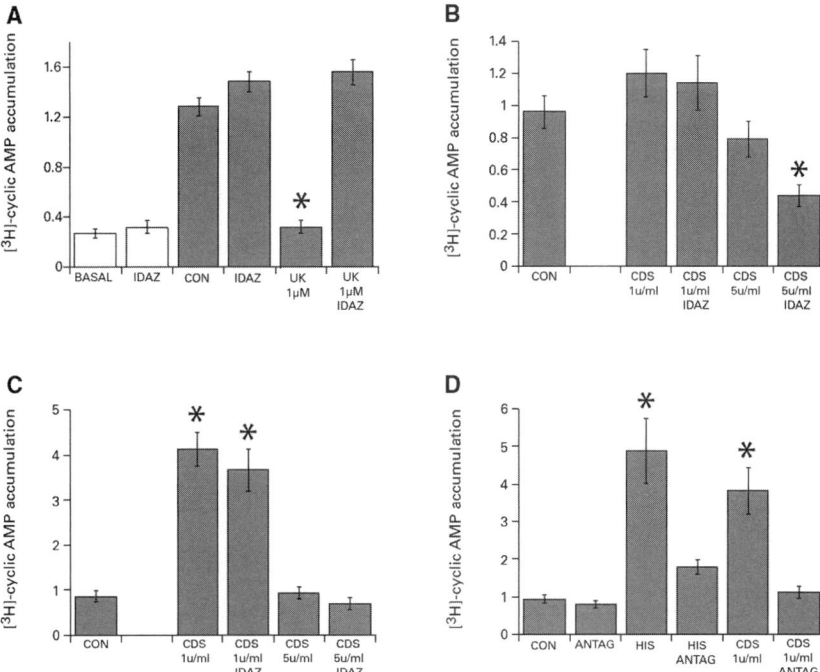

FIGURE 1. The effects of brain methanolic CDS and lung methanolic CDS on [^{3}H]-cyclic AMP accumulation in the guinea pig cerebral cortex. (**A**) Basal and forskolin-stimulated [^{3}H]-cyclic AMP accumulation (CON) is compared in the presence and absence of 1 μM idazoxan (IDAZ). The effect of 1 μM UK-14304 (with and without IDAZ) on forskolin-stimulated [^{3}H]-cyclic AMP accumulation is also shown. (**B**) The effect of brain methanolic CDS on forskolin-stimulated [^{3}H]-cyclic AMP accumulation (CON) in the presence and absence of 1 μM idazoxan. (**C**) The effect of lung methanolic CDS on forskolin-stimulated [^{3}H]-cyclic AMP accumulation (CON) in the presence and absence of 1 μM idazoxan. (**D**) The effect of 100 μM histamine and lung methanolic CDS on forskolin-stimulated [^{3}H]-cyclic AMP accumulation (CON) in the presence and absence of a combination of 1 μM mepyramine and 100 μM cimetidine (ANTAG). The results have been expressed as the percentage conversion of [^{3}H]-adenine into [^{3}H]-cyclic AMP accumulation, representing the mean ± SEM of three to five separate experiments conducted in duplicate. * Significant difference ($P < 0.05$) between forskolin-stimulated [^{3}H]-cyclic AMP accumulation (CON) and the effect of brain methanolic CDS, lung methanolic CDS, UK-14304, and histamine.

methanolic CDS extract failed to affect forskolin-stimulated [^{3}H]-cyclic AMP accumulation (FIG. 1B). Although idazoxan (1 μ M) did not alter the effect of 1 unit/mL brain methanolic CDS extract on forskolin-stimulated [^{3}H]-cyclic AMP accumulation, it uncovered an inhibitory effect of 5 units/mL of brain methanolic CDS extract on [^{3}H]-cyclic AMP accumulation (FIG. 1B). Lung methanolic CDS extract (1 unit/mL) did not affect basal [^{3}H]-cyclic AMP accumulation (control, 0.27 ± 0.04% conversion of [^{3}H]-adenine, n = 8; plus extract, 0.37 ± 0.05% conversion of [^{3}H]-adenine, n = 8). But, the lung CDS extract (1 unit/mL) significantly potentiated (approximately fourfold) forskolin-stimulated [^{3}H]-cyclic AMP accumulation (FIG. 1C). In marked contrast, 5 units/mL lung methanolic CDS extract did not significantly alter forskolin-stimulated [^{3}H]-cyclic AMP (FIG. 1C). Idazoxan (1 µM) failed to alter the effect of either 1 unit/mL or 5 units/mL lung methanolic CDS extract on forskolin-stimulated [^{3}H]-cyclic AMP accumulation (FIG. 1C). Thus, neither of the methanolic CDS extracts mimicked the effect of UK-14304 on forskolin-stimulated [^{3}H]-cyclic AMP accumulation.

Histamine is known to be present in methanolic CDS extracts of bovine lung[19] and has been reported to potentiate agonist-induced [^{3}H]-cyclic AMP accumulation in guinea pig cerebral cortex slices.[20] Therefore, we examined whether this amine could account for the potentiation of forskolin-stimulated [^{3}H]-cyclic AMP accumulation produced by lung methanolic CDS extract. Histamine (100 µM) failed to affect basal [^{3}H]-cyclic accumulation (data not shown) but significantly potentiated (approximately fourfold) forskolin-stimulated [^{3}H]-cyclic AMP accumulation (FIG. 1D). A combination of 1 µM mepyramine and 100 µM cimetidine did not alter basal [^{3}H]-cyclic AMP accumulation (FIG. 1D) but significantly reduced the enhancements of forskolin-stimulated [^{3}H]-cyclic AMP accumulation induced by histamine (100 µM) and lung methanolic CDS extract (1 unit/mL) (FIG. 1D). Thus, histamine seems to account for the ability of the lung extract to potentiate forskolin-stimulated [^{3}H]-cyclic AMP accumulation in the guinea pig cerebral cortex.

Effect of Clonidine and CDS on Electrically Evoked Contractions of the Rat Isolated Vas Deferens

FIGURE 2A shows that brain and lung methanolic CDS extracts produced biphasic effects on electrically evoked contractions of the rat isolated vas deferens. Low concentrations (0.05 unit/mL) caused a statistically significant ($P < 0.05$) reduction in electrically evoked contractions (brain CDS, 19.1 ± 3.1%, n = 5; lung CDS, 15.2 ± 2.3%, n = 6). Higher concentrations led to enhanced responses (brain CDS, 1.7 units/mL: 32.1 ± 12.4%, n = 5; lung CDS, 4 units/mL: 50.1 ± 2.1%, n = 6). Neither extract caused a contraction of the rat vas deferens at the concentrations examined. In contrast, clonidine produced concentration-dependent inhibition of electrically-evoked contractions (pD_2, 8.62 ± 0.04, n = 5) with the highest concentration (10 nM) abolishing the responses (FIG. 2B, open circles). Idazoxan (1 µM) blocked responses to 10nM clonidine (n = 4) but failed to alter significantly either the inhibitory response (0.1 unit/mL: control, 19.6 ± 4.1%; antagonist present, 28.5 ± 6.6%; n = 5) or excitatory response (1 unit/mL: control, 22.3 ± 4.0%; antagonist present, 7.1 ± 8.0%; n = 5) of the brain methanolic CDS extract.

FIGURE 2B shows the effect of clonidine on electrically evoked contractions in the absence and in the presence of 1.7 units/mL brain methanolic CDS extract and 4 units/mL lung methanolic CDS extract. The potency of clonidine (pD_2, 8.62 ± 0.06; n = 5) in the rat vas deferens was not significantly altered by 1.7 units/mL brain methanolic CDS extract (pD_2, 8.27 ± 0.12; n = 5) but was significantly reduced ($P < 0.05$) by 4 units/mL lung methanolic CDS extract (pD_2, 8.13 ± 0.10; n = 6).

Effect of UK-14304 and CDS on the Porcine Isolated Palmar Lateral Vein

In the porcine isolated palmar vein, a vessel with a high density of α_2-adrenoceptors,[17] UK-14304 caused concentration-dependent contractions (pD_2, 7.75 ± 0.14;

FIGURE 2. The effect of brain and lung methanolic CDS extract against electrically evoked contractions of the rat isolated vas deferens. Shown are (**A**) the effects of CDS extracts alone and (**B**) the effect of clonidine, in the absence or presence of either 1.7 unit/mL brain methanolic CDS extract or 4 units/mL lung methanolic CDS extract. Contractions were elicited by transmural electrical stimulation (0.5 millisecond duration, 0.1 Hz, 200 mA). The effects of the extracts and clonidine have been calculated as a percentage of the control response and are shown as the mean ± SEM of five or six separate observations.

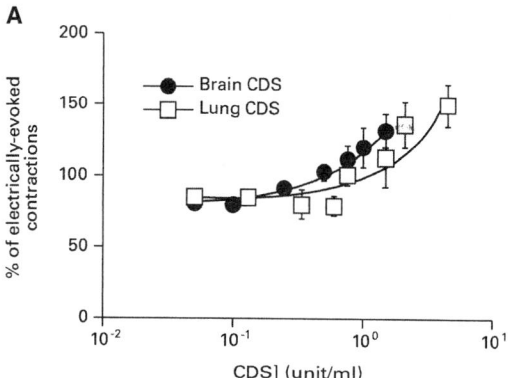
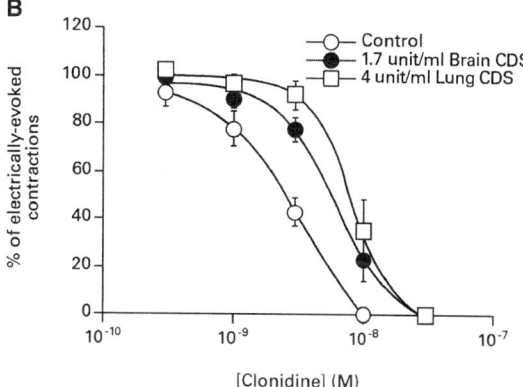

maximum response of 71.8 ± 9.1%; n = 5) of the contraction to 60 mM KCl. The effects of UK-14304 were unaffected by 0.1 µM prazosin but were inhibited by 0.1 µM rauwolscine (FIG. 3A). In a separate series of experiments the response to 0.3 µM UK-14304 (56.3 ± 5.6% of 60 mM KCl; n = 4) was unaffected by the presence of 1 µM mepyramine (55.1 ± 10.5% of 60 mM KCl; n = 4), whereas the contraction to 30 µM histamine (40.8 ± 11.5% of 60 mM KCl; n = 4) was abolished by this antagonist.

FIGURE 3B shows that lung methanolic CDS extract (0.02 1 unit/mL) caused concentration-dependent contractions of the porcine isolated palmar lateral vein in the presence of 1 µM mepyramine. Neither 0.1 µM prazosin nor 0.1 µM rauwolscine significantly affected the response to the lung methanolic CDS extract.

Effect of Harmane in the Rat Vas Deferens and Porcine Isolated Palmar Lateral Vein

Harmane is an indole-based derivative that has recently been advanced as a possible candidate for CDS.[6] Harmane (1–30 µM) did not elicit a contraction of the porcine isolated palmar lateral vein (FIG. 4A), but the highest concentration caused a threefold rightward displacement of the concentration response curve for the

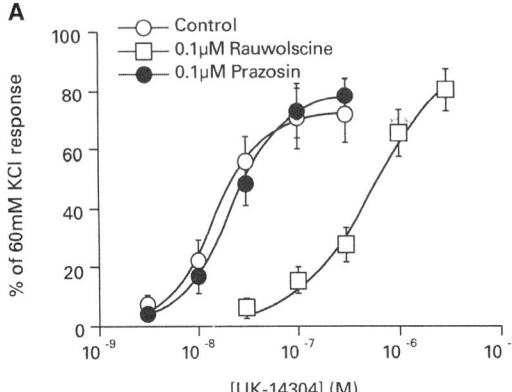

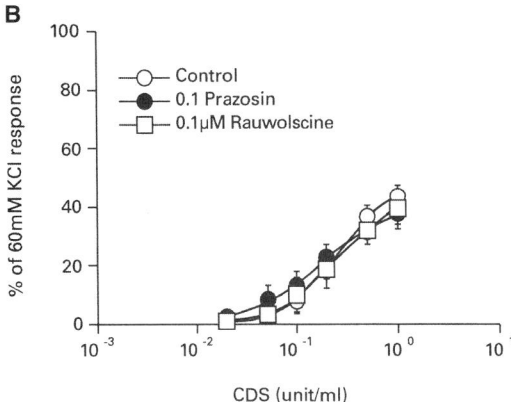

FIGURE 3. The effect of (**A**) UK-14304 and (**B**) lung methanolic CDS extract on the porcine isolated palmar lateral vein, in the absence or presence of either 0.1 µM prazosin or 0.1 µM rauwolscine. Responses have been calculated as a percentage of the contraction to 60 mM KCl and are shown as the mean ± SEM of five observations.

contractile effect of UK-14304. In the rat isolated vas deferens, harmane caused a concentration-dependent enhancement of electrically evoked contractions, with the maximum effect equivalent to a 95.1 ± 16.1% (n = 6) increase in the neurogenic response (FIG. 4B). The inhibitory effect of clonidine on neurogenic responses was displaced threefold in the presence of 30 µM harmane.

DISCUSSION

CDS was originally described as an endogenous, noncatecholamine ligand for α_2-adrenoceptors.[1] Over the past 15 years, however, much of the research on CDS has been directed towards its potential as a ligand for imidazoline binding sites, which could then account for its nonadrenoceptor actions and those of various imidazoline-based compounds.[4,9,10] To investigate functional actions of CDS pharmacologically, it is necessary to have access to well-characterized selective antagonists. For example, using strict pharmacologic criteria, Eglen and colleagues[4] were able to discount the

FIGURE 4. Comparison of harmane, UK-14304, and clonidine at peripheral α_2-adrenoceptors. (**A**) The effect of UK-14304 and harmane on porcine isolated palmar lateral vein and the effect of UK-14304 in the presence of 30 μM harmane. Responses have been calculated as a percentage of the response to 60 mM KCl. All responses shown are the mean ± SEM of six observations. (**B**) The effect of clonidine and harmane on electrically evoked contractions of the rat isolated vas deferens and the effect of clonidine in the presence of 30 μM harmane. Contractions were elicited by transmural electrical stimulation (0.5 millisecond duration, 0.1 Hz, 200 mA) and responses are expressed as a percentage of the response before the addition of the agonist.

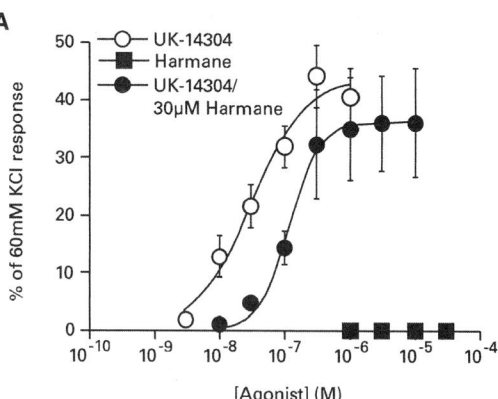
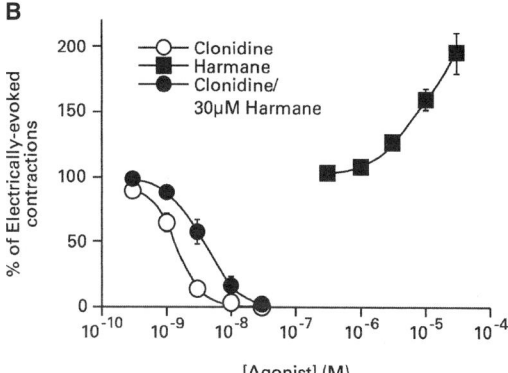

possibility that agmatine was responsible for the CDS activity originally described by Atlas and Burstein.[1] Although a suitable antagonist (KU 14R) has been identified for the imidazoline I_3 site in pancreatic islet cells,[21] only α_2-adrenoceptors have been sufficiently well characterized to permit detailed pharmacologic evaluation of biologic responses to extracts containing CDS activity. Thus, the principal aim of this study was to provide confirmation of earlier reports[7,8] that CDS is an endogenous, noncatecholamine ligand for α_2-adrenoceptors.

Three functional models of α_2-adrenoceptors have been used. In the guinea pig cerebral cortex and porcine palmar lateral vein, UK-14304, a selective α_2-adrenoceptor agonist,[22] reduced forskolin-stimulated [^{3}H]-cyclic AMP accumulation and elicited contractions, respectively. In the rat vas deferens, clonidine, an α_2-adrenoceptor agonist, inhibited electrically evoked contractions. For each preparation, evidence for activation of α_2-adrenoceptors was provided by the ability of idazoxan or rauwolscine, α_2-adrenoceptor antagonists,[23,24] to inhibit the responses.

Pharmacologic data from several studies indicate the presence of α_{2A}-adrenoceptors on the porcine palmar lateral vein[17] and α_{2D}-adrenoceptors on the prejunctional nerves of rat vas deferens.[25] In the guinea pig cerebral cortex, however, the subtype of α_2-adrenoceptor present is less clear. Our choice of this tissue was based on the presence of α_2-adrenoceptor binding sites[26] and the observation by Uhlen and Wikberg[27] that this receptor produces inhibition of forskolin-stimulated [^{3}H]-cyclic AMP accumulation in the guinea pig isolated spinal cord. The inhibition of forskolin-stimulated [^{3}H]-cyclic AMP accumulation by UK-14304 in our preparation (approximately 90%) was significantly greater than that observed in either the guinea pig isolated spinal cord or rat cerebral cortex,[27,28] thereby affording a sensitive, small-volume model for detecting agonist activity of the extracts. Although the pharmacologic characteristics of the α_2-adrenoceptor in the guinea pig cerebral cortex were not examined in our study, Trendelenburg and coworkers[29] have reported that α_{2D}-adrenoceptors mediate inhibition of [^{3}H]-noradrenaline release in this preparation. Thus, the present study covers the activity of CDS at α_{2A}- and α_{2D}-adrenoceptors. Piletz et al.[3] have previously shown that CDS-containing extracts from bovine hypothalamus can interact with all four subtypes of α_2-adrenoceptors.

Comparison of the effects of CDS-containing methanolic extracts of bovine brain and lung with α_2-adrenoceptor agonists revealed significant differences. The concentration of CDS employed (0.1–4 units/mL) was based on the ability of 1 unit/mL to occupy 50% of α_2- adrenoceptor sites labeled by [^{3}H]-clonidine. Although the lung methanolic CDS extract produced a contraction similar to UK-14304 and low concentrations of the extracts mimicked clonidine in the rat vas deferens, neither of these responses was inhibited by selective α_2-adrenoceptor antagonists. In the case of isolated cerebral cortex slices neither extract mimicked the effect of α_2-adrenoceptor agonists, nor were their effects reversed following exposure to idazoxan, which is taken as evidence against activation of α_2-adrenoceptors. Although high concentrations of brain methanolic CDS extract reduced forskolin-stimulated [^{3}H]-cyclic AMP accumulation (see FIG. 1B), this effect was enhanced (rather than reversed) by idazoxan. The basis of this effect is not known. Second, the enhancement of neurogenic responses produced by higher concentrations of the brain and lung extract in the vas deferens was also insensitive to idazoxan. Although the potency of clonidine against neurogenic responses was significantly reduced in the presence of 4 units/mL lung methanolic CDS extract, it is unclear whether this reduction occurs simply because the extract can enhance electrically evoked contractions or is evidence of antagonist activity of CDS at α_2-adrenoceptors.

The finding that the CDS extracts were inactive at prejunctional α_2-adrenoceptors in the rat vas deferens makes it unlikely that it possesses agonist activity in other models of α_2-adrenoceptors. The receptor in rat vas deferens has a high receptor reserve and is responsive to even weak α_2-adrenoceptors agonists.[30] Taken together, our findings indicate that neither lung nor brain methanolic CDS extracts have the potential to activate α_2-adrenoceptors and cast doubts on one of the central tenants of research into CDS, namely that CDS represents an endogenous, noncatecholamine agonist for α_2-adrenoceptors.[4,9,10] Thus, our observations on the rat vas deferens provide no support for the seminal findings by Diamant and Atlas[7] that brain CDS (approximately 8 units/mL) inhibited neurogenic contractions of the rat vas deferens through a phentolamine- and yohimbine-sensitive (α_2-adrenoceptor) mechanism. There are two possible explanations for this discrepancy between studies. First, Diamant and Atlas[7] used higher concentrations of CDS than those examined in the present study. We found, however, that 2 to 4 units/mL of either extract enhanced (rather than inhibited) neurogenic contractions; we avoided higher concentrations because of the presence of monovalent cations (see Singh et al.[19]). Alternatively, the methanolic extracts prepared by Atlas and Burstein[1] may have been contaminated with catecholamines able to activate pre-junctional α_2-adrenoceptors. This possibility was originally discounted by Atlas and colleagues on the basis of the failure of their extract to interact with either α_1- or β-adrenoceptor binding sites. We have shown, however, that catecholamines possess markedly lower potency (1/100) at α_1-adrenoceptor binding sites than at α_2-adrenoceptor binding sites.[31] It seems unlikely, therefore, that the radio-receptor method employed by Atlas and colleagues could have detected contamination even by high concentrations of catecholamines. The possibility of catecholamine contamination of extracts was considered at the beginning of our study of CDS, and we took steps to minimize this problem. We opted to use electrochemical detection to exclude the involvement of catecholamines,[19] a method sensitive enough to detect catecholamines at levels one tenth of those required to interact with α_2-adrenoceptor binding sites labeled by [^{3}H]-clonidine.[31]

The failure to detect CDS agonistic activity at α_2-adrenoceptors poses a second problem for the interpretation of an earlier study from our laboratory. Based on the profile of the interaction of the extract with high- and low-affinity states of α_2-adrenoceptors, we previously argued that bovine lung and brain CDS exhibited an agonist-like profile.[32] Significantly, however, Chan and coworkers[33] have reported that methanolic extracts of bovine brain containing CDS also failed to activate α_2-adrenoceptors on islet of Langerhans. At present we have no convincing explanation for the failure of the radioligand model to predict accurately the biologic activity of the extracts, although it is clear that other substances in the extracts have the potential to mask the biologic activity of CDS. For example, the lung extract potentiates (rather than inhibits) forskolin-stimulated [^{3}H]-cyclic AMP accumulation in the guinea pig cerebral cortex. This effect of the extract is similar to that noted for histamine, a recognized contaminant,[19] and, significantly, was prevented by a combination of the histamine receptor antagonists mepyramine and cimetidine. In the case of the rat vas deferens, it is intriguing that harmane, a putative endogenous agonist for central imidazoline receptors,[6] mimicked the effect of the extract on the rat vas deferens (see FIGS. 2 and 4). The possibility of yet another contaminant is also indicated by the results on the porcine isolated palmar lateral vein, where neither histamine nor harmane could account for the non–α_2-adrenoceptor vasoconstriction produced by the lung extract. Clearly, further experiments with purified extracts are needed, perhaps based on defined cells rather than on a heterogeneous tissue (see Parker et al.[34]), to examine the basis of the interaction of CDS with α_2-adrenoceptors.

In summary, we have shown that crude methanolic extracts of bovine brain and lung containing CDS fail to activate either α_{2A}- or α_{2D}-adrenoceptors in the porcine isolated palmar lateral vein, guinea pig cerebral cortex, or rat vas deferens. Thus, the seminal observation by Atlas and coworkers that brain CDS can activate α_2-adrenoceptors,[7,8] which provided the springboard for much of the work re-examining the properties of imidazoline derivatives, has not been confirmed.

REFERENCES

1. ATLAS, D. & Y. BURSTEIN. 1984. Isolation and partial purification of a clonidine-displacing substance. Eur. J. Biochem. **144:** 287–293.

2. PARINI, A., I. COUPRY, R.M. GRAHAM, et al. 1989. Characterization of an imidazoline/gaunidinium receptive site distinct from the α_2-adrenergic receptor. J. Biol. Chem. **264:** 11874–11878.
3. PILETZ, J.E., D.N. CHIKKALA & P. ERNSBERGER. 1995. Comparison of the properties of agmatine and endogenous clonidine-displacing substance at imidazoline and α_2-adrenoceptors. J. Pharmacol. Exp. Ther. **272:** 581–587.
4. EGLEN, R.M., A.L. HUDSON, D.A. KENDALL, et al. 1998. "Seeing through a glass darkly": casting light on imidazoline 'I' sites. Trends Pharmacol. Sci. **19:** 381–390.
5. LI, G., S. REGUNATHAN, C.J. BARROW, et al. 1994. Agmatine: an endogenous "clonidine-displacing substance" in the brain. Science **263:** 966–969.
6. MUSGRAVE, I.F. & E. BADOER. 2000. Harmane produces hypotension following microinjection into the RVLM: possible role of I_1-imidazoline receptors. Br. J. Pharmacol. **129:** 1057–1059.
7. DIAMANT, S. & D. ATLAS. 1986. An endogenous brain substance, CDS (clonidine-displacing substance) inhibits the twitch response of rat vas deferens. Biochem. Biophys. Res. Comm. **134:** 184–190.
8. DIAMANT, S., A. ELDOR & D. ATLAS. 1987. A low molecular weight brain substance interacts similarly to clonidine with α_2-adrenoceptors of human platelets. Eur. J. Pharmacol. **144:** 247–255.
9. ATLAS, D. 1991. Clonidine displacing substance (CDS) and its putative imidazoline receptors. Biochem. Pharmacol. **41:** 1541–1549.
10. REGUNATHAN, S. & D.J. REIS. 1996. Imidazoline receptors and their endogenous ligands. Ann. Rev. Pharmacol. Toxicol. **36:** 511–544.
11. RUFFOLO, R.R., P. RICE, P.N. PATIL, et al. 1983. Differences in the applicability of the Easson-Stedman hypothesis to α_1- and α_2-adrenergic effects of phenethylamines and imidazolines. Eur. J. Pharmacol. **86:** 471–475.
12. RICE, P.J., A. HAMADA, D.D. MILLER, et al. 1987. Asymmetric catecholimidazoline and catecholamides: affinity and efficacy relationships at α-adrenoceptors in rat aorta. J. Pharmacol. Exp. Ther. **242:** 121–130.
13. MCGRATH, J.C., C.M. BROWN, C.J. DALY, et al. 1995. The relationship between the adrenoceptor and non-adrenoceptor effects of imidazoline and imidazoline containing compounds. Ann. N. Y. Acad. Sci. **736:** 591–605.
14. BYLUND, D.B., D.C. EIKENBURG, J.P. HIEBLE, et al. 1994. International Union of Pharmacology nomenclature on adrenoceptors. Pharmacol. Rev. **46:** 121–136.
15. MACKINNON, A.C., M.J. SPEDDING & C.M. BROWN. 1994. α_2-Adrenoceptors: more subtypes but few functional differences. Trends Pharmacol. Sci. **15:** 119–123.
16. MCGRATH, J.C. 1984. α-Adrenoceptor antagonism by aopyohimbine and some observations of α-adrenoceptors in the rat anoccoygeus and vas deferens. Br. J. Pharmacol. **82:** 769–782.
17. WRIGHT, I.K., D.A. KENDALL & V.G. WILSON. 1995. α_2-Adrenoceptor-mediated inhibition of forskolin-stimulated cyclic AMP accumulation in porcine isolated palmar lateral vein. Naunyn Schmiedeberg's Arch. Pharmacol. **352:** 113–120.
18. DELEAN, A., P.J. MUNSON & D. ROBARD. 1978. Simultaneous analysis of families of sigmoidal curves: applications to bioassay, radioligand assay and physiological dose response curves. Am. J. Physiol. **235:** E97–E102.
19. SINGH, G., J.F. HUSSAIN, A. MACKINNON, et al. 1995. Further studies on crude, methanolic extracts of bovine brain and lung–evidence for the presence of a non-catecholamine, clonidine-displacing substance. Naunyn Schmideberg's Arch. Pharmacol. **351:** 17–26.
20. DONALDSON, J., A.M. BROWN & S.J. HILL. 1988. Influence of rolipram on the cyclic 3′,5′ adenosine monophosphate response to histamine and adenosine to slices of guinea-pig cerebral cortex. Biochem. Pharmacol. **37:** 715–723.
21. CHAN, S.L.F., A.L. PALLETT, J. CLEWS, J., et al. 1998. Characterization of new efaroxan derivatives for use in purification if imidazoline-binding sites. Eur. J. Pharmacol. **355:** 67–76.
22. CAMBRIDGE, D. 1981. UK-14304, a potent and selective α^2-agonist for the characterisation of α-adrenoceptor subtypes. Eur. J. Pharmacol. **72:** 413–415.

23. MALLARD, N.J., A.L. HUDSON & D.J. NUTT. 1992. Characterization and autoradiographical localization of non-adrenoceptor, idazoxan binding sites in the rat brain. Br. J. Pharmacol. **106:** 1019–1027.
24. MCGRATH, J.C., C.M. BROWN & V.G. WILSON. 1989. Alpha-adrenoceptors: a critical review. Med. Res. Rev. **9:** 408–533
25. SMITH, K., S. CONNAUGHTON & J.R. DOCHERTY. 1992. Investigation of pre-junctional α_2-adrenoceptors in the rat atrium, rat vas deferens and rat submandibular gland. Eur. J. Pharmacol. **211:** 251–256.
26. HUSSAIN, J.F., D.A. KENDALL & V.G. WILSON. 1993. Species selective binding of [^{3}H]-idazoxan to α_2-adrenoceptors and non-adrenoceptor, imidazoline binding sites in the central nervous system. Br. J. Pharmacol. **109:** 831–837.
27. UHLEN, S. & J.E.S. WIKBERG. 1989. α_2-Adrenoceptors mediate inhibition of cyclic AMP production in the spinal cord after stimulation of cyclic AMP with forskolin but not after stimulation with capsaicin or vasoactive intestinal peptide. J. Neurochem. **52:** 761–767.
28. DUMAN, R.S. & S.J. ENNA. 1986. A procedure for measuring α_2-adrenergic receptors mediated inhibition of cyclic AMP accumulation in rat brain slices. Brain Res. **384:** 391–394.
29. TRENDELENBURG, A.-U., N. LIMBERGER & K. STARKE. 1995. Subclassification of presynaptic α_2-autoreceptors in guinea-pig atria and brain. Naunyn Schmideberg's Arch. Pharmacol. **352:** 49–57.
30. ALI, A., H.-Y. CHENG, K.N. TING, et al. 1998. Rilmenidine reveals differences in the pharmacological characteristics of pre-junctional α_2-adrenoceptors in the guinea-pig, rat and pig. Br. J. Pharmacol. **125:** 127–135.
31. HUSSAIN, J.F., C.M. BROWN, D.A. KENDALL, et al. 1991. The activity of a crude extract of bovine adrenal medulla at α_2-adrenoceptors and a non-adrenoceptor, imidazoline binding site can be accounted for by adrenaline. Br. J. Pharmacol. **104:** 79P.
32. PINTHONG, D., V.G. WILSON & D.A. KENDALL. 1995. Comparison of the interaction of crude methanolic extracts of bovine lung and brain and agmatine with α_2-adrenoceptors. Br. J. Pharmacol. **115:** 689–695.
33. CHAN, S.L.F., D.A. ATLAS, R.F.L. JAMES, et al. 1997. The effect of the putative, endogenous imidazoline receptor ligand clonidine-displacing substance on insulin secretion from rat and human islet of Langerhans. Br. J. Pharmacol. **120:** 926–932.
34. PARKER, C.A., A.L. HUDSON, D.J. NUTT, et al. 2000. Isolation of RP-HPLC pure clonidine-displacing substance from NG 108-15 cells. Eur. J. Pharmacol. **387:** 27–30.

Complex Interaction of α_2-Adrenoceptor Binding Sites with Bovine Brain and Lung Extracts Containing Clonidine-Displacing Substance

D. PINTHONG, D.A. KENDALL, AND V.G. WILSON

School of Biomedical Sciences, The Medical School, Queen's Medical Centre, Clifton Boulevard, Nottingham NG7 2UH, UK

ABSTRACT: Previous studies have established that methanolic extracts of bovine brain and lung possess CDS activity with an agonist-like profile at α_2-adrenoceptor binding sites (i.e., greater potency against [^{3}H]-clonidine sites than against [^{3}H]-RX-821001 sites). Following prolonged reflux in ethylacetate, monovalent cations and histamine were removed from the lung extract, and the resulting extract exhibited similar potency against both radioligands, indicative of an antagonist-like profile. These observations help explain the absence of biologic activity at α_2-adrenoceptors in the methanolic extracts as reported in our companion paper.

KEYWORDS: clonidine-displacing substance; α_2-adrenoceptor binding sites

INTRODUCTION

We have previously demonstrated that methanolic extracts of bovine brain and lung selectively displace [^{3}H]-clonidine from α_2-adrenoceptor binding sites on bovine cerebral cortex membranes, evidence for a clonidine-displacing substance (CDS).[1] A more detailed examination of this interaction revealed that both tissue extracts possessed higher affinity for α_2-adrenoceptor sites labeled by [^{3}H]-clonidine, the so-called high-affinity or agonist sites, compared with sites labeled by the selective α_2-adrenoceptor antagonist, [^{3}H]-RX-821002.[2] In keeping with the original description of CDS, and observations on the rat isolated vas deferens[3] and human platelets,[4] this finding suggested that the extracts possessed a noncatecholamine substance with agonist activity at α_2-adrenoceptors. Subsequent experiments with both extracts in a variety of functional preparations, including the rat isolated vas deferens, failed to demonstrate agonist activity, however.[5]

One possible explanation for these conflicting findings is the presence of high concentrations of sodium ions and histamine in the CDS extracts. These contaminants are known to interact selectively with high-affinity α_2-adrenoceptors labeled

---

Address for correspondence: Vince G. Wilson, School of Biomedical Sciences, The Medical School, Queen's Medical Centre, Clifton Boulevard, Nottingham NG7 2UH, UK. Voice: 00 44 115 9709472; fax: 00 44 115 9709259.
e-mail: Vince.wilson@nottingham.ac.uk

Ann. N.Y. Acad. Sci. 1009: 216–221 (2003). © 2003 New York Academy of Sciences.
doi: 10.1196/annals.1304.026

by [3H]-clonidine.[6] In the present study, we have examined the effect of prolonged reflux of methanolic extracts with ethylacetate on the content of known contaminants and subsequent interaction with α_2-adrenoceptor binding sites.

METHODS

Methanolic extracts of bovine brain and lung were prepared as previously described,[1] and the lyophilsylate was refluxed in ethylacetate for 72 hours, as shown in FIGURE 1. Step-1 methanolic (Meth) extracts as well as step-2 methanolic-ethylacetate (Meth EA) extracts from the lung and brain were reconstituted in distilled water. These reconstituted extracts were used to examine interactions with α_2-adrenoceptor binding sites on bovine cerebral cortex membranes labeled by 1 nM [3H]-clonidine or 0.3 nM [3H]-RX-821002.[2] Nonspecific binding was determined by the presence of 0.1 mM noradrenaline, usually 10% to 20% of the total binding. The effects of UK-14304 and RX-811059, agonist and antagonist, respectively, were also examined against the two radioligands. One unit of CDS was defined as the volume of extract in 0.5 mL assay volume that reduced specific binding of 1 nM [3H]-clonidine by 50%. Log K_i was the concentration of the agent causing 50% reduction in specific binding of the radioligand.

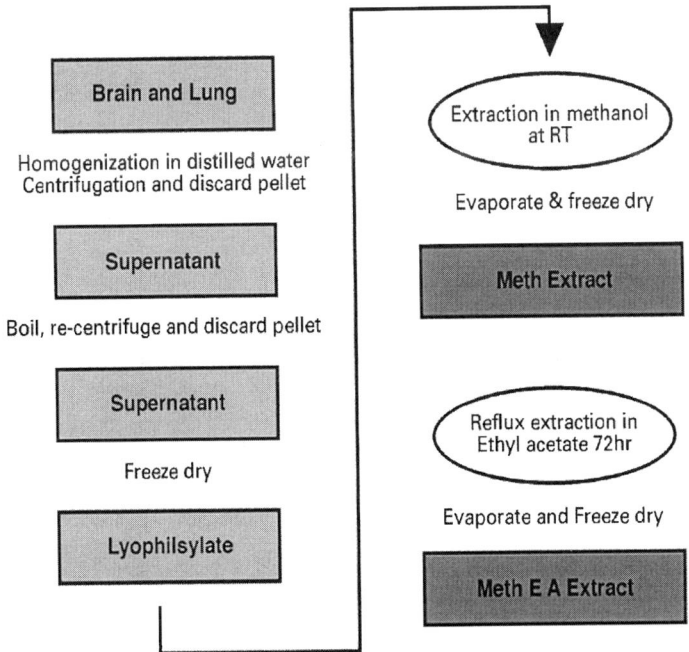

FIGURE 1. The extraction procedure for methanolic (Meth) and methanolic-ethylacetate (Meth EA) extracts of bovine brain and lung.

RESULTS

Methanolic extracts of the brain and lung inhibited [^{3}H]-clonidine binding to bovine cerebral cortex membranes in a concentration-dependent manner, with a Hill slope not significantly different from unity. As shown in TABLE 1, bovine lung possessed approximately threefold more CDS activity than brain, based on the activity per unit weight. Neither extract exerted a significant effect on [^{3}H]-RX-821002 binding to bovine cerebral cortex membranes (IC_{50} > 100 µL/0.5 mL assay volume), giving rise to a RX/clonidine ratio greater than 5 (TABLE 1). The selective α_2-adrenoceptor agonist UK-14304 displaced both [^{3}H]-clonidine and [^{3}H]-RX-821002 from bovine cerebral cortex membranes with a RX/clonidine ratio of 10 (TABLE 1).

Methanolic-ethylacetate extracts of bovine brain and lung inhibited [^{3}H]-clonidine binding to bovine cerebral cortex membranes in a concentration-dependent manner, with a Hill slope not significantly different from unity. As shown in TABLE 1, bovine lung possessed approximately 10-fold more CDS activity than brain, based on the activity per unit weight. Both extracts also caused a significant displacement of [^{3}H]-RX-821002 binding to bovine cerebral cortex membranes, giving rise to a RX/clonidine ratio of less than 1 (TABLE 1). The selective α_2-adrenoceptor antagonist RX-811059 displaced both [^{3}H]-clonidine and [^{3}H]-RX-821002 from bovine cerebral cortex membranes with a RX/clonidine ratio of less than 1.

As shown in FIGURE 2 and TABLE 1, although the activity of the methanolic extract of bovine lung against [^{3}H]-clonidine was not altered by reflux in ethylacetate, the latter exhibited significantly greater activity against [^{3}H]-RX-821002 binding to bovine cerebral cortex membranes.

Reflux of the lung methanolic extract with ethylacetate for 3 days reduced the content of Na^+ ions from 1.4 ± 0.1 µmol/unit of CDS to less than 0.01 µmol/unit of CDS (n = 3) and reduced the content of K^+ ions from 1.2 ± 0.1 µmol/unit of CDS to less than 0.01 µmol/unit of CDS (n = 3). Qualitatively similar results were noted for the brain methanolic extract versus brain methanolic-ethylacetate extract. Also, the histamine content of the lung methanolic extract was reduced below the level of detection (a 100-fold reduction).

TABLE 1. IC_{50} values for drugs (negative log concentration) and tissue extracts (µL/mL) against α_2-adrenoceptor ligands (n = 4–8)

	[^{3}H]-Clonidine	[^{3}H]-RX-821002	RX/Clonidine Ratio	CDS Activity (units/g tissue)
UK-14304	8.56 ± 0.04	7.51 ± 0.01	10	—
RX-811059	8.73 ± 0.11	9.04 ± 0.02	0.5	—
Brain Meth CDS	18.6 ± 1.7	>100	>5	4.8 ± 0.5
Lung Meth CDS	6.8 ± 1.0	>100	>16	18.6 ± 2.1
Brain Meth EA CDS	58.1 ± 13.3	44.6 ± 12.2	0.7	1.6 ± 0.5
Lung Meth EA CDS	6.7 ± 1.9	4.9 ± 1.5	0.7	17.3 ± 4.7

CDS, clonidine-displacing substance; Meth, methanolic; Meth EA, methanolic-ethylacetate.

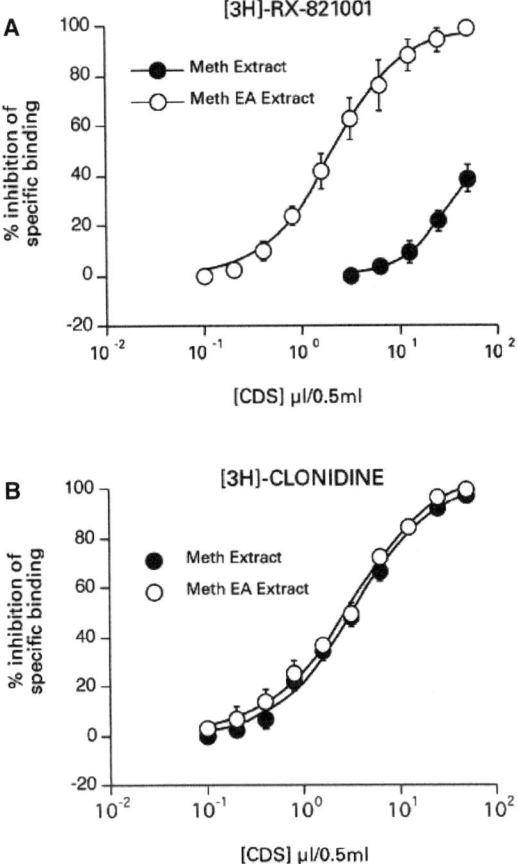

FIGURE 2. Comparison of the effect of methanolic (Meth) and methanolic-ethylacetate (Meth EA) extracts of bovine lung against α_2-adrenoceptor binding sites labeled by 1 nM [^{3}H]-clonidine and 0.3 nM [^{3}H]-RX-821102. The values shown are the mean ± SEM of four to six observations with separate batches of the extract.

DISCUSSION

We have demonstrated that prolonged reflux in ethylacetate of methanolic extracts of bovine lung and brain removed monovalent cations and histamine, but the extracts retained significant CDS activity. In the case of bovine brain extracts, this procedure resulted in a loss of activity against [^{3}H]-clonidine binding sites (approximately 60%; TABLE 1), but for lung extracts CDS activity was largely unchanged (FIG. 2). The use of ethylacetate to purify CDS differs from procedures used in several earlier studies that relied on a variety of chromatographic approaches[3,4,7,8] but supports the view that CDS is relatively stable and unrelated to the presence of monovalent cations.[1] In light of the differential effect of ethylacetate extraction on brain and lung CDS activity, the possibility exists that more than a single substance may be responsible for the effects noted.

As previously described,[2] the methanolic extracts of both tissues exhibited a higher affinity for the [3H]-clonidine binding to α_2-adrenoceptor binding sites on bovine cerebral cortex compared to sites labeled by [^{3}H]-RX-821002 (FIG. 1). This profile is similar to that observed with the selective α_2-adrenoceptor agonist UK-14304[9] and suggests that CDS prefers the high-affinity agonist form of the binding site. After prolonged reflux with ethylacetate, however, the extract of both tissues (Meth EA CDS) possessed increased activity against [^{3}H]-RX-821001, such that the order of potency against the two radioligands was similar to that noted with RX-811059, a selective α_2-adrenoceptor antagonist.[10] Significantly, a 72-hour reflux of a solution containing UK-14304 led to reduced activity of the α_2-adrenoceptor agonist (data not shown), even though the profile of CDS after its 7-hour reflux was not lowered against [^{3}H]-clonidine and [^{3}H]-RX821001. Thus, the interaction between these extracts and α_2-adrenoceptor binding sites is complex and may not predict biologic activity in a straightforward manner. This point is underlined by the failure of methanolic extracts of bovine brain and lung to mimic the reported agonist activity of either UK-14304 or clonidine in the rat isolated vas deferens, the porcine isolated palmar vein, and guinea pig cerebral cortex.[5]

To date, most binding studies of CDS have assessed either α_2-adrenoceptors or nonadrenoceptor imidazoline binding sites (NAIBS).[1,3,4,7,8] The studies of the α_2-adrenoceptor have usually involved only [^{3}H]-clonidine. Diamant and colleagues,[8] however, described the interaction between brain-derived CDS and platelet α_2-adrenoceptors labeled with the antagonist [^{3}H]-rauwolscine. In that study, the extract competed with [^{3}H]-rauwolscine with similar potency to that observed against [^{3}H]-clonidine in the bovine cerebral cortex. Thus, the extract failed to discriminate between the presumed high-affinity and low-affinity sites for α_2-adrenoceptors and, as such, behaved in a manner comparable to that observed for the methanolic-ethylacetate extracts of lung and brain in this study. At present we have not identified the factors present in methanolic extracts, but something must be absent in the methanolic-ethylacetate preparations, because they had increased potency at α_2-adrenoceptors labeled by [^{3}H]-RX-821002. Further experiments are needed to assess whether the ethylacetate purification step is associated with a change in biologic activity of the CDS-containing extract.

REFERENCES

1. SINGH, G., J.F. HUSSAIN, A. MACKINNON, et al. 1995. Further studies on crude, methanolic extracts of bovine brain and lung–evidence for the presence of a non-catecholamine, clonidine-displacing substance. Naunyn Schmiedeberg's Arch. Pharmacol. **351:** 17–26.
2. PINTHONG, D., V.G. WILSON & D.A. KENDALL. 1995. Comparison of the interaction of crude methanolic extracts of bovine lung and brain and agmatine with α_2-adrenoceptors. Br. J. Pharmacol. **115:** 689–695.
3. DIAMANT, S. & D. ATLAS. 1986. An endogenous brain substance, CDS (clonidine-displacing substance) inhibits the twitch response of rat vas deferens. Biochem. Biophys. Res. Comm. **134:** 184–190.
4. DIAMANT, S., A. ELDOR & D. ATLAS. 1987. A low molecular weight brain substance interacts similarly to clonidine with α_2-adrenoceptors of human platelets. Eur. J. Pharmacol. **144:** 247–255.

5. PINTHONG, D., D.A. KENDALL, S.J. MACLENNAN, *et al.* 2003. No evidence for activation of α_2-adrenoceptors by methanolic extracts of bovine brain and lung containing clonidine-displacing substance. Ann. N.Y. Acad. Sci. This volume.
6. WILSON, A.L., K. SEIBERT, S. BRANDON, *et al.* 1991. Monovalent cation and amiloride analog modulation of adrenergic ligand binding to the unglycosylated a2B-adrenergic receptor subtype. Mol. Pharmacol. **39:** 481–486.
7. ERNSBERGER, P., M.P. MEELEY & D.J. REIS. 1988. An endogenous substance with clonidine-like properties: selective binding to imidazole sites in the ventrolateral medulla. Brain Res. **441:** 309–318.
8. MEELEY, M.P., M.L. HENSLEY, P. ERNSBERGER, *et al.* 1992. Evidence for a bioactive clonidine-displacing substance in peripheral tissues and serum. Biochem. Pharmacol. **44:** 733–740.
9. CAMBRIDGE, D. 1981. UK-14304, a potent and selective α_2-agonist for the characterisation of α-adrenoceptor subtypes. Eur. J. Pharmacol. **72:** 413–415.
10. MALLARD, N.J., A.L. HUDSON & D.J. NUTT. 1992. Characterization and autoradiographical localization of non-adrenoceptor, idazoxan binding sites in the rat brain. Br. J. Pharmacol. **106:** 1019–1027.

Endogenous Imidazoline Receptor Ligands Relax Rat Aorta by an Endothelium-Dependent Mechanism

IAN F. MUSGRAVE,[a] ANDREA VAN DER ZYPP,[b] MATHEW GRIGG,[c] AND COLIN J. BARROW[c]

[a]*Department of Clinical and Experimental Pharmacology, University of Adelaide, Adelaide 5005, Australia*

[b]*Department of Medical Laboratory Science, RMIT University, Melbourne 3001, Australia*

[c]*Department of Chemistry, University of Melbourne, Melbourne 3001, Australia*

> ABSTRACT: Agmatine and harmane have been proposed as endogenous ligands of imidazoline receptors. Agmatine has been reported to activate nitric oxide synthetase (NOS) in endothelial cells, so we sought to determine if agmatine or harmane and an analogue of harmane, propyl harmane, produced vasodilatation through an endothelium-dependent mechanism. The experiments were performed in endothelium-denuded and intact rat aortic rings preconstricted with phenylephrine (0.1 μM). Agmatine (0.3–1000 μM), harmane, and propyl harmane (0.3–100 μM) relaxed endothelium-intact rings in a concentration-dependent manner. Removal of endothelium inhibited the relaxant effect of agmatine, harmane, and propyl harmane. The NOS inhibitor L-NIO (100 μM) inhibited the relaxant effect of agmatine and harmane. The I_1-receptor antagonist AGN (100 μM) partly inhibited the effect of harmane but not that of agmatine. These results suggest that the endogenous imidazoline ligands are capable of stimulating NOS largely by an I_1-receptor–independent mechanism.
>
> KEYWORDS: agmatine; harmane; vasodilatation; nitric oxide; imidazoline receptors

INTRODUCTION

The polyamine agmatine and the β-carboline harmane have been proposed as endogenous ligands of imidazoline receptors.[1,2] Establishing physiologic roles for these compounds has been difficult, however. Unlike other imidazoline ligands, agmatine has no effect on blood pressure when microinjected into the rostrolateral ventrolateral medulla (RVLM).[3] In contrast, agmatine administered peripherally produces a significant hypotensive response, mediated at least in part by vasodilatation.[4,5] These results, along with the findings that agmatine is present in the circulation and in

---

Address for correspondence: Ian F. Musgrave, Department of Clinical and Experimental Pharmacology, University of Adelaide, Adelaide 5005, Australia. Voice: (+61) 8 8303 3905; fax: (+61) 8 8224 0685.
e-mail: ian.musgrave@adelaide.edu.au

Ann. N.Y. Acad. Sci. 1009: 222–227 (2003). © 2003 New York Academy of Sciences.
doi: 10.1196/annals.1304.027

endothelial cells and that agmatine modulates the growth of vascular smooth muscle, suggest that agmatine may play a role in tonically controlling vascular resistance.

This likelihood is further re-enforced by the finding that agmatine is also an inhibitor of nitric oxide synthetase[6,7] (NOS), and inhibition of NOS seems to underlie agmatine's anti-ischemic activity.[8] Paradoxically, agmatine has been reported to activate NOS in endothelial cells,[9] and its ability to stimulate locus coeruleus neurons appears to be caused by the stimulation of NOS.[10] Thus the ability of agmatine to produce vasodilatation may be a balance between its ability to activate and inhibit NOS.

In contrast to agmatine, harmane does produce hypotension when injected into the RVLM[11]; however, the effect of harmane on blood vessels is not known. If harmane, like agmatine, were an endogenous imidazoline ligand, then one would expect it to act in a manner similar to agmatine. The aim of these experiments was to determine if agmatine could relax blood vessels through endothelium-dependent mechanisms and whether this relaxation was caused by activation of NOS. In addition we wished to determine if harmane, another candidate endogenous ligand, and a more I_1-selective analogue, propyl harmane, were able to relax blood vessels in a similar manner. We also sought to determine the role of I_1-imidazoline receptors in the activation of endothelial NOS.

METHODS

Tissue Preparation

Aortas were isolated from male Sprague–Dawley rats 8 weeks of age weighing 180–220 g. After the animals were killed by decapitation, the thoracic aorta was removed and cleaned free of fat and connective tissue and then cut into ring segments 4 mm in length. Each ring was then placed in an organ bath containing 1.0 mL of physiologic salt solution PSS of the following composition (in mM): NaCl 118, KCl 4.7, KH_2PO_4 1.03, $NaHCO_3$ 25, D-glucose 11.1, $MgSO_4$ 1.2, $CaCl_2$ 1.8, EDTA 0.067, and ascorbic acid 0.14. Where necessary, the endothelium was removed by gentle rubbing of the luminal surface with a stainless steel rod. Rings were mounted between two stainless steel hooks through the lumen with the lower hook connected to a tissue holder and the upper to an isometric force displacement transducer. Rings were washed thoroughly by replacing the PSS repeatedly and were then allowed to equilibrate for a period of 45 minutes under 2 g of resting tension. Supply reservoirs and organ baths were maintained at 37°C and were gassed with 95% O_2 and 5% CO_2.

Tissue Viability Assessment

Following the 45-minute equilibration period, the viability of the tissues was assessed. Tissues that failed to produce a 0.5-g increase in tension to phenylephrine 0.1 µM were rejected. The presence of the endothelium was assessed by examining the relaxation to acetylcholine 10 µM in the presence of phenylephrine. The tissue bathing solution was then replaced repeatedly with fresh, drug-free PSS until a stable baseline tension was achieved. The tension was then readjusted to 2 g.

Vasorelaxation Studies

After assessment of tissue viability, a further equilibration period of 45 minutes occurred. Then tissues were constricted with phenylephrine (0.1 μM). After the phenylephrine response had reached a stable plateau, imidazoline-receptor ligands were added in a cumulative fashion. The imidazoline-receptor ligands used were agmatine (relatively selective for I_1-receptors), harmane (nonselective), propyl harmane (relatively selective for I_1-receptors), and moxonidine (relatively selective for I_1-receptors). The $-\log EC_{50}$ was defined as the negative log of the concentration of drug that reduced the phenylephrine constriction to 50% of the original.

When other drugs were present, they or their vehicles were added 45 minutes before the imidazoline receptor ligands. Drugs used were the NOS inhibitor L-N5-(-1-iminoethyl) ornithine (NIO), and the relatively selective I_1-receptor antagonist AGN 192403 (AGN).

Drug Sources

Agmatine, phenylephrine hydrochloride, and moxonidine were obtained from Sigma (St. Louis, MO). L-N5-1-iminoethyl ornithine HCl (L-NIO) was obtained from Cayman Chemicals (Ann Arbor, MI). Harmane and propyl harmane were synthesized by Matthew Grigg.

Statistical Analysis

All values are given as the means ± SEM; n indicates the number of observations. Differences between curves were analyzed using a repeated-measures analysis of variance. The differences between $-\log EC_{50}$ values for relaxation by drugs in the presence and absence of endothelium or NOS inhibitors were analyzed using a Student's t-test. A P value of less than 0.05 was considered to be significant. Curve fitting and statistical testes were performed using GraphPad (GraphPad Software Inc, San Diego, CA). Although multiple aortic rings were obtained from one rat, each ring was used for a different drug group.

Animal Statement

The investigation conforms to the Australian code of practice for the care and use of animals for scientific purposes published by the National Health and Medical Research Council.

RESULTS

Agmatine (3–1000 μM), harmane (0.1–10 μM), and propyl harmane (0.1–10 μM) produced significant concentration-dependent vasodilatation of phenylephrine (0.1 μM) precontracted rat aorta segments (FIG. 1, TABLE 1). Removal of endothelium resulted in a significant rightward shift in the concentration response curve for agmatine, harmane, and propyl harmane (FIG. 1, TABLE 1). In the presence of the NOS inhibitor NIO (100 μM), the concentration response curves to both agmatine (3–1000 μM) and harmane (0.1–10 μM) were shifted significantly to the right (TABLE 1).

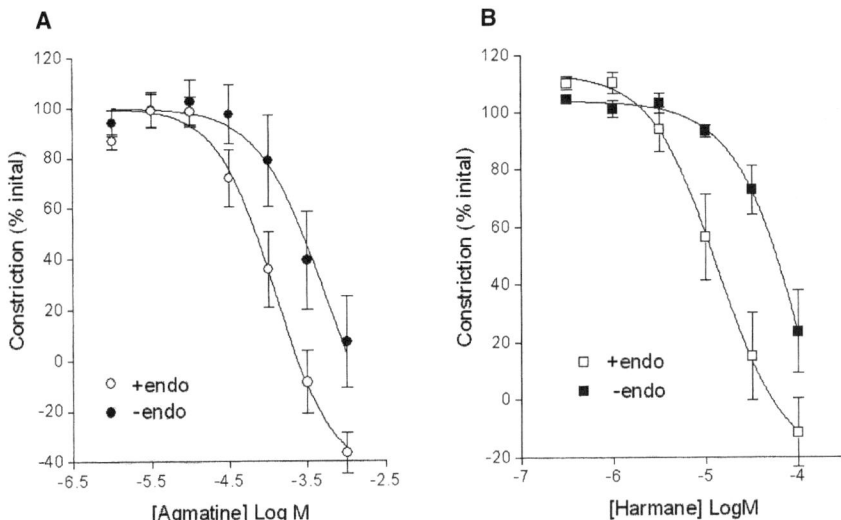

FIGURE 1. (**A**) The effect of agmatine (3–1000 µM) on rat aortic rings precontracted with phenylephrine (0.1 µM). Agmatine produced a concentration-dependent relaxation that was shifted to the right by endothelium removal (−log EC_{50} values: 3.9 ± 0.1 versus 3.2 ± 0.1; $P < 0.05$, n = 5). (**B**) The effect of harmane (0.1–10 µM) on rat aortic rings precontracted with phenylephrine (0.1 µM). Harmane produced a concentration-dependent relaxation that was shifted to the right by endothelium removal (−log EC_{50} values: 4.9 ± 0.1 versus 3.8 ± 0.6; $P < 0.05$, n = 6). Mean values ± SEM are shown. Curve fitting was performed with GraphPad Prism 3.02.

The I_1-selective imidazoline agonist moxonidine (1–100 µM) produced no relaxation either in the presence or absence of endothelium (TABLE 1). The selective I_1-antagonist AGN (100 µM) produced a small but significant rightward shift of the relaxation produced by harmane (−log EC_{50} values: 4.9 ± 0.1 harmane versus 4.6 ± 0.6, harmane and AGN; $P < 0.05$, n = 6). AGN had no effect on agmatine-induced relaxation (−log EC_{50} values: 3.9 ± 0.1 agmatine versus 3.9 ± 0.1, agmatine and AGN).

DISCUSSION

Agmatine produced concentration-dependent relaxation in rat aorta precontracted with phenylephrine. This finding is consistent with the reports of agmatine producing vasodilatation in intact animals.[4,5] This vasodilatation was partially blocked by removal of endothelium and incubation of aorta with a concentration of the NOS inhibitor NIO that completely blocked the relaxation produced by acetylcholine. This finding suggests that some of the vasodilatation produced by agmatine is caused by activation of endothelial NOS. These results are consistent with the findings of Morrissey et al.,[9] who found that micromolar concentrations of agmatine activated NO production from

TABLE 1. Comparison of $-\log EC_{50}$ values with the $-\log K_i$ values

Compound	$-\log K_i$ (M)		$-\log EC_{50}$ (M)		
	I_1	I_2	+Endo	−Endo	+NIO
Harmane	6.3	6.3	4.9 ± 0.1 (6)	3.8 ± 0.6 (6)*	4.1 ± 0.6 (4)*
Propyl harmane	6.5	4.0	4.9 ± 0.1 (6)	4.0 ± 0.1 (6)*	—
Moxonidine	6.6		NA	NA (5)	—
Agmatine	7.5	4.1	3.9 ± 0.1 (5)	3.2 ± 0.1 (5)*	3.1 ± 0.6 (3)*

Comparison of $-\log EC_{50}$ values for relaxation produced by imidazoline ligands in the presence and absence of either endothelium or the NOS inhibitor NIO with the $-\log K_i$ values of these ligands for the I_1-imidazoline receptor. Mean values ± SEM are shown, figures in brackets are n values.

ABBREVIATIONS: NA, not applicable because no relaxation was produced; —, experiment not performed.
SOURCE: $-\log K_i$ values for harmane, propyl harmane, and moxonidine are from Musgrave, Grigg, and Barrow (unpublished data). $-\log K_i$ value for agmatine is from Piletz, J.E., et al. 1996. J. Pharmacol. Exp. Ther. 279: 694–702.
* Significantly different from endothelium intact or vehicle pretreated tissues ($P < 0.05$).

cultured human endothelial cells. Inhibition of NOS by agmatine has been reported[6,7]; however, the IC_{50} for inhibiting the endothelial isoform of NOS is 7.5 mM, approximately 30 times greater than the EC_{50} for endothelial-dependent vasodilatation. Thus it seems that relatively low concentrations of agmatine may tonically control vascular tone. Circulating agmatine levels are probably too low to have a significant effect. Agmatine is present in endothelial cells,[12] however, and may play an autocrine role.

Harmane, and a more I_1-selective analogue, propyl harmane (Musgrave, Grigg, and Barrow, unpublished results) also produced significant vasodilatation. Like agmatine, this vasodilatation was partially blocked by removal of endothelium and incubation of aorta with the NOS inhibitor NIO. This finding suggests that, as for agmatine, some of the vasodilatation produced by harmane is caused by activation of endothelial NOS.

The identity of the receptors through which harmane and agmatine act is uncertain. The selective I_1-receptor agonist moxonidine did not produce any vasodilatation; indeed, it produced a small vasoconstriction, possibly by activation of α_2-adrenoceptors. The selective I_1-receptor antagonist AGN did not affect the vasodilatation produced by agmatine and had a small effect on the vasodilatation produced by harmane. Furthermore, the EC_{50}s of these compounds do not correlate with their pK_is at I_1-receptors, nor is their order of potency in vasodilatation consistent with their order of potency at the I_1-receptor (TABLE 1). Taken together, this evidence suggests that I_1-receptors play only a small role in the vasodilatation produced by these compounds. I_1-receptors have been reported to be responsible for the hemodynamic effects of agmatine, including vasodilatation,[5] because these effects were completely blocked by efaroxan but not by idazoxan or yohimbine. The extent to which the vasodilatation in this study was centrally mediated is not clear, however. Also, although efaroxan is relatively selective for I_1-receptors, it is not as selective as AGN. The agmatine-induced stimulation of NOS in human endothelial cells was blocked by idazoxan, but this finding does not allow discrimination between I_1- and I_2- receptors.

Both endogenous imidazoline receptor ligands produce vasodilatation by an endothelium-dependent mechanism and by a direct action on vascular smooth muscle. The receptor underlying this relaxation is unclear, but the fact that two structurally dissimilar imidazoline ligands have the same effect suggests that they are acting on the same receptors. For the endothelial cells, this may be the I_2-receptor, because endothelial cells are known to have I_2- rather than I_1-receptors,[12] and the order of potency and EC_{50} values of agmatine and propyl harmane are more consistent with I_2-receptors. The situation for the vascular smooth muscle cells is more complex: whereas these cells have I_2-receptors,[12] both agmatine[13] and harmane[14] have been reported to block L-type calcium channels with IC_{50}s similar to the EC_{50}s of these compounds for vasodilatation of endothelium-denuded aorta. Thus further investigation of the receptors underlying the effects of agmatine and harmane is required.

In conclusion, both agmatine and harmane produce concentration-dependent relaxation of rat aorta. This relaxation is partly endothelium- and NOS-dependent. I_1-receptors seem to play little role in this vasorelaxation.

ACKNOWLEDGMENTS

This research was supported by the Australian National Health and Medical Research council grant 981113.

REFERENCES

1. LI, G., et al. 1994. Agmatine: an endogenous clonidine-displacing substance in the brain. Science **263**: 966–969.
2. HUDSON, A.L., et al. 1999. Harmane, norharmane and tetrahydro β-carboline have high affinity for rat imidazoline binding sites. Br. J. Pharmacol. **126**: 2P.
3. SUN, M.K., et al. 1995. Cardiovascular responses to agmatine, a clonidine-displacing substance, in anesthetized rat. Clin. Exp. Hypertens. **17**: 115–128.
4. GAO, Y., et al. 1995. Agmatine: a novel endogenous vasodilator substance. Life Sci. **57**: L83–L86.
5. LI, Q. & R.R. HE. 2001. Hemodynamic effects of agmatine in Dahl salt-sensitive hypertensive and Dahl salt-resistant rats. Sheng Li Xue Bao **53**: 355–360.
6. GALEA, E., et al. 1996. Inhibition of mammalian nitric oxide synthases by agmatine, an endogenous polyamine formed by decarboxylation of arginine. Biochem. J. **316**: 247–249.
7. AUGUET, M., et al. 1995. Selective inhibition of inducible nitric oxide synthase by agmatine. Jpn. J. Pharmacol. **69**: 285–287.
8. FENG, Y., et al. 2002. Agmatine suppresses nitric oxide production and attenuates hypoxic-ischemic brain injury in neonatal rats. Pediatr. Res. **52**: 606–611.
9. MORRISSEY, J.J. & S. KLAHR. 1997. Agmatine activation of nitric oxide synthase in endothelial cells. Proc. Assoc. Am. Physicians **109**: 51–57.
10. RUIZ-DURANTEZ, E., et al. 2002. Effect of agmatine on locus coeruleus neuron activity: possible involvement of nitric oxide. Br. J. Pharmacol. **135**: 1152–1158.
11. MUSGRAVE, I.F. & E. BADOER. 2000. Harmane produces hypotension following microinjection into the RVLM: possible role of I(1)-imidazoline receptors. Br. J. Pharmacol. **129**: 1057–1059.
12. REGUNATHAN, S., et al. 1996. Imidazoline receptors and agmatine in blood vessels: a novel system inhibiting vascular smooth muscle proliferation. J. Pharmacol. Exp. Ther. **276**: 1272–1282.
13. LI, Q., et al. 2002. Effect of agmatine on L-type calcium current in rat ventricular myocytes. Acta Pharmacol. Sin. **23**: 219–224.
14. SHI, C.C., et al. 2001. Comparative study on the vasorelaxant effects of three harmala alkaloids in vitro. Jpn. J. Pharmacol. **85**: 299–305.

I_1 Imidazoline Receptors Involved in Cardiovascular Regulation

Where Are We and Where Are We Going?

P. BOUSQUET, H. GRENEY, V. BRUBAN, S. SCHANN, J.D. EHRHARDT, L. MONASSIER, AND J. FELDMAN

INSERM E0333, Faculté de Médecine, Université Louis Pasteur, 67000 Strasbourg, France

ABSTRACT: Clonidine-like drugs (hybrid drugs) reduce blood pressure by acting centrally at both α_2-adrenergic receptors (α_2AR) and I_1 receptors (I_1R). Some attempts at cloning I_1R have failed, probably because of the lack of selectivity of the ligands. Recently, compounds acting exclusively at I_1R were synthesized: LNP 911, LNP509, and S23515. For example, LNP911 has a K_d value of 1.7 nmol/L at I_1R. LNP509 and S23515 reduce blood pressure when injected centrally in anesthetized animals, whereas S23757 behaves as an antagonist of hypotensive imidazolines. LNP509 reduces blood pressure even in genetically engineered mice lacking functional α_2AR. An exclusive action at central I_1R is therefore sufficient to modify blood pressure. With the help of drugs selective for I_1R and α-methylnoradrenaline, selective for α_2AR, we showed that imidazoline and α_2-adrenergic mechanisms interact synergistically in controlling the blood pressure. Such a synergism may explain the very powerful hypotensive effects of hybrid drugs. The new ligands selective for I_1R will be very helpful to investigate the molecular features and the signaling system of I_1R.

KEYWORDS: imidazolines; blood pressure; central nervous system; I_1-receptors

INTRODUCTION

Imidazolines and similar centrally acting drugs are antihypertensive agents that inhibit the activity of the sympathetic nervous system.[1] Their site of action is located in the central nervous system, more specifically in the medulla oblongata, which is located in the lateral reticular nucleus of the rostroventral medulla.[2] Imidazolines and related hypotensive substances are highly effective drugs. However, the first generation frequently had bothersome adverse effects, although they were generally not very severe. Pharmacologists and chemists interested in these drugs had to answer at least two important questions: (1) What is the pharmacological mechanism underlying the hypotensive action of these products? (2) From a mechanistic point of view, would it be possible to differentiate the hypotensive effect from the most common adverse effect, that is, sedation?

Address for correspondence: P. Bousquet, INSERM E0333, Faculté de Médecine, Université Louis Pasteur, 67000 Strasbourg, France. Voice: (+33) 3 90 24 33 90; fax: (+33) 3 90 24 33 88.
e-mail: Pascal.Bousquet@medecine.u-strasbg.fr

MECHANISM OF ACTION

It was established very early that imidazolines and molecules with imidazoline-like structures were able to lower blood pressure by an effect on their site of action in the medulla, although catecholamines and phenylethylamines were incapable of producing such an effect at the same site.[3] This structure-activity relationship factor showed that activation of α-adrenergic receptors was not the prime mechanism of this action. On the basis of this observation, the existence of a nonadrenergic receptor specifically acted upon by imidazolines was suggested. The identification and biochemical characterization of these receptors was somewhat delayed by the fact that all the available ligands were "hybrid." That is, they bound not only to α_2-adrenergic receptors and sometimes α_1-adrenergic receptors, but also to specific, nonadrenergic imidazoline receptors. This was particularly true in the case of clonidine.[4-6] Compounds belonging to the second generation—including rilmenidine and moxonidine—exhibit a certain selectivity for nonadrenergic receptors. Compared with clonidine, their selectivity has approximately 3 to 10 times greater affinity for imidazoline receptors over α_2-adrenergic receptors.[7] This selectivity is the result of a lower affinity for α_2-adrenergic receptors. Nevertheless, this means that, although selective, some binding to adrenergic receptors does occur. Therefore, these second generation centrally-acting drugs show sufficiently poor affinity and weak activity at α_2-adrenergic receptors for side effects associated with the activation of α_2-adrenergic receptors to be adequately diminished in terms of both frequency and severity compared with the earlier generation of drugs. This is notably true in the case of the sedative effect, dry mouth, bradycardia, and even the rebound effect upon withdrawal, which is not observed with rilmenidine and moxonidine.[1]

Using these pharmacologic tools, it was possible to distinguish two or even three subtypes of imidazoline receptors. Subtype I_1, involved in cardiovascular effects, is sensitive to clonidine and idazoxan (an antagonist of central antihypertensive effects), whereas subtype I_2 is insensitive to clonidine but sensitive to idazoxan. The I_2 imidazoline receptor was identified at a site for monoamine oxidase regulation.[8,9] As for subtype I_3, it is currently the most puzzling subtype; its existence was suggested on the basis of functional studies demonstrating that certain imidazolines exerted a regulatory action on the pancreatic secretion of insulin. These pharmacologic effects fail to correspond with the pharmacology of either I_1 or I_2 imidazoline receptors.[10] However, so far it has been impossible to detect any novel nonadrenergic-specific binding of imidazoline-like or related compounds in the pancreas. Ongoing research work in this exciting field is designed to achieve this end. The remainder of this update will be devoted solely to describing advances made concerning receptors involved in the regulation of sympathetic tone, namely I_1 imidazoline receptors.

I_1 imidazoline receptors have been identified in several different species, and in several different tissues, organs, and cell lines. We have shown that they are present at a fairly high density in the region of the medulla oblongata that contains the site of hypotensive action for imidazoline-like and related drugs. We also demonstrated that they are located on the plasma membrane of neurons.[11]

Various teams have attempted to clone the receptors. For the moment, these have not been entirely successful, probably because the receptor protein is unstable in the case of attempts that require purification of the receptor, and because the molecular tools are not sufficiently selective in the case of attempted cloning that relies on expression. New cloning strategies are being developed. There are several experimental arguments in favor of coupling the receptor to one or more G proteins. Two mechanisms of signal transduction associated with I_1 imidazoline receptors have recently been identified: activation of phosphatidylcholine-sensitive phospholipase C and inhibition of adenylcyclase.[12,13]

Much information has already been obtained concerning I_1 imidazoline receptors. However, ligands that would only bind to and therefore only act upon these receptors—specifically avoiding α_2-adrenergic receptors—have been sadly lacking not only for use in the continued analysis of this nonadrenergic receptor system, but also for the exploration of potential new therapeutic agents that would rely exclusively on I_1 imidazoline receptors.

The synthesis of pyrroline analogues of imidazolines and reference oxazolines led to an appreciable increase in selectivity for I_1 receptors over α_2- and I_2-receptors. A few of these compounds are: S23515, S23757, LNP509, and LNP911. TABLE 1 indicates the affinities of these compounds for I_1, I_2 and α_2-adrenergic receptors and their selectivity ratios.[14–16] These compounds are the first imidazoline analogues described that are devoid of any significant affinity for α_2-adrenergic receptors, and we have confirmed that they do not exhibit any agonist or antagonist activity at these receptors.

The LNP911 compound has a nanomolar affinity for the I_1-receptors and no detectable affinity for α_2- and I_2- receptors. It has been labeled with ^{125}-iodine; and this radiolabeled ligand is the first to be truly selective for I_1-receptors.[16] An azido-derivative has also been synthesized as a photo-affinity ligand for I_1-receptors and proved able to bind to them in an irreversible manner.

Hence, these compounds are powerful tools that are already being used for the further exploration and identification of these original receptors, and especially for further attempts at cloning as well as in drug design strategies.[15]

Some other selective compounds have allowed us to answer one crucial question concerning this research topic: are imidazoline analogues that are totally without effect on adrenergic receptors capable of affecting blood pressure? We recently reported that compounds S23515 and LNP509 induce a dose-dependent hypotensive effect in the anaesthetized rabbit when they are administered directly into the vicinity of the medulla oblongata, that is, intracisternally (FIG. 1).[14,17] These drugs do not cross the blood-brain barrier and must be injected directly into the brain. We also showed that LNP509 is as active in genetically modified D79N mice (whose α_{2A}-adrenergic receptors have undergone mutation so that they are no longer functional)

TABLE 1. Affinities of the selective ligands K_i ± SEM (nmol/L)

	α_1AR	α_2AR	I_1R
LNP509	>10,000	>10,000	538 ± 163
S23515	1710 ± 474	>10,000	6.40 ± 1.94
S23757	>10,000	>10,000	5.30 ± 1.48
LNP911	>10,000	>10,000	0.2 ± 0.1

AR, adrenergic receptor; I_1R, I_1 imidazoline receptor.

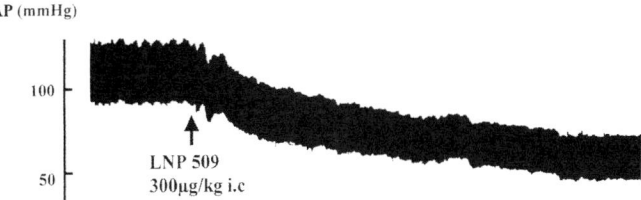

FIGURE 1. Blood pressure effect of LNP 509 injected intracisternally in an anesthetized rabbit.

as in wild type mice (that is, those having normally functioning α_{2A}-adrenergic receptors).[17]

S23757, which has no effect by itself on blood pressure when used under the same experimental conditions, completely prevents the hypotensive action of both S23515 and LNP509. S23757 is the first antagonist that is truly selective towards imidazoline receptors; it has no inhibitory effect whatsoever on the hypotensive effect of a purely α_2-adrenergic agonist, α-methylnoradrenaline.[14]

More recently, we synthesized other imidazoline, oxazoline and pyrroline analogues that also proved to be highly selective for imidazoline receptors but are more lipophilic. As expected, some of them, such as LNP640, are active when injected systemically, indicating an ability to cross the blood brain barrier.

Several experimental findings indicated that imidazoline and α-adrenergic systems might interact synergistically in the central regulation of cardiovascular function and the action of hybrid drugs. We tested this hypothesis using these new molecular tools. Thus, in the anesthetized rabbit, the sequential administration of a low dose of LNP509, without any effect by itself, followed 10 minutes later by a low dose of α-methylnoradrenaline, with very little effect, produced a very marked fall in blood pressure. The drugs were administered intracisternally in these experiments, α-methylnoradrenaline being used as the reference "pure" α_2-adrenergic agonist. As expected, this synergistic interaction was not found in the D79N mouse whose α_{2A}-adrenergic receptors are non-functional.[17]

Interestingly, the central hypotensive effect of rilmenidine was only obtained at high doses in the D79N mice and the effect was less pronounced than in the control wild-type mice. Only the imidazoline receptor-mediated effect persisted in D79N mice; in this case, the synergistic interaction induced in normal animals only by the hybrid drugs, such as rilmenidine, did not occur in D79N mice. It is evident from these data that rilmenidine has sufficiently weak α_{2A}-adrenergic activity so that it has few adverse effects at the recommended doses, but is adequate to trigger the synergistic interaction that is responsible for its marked hypotensive effect.

ADDITIONAL EFFECTS

Second generation central antihypertensives have remarkable antiarrhythmic effects in experimental models of ventricular arrhythmia associated with sympathetic hyperactivity.[18] They are also capable of producing an appreciable improvement in hemodynamic parameters in models of left ventricular dysfunction (certain forms of chronic heart failure). Some have a beneficial effect on survival in the models previously mentioned.[19] Such additional effects are extremely interesting and need to be confirmed, particularly in humans. Clinical trials are being designed with the aim of achieving these data. Some drugs that are selective for imidazoline receptors, such as LNP509, retain these cardiac activities, and therefore it should be possible to develop new, well tolerated drugs such as:

- antihypertensive agents with additional cardiac effects;
- antiarrhythmics at non-hypotensive doses;
- drugs that can be used in the treatment of heart failure at non-hypotensive doses.

CONCLUSION

A great many new facts have recently come to light concerning both the mechanism of action and clinical efficacy of imidazoline-like drugs. New pharmacological tools and modern animal models have made it possible to develop compounds that are highly selective towards specific nonadrenergic imidazoline receptors, which, in turn, have led to the resolution of four important questions:

- The activation of I_1 imidazoline receptors in the medulla oblongata is by itself sufficient to lower blood pressure. S23515, LNP509, and LNP640 are highly selective for I_1 receptors, and decrease blood pressure and the heart rate. All of these drugs act centrally, but only LNP640 is able to cross the blood-brain barrier.

- Selective compounds are now available that are very useful to further investigate the I_1 imidazoline receptors. LNP911 has a nanomolar affinity for I_1 imidazoline receptors and no detectable affinity at α_2-adrenergic receptors; its azido-derivative is a photo-affinity ligand with similar binding features, except that it binds to the I_1-receptors in a non-reversible manner. S23757 is the first antagonist of the I_1 receptor-mediated cardiovascular effects with no detectable affinity and activity at α_2-adrenergic receptors.

- The imidazolinergic system and α_2-adrenergic system act synergistically in the processes of regulating vasomotor sympathetic tone.

- The residual α_2-adrenergic activity of the second generation drugs, such as rilmenidine, is enough to exert this synergistic effect and also sufficiently weak to be much better tolerated than the drugs of the first generation.

REFERENCES

1. BOUSQUET, P. & J. FELDMAN. 1999. Drugs acting on imidazoline receptors: a review of their clinical pharmacology, their use in blood pressure control and their potential interest in cardioprotection. Drugs **58:** 799–812.
2. BOUSQUET, P., J. FELDMAN, R. BLOCH, *et al*. 1981. The nucleus reticularis lateralis: a region highly sensitive to clonidine. Eur. J. Pharmacol. **69:** 389–392.

3. BOUSQUET, P., J. FELDMAN & J. SCHWARTZ. 1984. Central cardiovascular effects of α-adrenergic drugs: difference between catecholamines and imidazolines. J. Pharmacol. Exp. Ther. **230:** 232–236.
4. BRICCA, G., M. DONTENWILL, A. MOLINES, et al. 1989. The imidazoline preferring receptors: binding studies in bovine, rat and human brainstem. Eur. J. Pharmacol. **62:** 1–9.
5. BRICCA, G., H. GRENEY, J. ZHANG, et al. 1994. Human brain imidazoline receptors: Further characterization with [^{3}H]clonidine. Eur. J. Pharmacol. **266:** 25–33.
6. ERNSBERGER, P., M.P. MEELEY, J.J. MANN, et al. 1987. Clonidine binds to imidazole binding sites as well as α_2-adrenoceptors in the ventrolateral medulla. Eur. J. Pharmacol. **134:** 1–13.
7. BRICCA, G., M. DONTENWILL, A. MOLINES, et al. 1989. Rilmenidine selectivity for imidazoline receptors in human brain. Eur. J. Pharmacol. **163:** 373–377.
8. PARINI, A., I. COUPRY, R.M. GRAHAM, et al. 1989. Characterization of an imidazoline/guanidinium receptive site distinct from the α_2-adrenergic receptor. J. Biol. Chem. **264:** 11874–11878.
9. LIMON, I., I. COUPRY, S.M. LANIER, et al. 1992. Purification and characterization of mitochondrial imidazoline-guanidinium receptive site from rabbit kidney. J. Biol. Chem. **267:** 21645–21649.
10. MORGAN, N.G. & S.L. CHAN. 2001. Imidazoline binding sites in the endocrine pancreas: can they fulfil their potential as targets for the development of new insuline secretagogues? [Review] Curr. Pharm. Res. **14:** 1413–1431.
11. HEEMSKERK, F.M.J., M. DONTENWILL, C. VONTHRON, et al. 1998. [^{125}I]para-iodoclonidine reveals a new subtype of imidazoline specific sites in synaptosomal plasma membranes of the bovine brainstem. J. Neurochem. **71:** 2193–2202.
12. SEPAROVIC, D., M. KESTER, M.A. HAXHIU, et al. 1997. Activation of phosphatidylcholine-selective phospholipase C by I_1-imidazoline receptors in PC12 cells and rostral ventrolateral medulla. Brain Res. **749:** 335–339.
13. GRENEY, H., P. RONDE, C. MAGNIER, et al. 2000. Coupling of I_1-imidazoline receptors to the cAMP pathway: studies with a highly selective ligand, benazoline. Mol. Pharmacol. **57:** 1142–1151.
14. BRUBAN, V., J. FELDMAN, H. GRENEY, et al. 2001. Respective contribution of α–adrenergic and non-adrenergic mechanisms in the hypotensive effect of imidazoline-like drugs. Br. J. Pharmacol. **133:** 261–266.
15. SCHANN, S., V. BRUBAN, K. POMPERMAYER, et al. 2001. Synthesis and biological evaluation of pyrrolinic isosteres of rilmenidine. Discovery of cis/trans-Dicyclopropylmethyl-(4,5-dimethyl–4,5-dihydro-3H-pyrrol-2-yl)-amine (LNP 509), an I_1 imidazoline receptor selective ligand with hypotensive activity. J. Med. Chem. **44:** 1588–1593.
16. GRENEY, H., D. UROSEVIC, S. SCHANN, et al. 2002. [(125)I]2-(2-Chloro-4-iodo-phenylamino)-5-methyl-pyrroline (LNP 911), a high-affinity radioligand selective for I(1) imidazoline receptors. Mol. Pharmacol. **62:** 181–191.
17. BRUBAN, V., V. ESTATO, S. SCHANN, et al. 2002. Evidence for synergy between α_2-adrenergic and nonadrenergic mechanisms in central blood pressure regulation. Circulation **105:** 1116–1121.
18. ROEGEL, J.C., N. YANNOULIS, W. DE JONG, et al. 1998. Preventive effect of rilmenidine on the occurrence of neurogenic ventricular arrhythmias in rabbits. J. Hypertension **16**(suppl 3): S39–S43.
19. THOMAS, L., B. GASSER, P. BOUSQUET, et al. 2003. Haemodynamic and cardiac antihypertrophic actions of clonidine in Goldblatt one kidney, one clip rats. J. Cardiovasc. Pharmacol. **41:** 203–209.

Are Centrally Acting Imidazoline Agents Appropriate Therapy for Renovascular Hypertension?

GEOFFREY A. HEAD AND SANDRA L. BURKE

Neuropharmacology Laboratory, Baker Heart Research Institute, Melbourne, Victoria, Australia

> ABSTRACT: An increased role of the sympathetic nervous system has been suggested to be a major contributor to the chronic elevation of BP in renovascular hypertension. We assessed the effects of rilmenidine, a centrally acting antihypertensive imidazoline agent, on BP and renal sympathetic nerve activity (RSNA) in 2K1C renovascular hypertensive conscious rabbits. Rabbits were made hypertensive with a renal clip or were sham-operated and were studied 3 and 6 weeks later. Acute treatment with rilmenidine reduced BP to a greater extent in the hypertensive rabbits. Although rilmenidine reduced the heart rate by the same extent in all groups, rilmenidine produced much less inhibition of RSNA in the hypertensive animals. These studies suggest that the contribution of the sympathetic nervous system is greater in 2K1C hypertension and that imidazoline agents may be beneficial in treating renovascular hypertension.
>
> KEYWORDS: rilmenidine; centrally acting antihypertensive agents; renovascular hypertension; renal sympathetic nerve activity; blood pressure; heart rate

INTRODUCTION

There is little doubt that in the longer term, the level of blood pressure (BP) relies on the kidney, and specifically on the relationship between renal perfusion pressure and urinary Na^+ excretion, and thus body fluid balance. Guyton[1] suggests that hypertension can develop only when there is a shift in the pressure–natriuresis relationship towards a higher pressure and that this mechanism underlies all forms of hypertension in humans and experimental animals. The sensitivity of the pressure–natriuresis mechanism is altered by a number of hormonal regulatory systems, of which the renin/angiotensin system is most important because it is nonadapting.[2] The importance of the sympathetic nervous system in short-term regulation of BP is well accepted, because autonomic baroreflexes and the influence of command signals from higher brain centers on these sympathetic reflexes dominate the moment-to-moment control of BP. The question of whether neural systems participate in long-term regulation of BP has long been debated[3]; this question is important, because

---

Address for correspondence: Geoffrey A. Head, Ph.D., B.Sc. (Hons), Principal Research Fellow, Head, Neuropharmacology Laboratory, Baker Heart Research Institute, P.O. Box 6492, St. Kilda Road, Central, Melbourne, Victoria 8008 Australia. Voice: (+61) 3 85321332; fax: (+61) 3 85321100. e-mail: geoff.head@baker.edu.au

there is increasing evidence that sympathetic activity has a role in a number of disease states such as hypertension, congestive heart failure, and renal failure.[4] Studies from Esler and coworkers[5] have demonstrated that noradrenaline release from renal nerves is elevated in young patients with borderline hypertension and that they also have altered spillover of central monoamine neurotransmitters from subcortical regions of the brain. There seems to be a major contribution from the sympathetic nervous system in many experimental models of hypertension, including genetic forms, such as the spontaneously hypertensive rat (SHR),[6] and in hypertension induced by blockade of nitric oxide.[7] Neonatal sympathectomy in SHRs produces a long-term BP reduction,[8] and interruption of central nervous system neuromodulators or lesions of specific areas involved in sympathetic regulation prevents genetic hypertension and also deoxycorticosterone acetate (DOCA)-salt hypertension.[9–11]

Although the importance of the sympathetic nervous system in human essential hypertension is well established, its role in secondary forms of hypertension such as renovascular disease is not so clear, as suggested in a recent review by Grassi and Esler.[12] Renovascular hypertension is primarily caused by renal ischemia, which evokes a number of changes including the release of renin from juxtaglomerular cells in the kidney and also blood volume changes.[13] The latter mechanism is thought to be particularly important in some forms of renal hypertension, such as the 1K1C model in which total kidney filtration is compromised and blocking the renin/angiotensin/aldosterone system seems to have little effect.[14–16] By contrast, in the 2K1C model with only 1 kidney ischemic, in which renal function is less compromised because of the intact kidney, the renin/angiotensin system is essential for maintaining the high BP.[14,15] Although the incidence of renal hypertension in the community is relatively low (2%–4%), its importance is increasing as the population ages and the incidence of renal artery atherosclerotic lesions becomes more prevalent.[17] Indeed, it has been shown that the incidence of atherosclerotic renal disease in elderly patients with heart failure is as high as 34%.[18] Thus it is timely to examine whether centrally acting sympatholytic agents, such as clonidine, or the second-generation agents, such as rilmenidine or moxonidine, that are selective for imidazoline receptors are appropriate therapy for this form of hypertension. This review briefly examines the evidence for a significant contribution of the sympathetic nervous system to renovascular hypertension and evaluates the appropriateness of centrally acting agents as a form of therapy. We focus on the renin/angiotensin-dependent form of the disease, because this is the model in which we have been investigating this question.

SYMPATHETIC NERVOUS SYSTEM AND RENOVASCULAR HYPERTENSION

Clinical Studies

In humans, the techniques for measuring sympathetic activity directly have been limited to skeletal muscle sympathetic activity. Miyajima and colleagues[19] found that sympathetic activity was increased in renovascular hypertensive patients. By contrast Grassi and colleagues[20] found that muscle sympathetic activity was normal and less than that observed in age-matched patients with essential hypertension. Apart from the difficulty of comparisons between patient groups, direct sympathetic recording of muscle quantifies only the frequency of sympathetic bursts rather than the magnitude of the burst. Furthermore, the differential regulation of regional sympathetic activity means that activity in one bed may not be reflected in other beds. Indirect measures of sympathetic activity have been developed, such as the noradrenaline spillover technique which involves the infusion of a small amount of radiolabeled noradrenaline.[21] Examination of total noradrenaline spillover as an index of global sympathetic activity has yielded conflicting results in patients with renovascular hypertension: initial results suggested an increased sympathetic activity,[22] whereas a later study from the same group showed no difference compared with normotensive persons.[23] The explanation given was that the hypertension was of different durations, a factor that is particularly important in this context, in which the disease has several quite different stages.[12,13]

The advantage of the noradrenaline spillover technique is that it has been possible to sample from regional veins and gauge an estimation of sympathetic activity to a variety of organs independently. In a relatively small study in patients with renovascular hypertension, Friberg and colleagues[24] found no evidence for increased renal nerve activity in the affected kidney, despite the marked renin production. Another study from this group, however, has shown an increased sympathetic activity to the heart in patients with renovascular hypertensive patients.[23] Thus, there is some evidence suggesting increased sympathetic activity, but the findings are not really convincing, although the balance of evidence suggests that the contribution of the sympathetic nervous system is likely to be increased rather than decreased.[13,25,26] Perhaps the most convincing evidence has come from Mathias and colleagues[25,27] who found that clonidine lowered BP substantially and for a prolonged period even in patients whose disease had been refractory to multiple antihypertensive drug therapy. Levels of plasma renin activity (PRA) were unchanged after clonidine administration, but plasma noradrenaline levels fell. These studies suggest that there was profound support of the hypertension by the sympathetic nervous system and that centrally acting agents may be appropriate for its treatment.

Experimental Studies

Although the findings in humans as to whether the sympathetic nerve activity contributes to renovascular hypertension have not been conclusive, studies in experimental models of renovascular hypertension give more consistent results.[28] A greater depressor response to ganglion blockade has been observed in renal wrap hypertensive rats, and a neuropeptide Y antagonist has been shown to attenuate the development of 2K1C hypertension in rats.[29] Kagiyama and colleagues[30] found that antisense inhibition of the brain renin-angiotensin system decreased BP and plasma epinephrine and proposed that the mechanism of maintenance of high BP in chronic 2K1C hypertension involves high levels of angiotensin II in the hypothalamus activating the paraventricular nucleus to increase sympathetic outflow. Studies in the rabbit by Cox and Bishop[31] showed that during 10 days of intravenous (i.v.) angiotensin II infusion the hypertension was initially caused by angiotensin-mediated vasoconstriction, but this vasoconstriction subsided and was replaced by a greater neurogenic component as determined by the depressor effect of ganglionic blockade. Lesions of specific brain areas important for the regulation of sympathetic activity lower BP in various forms of renovascular hypertension.[32–34] Thus a contribution of the sympathetic nervous system seems essential for the development of renal hypertension, suggesting that sympathetic activity would be expected to be increased. The expected greater sympathetic activity in renovascular hypertension has been surprisingly difficult to establish, however, because of the use of indirect measures, such as peripheral noradrenaline kinetics, which have yielded conflicting findings.[35,36] Tanaka and colleagues[35] showed that norepinephrine turnover in the cardiovascular tissues in the 2K1C group was similar to that found in the control group. By contrast, Kumagai and colleagues[36] showed a threefold higher level of plasma norepinephrine in 2K1C hypertensive rabbits than in sham-operated animals.

ROLE OF RENAL SYMPATHETIC NERVES

Changes in sympathetic nervous activity to each vascular bed are not uniform and vary widely in response to different afferent signals. Thus, not all sympathetic outflow may be relevant to the development of hypertension. It has been recognized that the most important sympathetic outflow to the long-term regulation of BP and also to hypertension is renal sympathetic nerve activity (RSNA), because these nerves affect renal hemodynamics, tubular function, and renal renin release.[4] All these effects have the potential to contribute to the initiation, development, and maintenance of hypertension.[37] Chronic alterations in renal adrenergic activity, by infusion of noradrenaline at doses that increase PRA but do not alter renal hemodynamics, shift the pressure–natriuresis relationship towards increased BP, and, if given chronically, produce sustained hypertension.[38] These effects were achieved with low doses of noradrenaline that had little or no effect on renal hemodynamics but were associated with changes in PRA. Sustained increases in adrenergic activity had no effect on BP if the activity of the renin/angiotensin system was clamped. The adrenergic pressor effect in the kidney is probably mediated by renin release, because renal denervation prevents or delays most forms of hypertension including SHRs, aortic coarctation, obesity hypertension, and DOCA salt.[37] Taken together, these observations suggest that activation of the renin/angiotensin system can play an important role in the development of hypertension secondary to activation of the sympathetic nervous system.

Few studies have directly measured sympathetic activity, mainly because of technical problems associated with chronic nerve recording and an inability to compare measures within and among different groups. The difficulty is that measurement of activity from an implanted electrode is influenced by the physical characteristics of the electrode, which differ in each implantation. Thus comparisons in μV between different animals are not meaningful, and there has been no consensus as to how sympathetic activity contributes to renovascular hypertension. We have largely solved these problems in an experimental rabbit preparation where we have shown that long-term recording (up to 6 weeks) of nerve activity is possible by using a calibration method involving testing each animal with a maximal sympathetic discharge associated with the nasopharyngeal reflex.[39] This method enables comparisons among different groups of rabbits and also within the same animal over an extended recording period of several weeks.[39]

We have determined the change in RSNA in 2K1C hypertension in conscious rabbits at 3 weeks and 6 weeks and compared it with sham-clipped normotensive rabbits of either sex whose weight ranged from 2.4 to 3.2 kg. All rabbits underwent an initial

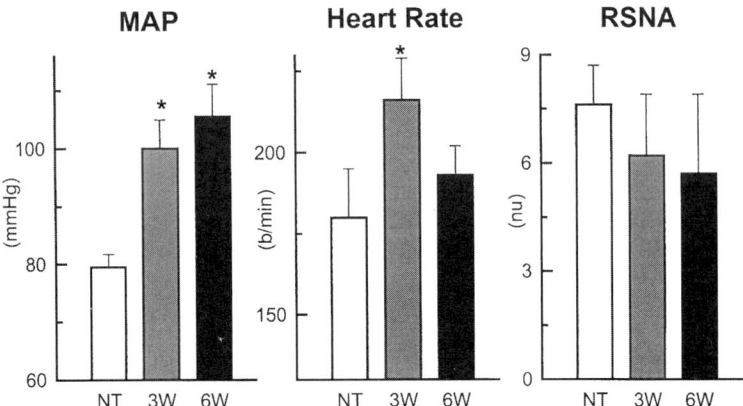

FIGURE 1. Mean arterial pressure, heart rate (beats per minute), and renal sympathetic nerve activity measured in normotensive rabbits (*open bars*, n = 8) and in hypertensive rabbits at 3 weeks (*gray bars*, n = 8) and 6 weeks (*black bars*, n = 8) after renal clipping. Error bars are SEM indicating between animal variance, * $P < 0.05$ for comparison with normotensive response. MAP, mean arterial pressure in mm Hg; NT, normotensive; RSNA, renal sympathetic nerve activity in normalized units; 3W, 3 weeks; 6W, 6 weeks.

operation performed under halothane anesthesia to insert a silver clip fitted on the right renal artery (hypertensive group) or a similar procedure in which the clip was removed immediately (sham group). Two weeks later, half the hypertensive and half the sham-operated animals underwent a second operation in which a stainless-steel chronic recording electrode was implanted on the left renal sympathetic nerve.[40] The remaining hypertensive and sham-operated animals received the electrode at least 5 weeks after the clip implantation. The experiment was conducted at least 6 days after implantation of the renal electrode (i.e., either 3 or 6 weeks after insertion of the clip). At this time arterial BP was measured from the central ear artery, and RSNA measurements were amplified using a low-noise differential preamplifier and amplifier combination, rectified and integrated with a 20-millisecond time constant. Background electrode noise was estimated in the silent periods between bursts and was subtracted from all RSNA values. RSNA was normalized to the maximum 2 seconds of RSNA evoked by 50-mL smoke (response = 100 units). At 3 weeks and 6 weeks mean arterial pressure (MAP) was elevated by 26% and 33%, respectively (FIG. 1). Heart rate was slightly greater, by 36 beats per minute at 3 weeks ($P = 0.05$) but not at 6 weeks. RSNA tended to be slightly less in the hypertensive groups but was not significantly different from that in sham-operated normotensive animals (FIG. 1). We did not observe an increase in RSNA, a finding that is consistent with other studies.[41]

EFFECT OF CENTRALLY ACTING AGENTS IN RENOVASCULAR HYPERTENSION

Despite increasing suggestions that sympatholytic agents such as the centrally acting clonidine like drugs may be useful in the treatment of renovascular hypertension,[28] few studies have explored this interaction. Sattar and colleagues[42] have shown that a specific clonidine analogue normalizes BP in 2K1C hypertensive rats. Clonidine itself reverses the development of low-dose angiotensin II–induced hypertension.[43] This model of hypertension does not affect the plasma angiotensin II and is analogous to the chronic phase of renovascular hypertension. Armah and colleagues[44] have reported that moxonidine and clonidine lower BP in renal hypertensive rats and dogs. There have been no studies examining the second-generation agent rilmenidine in renovascular hypertension. Furthermore, there have been no comparisons with control animals to determine whether the responses are greater or less than one would expect in the absence of high BP.

We examined whether there is evidence for an increased role of the sympathetic nervous system by giving an intravenous dose of rilmenidine to normotensive, 3-week and 6-week 2K1C hypertensive rabbits (FIG. 2). The dose of 300 µg/kg is equivalent to the ED_{90} dose as previously described.[45] The fall in BP was substantially greater in the hypertensive groups (-16.6 ± 0.9 mm Hg, n = 16) compared with the normotensive rabbits (-10.7 ± 0.9 mm Hg, n = 8, $P < 0.001$). The bradycardia was similar in all three groups of rabbits. However, the sympatho-inhibition in the hypertensive animals was markedly less than in the normotensive rabbits (FIG. 2). RSNA fell by

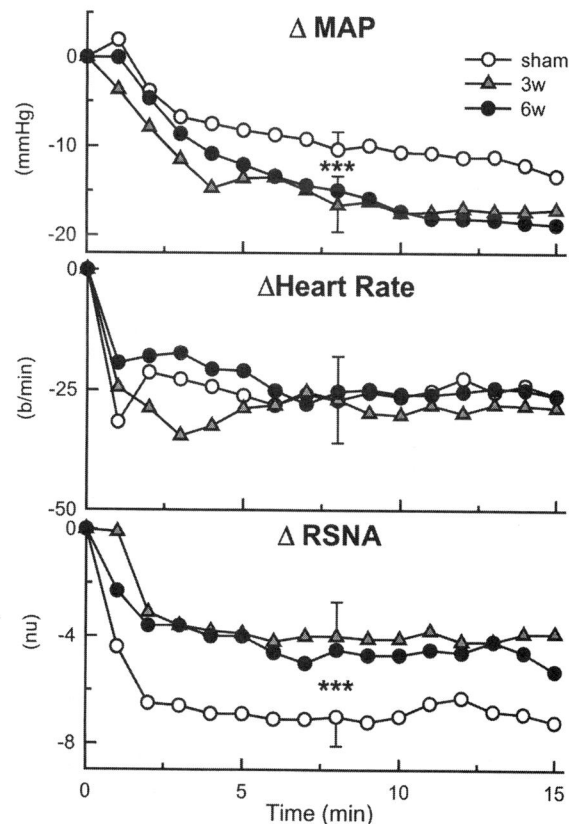

FIGURE 2. Changes in mean arterial pressure, heart rate (beats per minute), and renal sympathetic nerve activity following intravenous dose of rilmenidine (300 µg/kg) in normotensive sham-operated rabbits (*open circles*, n = 8), 3-week hypertensive rabbits (*filled triangle*, n = 8), and 6-week hypertensive rabbits (*filled circle*, n = 8) rabbits. Error bars are SEM indicating between animal variance. *** $P < 0.001$ for comparison of sham with each hypertensive group. ΔMAP, change in mean arterial pressure in mm Hg; ΔRSNA, change in renal sympathetic nerve activity in normalized units; 3W, 3-week; 6W, 6-week.

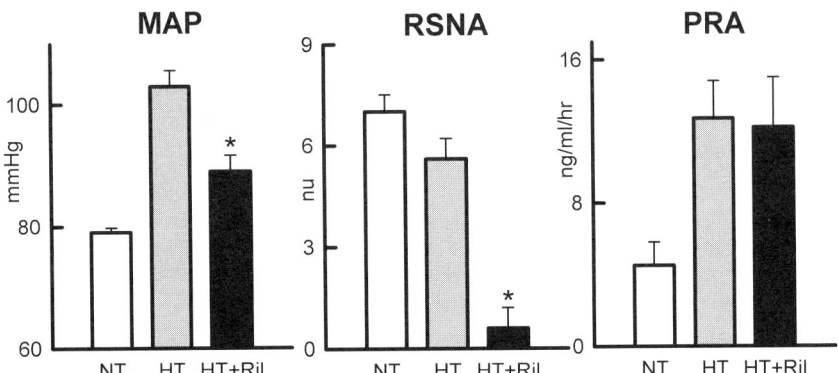

FIGURE 3. Mean arterial pressure, renal sympathetic nerve activity, and plasma renin activity measured in normotensive rabbits (*open bars*), 6-week hypertensive rabbits (*gray bars*), and 6-week hypertensive rabbits during treatment with 300 μg/kg rilmenidine (*black bars*). Error bars are SEM indicating between animal variance, * $P < 0.05$ for comparison with normotensive response. HT, hypertensive; MAP, mean arterial pressure in mm Hg; NT, normotensive; PRA, plasma renin activity in ng/mL/hour; RSNA, renal sympathetic nerve activity in normalized units.

6.9 ± 0.4 normalized units in the sham-operated animals and by 4.0 and 4.7 normalized units in the 3-week and 6-week hypertensive rabbits ($P < 0.001$, FIG. 2). The acute depressor effect of rilmenidine was likely to be mediated by the reduction in RSNA, but there was no change in PRA (FIG. 3).

These studies suggest that the contribution of the sympathetic nervous system has increased in renovascular hypertension, a finding that is consistent with previous studies mentioned. What is surprising, however, is the lack of enhanced sympathetic activity to the kidney (effectively no change) and a reduced inhibition of RSNA by rilmenidine. It is possible that the sympathetic drive to other beds is enhanced in renovascular hypertension, but the evidence is not convincing except for the cardiac sympathetic, which is unlikely to account for the enhanced rilmenidine effect on BP (i.e., there were no differences in heart rate responses to rilmenidine). Another possibility is that the responsiveness to neural activity is enhanced. Using our data, we can quantify a sympathetic neuroeffector feed forward gain by calculating the change in BP per change in RSNA. We found that this gain increased from 2 to 4 by 3 weeks and to 9 by 6 weeks of 2K1C hypertension, corresponding to a fivefold increase in neuroeffector gain in the model of hypertension. Thus, whereas levels of RSNA are reduced or similar to controls, the relative contribution of the sympathetic nervous system to the maintenance of BP is dramatically amplified in hypertension.

CONCLUSION

There is a consistent view expressed in the literature that the sympathetic nervous system makes an important contribution to the development and maintenance of renovascular hypertension. Studies, however, have not consistently been able to show that this contribution results from an increase in sympathetic activity, in part because of the differing phases of the disease and also because of the slowly resetting baroreflex mechanisms that suppress sympathetic activity in the face of high BP and can take up to 6 weeks to normalize.[46] Our studies have demonstrated that centrally acting agents such as rilmenidine are appropriate for the treatment of renovascular hypertension and are significantly more effective than in normal animals. Furthermore the enhanced depressor effects of sympathetic blockade in this model suggest that there may be a major shift in the neuroeffector gain. The mechanism responsible for this change is not clear, but this process is undoubtedly important in the development of renovascular hypertension and key to our understanding of how the central nervous system takes back control of BP in the presence of an ischemic kidney.

REFERENCES

1. GUYTON, A.C. 1990. The surprising kidney-fluid mechanism for pressure control—its infinite gain! Hypertension **16**: 725–730.
2. OLSEN, M.E., J.E. HALL, J.P. MONTANI, *et al.* 1984. Angiotensin II natriuresis and antinatriuresis: role of renal artery pressure in anaesthetized dogs. J. Hypertens. Suppl. **2**: S347–S350.
3. BROOKS, V.L. & J.W. OSBORN. 1995. Hormonal-sympathetic interactions in long-term regulation of arterial pressure: an hypothesis. Am. J. Physiol. **268**: R1343–R1358.
4. LOHMEIER, T.E. 2001. The sympathetic nervous system and long-term BP regulation. Am. J. Hypertens. **14**: 147S–154S.
5. ESLER, M. 1995. Sympathetic nervous system: contribution to human hypertension and related cardiovascular diseases. J. Cardiovasc. Pharmacol. **26**: S24–S28.
6. JUDY, W.V., A. WATANABE, D.P. HENRY, *et al.* 1976. Sympathetic nerve activity: role in regulation of BP in the spontaneously hypertensive rat. Circ. Res. **38**: II-21–II-29.
7. FITZGERALD, S.M. & M.W. BRANDS. 2002. Hypertension in L-NAME-treated diabetic rats depends on an intact sympathetic nervous system. Am. J. Physiol. **282**: R1070–R1076.
8. GRISK, O., I. KLOTING, J. EXNER, *et al.* 2002. Long-term arterial pressure in spontaneously hypertensive rats is set by the kidney. J. Hypertens. **20**: 131–138.
9. ITO, S., K. KOMATSU, K. TSUKAMOTO, *et al.* 2000. Excitatory amino acids in the rostral ventrolateral medulla support BP in spontaneously hypertensive rats. Hypertension **35**: 413–417.
10. COLOMBARI, E., M.A. SATO, S.L. CRAVO, *et al.* 2001. Role of the medulla oblongata in hypertension. Hypertension **38**: 549–554.
11. KUBO, T., R. FUKUMORI, M. KOBAYASHI, *et al.* 1998. Evidence suggesting that lateral parabrachial nucleus is responsible for enhanced medullary cholinergic activity in hypertension. Hypertens. Res. **21**: 201–207.
12. GRASSI, G. & M. ESLER. 2002. The sympathetic nervous system in renovascular hypertension: lead actor or 'bit' player? J. Hypertens. **20**: 1071–1073.
13. MARTINEZ-MALDONADO, M. 1991. Pathophysiology of renovascular hypertension. Hypertension **17**: 707–719.
14. VOLPE, M., G. ODELL, H.D. KLEINERT, *et al.* 1985. Effect of atrial natriuretic factor on BP, renin, and aldosterone in Goldblatt hypertension. Hypertension **7**: I43–I48.
15. WANG, H., T.H. GU, W.H. PAN, *et al.* 1987. BP response of two types of Goldblatt hypertensive rats to enalapril. J. Cardiovasc. Pharmacol. **10**: S119–S121.
16. AKAHOSHI, M. & O.A. CARRETERO. 1989. Body fluid volume and angiotensin II in maintenance of one-kidney, one clip hypertension. Hypertension **14**: 269–273.
17. ZOCCALI, C., F. MALLAMACI & P. FINOCCHIARO. 2002. Atherosclerotic renal artery stenosis: epidemiology, cardiovascular outcomes, and clinical prediction rules. J. Am. Soc. Nephrol. **13** (Suppl 3): S179–S183.

18. MACDOWALL, P., P.A. KALRA, D.J. O'DONOGHUE, *et al.* 1998. Risk of morbidity from renovascular disease in elderly patients with congestive cardiac failure. Lancet **352:** 13–16.
19. MIYAJIMA, E., Y. YAMADA, Y. YOSHIDA, *et al.* 1991. Muscle sympathetic nerve activity in renovascular hypertension and primary aldosteronism. Hypertension **17:** 1057–1062.
20. GRASSI, G., B.M. CATTANEO, G. SERAVALLE, *et al.* 1998. Baroreflex control of sympathetic nerve activity in essential and secondary hypertension. Hypertension **31:** 68–72.
21. ESLER, M., A. ZWEIFLER, O. RANDALL, *et al.* 1977. Agreement among three different indices of sympathetic nervous system activity in essential hypertension. Mayo Clin. Proc. **52:** 379–382.
22. GAO, S.A., M. JOHANSSON, B. RUNDQVIST, *et al.* 2002. Reduced spontaneous baroreceptor sensitivity in patients with renovascular hypertension. J. Hypertens. **20:** 111–116.
23. PETERSSON, M.J., B. RUNDQVIST, M. JOHANSSON, *et al.* 2002. Increased cardiac sympathetic drive in renovascular hypertension. J. Hypertens. **20:** 1181–1187.
24. FRIBERG, P., R. VOLKMANN, G. JENSEN, *et al.* 1991. Norepinephrine overflow and renin pattern of the individual kidney in patients with unilateral renal artery stenosis. Hypertension **17:** 1003–1009.
25. MATHIAS, C.J., J.S. KOONER & S. PEART. 1987. Neurogenic components of hypertension in human renal artery stenosis. Clin. Exp. Hypertens. [A] **9**(Suppl 1): 293–306.
26. TUNCEL, M., R. AUGUSTYNIAK, W. ZHANG, *et al.* 2002. Sympathetic nervous system function in renal hypertension. Curr. Hypertens. Rep. **4:** 229–236.
27. MATHIAS, C.J., A.H. WILKINSON, F.A. PIKE, *et al.* 1983. Clonidine in unilateral renal artery stenosis and unilateral renal parenchymal disease–similar antihypertensive but different renin suppressive effects. J. Hypertens. Suppl. **1:** 123–125.
28. JOHANSSON, M. & P. FRIBERG. 2000. Role of the sympathetic nervous system in human renovascular hypertension. Curr. Hypertens. Rep. **2:** 319–326.
29. SHIN, L.H., P.S. DOVGAN, T.J. NYPAVER, *et al.* 2000. Role of neuropeptide Y in the development of two-kidney, one-clip renovascular hypertension in the rat. J. Vasc. Surg. **32:** 1015–1021.
30. KAGIYAMA, S., A. VARELA, M.I. PHILLIPS, *et al.* 2001. Antisense inhibition of brain renin-angiotensin system decreased BP in chronic 2-kidney, 1 clip hypertensive rats. Hypertension **37:** 371–375.
31. COX, B.F. & V.S. BISHOP. 1991. Neural and humoral mechanisms of angiotensin-dependent hypertension. Am. J. Physiol. **261:** H1284–H1291.
32. FINK, G.D., C.M. PAWLOSKI, L.E. OHMAN, *et al.* 1991. Lateral parabrachial nucleus and angiotensin II-induced hypertension. Hypertension **17:** 1177–1184.
33. FINK, G.D., C.A. BRUNER & M.L. MANGIAPANE. 1987. Area postrema is critical for angiotensin-induced hypertension in rats. Hypertension **9:** 355–361.
34. MORTENSEN, L.H., L.E. OHMAN & J.R. HAYWOOD. 1994. Effects of lateral parabrachial nucleus lesions in chronic renal hypertensive rats. Hypertension **23:** 774–780.
35. TANAKA, T., A. SEKI, J. FUJII, *et al.* 1982. Norepinephrine turnover in the cardiovascular tissues and brain stem of the rabbit during development of one-kidney and two-kidney Goldblatt hypertension. Hypertension **4:** 272–278.
36. KUMAGAI, H., H. SUZUKI, M. ICHIKAWA, *et al.* 1995. Different responses of renal blood flow and sympathetic nerve activity to captopril and nicardipine in conscious renal hypertensive rabbits. J. Cardiovasc. Pharmacol. **25:** 57–64.
37. DIBONA, G.F. & U.C. KOPP. 1997. Neural control of renal function. Physiol. Rev. **77:** 75–197
38. REINHART, G.A., T.E. LOHMEIER & C.E. HORD. 1995. Hypertension induced by chronic renal adrenergic stimulation is angiotensin dependent. Hypertension **25:** 940–949.
39. BURKE, S.L. & G.A. HEAD. 2003. Method for in-vivo calibration of renal sympathetic nerve activity in rabbits. J. Neurosci. Methods. **127:** 63–74.
40. DORWARD, P.K., W. RIEDEL, S.L. BURKE, *et al.* 1985. The renal sympathetic baroreflex in the rabbit. Arterial and cardiac baroreceptor influences, resetting, and effect of anesthesia. Circ. Res. **57:** 618–633.

41. BELL, L., D.J. WILSON, L.M. QUANDT, *et al.* 1995. Renal sympathetic and heart rate baroreflex function in conscious and isoflurane anaesthetized normotensive and chronically hypertensive rabbits. Clin. Exp. Pharmacol. Physiol. **22:** 701–710.
42. SATTAR, M.A., A.P.M. YUSOF, E.K. GAN, *et al.* 2000. Acute renal failure in 2K2C Goldblatt hypertensive rats during antihypertensive therapy: comparison of an angiotensin AT(1) receptor antagonist and clonidine analogues. J. Autonom. Pharmacol. **20:** 297–304.
43. GORBEA-OPPLIGER, V.J. & G.D. FINK. 1994. Clonidine reverses the slowly developing hypertension produced by low doses of angiotensin II. Hypertension **23:** 844–847.
44. ARMAH, B.I., E. HOFFERBER & W. STENZEL. 1988. General pharmacology of the novel centrally acting antihypertensive agent moxonidine. Arzneimittel Forschung Drug Reseach **38:** 1426–1434.
45. CHAN, C.K.S. & G.A. HEAD. 1996. Relative importance of central imidazoline receptors for the antihypertensive effects of moxonidine and rilmenidine. J. Hypertens. **14:** 855–864.
46. HEAD, G.A. & S.L. BURKE. 2001. Renal and cardiac sympathetic baroreflexes in hypertensive rabbits. Clin. Exp. Pharmacol. Physiol. **28:** 972–975.

Cardiac Effects of Moxonidine in Spontaneously Hypertensive Obese Rats

S. MUKADDAM-DAHER,[a] A. MENAOUAR,[a] R. EL-AYOUBI,[a] J. GUTKOWSKA,[a] M. JANKOWSKI,[a] R.A. VELLIQUETTE,[b] AND P. ERNSBERGER[b]

[a]*CHUM-Research Center, Université de Montréal, Montreal, QC, Canada*
[b]*Department of Nutrition, Case Western Reserve University, Cleveland, Ohio 44106, USA*

ABSTRACT: Moxonidine, an imidazoline receptor agonist that acts centrally to inhibit sympathetic activity, has been shown to reduce effectively blood pressure, fasting insulin levels, and free fatty acids. In this study, we investigated the long-term effects of moxonidine treatment on cardiac natriuretic peptides (ANP and BNP) in Spontaneously Hypertensive Obese Rats (SHROBs), a rat model that resembles human Syndrome X. SHROBs expressing spontaneous hypertension, insulin resistance, and genetic obesity (weight 590 ± 20 g, at 30 weeks) received moxonidine in chow at 4 mg/kg/day for 15 days. Moxonidine significantly reduced not only systolic blood pressure (187 ± 6 versus 156 ± 5 mm Hg, $P < 0.05$) but also plasma ANP (1595 ± 371 versus 793 ± 131 pg/mL, $P < 0.05$) and BNP (22 ± 3 versus 14 ± 1 pg/mL, $P < 0.04$), without influencing cardiac content of either peptide. Semi-quantitative PCR revealed that atrial ANPmRNA/GAPDHmRNA decreased to 39% ± 10% of pair-fed controls, $P < 0.03$. In left ventricles, moxonidine also decreased ANP mRNA to 69% ± 7% and BNP mRNA to 74% ± 6% of control, $P < 0.02$, but right ventricular ANP and BNP mRNA were not affected. These findings indicate that chronic inhibition of sympathetic activity with moxonidine in SHROB is associated with decreased ventricular natriuretic peptide transcription, consistent with the cardioprotective effects of moxonidine given the role of ANP and BNP as markers of cadiac disease. Moxonidine also improves the metabolic profile in these rats, thus it may be considered the drug of choice in treatment of metabolic syndrome X.

KEYWORDS: spontaneously hypertensive obese rats (SHROBs); metabolic syndrome X; LVH; moxonidine; natriuretic peptides

INTRODUCTION

Obesity is often associated with cardiovascular and metabolic disorders, such as hypertension, hyperglycemia, and dyslipidemia. This cluster of abromalities is referred to as metabolic syndrome X, insulin resistance syndrome, or the "deadly quartet" and leads to a threefold increase in coronary heart disease risk. This syndrome is also a risk factor for left ventricular hypertrophy (LVH).[1]

Address for correspondence: Suhayla Mukaddam-Daher, Ph.D., Laboratory of Cardiovascular Biochemistry, CHUM Research Center, Hotel-Dieu Hospital (6-816), 3840 St-Urbain Street, Montreal (Quebec), Canada, H2W 1T8. Voice: (514) 890-8000, ext: 12757; fax: (514) 412-7199.
e-mail: suhayla.mukaddam-daher@umontreal.ca

Ann. N.Y. Acad. Sci. 1009: 244–250 (2003). © 2003 New York Academy of Sciences.
doi: 10.1196/annals.1304.030

LVH develops in response to increased sympathetic outflow to the heart as well as to obesity- and hypertension-stimulated neurohormones, such as norepinephrine, angiotensin II, aldosterone, endothelin, and cytokines such as TNF-α and interleukin 1β. In addition to their hemodynamic activity, these neurohormones are also growth factors that influence myocardial growth and composition.[2] At the cellular level, cardiomyocyte hypertrophy is characterized by increased protein synthesis and cell size and is preceded by the induction of immediate early (e.g., *c-fos*, *c-jun*) and fetal genes, including contractile (α-actin and β-myosin heavy-chain gene expression) and noncontractile (atrial natriuretic peptide, ANP) protein genes.[3–5] At early to intermediate stages, myocardial growth parallels progressive alteration in tissue composition, with expansion of interstitial fibroblast compartment and enhanced collagen deposition as the most evident consequences. Although this process may provide a skeletal support for the myocardium and allows the heart to withstand the increased intracardiac pressures associated with overload, increased interstitial collagen might lead to abnormalities in conduction, thus predisposing to arrythmias.[2,3] Fortunately, hypertrophy can often be reversed by some, but not all, antihypertensives.

A common feature in obesity and hypertension is sympathetic hyperfunction. Sympathetic overactivity is also a major contributor to metabolic syndrome X.[6] The level of sympathetic drive to the heart is a major determinant of prognosis in patients with hypertension and heart failure, and a decrease in heart rate and nerve activity might be beneficial for long-term prognosis in these patients. In fact, the therapeutic value of sympathetic nervous inhibition is already established. Direct inhibition of peripheral α_1-adrenergic and β-adrenergic receptors and central activation of α_2-adrenergic receptors are routine ways to reduce high blood pressure by lowering peripheral sympathetic nervous activity. In hypertensive obese patients and in patients with metabolic syndrome X, where insulin resistance represents a primary physiologic defect, treatment is more complex. Nonpharmacologic interventions, such as weight loss and increased physical activity, can be effective in reducing insulin resistance. In addition, the primary target of pharmacologic antihypertensive therapy should include LVH regression, as well as improving, or at least not worsening, insulin sensitivity and lipid metabolism. In this case, selective α_1-blockers and angiotensin-converting enzyme inhibitors have a favorable metabolic profile, producing increases in insulin sensitivity. Calcium-channel blockers are considered neutral, but most β-adrenergic blockers are avoided because of their adverse metabolic effects on lipids or insulin sensitivity and because they can cause further weight gain. Thiazide diuretics induce dyslipoproteinemia and stimulate the sympathetic nervous system.[7]

Recently, a new class of centrally acting antihypertensive drugs, moxonidine and rilmenidine, has been developed. These agents reduce blood pressure by selective activation of the nonadrenergic imidazoline I_1-receptors in the CNS[8,9] with little effect at the central α_2-adrenergic receptors, thus having an improved side-effect profile. Acute and long-term hemodynamic studies show that moxonidine reduces arterial pressure by lowering systemic vascular resistance while sparing heart rate, cardiac output, and stroke volume. Moxonidine inhibits sympathetic tone in hypertensive patients and animals and in heart-failure rats.[10,11] In addition to its centrally mediated effects, moxonidine exerts direct actions on I_1-receptors in the kidney to cause diuresis and natriuresis,[12,13] both mechanisms leading to acute and long-term control of pressure.

Studies from this laboratory have shown that acute intravenous moxonidine administration to normotensive rats[14] and spontaneously hypertensive rats (SHRs)[15] reduces blood pressure, increases plasma ANP, and stimulates urine flow and excretion of sodium, potassium, and cGMP, an index of ANP activity. The latter finding implicates ANP in the acute renal effects of moxonidine. Furthermore, 1-week treatment of SHRs with moxonidine results in blood pressure reduction associated with increased atrial synthesis and release of the cardiac natriuretic peptides, ANP and brain natriuretic peptide (BNP).[16] Natriuretic peptides are increased in response to, and act to counteract the effects of, activated renin-angiotensin and sympathetic systems, through their sympatholytic, antifibrotic, and antiproliferative effects.[17–21] Because the expression of ANP and BNP is increased in human cardiac disorders leading to elevated circulating ANP and BNP, increased ANP and BNP plasma levels are often used as tools for the diagnosis and prognosis of cardiac disorders. Plasma BNP levels are normally lower than ANP levels but increase by 100-fold in heart failure, where BNP plasma levels provide an index of cardiac dysfunction.

EXPERIMENTAL PROTOCOL

In the following studies, the effect of chronic moxonidine on cardiac natriuretic peptides was investigated in spontaneously hypertensive obese rats (SHROBs), also known as Koletsky strain rats (SHROB/Kol).[22] The SHROB has monogenetic obesity superimposed on a hypertensive genetic background. The obesity mutation is a recessive trait, designated fa^k, which is a non-sense mutation of leptin receptor gene resulting in a premature stop codon in the leptin receptor extracellular domain.[23]

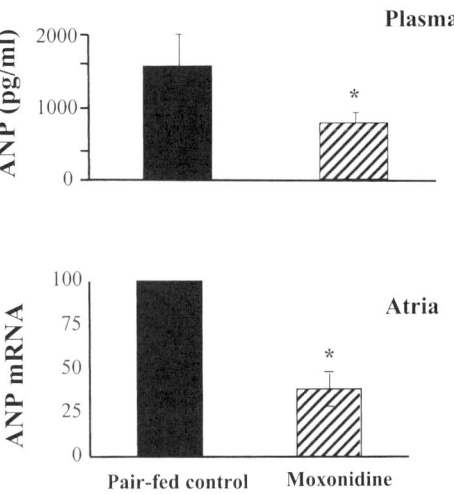

FIGURE 1. Moxonidine treatment reduced plasma ANP in SHROB as compared to pair-fed controls. * $P < 0.04$.

This mutation renders the SHROB incapable of central and peripheral responses to leptin. The SHROB is a unique animal model with phenotypic features that strongly resemble metabolic syndrome X, expressing spontaneous hypertension, insulin resistance, genetic obesity, hypertriglyceridemia, and proteinuria. The SHROBs have significantly higher plasma insulin, glucagon, insulin/glucagon molar ratio, and free fatty acid concentrations compared with lean littermates.[22]

Homozygous male and female SHROBs (fa^k/fa^k; weight: 590 ± 20 g, 30 weeks old) were housed individually and were provided food (Tek lab formula 8664) and water *ad libitum* and were maintained at a constant temperature of 21°C. Rats received moxonidine (4 mg/kg/d) in lab chow for 15 days. Blood pressure was measured in all animals by the tail cuff method.[24] The rats were euthanized, blood was collected, and hearts were excised, cleaned from fat tissue, immediately frozen in liquid N_2, and stored at −80°C for later measurement of natriuretic peptides.[16,25]

RESULTS

Compared with pair-fed controls (n = 10), moxonidine treatment (n = 15) in SHROBs significantly reduced systolic blood pressure (187 ± 6 versus 156 ± 5 mm Hg, $P < 0.05$). This antihypertensive action was associated with decreased plasma ANP (1595 ± 371 versus 793 ± 131 pg/mL, $P < 0.04$) (FIG. 1) and BNP (22 ± 3 versus 14 ± 1 pg/mL, $P < 0.04$). Moxonidine treatment had no effect on cardiac content of ANP and BNP in either compartment, but the reduced plasma levels paralleled reduced synthesis. FIGURE 1 shows that atrial ANP mRNA significantly ($P < 0.03$) decreased to 39% ± 10% of untreated control levels (defined as 100%), whereas atrial BNP mRNA was not changed (data not shown). Similarly, in left ventricles, ANP mRNA decreased to 69% ± 7% ($P < 0.02$) (FIG. 2), and BNP mRNA decreased to 74% ± 6% of control levels ($P < 0.02$) (FIG. 3). Right ventricular ANP and BNP mRNA were not affected by moxonidine treatment.

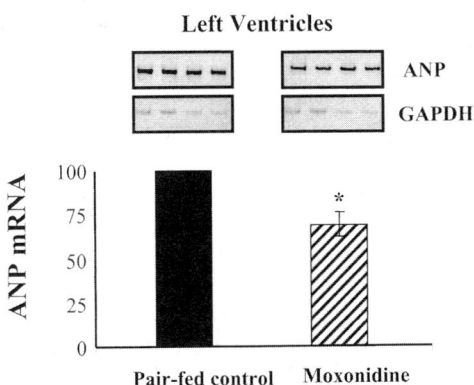

FIGURE 2. Semi-quantitative PCR measurement of left ventricular ANP mRNA. Values are normalized to corresponding GAPDH mRNA. Data are presented as percent of untreated controls (100%). * $P < 0.02$.

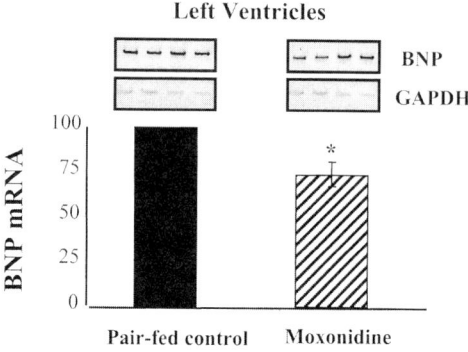

FIGURE 3. Semi-quantitative PCR measurement of left ventricular BNP mRNA. Values are normalized to corresponding GAPDH mRNA. Data are presented as percent of untreated controls (100%). * $P < 0.02$.

DISCUSSION

The ANP gene is expressed in the atria and ventricles during fetal life. In the adult heart, ventricular ANP is reduced, and the atria remain the primary site of ANP synthesis. In response to cardiac overload, however, diverse and distinct hormonal stimuli activate several autocrine and paracrine factors to influence expression of these peptides.[4,5] Through activation of protein kinase C, these factors may induce a program of embryonic gene expression, including the natriuretic peptide gene.[3] Thus, increased synthesis of natriuretic peptides in left ventricles is used as a marker of severity of cardiac hypertrophy. Accordingly, the results of the present study showing decreased synthesis of natriuretic peptides with chronic moxonidine treatment reflects a beneficial effect of the drug on the SHROB heart.

These findings are in agreement with previous reports that moxonidine reduces LVH in patients and rats.[26,27] In rats after myocardial infarction, moxonidine treatment suppressed sympathetic activation, prevented cardiac hypertrophy, and restored interstitial collagen content to sham-values.[10] In SHRs, moxonidine normalized myocardial fibrosis and capillarization to normotensive levels.[27]

The mechanisms of cardioprotection by moxonidine were not investigated in the present study. In addition to central imidazoline I_1-receptors, moxonidine may directly activate I_1-receptors in the heart.[28] We have previously reported ample evidence that cardiac imidazoline receptors are functional and may be involved in the release of ANP.

Velliquette et al[29] have shown that chronic inhibition of sympathetic activity with moxonidine in SHROBs, as evidenced by significant reduction in urinary excretion of epinephrine and norepinehrine, is associated with improved glucose tolerance, reduced plasma insulin and insulin-to-glucose ratio, and lower levels of free fatty acids. A single agent, moxonidine, reduces blood pressure and improves insulin sensitivity and lipid profile; as shown in the present study, moxonidine is cardioprotective in this model. Accordinly, moxonidine may be the drug of choice in the treatment of metabolic syndrome X and in obesity-related cardiac dysfunction.

ACKNOWLEDGMENTS

This work was supported by grants from The Canadian Institutes for Health Research (MOP-57714) and the Heart and Stroke Foundation of Canada (to SMD & JG) and from the National Insititues of Health HL44514 (to PE).

REFERENCES

1. DAVIS, C.L., G. KAPUKU, H. SNIEDER, et al. 2002. Insulin resistance syndrome and left ventricular mass in healthy young people Am. J. Med. Sci. **324:** 72–75.
2. WEBER, K.T., Y. SUN & E. GUARDA. 1994. Structural remodeling in hypertensive heart disease and the role of hormones. Hypertension **23:** 869–877.
3. CHIEN, K.R., K.U. KNOWLTON, H. ZHU, et al. 1991. Regulation of cardiac gene expression during myocardial growth and hypertrophy: molecular studies of an adaptive physiologic response. FASEB J. **5:** 3037–3046.
4. DEBOLD, A.J., B.G. BRUNEAU & M.L. KUROSKI DE BOLD. 1996. Mechanical and neuroendocrine regulation of the endocrine heart. Cardiovasc. Res. **31:** 7–18.
5. MORGAN, H.E. & K.M. BAKER. 1991. Cardiac hypertrophy. Mechanical, neural, and endocrine dependence. Circulation **83:** 13–25.
6. LANDSBERG, L. 1999. Role of the sympathetic adrenal system in the pathogenesis of the insulin resistance syndrome. Ann. N. Y. Acad. Sci. **892:** 84–90.
7. PISCHON, T. & A.M. SHARMA. 2002. Recent developments in the treatment of obesity-related hypertension. Curr. Opin. Nephrol. Hypertens. **11:** 497–502.
8. BOUSQUET, P., J. FELDMAN & J. SCHWARTZ. 1984. Central cardiovascular effects of alpha adrenergic drugs: differences between catecholamines and imidazolines. J. Pharmacol. Exp. Ther. **230:** 232–236.
9. ERNSBERGER, P. 2000. Pharmacology of moxonidine: an I_1-imidazoline receptor agonist. J. Cardiovasc. Pharmacol. **35:** S27–S41.
10. VAN KERCKHOVEN, R., T.A. VAN VEEN, F. BOOMSMA, et al. 2000. Chronic administration of moxonidine suppresses sympathetic activation in a rat heart failure model. Eur. J. Pharmacol. **397:** 113–120.
11. DICKSTEIN, K., C. MANHENKE, T. AARSLAND, et al. 2000. The effects of chronic, sustained-release moxonidine therapy on clinical and neurohumoral status in patients with heart failure. Int. J. Cardiol. **75:** 167–176.
12. PENNER, S.B. & D.D. SMYTH. 1995. The role of the peripheral sympathetic nervous system in the natriuresis following central administration of an I_1 imidazoline agonist, moxonidine. Br. J. Pharmacol. **116:** 2631–2636.
13. EVANS, R.G. 1996. Current status of putative imidazoline (I_1) receptors and renal mechanisms in relation to their antihypertensive therapeutic potential. Clin. Exp. Pharmacol. Physiol. **23:** 845–854.
14. MUKADDAM-DAHER, S. & J. GUTKOWSKA. 2000. Atrial natriuretic peptide is involved in renal actions of moxonidine. Hypertension **35:** 1215–1220.
15. MUKADDAM-DAHER, S. & J. GUTKOWSKA. 1999. The renal actions of moxonidine are mediated by atrial natriuretic peptide and involve the opioid receptors. Ann. N. Y. Acad. Sci. **881:** 385–387.
16. MENAOUAR, A., R. EL-AYOUBI, M. JANKOWSKI, et al. 2002. Chronic imidazoline receptor activation in spontaneously hypertensive rats. Am. J. Hypertens. **15:** 803–838.
17. MELO, L.G., A.T. VERESS, U. ACKERMANN, et al. 1999. Chronic hypertension in ANP knockout mice: contribution of peripheral resistance. Regul. Pept. **79:** 109–115.
18. TAMURA, N., Y. OGAWA, H. CHUSHO, et al. 2000. Cardiac fibrosis in mice lacking brain natriuretic peptide. Proc. Natl. Acad. Sci. U. S. A. **97:** 4239–4244.
19. CALDERONE, A., C.M. THAIK, N. TAKAHASHI, et al. 1998. Nitric oxide, atrial natriuretic peptide, and cyclic GMP inhibit the growth-promoting effects of norepinephrine in cardiac myocytes and fibroblasts. J. Clin. Invest. **101:** 812–818.
20. CAO, L. & D.G. GARDNER. 1995. Natriuretic peptides inhibit DNA synthesis in cardiac fibroblasts. Hypertension **25:** 227–234.

21. HORIO, T., T. NISHIKIMI, F. YOSHIHARA, *et al.* 2000. Inhibitory regulation of hypertrophy by endogenous atrial natriuretic peptide in cultured cardiac myocytes. Hypertension **35:** 19–24.
22. ERNSBERGER, P., R.J. KOLETSKY & J.E. FRIEDMAN. 1999. Molecular pathology in the obese spontaneous hypertensive Koletsky rat: a model of syndrome X. Ann. N. Y. Acad. Sci. **892:** 272–288.
23. TAKAYA, K., Y. OGAWA, J. HIRAOKA, *et al.* 1996. Nonsense mutation of leptin receptor in the obese spontaneously hypertensive Koletsky rat. Nat. Genet. **14:** 130–131.
24. ERNSBERGER, P., T. ISHIZUKA, S. LIU, *et al.* 1999. Mechanisms of antihyperglycemic effects of moxonidine in the obese spontaneously hypertensive Koletsky rat (SHROB). J. Pharmacol. Exp. Ther. **288:** 139–147.
25. GUTKOWSKA, J. 1987. Radioimmunoassay for atrial natriuretic factor. Int. J. Rad. Appl. Instrum. **14:** 323–331.
26. MALL, G., D. GREBER, H. GHARENHBAGHI, *et al.* 1991. Effects of nifedipine and moxonidine on cardiac structure in spontaneously hypertensive rats (SHR)–stereological studies on myocytes, capillaries, arteries, and cardiac interstitium. Basic Res. Cardiol. **86**(Suppl 3): 33–44.
27. OLLIVIER, J.P. & M.O. CHRISTEN. 1994. I_1-imidazoline-receptor agonists in the treatment of hypertension: an appraisal of clinical experience. J. Cardiovasc. Pharmacol. **24:** S39–S48.
28. EL-AYOUBI, R., J. GUTKOWSKA, S. REGUNATHAN, *et al.* 2002. Imidazoline receptors in the heart: characterization, distribution, and regulation. J. Cadiovasc. Pharmacol. **39:** 875–883.
29. VELLIQUETTE, R.A., R.J. KOLETSKY & P. ERNSBERGER. 2002. Plasma glucagon and free fatty acid responses to a glucose load in the obese spontaneous hypertensive rat (SHROB) model of metabolic syndrome X. Exp. Biol. Med. **227:** 164–170.

The Role of I_1-Imidazoline Receptors and α_2-Adrenergic Receptors in the Modulation of Glucose and Lipid Metabolism in the SHROB Model of Metabolic Syndrome X

RICHARD J. KOLETSKY, RODNEY A. VELLIQUETTE, AND PAUL ERNSBERGER

Department of Nutrition, Case Western Reserve University School of Medicine, Cleveland, Ohio 44106-4906, USA

ABSTRACT: Hypertension is commonly accompanied by obesity, hyperlipidemia, and insulin resistance in humans, a cluster of abnormalities known as metabolic syndrome X. With the notable exception of inhibitors of the renin-angiotensin system, which have mildly beneficial effects on insulin resistance, most antihypertensive agents worsen one or more components of metabolic syndrome X. Second-generation centrally acting antihypertensive agents such as rilmenidine and moxonidine have mixed effects on components of metabolic syndrome X, which might reflect in part actions on two different receptors: I_1-imidazoline and α_2-adrenergic. Using a rat model of metabolic syndrome X, we sought to separate the influence of these two receptors on glucose and lipid metabolism by using selective antagonists. Rilmenidine and moxonidine acutely raised glucose and lowered insulin, thereby further worsening glucose tolerance. These effects were entirely mediated by α_2-adrenergic receptors. Rilmenidine and moxonidine also lowered glucagon, an effect that was mediated solely by I_1-imidazoline receptors since it was potentiated by α_2-blockade, but eliminated in the presence of I_1-antagonists. Lowering of triglyceride and cholesterol levels followed the same pattern as glucagon, implicating I_1-imidazoline receptors in lipid-lowering actions. Chronic treatment with moxonidine reproduced the beneficial effects on glucagon and lipids while the acute hyperglycemic response did not persist. Thus, α_2-adrenergic receptors mediate an acute deterioration of glucose tolerance, whereas in contrast I_1-imidazoline receptors appear to mediate the persistent long-term improvements in glucose tolerance. The therapeutic action of I_1-imidazoline agonists may be primarily mediated through reduced glucagon secretion.

KEYWORDS: insulin resistance; hyperlipidemia; hypertension; obesity; metabolic syndrome X; imidazoline receptors; adrenergic receptors; diabetes mellitus

INTRODUCTION

Obesity, hypertension, hyperlipidemia and hyperinsulinemia cluster together as components of Metabolic Syndrome X, leading to increased morbidity and mortality

Address for correspondence: Paul Ernsberger, Ph.D., Department of Nutrition, Case Western Reserve University School of Medicine, 10900 Euclid Avenue, Cleveland, OH 44106-4906, USA. Voice: 216-368-4738; fax: 216-368-4752.
e-mail: pre@po.cwru.edu

Ann. N.Y. Acad. Sci. 1009: 251–261 (2003). © 2003 New York Academy of Sciences.
doi: 10.1196/annals.1304.031

from cardiovascular disease.[1] The link between insulin, insulin resistance, and hypertension has been the subject of intense investigation. Insulin causes sodium retention and can modulate sympathetic nervous system activity. Insulin may also alter hemodynamic factors in the vascular bed, leading to the development of both hypertension and atherosclerosis.[2]

In selecting pharmacological agents for treating obese hypertension, one should consider the potential benefits and potential drawbacks regarding each component of this common syndrome. Diuretics, while decreasing intravascular volume and cardiac output, can increase sympathetic activity as well as activate the renin angiotensin system.[3] Additionally, diuretics can worsen glucose tolerance and increase lipid levels. Beta blockers antagonize sympathetic nervous system (SNS) activity, and, while helpful in treating heart disease, can cause both weight gain and worsen diabetes in addition to leading to unfavorable changes in the plasma lipid profile.[3] Calcium channel blockers can cause fluid retention and lead to more weight gain.[3] Angiotensin-converting enzyme (ACE) inhibitors and angiotensin receptor blockers (ARB) have been shown to slightly improve insulin resistance and are neutral with regard to lipids and body weight.[4] Thus, ACEs and ARBs are increasingly seen as treatments of choice for hypertensive patients with metabolic syndrome. Peripheral α_1-adrenergic antagonists have been associated with modest improvements in glucose tolerance and lipid profiles, but are seldom used because of severe side effects such as orthostatic hypotension leading to syncope and sexual dysfunction.[3]

Centrally acting agents in the α_2AR agonist class are effective in lowering blood pressure, but are poorly tolerated due to dry mouth, somnolence, and, in the case of clonidine, rebound hypertension on withdrawal.[5] α_2AR agonists have been shown to reduce insulin secretion and thereby worsen glucose tolerance.[6–9] Few data are available on lipid changes or body weight. In animals, clonidine increases food intake and body weight.[10]

Thus, no current antihypertensive agent is clearly beneficial and indeed most have some harmful effects on the various metabolic abnormalities in syndrome X.[11] Current treatments for components of metabolic syndrome X can also interfere with the treatment of other components. For example, sympathomimetic agents such as amphetamines and sibutramine are used to treat obesity but may elevate blood pressure, particularly with long-term therapy.[12] Thus, it would be preferable to give an agent that had a positive impact on more than one aspect of the overall syndrome and find a single antihypertensive agent that does not cause weight gain, improves insulin resistance, and lowers lipid levels.

Second-generation centrally acting hypertensive agents have been developed which interact not only with α_2AR but also with a novel site known as the I_1-imidazoline receptor (I_1R).[13] The various effects of these agents on syndrome X, beneficial or harmful, may be mediated through differences in specific receptor action. α_2AR agonists have been associated with worsening glucose tolerance, while I_1R agonists have beneficial effects to lower insulin resistance and improve glucose tolerance. Besides central sympatholytic action, there is increasing evidence for direct actions of imidazoline agonists in the liver and pancreas.[14] A controlled clinical trial has shown that moxonidine improves insulin sensitivity in a subgroup of human hypertensives with insulin resistance.[15]

The SHROB rat is known as the obese, spontaneously hypertensive or Koletsky rat. The SHROB model of syndrome X includes obesity, hypertension, hyperlipidemia, hyperinsulinemia, and hyperglucagonemia.[16] The α_2AR and I_1 agonist, moxonidine, has multiple beneficial effects on the various metabolic abnormalities found in this syndrome. Some of the effects are mediated through enhancement of insulin release from the pancreas and improvements in insulin action via increases in insulin receptor action and post-receptor signaling pathways.[17]

The multiple beneficial effects of moxonidine in syndrome X may be mediated by favorable changes in insulin and possibly glucagon as well. In this study we examined the different influences of α_2AR and I_1R on glucose homeostasis to determine which receptor was responsible for the observed effects.

METHODS

Animals

SHROB rats (fa^k/fa^k) were bred in a closed colony from brother-sister mating of heterozygous carriers (Fa^k/fa^k), since obese animals or either sex cannot reproduce.[18]

Drug Treatment

All drugs were administered after an 18-h overnight fast. Tail blood was taken at baseline and 1, 2, and 4 h after i.p. injection. In blocking experiments, antagonists were mixed together with agonists and administered as one bolus. To test whether acute I_1R activation modulated glucose tolerance, we injected SHROB with moxonidine (0.5 mg/kg), moxonidine + rauwolscine (0.5 + 7.5 mg/kg) or saline solution followed by a glucose challenge. An oral glucose tolerance test (OGTT) was performed 15 min postinjection.

To test progressive changes in glucose and insulin during the course of chronic treatment, 8 SHROBs and 8 SHRs were given moxonidine orally by adding it to powdered rat chow prior to pelleting. Food was removed each day at 12 PM and a single tail blood sample (0.2 mL) was taken at 4 PM prior to reintroduction of food. Blood glucose and plasma insulin were determined as described below.

Oral Glucose Tolerance Test (OGTT)

As previously described,[17] rats were given, by oral gavage, a 50% glucose solution at a dose of 6 g/kg body weight. Blood (0.2 mL) was obtained from the tail vein of conscious animals at baseline and 30, 60, 120, 240, and 360 min after the glucose load. Plasma glucose, insulin, and glucagon were determined at each time point.

Biochemical Measurements

Glucose in whole blood or plasma was determined by colorimetric glucose oxidase assay, and the remaining sample frozen at −70°C until assayed for insulin and glucagon. Insulin, and glucagon radioimmunoassays were conducted in duplicate and used rat insulin and glucagon standards (Linco, St. Charles, MO).

Statistics

Results are presented as means ± standard error of the mean. Comparisons between groups were made using one- or two-way analysis of variance (ANOVA) or analysis of variance with repeated measures (REMANOVA) using Prism (Graph Pad Software, San Diego, CA) with post-hoc analyses by Neuman-Keuls test.

RESULTS

Chronic administration of moxonidine improves glucose tolerance in SHROBs.[17–19] We tested whether moxonidine has an immediate impact on glucose tolerance (FIG. 1). SHROBs show fasting normoglycemia with impaired glucose tolerance, as previously reported.[16] Moxonidine alone caused further deterioration of glucose tolerance. When moxonidine was given with rauwolscine, producing α_2AR blockade, glucose tolerance improved relative to moxonidine alone and even in comparison to saline-treated controls. Thus, the α_2AR component worsens, and the I_1R component of moxonidine improves, the blood glucose response during an oral glucose challenge (FIG. 1).

To further examine the roles of these two receptors during glucose tolerance, insulin levels were measured following administration of saline, moxonidine alone, and moxonidine with rauwolscine (FIG. 2). Control SHROB rats showed the expected biphasic insulin response to oral glucose, with a modest early phase and an exaggerated late phase. Moxonidine eliminated the early phase of insulin secretion, even producing a decline in insulin levels during the first 2 hours. The late phase of

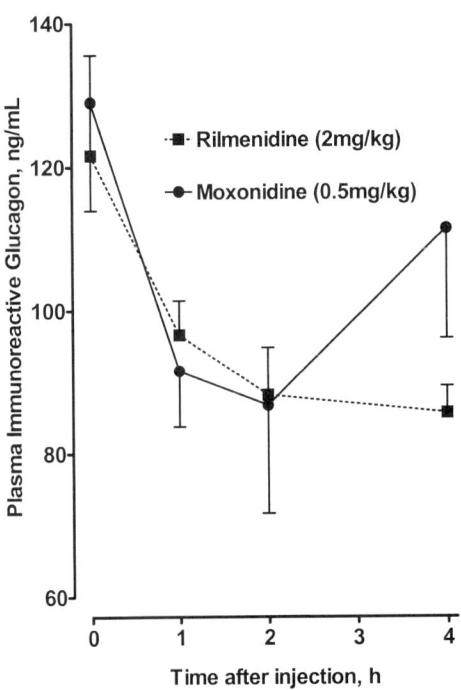

FIGURE 1. Serial plasma glucose levels were measured after an oral glucose load which was preceded 15 min earlier by an injection of either saline, moxonidine, or a combination of moxonidine and rauwolscine. SHROB rats show fasting normoglycemia with impaired glucose tolerance. Moxonidine alone caused further deterioration of glucose tolerance. When moxonidine was given with rauwolscine, producing α_2AR blockade, glucose tolerance improved relative to moxonidine alone and even in comparison to saline-treated controls.

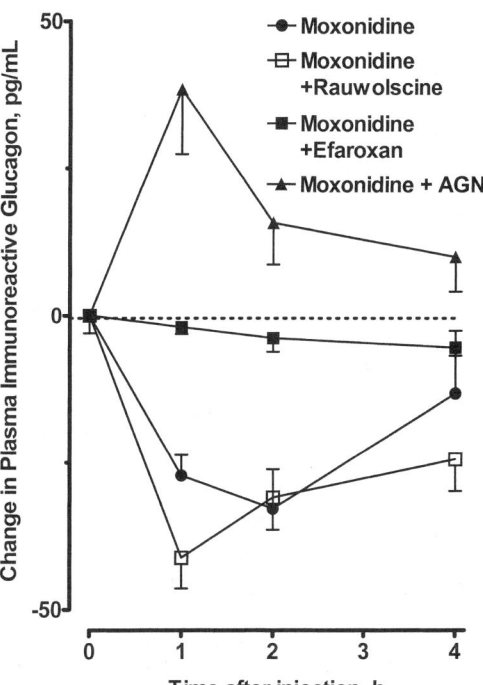

FIGURE 2. Insulin levels were measured during oral glucose loading preceded by either saline, moxonidine, or a combination of moxonidine and rauwolscine. After saline injection, SHROB rats showed the expected biphasic insulin response to oral glucose, with a modest early phase and an exaggerated late phase. Moxonidine eliminated the early phase of insulin secretion, even producing a decline in insulin levels during the first two hours. The late phase of insulin secretion was slightly potentiated, as indicated by an increased area under the curve for 2 to 4 h after glucose, suggesting a rebound effect. When moxonidine was given with rauwolscine to produce α_2AR blockade, the early phase of insulin secretion was maintained, while the late phase developed sooner and peaked at 4 h.

insulin secretion was slightly potentiated, as indicated by an increased area under the curve for 2 to 4 h after glucose, suggesting a rebound effect. When moxonidine was given with rauwolscine to produce α_2AR blockade, the early phase of insulin secretion was maintained, while the late phase developed sooner and peaked at 4 h. Total insulin secretion was increased by combined treatment with moxonidine and rauwolscine, as indicated by an increased area under the curve. These data all suggest that α_2AR strongly suppress and I_1R modestly potentiate the insulin response to a glucose challenge in a model of metabolic syndrome X.

Multiple mechanisms may be responsible for the improvement in glucose tolerance following activation of I_1R. The increase in insulin secretion can only partially account for the reduced excursion of glucose following an oral load. Because SHROBs have recently been shown to have elevated glucagon levels which may contribute to their insulin resistance,[20] we speculated that alterations in glucagon dynamics might contribute the changes seen in response to activation of I_1R.

We determined the immediate influence of moxonidine on glucagon levels during an oral glucose tolerance test (FIG. 3). Glucagon levels rose dramatically in response to oral glucose in control SHROB rats, a paradoxical response we have documented previously.[20] Moxonidine, given 15 min prior to the glucose load, blunted the rise in glucagon elicited by the glucose load as indicated by a reduced area under the curve

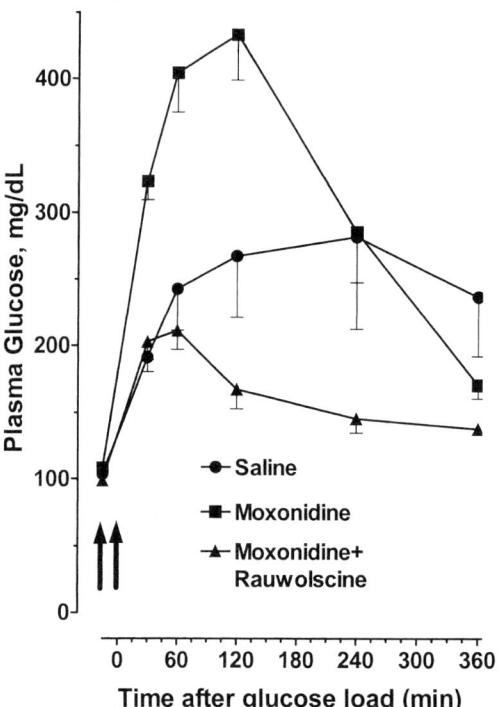

FIGURE 3. Glucagon levels during an oral glucose tolerance test rose dramatically in saline-treated SHROB. Moxonidine, given 15 min prior to the glucose load, blunted the rise in glucagon elicited by the glucose load as indicated by a reduced area under the curve ($P < 0.01$). Selective blockade of α_2AR with rauwolscine allowed moxonidine to reduce the net secretion of glucagon even further.

($P < 0.01$). Finally, selective blockade of α_2AR with rauwolscine reduced the net secretion of glucagon even further. Thus, rauwolscine actually potentiated moxonidine's ability to suppress plasma glucagon. This finding supports a role for α_2AR in the facilitation of glucagon secretion and implicates I_1R in the inhibition of glucagon secretion.

Next, we sought to determine the direct effect of α_2AR and I_1R stimulation on glucagon levels. After an overnight fast, moxonidine and rilmenidine, two selective I_1R agonists, immediately lowered plasma glucagon levels for up to four hours in SHROB rats (FIG. 4).

TABLE 1 summarizes the acute metabolic effects of moxonidine. The immediate response to moxonidine, mediated through α_2AR, are to raise blood glucose and lower insulin levels. These α_2AR-mediated actions may worsen diabetic control in the short term. Combined α_2AR and I_1R antagonism blocked the fall in glucagon, while selective α_2AR antagonism potentiated the fall in glucagon. This suggests that the glucagon-lowering effects of moxonidine are I_1R-specific, but are counteracted acutely by α_2AR effects. Also summarized in TABLE 1 is recent work showing lipid-lowering actions of moxonidine and rilmenidine, which are mediated by I_1R.[14]

TABLE 2 summarizes the chronic effects of moxonidine. In contrast to acute

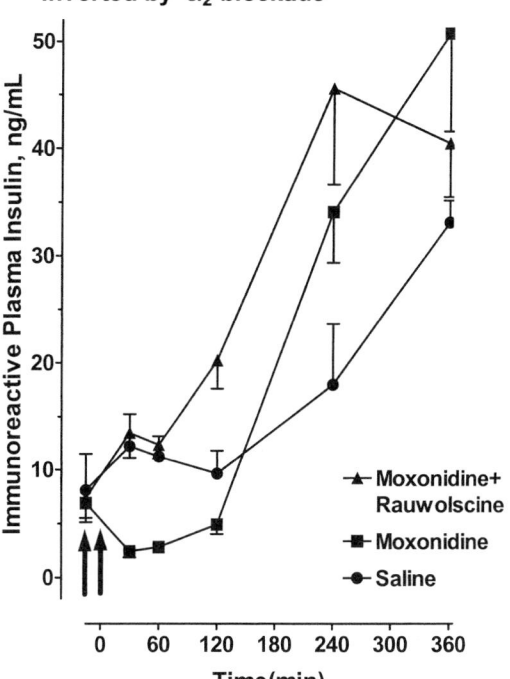

FIGURE 4. Glucagon levels after an overnight fast were immediately lowered by injection of moxonidine or rilmenidine, two selective I_1R agonists. The effect persisted for up to 4 hours in SHROB rats.

changes, the chronic administration of moxonidine improves glucose tolerance, increases insulin levels, and lowers glucagon levels as well as lowering lipid levels through activation of I_1R. The receptor responsible for the chronic improvements in these parameters is the I_1R and not the α_2AR. Thus, chronically, the beneficial effects of moxonidine's I_1R activation overcome the adverse α_2AR actions that are seen acutely.

TABLE 1. Summary of the effects of acute moxonidine or rilmenidine on parameters of metabolic syndrome X

Parameters	Moxonidine	Rilmenidine
Blood pressure	↓	↓
Blood glucose	↑	↑
Plasma insulin	↓	↓
Plasma glucagon	↓	↓
Plasma triglycerides	↓	↓
Plasma cholesterol	↓	↓

TABLE 2. Receptors responsible for acute effects of moxonidine on fasting parameters of metabolic syndrome X

Parameters	I_1 Responsible	α_2 Responsible
Reduced blood pressure	Yes	Yes
Hyperglycemia	No	Yes
Hypoinsulinemia	No	Yes
Hypoglucagonemia	Yes	No
Reduced triglycerides	Yes	No
Reduced cholesterol	Yes	No

DISCUSSION

There is mounting evidence that diabetes is a dual disorder of islet cell dysfunction involving insulin and glucagon.[21] Insulin is a hormone that promotes energy storage and is glycogenic, anti-gluconeogenic, and anti-lipolytic. Glucagon opposes the actions of insulin, resulting in mobilization of nutrients for energy production. The two hormones act in concert to control the direction of nutrient metabolism for either immediate utilization for energy or to store for later use. These effects are prominent in the liver, but the pancreas and peripheral tissue such as muscle and fat may be involved too.

Resistance to insulin action is a key factor in the development of diabetes mellitus, Type 2. There are abnormalities in the pancreatic release of insulin in response to food intake as well as defects in both the hepatic and peripheral tissue responses to insulin. This leads to hyperinsulinemia and insulin resistance. Diabetes is also characterized by a state of relative hyperglucagonemia.[21] Glucagon levels rise promptly in response to hypoglycemia, promoting rapid glycocogenolyis in the liver and subsequent elevations in glucose levels. Glucagon levels normally fall in response to food intake. Diabetics have high levels of glucagon and are resistant to the suppressive effect of food intake or show paradoxical rises in glucagon in response to nutrients.[22] An excess of glucagon in the fasting state and in the postprandial state can contribute to hyperglycemia and create apparent insulin resistance. Thus, diabetes may be a bihormonal disease with high glucagon levels having a deleterious effect on metabolism that can exaggerate the consequences of insulin resistance. Developing drugs that alter glucagon action as well as improve insulin sensitivity will lead to new therapeutic drugs to treat syndrome X.

Our previous work has shown that SHROB rats have higher fasting plasma glucagon compared to lean SHRs, as well as having abnormal responses to an oral glucose challenge with an elevation in glucagon.[20] These abnormalities contribute to fasting hyperinsulinemia and glucose intolerance in syndrome X. Moxonidine has been shown to lower glucagon levels in SHROB rats and this may be in part responsible for the improvement in glucose tolerance and other favorable changes in correcting metabolic abnormalities in syndrome X. When moxonidine was compared with two other antihypertensive drugs after chronic treatment, one had no effect on

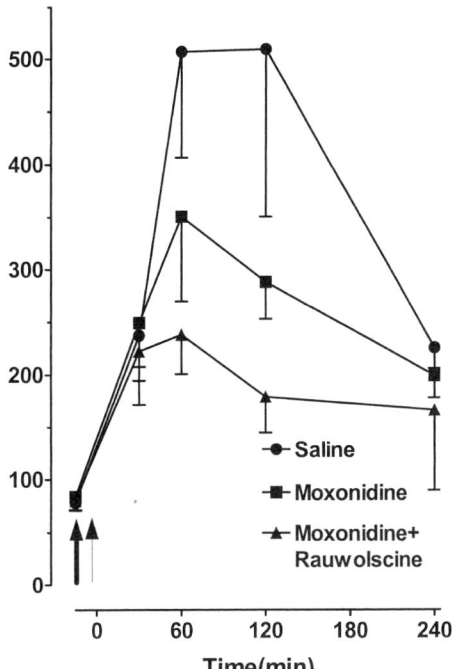

FIGURE 5. Glucagon levels were measured after the administration of various agents. Blockade of both I_1R and α_2AR with efaroxan abolished moxonidine's ability to lower glucagon. Selective blockade of I_1R with AGN192403 uncovered a stimulatory effect of moxonidine on glucagon levels, presumably mediated by unopposed activation of α_2AR. Rauwolscine, an α_2AR antagonist, produced an even greater fall in glucagon secretion when given with moxonidine.

glucagon and the other actually increased it.[23] Therefore, the effect of moxonidine on glucagon is not mediated by a fall in blood pressure.

The contrasting effects of αAR and I_1R are consistent with previous results showing treatment with moxonidine improves glucose tolerance. Any α_2AR agonist, including moxonidine, can, upon acute administration, worsen glucose tolerance, despite sympathoinhibitory and blood pressure–lowering actions. The I_1R agonist effects of moxonidine become more prominent chronically or following α_2AR blockade to improve various aspects of metabolic syndrome X. Thus, α_2AR and I_1R play different roles chronologically and by organ location and function. In the pancreas, the α_2AR reduces insulin secretion and slightly increases glucagon release.[24] The I_1R in the pancreas has the opposite effects, increasing insulin secretion and lowering glucagon levels to improve glucose tolerance. The hyperglucagonemia found in the SHROB rats could be responsible for some of its insulin resistance. Chronic moxonidine, acting on pancreatic I_1R, corrects this defect, as well as the aberrant glucagon responses to glucose load, all of which could have beneficial effects on metabolic syndrome X.

There are no α_2ARs in the liver.[25] I_1R agonists may act directly on the liver, or indirectly through hormone changes involving insulin or glucagon to decrease triglyceride production and lower lipid levels, thereby further correcting abnormalities in the metabolic syndrome X. The effects of I_1R agonists to alter energy metabolism in adipose tissue remain to be studied. I_1R are present in cardiac,[26] but not skeletal muscle,[27] and may therefore affect cardiac metabolism.

Moxonidine has the potential to be an effective monotherapy for metabolic syndrome X. Acutely, moxonidine improves several components of metabolic syndrome X, including hyperglucagonemia, but potent α_2AR actions to lower insulin and induce hyperglycemia mask these I_1R effects. Chronically, the I_1R effects predominate, leading to reduced insulin resistance, improved glucose tolerance and improved hyperlipidemia. A new imidazoline agonist with improved receptor specificity relative to moxonidine, acting specifically as a glucagon suppressor, may be the treatment of choice for hypertension-associated obesity, hyperlipidemia, or diabetes.

REFERENCES

1. REAVEN, G.M. 1993. Role of insulin resistance in human disease (syndrome X): an expanded definition. Annu. Rev. Med. **44:** 121–131.
2. SOWERS, J.R. 2001. Update on the cardiometabolic syndrome. Clin. Cornerstone **4:** 17–23.
3. IZZO, J.L., JR. & H.R. BLACK. 2003. Hypertension Primer. Lippincott, Williams & Wilkins. Dallas, TX.
4. BERNOBICH, E., L. DE ANGELIS, C. LERIN & G. BELLINI. 2002. The role of the angiotensin system in cardiac glucose homeostasis: therapeutic implications. Drugs **62:** 1295–1314.
5. REID, J.L., B.C. CAMPBELL & C.A. HAMILTON. 1984. Withdrawal reactions following cessation of central alpha-adrenergic receptor agonists. Hypertension **6:** II71–II75.
6. KLEIN, C., N. MORTON, S. KELLEY & S. METZ. 1985. Transdermal clonidine therapy in elderly mild hypertensives: effects on blood pressure, plasma norepinephrine and fasting plasma glucose. J. Hypertens. Suppl **3:** S81–S84.
7. GUTHRIE, G.P., JR., R.E. MILLER, T.A. KOTCHEN & S.H. KOENIG. 1983. Clonidine in patients with diabetes and mild hypertension. Clin. Pharmacol. Ther. **34:** 713–717.
8. WEBSTER, W.B., JR. & M.M. MCCONNAUGHEY. 1982. Clonidine and glucose intolerance. Drug Intell. Clin. Pharm. **16:** 325–328.
9. BARBIERI, C., C. FERRARI, R. CALDARA, G. TESTORI, G.A. DAL BO & A. BERTAZZONI. 1980. Clonidine-induced hyperglycemia: evidence against a growth hormone-mediated effect. J. Pharmacol. Exp. Ther. **214:** 433–436.
10. TSUJII, S. & G.A. BRAY. 1992. Food intake of lean and obese Zucker rats following ventricular infusions of adrenergic agonists. Brain Res. **587:** 226–232.
11. GOYAL, R.K. 1999. Hyperinsulinemia and insulin resistance in hypertension: differential effects of antihypertensive agents. Clin. Exp. Hypertens. **21:** 167–179.
12. BRAY, G.A. 2002. Sibutramine and blood pressure: a therapeutic dilemma J. Hum. Hypertens. **16:** 1–3.
13. ERNSBERGER, P., J.E. FRIEDMAN & R.J. KOLETSKY. 1997. The I_1-imidazoline receptor: from binding site to therapeutic target in cardiovascular disease. J. Hypertens. **15**(Suppl. 1): S9–S23.
14. VELLIQUETTE, R.A., A. DIVITO, S. PREVIS & P. ERNSBERGER. 2003. Lipid lowering actions of imidazolines reflects reduced hepatic lipid secretion and are mediated by I_1-imidazoline and not α_2-adrenergic receptors. [abstract]. FASEB J. **17:** A234.
15. HAENNI, A. & H. LITHELL. 1999. Moxonidine improves insulin sensitivity in insulin-resistant hypertensives. J. Hypertens. **17** Suppl **3:** S29-S35.
16. KOLETSKY, R.J., J.E. FRIEDMAN & P. ERNSBERGER. 2001. The obese spontaneously hypertensive rat (SHROB, Koletsky rat): a model of metabolic syndrome X. *In* Animal Models of Diabetes: A Primer, Vol. 2. A.A.F. Sima & E. Shafrir, Eds.: 143–158. Harwood. Singapore.
17. Ernsberger, P., T. ISHIZUKA, S. LIU, C.J. FARRELL, D. BEDOL, R.J. KOLETSKY & J.E. FRIEDMAN. 1999. Mechanisms of antihyperglycemic effects of moxonidine in the

obese spontaneously hypertensive Koletsky rat (SHROB). J. Pharmacol. Exp. Ther. **288:** 139–147.
18. ERNSBERGER, P., R.J. KOLETSKY & J.E. FRIEDMAN. 1999. Molecular pathology in the obese spontaneous hypertensive Koletsky rat: a model of syndrome X. Ann. N. Y. Acad. Sci. **892:** 272–288.
19. ERNSBERGER, P., R.J. KOLETSKY, L.A. COLLINS & D.L. BEDOL. 1996. Sympathetic nervous system in salt-sensitive and obese hypertension: amelioration of multiple abnormalities by a central symaptholytic agent. Cardiovasc. Drugs Ther. **10:** 275–282.
20. VELLIQUETTE, R.A., R.J. KOLETSKY & P. ERNSBERGER. 2002. Plasma glucagon and free fatty acid responses to a glucose load in the obese spontaneous hypertensive rat (SHROB) model of metabolic syndrome X. Exp. Biol. Med. **227:** 164–170.
21. UNGER, R.H. 1985. Glucagon physiology and pathophysiology in the light of new advances. Diabetologia **28:** 574–578.
22. SHAH, P., A. VELLA, A. BASU, R. BASU, W.F. SCHWENK & R.A. RIZZA. 2000. Lack of suppression of glucagon contributes to postprandial hyperglycemia in subjects with type 2 diabetes mellitus. J. Clin. Endocrinol. Metab **85:** 4053–4059.
23. VELLIQUETTE, R.A., R.J. KOLETSKY & P. ERNSBERGER. 2002. Contrasting effects of antihypertensive agents on glucose tolerance in an animal model of metabolic syndrome X [abstract]. FASEB J. **16:** A943.
24. HIROSE, H., H. MARUYAMA, K. ITOH, K. KOYAMA, K. KIDO & T. SARUTA. 1992. Alpha-2 adrenergic agonism stimulates islet glucagon release from perfused rat pancreas: possible involvement of alpha-2A adrenergic receptor subtype. Acta Endocrinol. (Copenh.) **127:** 279–283.
25. WANG, R.X. & L.E. LIMBIRD. 1997. Distribution of mRNA encoding three alpha 2-adrenergic receptor subtypes in the developing mouse embryo suggests a role for the alpha 2A subtype in apoptosis. Mol. Pharmacol. **52:** 1071–1080.
26. EL AYOUB I.R., J. GUTKOWSKA, S. REGUNATHAN & S. MUKADDAM-DAHER. 2002. Imidazoline receptors in the heart: characterization, distribution, and regulation. J. Cardiovasc. Pharmacol. **39:** 875–883.
27. PILETZ, J.E., J.C. JONES, H. ZHU, O. BISHARA & P. ERNSBERGER. 1999. Imidazoline receptor antisera-selected cDNA clone and mRNA distribution Ann. N. Y. Acad. Sci. **881:** 1–7.

Involvement of Forebrain Imidazoline and α_2-Adrenergic Receptors in the Antidipsogenic Response to Moxonidine

CARINA A.F. ANDRADE, LISANDRA B. OLIVEIRA, GIZELE MARTINEZ, DANIELA C.F. SILVA, LAURIVAL A. DE LUCA, JR., AND JOSÉ V. MENANI

Department of Physiology and Pathology, School of Dentistry, Paulista State University (UNESP), 14.801-903 Araraquara, SP, Brazil

ABSTRACT: We investigated the participation of central α_2-adrenoceptors and imidazoline receptors in the inhibition of water deprivation-induced water intake in rats. The α_2-adrenoceptor and imidazoline antagonist idazoxan (320 nmol), but not the α_2-adrenoceptor antagonist yohimbine, abolished the antidipsogenic effect of moxonidine (α_2-adrenoceptor and imidazoline agonist, 20 nmol) microinjected into the medial septal area. Yohimbine abolished the antidipsogenic effect of moxonidine intracerebroventricularly. Therefore, central moxonidine may inhibit water intake acting independently on both imidazoline receptors and α_2-adrenoceptors at different forebrain sites.

KEYWORDS: thirst; angiotensin II; dehydration; water intake

Activation of central α_2 adrenergic receptors by cerebral ventricle injections inhibits thirst induced by water deprivation,[1] but the inhibition of water intake by clonidine (α_2-adrenoceptor and imidazoline receptor agonist) injected into the medial septal area (MSA) is only partially reduced by idazoxan (α_2-adrenoceptor and imidazoline receptor antagonist) and yohimbine (α_2-adrenoceptor antagonist).[2] Moxonidine, an α_2-adrenoceptor and imidazoline receptor agonist that binds predominantly to imidazoline receptors, also reduces water deprivation-induced water intake when injected intracerebroventricularly.[3] In the present study, we investigated the effects of moxonidine alone or combined with idazoxan or yohimbine into the MSA and intracerebroventricularly (icv) on water deprivation-induced water intake.

Male Holtzman rats (280 to 300 g) with stainless steel cannulas stereotaxically implanted into the lateral ventricle or the MSA were used. Moxonidine (free base; 5 and 20 nmol; Solvay Pharma, Hannover, Germany), yohimbine (hydrochloride; 80 and 320 nmol; Research Biochemicals International [RBI], Natick, MA, USA), or idazoxan (hydrochloride; 320 nmol; RBI) was injected icv or into the MSA. The injection volume was 1 to 3 µL icv and 0.5 µL into the MSA. After 24 hours of water deprivation, idazoxan, yohimbine, or vehicle was injected icv or into the MSA. Fifteen minutes later, moxonidine or vehicle was injected icv or into the MSA. Water

Address for correspondence: José Vanderlei Menani, Ph.D., Department of Physiology and Pathology, School of Dentistry, UNESP Rua Humaitá, 1680, 14.801-903, Araraquara, SP, Brazil. Voice: (+55) 16 201-6486; fax: (+55) 16 201-6488.
e-mail: menani@foar.unesp.br

was returned to the animals 15 minutes after moxonidine and the intake was recorded during the next 60 minutes. At the end of the experiments, the brains were removed, cut in 50 μm-sections and analyzed to confirm the injection sites in the lateral ventricle and MSA. The results are reported as mean ± SEM. ANOVA and Newman-Keuls test were used for comparisons ($P < 0.05$).

Moxonidine (20 nmol) injected into the MSA reduced the water deprivation-induced water intake (FIG. 1). Idazoxan (320 nmol) injected into the MSA abolished the antidipsogenic effect of moxonidine into the same site (FIG. 1A), while yohimbine (320 nmol) produced no effect (FIG. 1B). Moxonidine (5 nmol) icv also reduced water intake and this effect was abolished by yohimbine (80 nmol; FIG. 2).

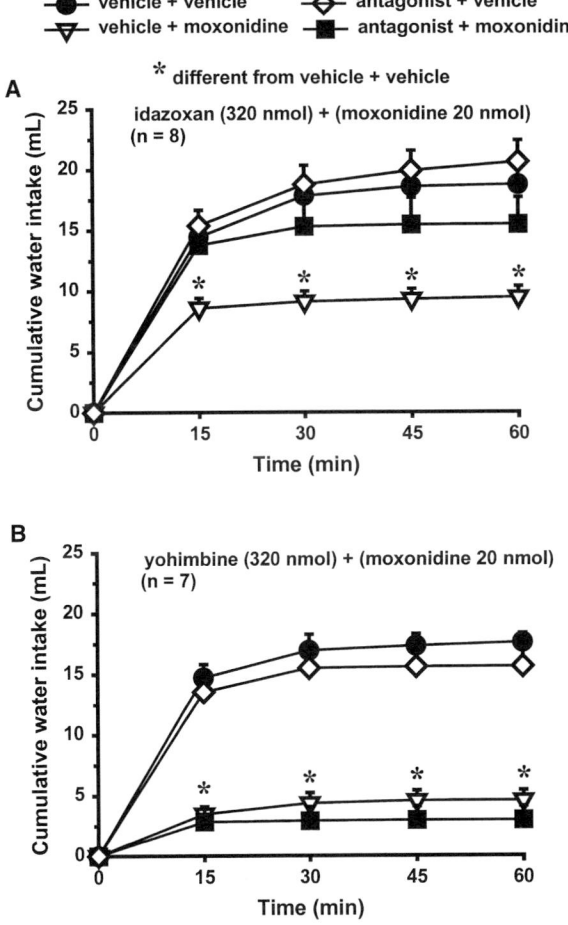

FIGURE 1. Cumulative 24-hour water deprivation-induced water intake in rats after treatment with **(A)** the mixed antagonist idazoxan and **(B)** the α_2-adrenoceptor antagonist yohimbine followed by the mixed agonist moxonidine microinjected into the MSA.

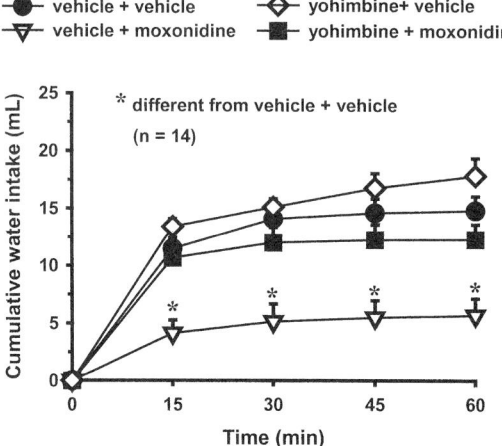

FIGURE 2. Cumulative 24-hour water deprivation-induced water intake in rats after treatment with yohimbine combined with moxonidine icv.

These results suggest that moxonidine may activate at least two different central receptors to inhibit water intake. Moxonidine injected icv activates α_2-adrenoceptors, while in the MSA moxonidine activates imidazoline receptors to inhibit water intake.

REFERENCES

1. SUGAWARA, A.M., T.T. MIGUEL, D.T. B. PEREIRA, et al. 2001. Effects of central imidazolinergic and alpha2-adrenergic activation on water intake. Braz. J. Med. Biol. Res. **34:** 1185–1190.
2. YADA, M.M., P.M. DE PAULA, J.V. MENANI, et al. 1997. Receptor-mediated effects of clonidine on need-induced 3% NaCl and water intake. Brain Res. Bull. **42:** 205–209.
3. MENANI, J.V., M.A. SATO, L. HAIKEL, et al. 1999. Central moxonidine on water and NaCl intake. Brain Res. Bull. **49:** 273–279.

Moxonidine Displays a Presynaptic Alpha-2-Adrenoceptor-Dependent Synergistic Sympathoinhibitory Action at Imidazoline-1 Receptors

ULRICH SCHÄFER,[a] CHRISTOF BURGDORF,[a] ASTRID ENGELHARDT,[a]
WALTER RAASCH,[b] THOMAS KURZ,[a] AND GERT RICHARDT[c]

[a]*Medizinische Klinik II, Universitätsklinikum Schleswig Holstein, Lübeck, Germany*

[b]*Institut für Experimentelle und Klinische Pharmakologie und Toxikologie, Universitätsklinikum Schleswig Holstein, Lübeck, Germany*

[c]*Herzzentrum, Segeberger Kliniken GmbH, Bad Segeberg, Germany*

ABSTRACT: The function of presynaptic imidazoline-1 receptors (I1-R) in the heart remains unclear. In rat hearts, UK14.304 and moxonidine reduced norepinephrine (NE) release. AGN192403 had no influence on NE, whereas rilmenidine, agmatine, rauwolscine, and efaroxan increased NE. These effects of moxonidine and rilmenidine were not affected by AGN192403 adminstration. Conversely, after pretreatment with UK14.304, only moxonidine displayed a pronounced inhibitory action on NE release (sensitive to AGN192403), indicating a synergistic inhibitory action at I1-R under conditions of a stimulated alpha2-adrenergic autoinhibition.

KEYWORDS: moxonidine; synergistic action; imidazoline-1-receptor; alpha-2-adrenoceptor

INTRODUCTION

There is a growing body of evidence that imidazolines mediate sympathoinhibition not only via activation of central nervous α_2-adrenoceptors (α_2-AR), but also via imidazoline-1 receptors (I_1-R).[1–3] Besides the most important regulatory location in the brainstem, additional inhibitory presynaptic actions on sympathetic nerve endings have been proposed. Recently, I_1-R have been identified in the heart,[4] but their functional relevance remains to be clarified.

METHODS

Concentration response curves on endogenous norepinephrine (NE) overflow, evoked by two sequential stimulations (S_1 = control and S_2 = pharmacologic inter-

Address correspondence to: Ulrich Schäfer, M.D., Medizinische Klinik II, Universitätsklinikum Schleswig Holstein, Ratzeburger Allee, 160 23538 Lübeck, Germany. Voice: (+49) 451/500-6105; fax: (+49) 451/500-6105.
e-mail: urs2001@med.cornell.edu

Ann. N.Y. Acad. Sci. 1009: 265–269 (2003). © 2003 New York Academy of Sciences.
doi: 10.1196/annals.1304.033

vention; each 1 min, 5 V, 6 Hz, 2 msec pulse width) of epicardial postganglionic sympathetic nerves in isolated buffer (modified Krebs-Henseleit solution; composition in mmol/L: Na+ 142, K$^+$ 4.0, Ca^{2+} 1.85, Mg^{2+} 1.1, Cl$^-$ 135, H$_2$PO$_4^-$ 0.22, HCO$_3^-$ 16.7, glucose 11, EDTA 0.027, 37.0°C) perfused rat (Wistar) hearts (flow: 8 mL/min/g), were performed for agmatine (AGM), UK14.304 (UK), rilmenidine (RIL), moxonidine (MOX), rauwolscine (RAU), AGN192403 (AGN), and efaroxan (EFA). To unmask an I$_1$-R-mediated effect of moxonidine and rilmenidine, hearts were pretreated in additional experiments with UK14,304 or rauwolscine, with or without AGN192403 or efaroxan, respectively. All experiments were performed in the presence of desipramine (DMI; 10^{-7} mol/L) to inhibit neuronal uptake and nonexocytotic release of NE. NE was measured by using a high-performance liquid chromatography (HPLC) electrochemical detection (detection 0.1 pmol per gram heart weight).

RESULTS

UK and MOX reduced stimulated NE overflow and AGN had no influence on NE release, whereas RIL, AGM, RAU, and EFA increased NE overflow (TABLE 1). MOX dose-dependently reduced stimulated NE overflow (LogEC$_{50}$: −6.15 ± 0.14). AGN192403, a selective antagonist at I$_1$-R, had no influence on the dose response curve of MOX (LogEC$_{50}$: −6.01 ± 0.25; FIG. 1). Conversely, RIL increased stimulated NE overflow (LogEC$_{50}$: −5.87 ± 0.17) and again AGN192403 had no influence on the dose response curve of RIL (LogEC$_{50}$: −5.04 ± 0.68; FIG. 1). To unmask an I$_1$-R–mediated effect (beyond α_2-adrenergic autoinhibition) of MOX and RIL, hearts were pre-exposed in additional experiments with the selective α_2-adrenergic ligands, UK and RAU, with or without AGN, respectively. After pretreatment with UK (10^{-5} mol/L; S1+S2; S1 = 167 ± 16 pmol/g; S2 = 139 ± 18 pmol/g; S2/S1 = 0.87 ± 0.1) the inhibitory action of MOX (10^{-6} mol/L) during S2 (UK: S1 = 191 ± 21 pmol/g; UK+MOX: S2 = 65 ± 9 pmol/g) was strongly augmented compared to control (S2/S1 = 0.33 ± 0.03; FIG. 1 and insert) and completely reversed with AGN (10^{-5} mol/L; FIG. 1 insert). Interestingly, RIL (10^{-6} mol/L and 10^{-5} mol/L; S2) in contrast to MOX, was not influenced by pretreatment with UK (10^{-5} mol/L; S1+S2). After pretreatment with RAU (10^{-5} mol/L), MOX (10^{-6} mol/L; S2) was unchanged (data not shown). Moreover, the inhibitory action of MOX (10^{-6} mol/L; S2) after pretreatment with UK (10^{-5} mol/L; S1+S2) was also totally inhibited by pretreatment (S1+S2) with indomethacin (10^{-7} mol/L; S2/S1 = 0.97 ± 0.02) as well as with D-609 (10^{-7} mol/L; S2/S1 = 1.03 ± 0.05), an inhibitor of phosphatidylcholine-selective phospholipase C (PC-PLC). Both compounds, indomethacin and D-609 by itself, were without effect on the release of NE (S2/S1: 1.01 ± 0.04 and 1.01 ± 0.05) during control experiments.

DISCUSSION

In summary, the imidazolines MOX and RIL show disparate effects on the release of NE. MOX displays an α_2-AR-agonistic and RIL an α_2-AR-antagonistic (or partial agonistic) activity with regard to electrically-stimulated NE release in this preparation. Under basal conditions, these effects are independent of I$_1$-R in cardiac tissue,

TABLE 1. Dose response relationship of UK14,304 (UK), moxonidine (MOX), rilmenidine (RIL), agmatine (AGM), AGN192403 (AGN), efaroxan (EFA), and rauwolscine (RAU) on endogenous norepinephrine overflow after stimulation of epicardial postganglionic sympathetic nerves

Concentration	Control		UK		MOX		RIL		AGM		AGN		EFA		RAU	
	S1	S2	S1	S2	S1	S2	S1	S2	S1	S2	S1	S2	S1	S2	S1	S2
NaCl	201 ±26	196 ±21														
10^{-9} mol/L															185 ±19	214 ±32
10^{-8} mol/L			256 ±21	225 ±17	388 ±22	365 ±25	240 ±28	228 ±24					150 ±13	216* ±20	234 ±28	386* ±22
10^{-7} mol/L			371 ±50	285* ±40	243 ±24	254 ±24	305 ±26	285 ±19			491 ±75	416 ±53	151 ±14	285* ±27	340 ±27	679* ±38
10^{-6} mol/L			249 ±18	123* ±9	296 ±24	212* ±13	335 ±21	413 ±17			223 ±13	236 ±22	190 ±12	545* ±73	373 ±47	737* ±64
10^{-5} mol/L			377 ±25	92* ±11	325 ±27	132* ±14	413 ±73	610* ±93	285 ±17	304 ±15	235 ±22	243 ±20	200 ±36	652* ±47	328 ±24	679* ±50
10^{-4} mol/L									284 ±20	298 ±19	443 ±49	485 ±44				
10^{-3} mol/L									280 ±12	327* ±18						

Norepinephrine release is induced by two electrical field stimulations (S1 and S2). The effect of each pharmacological intervention (S2) on norepinephrine release is intraindividually compared with the release during baseline condition (S1).
* Denotes statistical significance ($P > 0.05$) by unpaired t-test of S2 vs. S1 (untreated control).

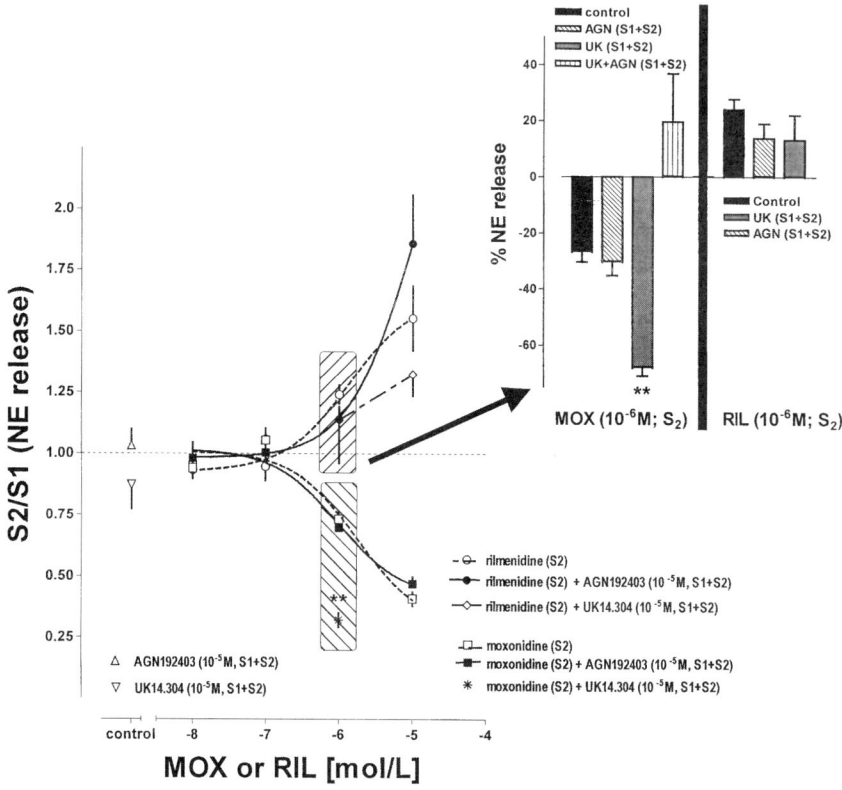

FIGURE 1. Influence of moxonidine (10^{-8} mol/L–10^{-4} mol/L; $n = 7$–12) and rilmendine (10^{-8} mol/L–10^{-4} mol/L; $n = 6$) on endogenous stimulated norepinephrine (NE) overflow (S2). In general, the effect of each pharmacologic intervention on norepinephrine release (S2) was intraindividually compared with the release during control condition (S1) and expressed as ratio of S2/S1 (% of control release). Statistical comparison of the effects of each single compound is in TABLE 1. The significant inhibitory effect of moxonidine (MOX) and the significant releasing effect of rilmenidine (RIL) was not influenced by AGN192403 (10^{-5} mol/L; drug administration during S1 and S2; $n = 5$–7). Conversely, after pretreatment with UK14.304 (10^{-5} mol/L; S2/S1 = 0.87), moxonidine (10^{-6} mol/L) markedly decreased NE release (S2/S1 = 0.33). The ratio of S2/S1 for AGN192403 ($n = 7$; NS) and UK14.304 ($n = 15$; NS) during control stimulation (drug administration at S1+S2) indicated stable experimental conditions. Depicted in the inserted graph (*arrow*), is the encircled section of moxonidine (10^{-6} mol/L) and rilmenidine (10^{-6} mol/L) during combination experiments with AGN192403 (10^{-5} mol/L; $n = 8$), UK14.304 (10^{-5} mol/L; $n = 8$), and UK14.304 combined with AGN192403 (10^{-5} mol/L; $n = 8$), respectively. Moxonidine displayed a strong synergistic inhibitory action after pretreatment with UK14.304, which could completely be reversed by AGN192403. ** Denotes statistical significance ($P > 0.01$) by unpaired *t*-test of moxonidine (at S2) + UK14.304 (S1+S2) versus control (UK14.304 at S1+S2).

demonstrating the prominent autoinhibitory presynaptic effect of α_2-AR as observed by others.[5–7] However, we also demonstrate that MOX, in contrast to RIL, strongly augments inhibition of NE release in an I_1-R-dependent pathway under conditions of a prestimulated α_2-adrenergic system. The observed difference between MOX and RIL could not be explained with the present data, but seems to comprise a different profile of receptor interaction. The existence of an allosteric modulation site at the level of the I_1-R, probably sensitive to moxonidine, has been proposed.[8] In addition, signaling pathways linked to I_1-R have been suggested to involve a PC-PLC[9] as well as the accumulation of free arachnidonic acid and the release of prostaglandins.[10] Indeed, the observed crosstalk between I_1-R and α_2-AR in this study was sensitive to indomethacin and D-609, indicating a pathway of prostaglandins and PC-PLC.

In conclusion, imidazoline derivatives might be of clinical interest under conditions of hyperadrenergic states (enhanced NE spillover), as is observed in hypertension, congestive heart failure, and myocardial infarction, with a consecutive autostimulation of presynaptic α_2-AR. In these circumstances, moxonidine might lead to a synergistic activation of I_1-R, inducing a marked sympathoinhibition.

REFERENCES

1. ERNSBERGER, P., R. GIULIANO, R.N. WILLETTE & D.J. REIS. 1990. Role of imidazole receptors in the vasodepressor response to clonidine analogs in the rostral ventrolateral medulla. J. Pharmacol. Exp. Ther. **253:** 408–418.
2. ERNSBERGER, P., T.H. DAMON, L.M. GRAFF, et al. 1993. Moxonidine, a centrally acting antihypertensive agent, is a selective ligand for I_1-imidazoline sites. J. Pharmacol. Exp. Ther. **264:** 172–182.
3. TOLENTINO-SILVA, F.P., M.A. HAXHIU, S. WALDBAUM, et al. 2000. α_2-Adrenergic receptors are not required for central anti-hypertensive action of moxonidine in mice. Brain Res. **862:** 26–35.
4. EL-AYOUBI, R., J. GUTKOWSKA, S. REGUNATHAN & S. MUKADDAM-DAHER. 2002. Imidazoline receptors in the heart: characterization, distribution, and regulation. J. Cardiovasc. Pharmacol. **39:** 875–883.
5. GAISER E.G., A.U. TRENDELENBURG & K. STARKE. 1999. A search for presynaptic imidazoline receptors at rabbit and rat noradrenergic neurones in the absence of α_2-autoinhibition. Naunyn Schmiedeberg's Arch. Pharmacol. **359:** 123–132.
6. MOLDERINGS G.J., F. HENTRICH & M. GÖTHERT. 1991. Pharmacological characterization of the imidazoline receptor which mediates inhibition of noradrenaline release in the rabbit pulmonary artery. Naunyn Schmiedeberg's Arch. Pharmacol. **344:** 630–638.
7. MOLDERINGS G.J. & M. GÖTHERT. 1995. Inhibitory presynaptic imidazoline receptors on sympathetic nerves in the rabbit aorta differ from I_1- and I_2-imidazoline binding sites. Naunyn Schmiedeberg's Arch. Pharmacol. **351:** 507–516.
8. MOLDERINGS, G.J., S. MENZEL, M. KATHMANN & M. GÖTHERT. 2000. Dual interaction of agmatine with the rat alpha(2D)-adrenoceptor: competitive antagonism and allosteric activation. Br. J. Pharmacol. **130:** 1706–1712.
9. SEPAROVIC, D., M. KESTER & P. ERNSBERGER. 1996. Coupling of I1-imidazoline receptors to diacylglyceride accumulation in PC12 rat pheochromocytoma cells. Mol. Pharmacol. **49:** 668–675.
10. ERNSBERGER, P., J.E. FRIEDMAN & R.J. KOLETSKY. 1997. The I1-imidazoline receptor: from binding site to therapeutic target in cardiovascular disease. J. Hypertens. Suppl. **15:** S9–23.

Norepinephrine Release Is Reduced by I_1-Receptors in Addition to α_2-Adrenoceptors

WALTER RAASCH, BRITTA JUNGBLUTH, ULRICH SCHÄFER, WALTER HÄUSER, AND PETER DOMINIAK

Institute of Experimental and Clinical Pharmacology and Toxicology, University Clinic Schleswig-Holstein, Campus Lübeck, Germany

ABSTRACT: In pithed spontaneous hypertensive rats, noradrenaline overflow was diminished by moxonidine even when α_2-adrenoceptors were blocked quantitatively using phenoxybenzamine, suggesting an I_1-receptor–mediated mechanism of noradrenaline release. This hypothesis was confirmed, since the noradrenaline overflow was (1) increased under α_2-adrenoceptors blockade by the mixed I_1/α_2-antagonists efaroxan or idazoxan, (2) still reduced by moxonidine when both α_2- and I_1-receptors were blocked, and (3) diminished by agmatine after pretreatment with phenoxybenzamine, but not with AGN192403. An indirect ganglionic I_1-receptor-mediated mechanism of noradrenaline release is supposed.

KEYWORDS: noradrenaline release; I_1-receptor; α_2-adrenoceptor; agmatine; electrical stimulation

INTRODUCTION

Imidazolines have been shown to modulate noradrenaline release via non I_1-/non I_2-presynaptic imidazoline receptors.[1] In contrast, these drugs were shown to inhibit noradrenaline release exclusively by activating prejunctional α_2-adrenoceptors (α_2-AR).[2] Such results have been based mainly on in vitro studies. The best way to demonstrate in vivo whether imidazoline binding sites would have some regulatory impact on noradrenaline release is to employ $\alpha_{2A/C}$-double knockout (KO) mice. Since this animal model was not available to us, we decided to overcome the limitation of a competitive blockade of α_2-adrenoceptors with rauwolscine (this α_2-AR antagonist was used in previous studies[3]) by performing experiments in pithed rats under irreversible α_2-AR blockade (by using phenoxybenzamine) or blockade of I_1-receptors (by using AGN192403). Thus, the aim of this study was to determine whether imidazoline binding sites contribute to the moxonidine-induced modification of noradrenaline release in vivo, and if so, to specify the subtype of imidazoline binding sites involved in mediating this effect.

MATERIALS AND METHODS

Animal Preparation

Spontaneously hypertensive rats (SHR; male, 200–250 g) were pithed following a standard protocol. Both the femoral vein (for drug administration) and the carotid artery (for measuring blood pressure and collecting blood) were catheterized.

Stimulation Experiments

Electrical stimulation of the thoracolumbar portion of the spinal cord was performed at 10 V (1 ms, 0.5 Hz, 3 min). Before stimulation, rats were pretreated with desipramine (0.5 mg/kg) and phenoxybenzamine (PBX; 10 mg/kg). SHR were pretreated facultatively with efaroxan (EFX; 1.0 mg/kg) or idazoxan (0.1 mg/kg). Moxonidine (MOX) or saline was infused over 10 min. Seven minutes after starting the infusion, rats were stimulated for 3 min as described above. During the last 30 sec of stimulation, blood (1 mL) was sampled from the carotid artery. Before infusing a higher dose of MOX, animals were allowed to recover for at least 10 min. To test the influence of agmatine on noradrenaline overflow, rats were pretreated for 10 min before agmatine infusion (6, 33, or 60 mg/kg) with either PBX (10 mg/kg) or AGN192403 (10 mg/kg).

Determination of Noradrenaline Overflow

Plasma noradrenaline as an index of sympathetic overflow was measured by high-pressure liquid chromatography and electrochemical detection.

RESULTS AND DISCUSSION

The adequacy of α_2-blockade was confirmed, since noradrenaline overflow was not enhanced any further by applying PBX concentrations >10 mg/kg (PBX 0, 3, 10, 30 mg/kg: 95 ± 8, 393 ± 38, 527 ± 82, 546 ± 76 pg/mL, respectively). In addition, the absence of any stimulation-evoked elevation of blood pressure (–3 ± 2 mm Hg) after 30 mg/kg PBX pretreatment is considered as evidence for a complete blockade of all α_2-ARs compared to PBX-free experiments (+17 ± 3 mm Hg). Furthermore, MOX did not increase blood pressure in the presence of PBX (TABLE 1). Finally, the stimulation-evoked blood pressure increase was abolished in the agmatine experiments under PBX, but not under AGN192403 treatment (FIG. 1).

Even though presynaptic α_2-ARs were blocked, MOX still reduced noradrenaline overflow (TABLE 1). Due to the affinity of MOX toward imidazoline receptors, the diminishing effect of MOX on noradrenaline overflow must arise via an interaction with imidazoline receptors.[1] However, MOX was characterized as an agonist at I_1-receptors rather than at non I_1-/non I_2-receptors, the latter of which were identified to be the presynaptically-located imidazoline receptors involved in regulation of noradrenaline release.[4] As such, our results conflict sharply with these findings[4] as well as the observation that MOX inhibits noradrenaline release from sympathetic nerve terminals solely via presynaptically-located α_2-ARs.[2] For strengthening the likelihood of an I_1-dependent mechanism in regulating noradrenaline overflow, we

TABLE 1. Influence of moxonidine on stimulated plasma noradrenaline concentrations (10 V, 0.5 Hz, 1 ms, 3 min) and stimulation-evoked elevation of diastolic blood pressure in the absence or presence of phenoxybenzamine (PBX, 10 mg/kg), or phenoxybenzamine (10 mg/kg) plus efaroxan (EFX, 1 mg/kg) and idazoxan (IDX, 0.1 mg/kg)

Pretreatment	Moxonidine (mg/kg)			
	0	0.18	0.6	1.8
	Plasma noradrenaline concentration (pg/mL)			
NaCl	88 ± 8	52 ± 6*	52 ± 5*	48 ± 5*
PBX	453 ± 60	275 ± 93*	134 ± 48*	96 ± 22*
PBX/EFX	1728 ± 64	1509 ± 148	1298 ± 155*	1200 ± 106*
PBX/IDX	1355 ± 194	973 ± 114	576 ± 196*	414 ± 42*
	Diastolic blood pressure (mm Hg)			
NaCl	30.3 ± 6.0	57.4 ± 11.2*	87.4 ± 15.5*	86.5 ± 15.2*
PBX	5.2 ± 2.2	8.8 ± 2.4	14.3 ± 5.6	14.1 ± 3.7
PBX/EFX	8.2 ± 6.7	10.5 ± 2.1	14.5 ± 4.1	15.0 ± 2.3
PBX/IDX	2.0 ± 4.9	0.7 ± 1.1	3.0 ± 2.6	8.7 ± 4.5

Values are expressed as means ± SEM; $n = 5-10$.
* $P < 0.05$ compared to moxonidine-free animals.

tested whether the mixed α_2-/I_1-antagonists EFX and IDX were able to reveal effects opposite to those of MOX. Continuing on with the MOX results, EFX (0.1, 1, 3 mg/g) and IDX (0.01, 0.1 mg/kg) by themselves both increased noradrenaline overflow dose-dependently during α_2-AR blockade (EFX: 1710 ± 48, 2131 ± 245, 2754 ± 214 pg/mL, IDX 990 ± 105, 1355 ± 194) compared to EFX/IDX-free controls (453 ± 40). In addition, MOX markedly diminished the EFX- or IDX-evoked increases in stimulated plasma noradrenaline concentration even under α_2-blockade (TABLE 1), which underlines the I_1-dependent mechanism of noradrenaline release. In order to reinforce once more the putative role of I_1-receptors in noradrenaline release in our in vivo model, agmatine was investigated regarding its potency in regulating noradrenaline overflow. Electrical stimulation caused an elevation of plasma noradrenaline in PBX- or AGN192403-pretreated animals. Noradrenaline overflow was markedly decreased by agmatine when α_2-ARs were blocked (FIG. 1), clearly emphasizing the relevance of imidazoline receptors. Confirming this mode of action, noradrenaline overflow was not affected by agmatine in the presence of the I_1-ligand AGN192403 (FIG. 1).

From our data on MOX, EFX, IDX and AGN192403, we have clear evidence that I_1-receptors might be involved. These data conflict sharply with in vitro findings, whereby the presynaptically-located non I_1-/ non I_2-imidazoline receptor was determined to regulate the release of noradrenaline.[1,4] This leads us to ask where the I_1-receptors that appear to be involved are located. A presynaptic location of these I_1-receptors on the sympathetic nerve terminals seems doubtful considering findings from isolated preparation experiments, so a ganglionic mechanism is therefore suggested due to the presence of I_1-receptors in ganglia and the ganglionic effects of

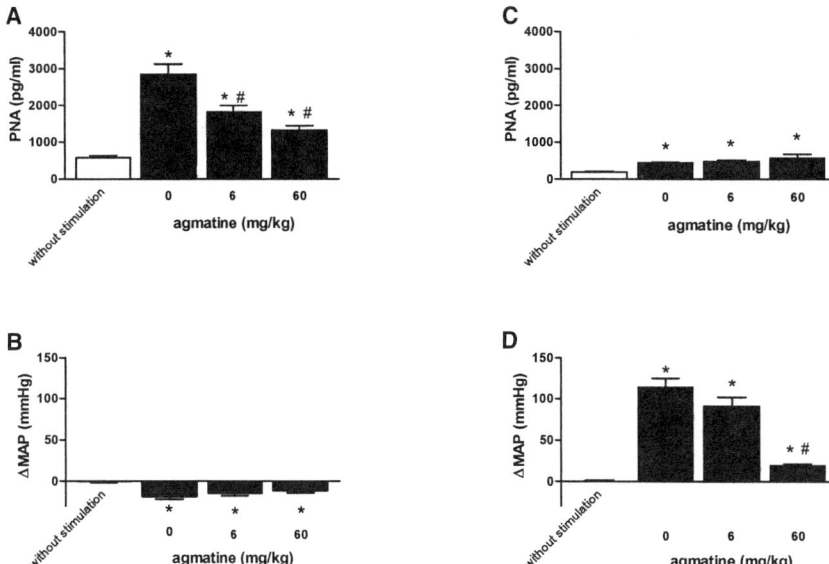

FIGURE 1. Influence of agmatine on plasma noradrenaline concentration (PNA) and mean arterial blood pressure (MAP) in the presence (*solid bars*) or absence (*open bars*) of preganglionic stimulation (20 V, 0.5 Hz, 1 ms, 0.5 min) in pithed spontaneous hypertensive rats pretreated with (**A, B**) desipramine/phenoxybenzamine (0.5/10 mg/kg) or (**C, D**) desipramine/AGN192403 (0.5/10 mg/kg). Values are expressed as means ± SEM of eight to ten experiments. * $P < 0.05$ compared to unstimulated agmatine-free controls. † $P < 0.05$ compared to stimulated agmatine-free controls.

agmatine.[5] Moreover, an indirect mechanism, probably via the cholinergic, histaminergic, or prostaglandin system is hypothesized, since the I_1-receptor was characterized as an excitatory rather than an inhibitory binding site. All these hypotheses require further clarification in future studies.

REFERENCES

1. GÖTHERT, M., M. BRUSS, H. BÖNISCH & G.J. MOLDERINGS. 1999. Presynaptic imidazoline receptors. New developments in characterization and classification. Ann. N. Y. Acad. Sci. **881:** 171–184.
2. SZABO, B., C. BOCK, U. NORDHEIM & N. NIEDERHOFFER. 1999. Mechanism of the sympathoinhibition produced by the clonidine-like drugs rilmenidine and moxonidine. Ann. N. Y. Acad. Sci. **881:** 253–264.
3. HÄUSER, W., J. GÜTTING, T. NGUYEN & P. DOMINIAK. 1995. Influence of imidazolines on catecholamine release in pithed spontaneously hypertensive rats. Ann. N. Y. Acad. Sci. **763:** 573–579.
4. LIKUNGU, J., G.J. MOLDERINGS & M. GÖTHERT. 1996. Presynaptic imidazoline receptors and alpha 2-adrenoceptors in the human heart: discrimination by clonidine and moxonidine. Naunyn Schmiedeberg's Arch. Pharmacol. **354:** 689–692.
5. RAASCH, W., U. SCHÄFER, J. CHUN & P. DOMINIAK. 2001. Biological significance of agmatine, an endogenous ligand at imidazoline binding sites. Br. J. Pharmacol. **133:** 755–780.

Normalization of Up-Regulated Cardiac Imidazoline I_1-Receptors and Natriuretic Peptides by Chronic Treatment with Moxonidine in Spontaneously Hypertensive Rats

R. EL-AYOUBI, A. MENAOUAR, J. GUTKOWSKA, AND S. MUKADDAM-DAHER

CHUM-Research Center, Université de Montréal, Montreal, Quebec, Canada

ABSTRACT: The effect of treatment with moxonidine (120 μg/kg/h sc, 4 weeks) on cardiac I_1-receptors and natriuretic peptide synthesis was evaluated in spontaneously hypertensive rats (SHR). I_1-receptor protein (85 kD) was up-regulated in SHR atria, and normalized in right and left atria by moxonidine. Similarly, moxonidine normalized atrial and ventricular atrial natriuretic peptide messenger RNA (mRNA) and brain natriuretic peptide mRNA. This study shows that cardiac I_1-receptors are functional, being regulated by hypertension and by chronic exposure to agonist, and that cardiac natriuretic peptides may be regulated by I_1-receptor-mediated mechanisms.

KEYWORDS: imidazoline receptors; moxonidine; natriuretic peptides

INTRODUCTION

Imidazoline I_1-receptors are non-adrenergic and non-cholinergic neurotransmitter receptors present in the brainstem, adrenal chromaffin cells, and kidneys. Activation of I_1-receptors is associated with blood pressure reduction, primarily by sympatho-inhibition[1,2]. In addition, we have recently identified imidazoline I_1-receptors in the heart atria and ventricles, and shown that heart imidazoline receptors are up-regulated in cardiovascular diseases, such as hypertension and heart failure,[3] implying that heart imidazoline receptors may be functional and involved in cardiovascular regulation.

Moxonidine, an antihypertensive imidazoline compound, reduces blood pressure by activation of central and peripheral imidazoline I_1-receptors and subsequent decrease of sympathetic nervous activity and stimulation of renal actions.[2] Acute moxonidine injections in normotensive Sprague-Dawley (SD) rats dose-dependently increase diuresis, natriuresis, and cyclic guanosine 3′,5′-monophosphate (cGMP) excretion as well as plasma levels of natriuretic peptides,[4] cardiac hormones that reduce blood pressure by several mechanisms, including vasodilation, diuresis, natriuresis, and sympathoinhibition.

Address correspondence to: Suhayla Mukaddam-Daher, Ph.D., Laboratory of Cardiovascular Biochemistry, CHUM Research Center, Hotel-Dieu Hospital, (6-816) 3840 St-Urbain Street, Montreal, Quebec, Canada, H2W 1T8. Voice: 514-890-8000, ext: 12757; fax: 514-412-7199.
e-mail: suhayla.mukaddam-daher@umontreal.ca

Ann. N.Y. Acad. Sci. 1009: 274–278 (2003). © 2003 New York Academy of Sciences.
doi: 10.1196/annals.1304.035

Based on the findings that cardiac natriuretic peptides may be involved in the acute activation of imidazoline receptors by moxonidine,[4] and that both imidazoline receptors and natriuretic peptide synthesis are increased in hearts of hypertensive rats,[3,5] the following studies were performed. We investigated the effect of a one-month treatment with moxonidine on imidazoline receptors and natriuretic peptide expression in hypertensive rat hearts, with the aim of demonstrating functionality of cardiac imidazoline I_1-receptors.

METHODS

Female spontaneously hypertensive rats (SHR; 12–14 weeks old) were treated during one month with two doses of moxonidine (60, 120 µg/kg/h) or saline vehicle, via Alzet osmotic minipumps (2ML4) implanted under the neck skin. Sprague-Dawley rats (200–225 g) (Charles River, St. Constant, QC) served as normotensive controls. Animals were housed in a temperature- and light-controlled room with food and water *ad libitum*. After one month of treatment, the rats were sacrificed by decapitation and the hearts were rapidly isolated, divided into four compartments, then flash frozen in liquid N_2 and stored at –80°C.

Imidazoline receptor regulation in cardiac atria and ventricles was analyzed by Western blot using a polyclonal imidazoline receptor antibody, as we have previously described.[3] Total RNA from ventricles and atria were extracted, then reverse-transcribed into cDNA and subjected to semiquantitative polymerase chain reaction (PCR), using specific primers for atrial natriuretic peptide (ANP), brain natriuretic peptide (BNP) and glyceraldehyde-3-phosphate dehydrogenase (GAPDH).[5] Values normalized to corresponding GAPDH are reported as percent of normotensive controls or vehicle-treated SHR controls.

RESULTS

Immunoblotting revealed that, compared to normotensive controls (100%), the intensity of the bands that correspond to 85 kD was increased ($135 \pm 3\%$; $n = 10$; $P < 0.001$) in SHR atria. Compared to vehicle-treated SHR (100%), treatment with 60 and 120 µg moxonidine significantly ($n = 6$–10; $P < 0.001$) decreased the intensity of the 85 kD band in right atria to $51 \pm 2\%$ and $47 \pm 3\%$, respectively. The bands that correspond to 29/30 kD were not altered in SHR with or without treatment (FIG. 1). The intensity of the bands corresponding to 29/30 and 85 kD proteins were not increased in hypertensive rat ventricles. One-month treatment with two doses of moxonidine had no effect on the 85 kD band, but was associated with reduced intensity of the bands corresponding to 29/30 kD to $89 \pm 2\%$ of vehicle-treated SHR ($n = 6$; $P < 0.002$).

ANP mRNA decreased in right atria and left ventricles to $68 \pm 2\%$ and $70 \pm 6\%$ of corresponding vehicle-treated hypertensive controls, respectively ($P < 0.001$). Similarly, right atrial and left ventricular BNP mRNA decreased to $46 \pm 1\%$ and $65 \pm 1\%$ ($P < 0.001$; FIG. 2). The levels of ANP and BNP mRNA were not significantly different from those measured in normotensive controls.

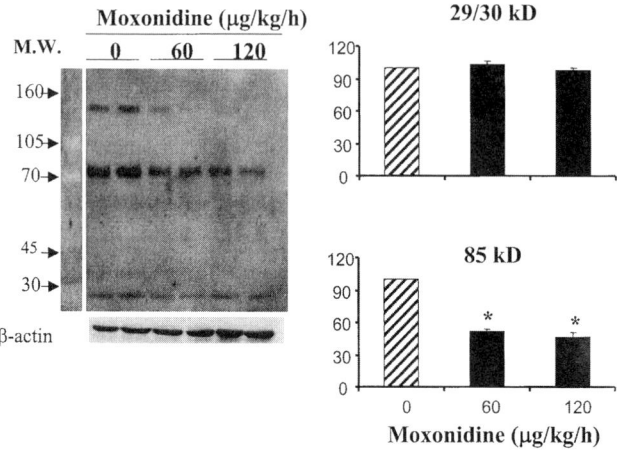

FIGURE 1. Western blot analysis of imidazoline receptor proteins in right atria in response to one-month treatment with two doses of moxonidine.

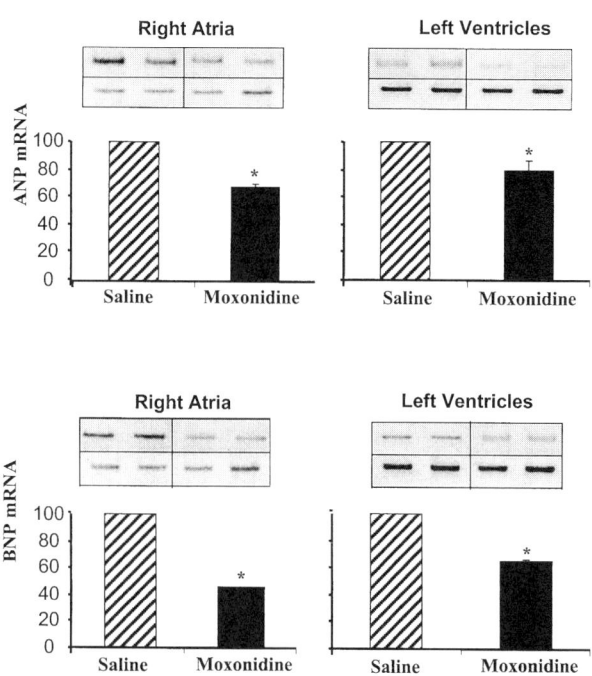

FIGURE 2. Effect of moxonidine treatment on natriuretic peptides ANP and BNP mRNA in right atria of SHR. Results are normalized to corresponding GAPDH and reported as percent of vehicle-treated SHR.

DISCUSSION

This study shows that chronic one-month treatment of hypertensive rats with moxonidine is associated with normalization of up-regulated imidazoline receptors and natriuretic peptide synthesis in cardiac atria and ventricles.

Imidazoline receptors of 29/30 kD, 45 kD, 85 kD, 176 kD proteins have been isolated from brainstem rostral ventrolateral medulla.[6] Similar proteins are also present in the heart.[3] However, it is not yet known which protein corresponds to the functional imidazoline I_1-receptor. Based on our present finding, we suggest that functional cardiac imidazoline I_1-receptors are tissue-specific, being differentially regulated in atria and ventricles by hypertension and chronic exposure to agonist. Whereas the 85 kD protein may correspond to the functional I_1-receptor in atria, it may be the 29/30 kD protein that is functional in ventricles. However, further studies are required to confirm this observation.

Previous studies from our laboratory and others have shown that natriuretic peptide synthesis is increased in hypertensive rat hearts.[3,7,8] In the present study, chronic treatment of SHR with 60 and 120 μg/kg/h moxonidine, over one month, is associated with significantly reduced ANP mRNA and BNP mRNA in right atria and left ventricles as compared to corresponding vehicle-treated SHR. The mechanisms of natriuretic peptide decrease by chronic moxonidine have not been investigated, but these changes parallel the changes in imidazoline receptor proteins; both are up-regulated in SHRs and down-regulated by moxonidine treatment. Therefore, based on the present findings and on our previous results that acute moxonidine injections increase circulating ANP levels, it appears likely that cardiac natriuretic peptides may be regulated by imidazoline I_1-receptor-mediated mechanisms.

ACKNOWLEDGMENTS

Moxonidine was generously provided by Solvay Pharma (Hannover, Germany). Studies are supported by the Canadian Institutes for Health Research, and the Heart and Stroke Foundation of Canada.

REFERENCES

1. BOUSQUET, P., J. FELDMAN & J. SCHWARTZ. 1984. Central cardiovascular effects of alpha adrenergic drugs: differences between catecholamines and imidazolines. J. Pharmacol. Exp. Ther. **230:** 232–236.
2. ERNSBERGER, P. 2000. Pharmacology of moxonidine: an I1-imidazoline receptor agonist. J. Cardiovasc. Pharmacol. **35:** S27–S41.
3. EL-AYOUBI, R., J. GUTKOWSKA, S. REGUNATHAN & S. MUKADDAM-DAHER. 2002. Imidazoline receptors in the heart: characterization, distribution, and regulation. J. Cardiovasc. Pharmacol. **39:** 875–883.
4. MUKADDAM-DAHER, S. & J. GUTKOWSKA. 2000. Atrial natriuretic peptide is involved in renal actions of moxonidine. Hypertension **35:** 1215–1220.
5. MENAOUAR, A., R. EL-AYOUBI, M. JANKOWSKI, *et al.* 2002. Chronic imidazoline receptor activation in spontaneously hypertensive rats. Am. J. Hypertens. **15:** 803–838.
6. ESCRIBA, P.V., M. SASTRE, H. WANG, *et al.* 1994. Immunodetection of putative imidazoline receptor proteins in the human and rat brain and other tissues. Neurosci. Lett. **178:** 81–84.

7. KUROSKI DE BOLD, M.L. 1998. Atrial natriuretic factor and brain natriuretic peptide gene expression in the spontaneous hypertensive rat during postnatal development. Am. J. Hypertens. **11:** 1006–1018.
8. RAIZADA, V., K. THAKORE, W. LUO, & P.G. MCGUIRE. 2001. Cardiac chamber-specific alterations of ANP and BNP expression with advancing age and with systemic hypertension. Mol. Cell. Biochem. **216:** 137–140.

Alpha$_{2A}$-Adrenergic Versus Imidazoline Receptor Controversy in Rilmenidine's Action

Alpha$_{2A}$-Antagonism in Humans Versus Alpha$_{2A}$-Agonism in Rabbits

GERHARD J. MOLDERINGS, HEINZ BÖNISCH, MICHAEL BRÜSS, AND MANFRED GÖTHERT

University of Bonn, Institute of Pharmacology and Toxicology, Bonn, Germany

ABSTRACT: At the α_{2A}-autoreceptors on the sympathetic nerve terminals of the human atrial appendages and rabbit pulmonary artery, rilmenidine and oxymetazoline exhibit different properties (antagonism and agonism, respectively). These opposite pharmacodynamic properties of α_2-adrenoceptor ligands seem to be due to substantial differences in the nucleotide and amino acid sequences between human and rabbit α_{2A}-adrenoceptors. Hence, the rabbit α_{2A}-adrenoceptor is not reliably predictive for the action of ligands at the human α_{2A}-adrenoceptor.

KEYWORDS: α_{2A}-adrenoceptor; rabbit; human; imidazoline receptor

INTRODUCTION

The mechanism by which imidazoline-like central antihypertensives such as rilmenidine lower blood pressure is still under debate. The original concept postulates activation of α_{2A}-adrenoceptors in the brain stem and on sympathetic nerve terminals to be the primary mechanism of action of these drugs (for review, see[1]). According to the more recent imidazoline receptor hypothesis, their hypotensive effect is substantially due to activation of I_1 imidazoline receptors in the rostral ventrolateral medulla (for review, see[2]). Most of the experiments aimed at elucidating the mechanism of imidazoline-like antihypertensive drugs, in particular, of rilmenidine, were performed with rabbits. A prerequisite for those experiments was the unproved assumption that the rabbit α_{2A}-adrenoceptor is reliably predictive as a model for the action of ligands at the human α_{2A}-adrenoceptor, although rilmenidine has been shown to exhibit no intrinsic activity at recombinant human α_{2A}-adrenoceptors.[3]

Address correspondence to: Gerhard J. Molderings, University of Bonn, Institute of Pharmacology and Toxicology, Reuterstr. 2b, D-53113 Bonn, Germany. Voice: (+49) 228 735421; fax (+49) 228 735404.
e-mail: molderings@uni-bonn.de

RESULTS AND DISCUSSION

Relation between the Molecular Structure of the Receptor and Its Pharmacological Characteristics

Although the presynaptic α_2-autoreceptors of the rabbit and human cardiovascular system have been basically subclassified as α_{2A}-adrenoceptors in functional experiments,[4,5] the actions of the α_2-adrenoceptor ligands rilmenidine and oxymetazoline at the presynaptic α_{2A}-autoreceptors of rabbit pulmonary arteries and human atrial appendages are markedly different: both compounds are full agonists at the rabbit α_{2A}-adrenoceptor but act as antagonists at the human α_{2A}-adrenoceptor.[5] In agreement with this observation, Jasper et al.[3] found rilmenidine to exhibit no, and oxymetazoline to have only low intrinsic activity at recombinant human α_{2A}-adrenoceptors.

These differences in the functional profile of human and rabbit α_{2A}-adrenoceptors are paralleled by substantial differences in the nucleotide and deduced amino acid sequences between both receptors. Comparison of the degree of homology between the amino acid sequences of α_{2A}-adrenoceptors of several mammalian species reveals an exceptional position of the rabbit (for sequence, see accession number AJ512644), because its degree of homology is 10% less than that of all other mammals among each other investigated so far (TABLE 1). To date a less degree of homology has only been found for the teleost fish, *Takifugu rubripes* (TABLE 1).

The differences in the deduced amino acid sequences of rabbit and human α_{2A}-adrenoceptors were most pronounced in the third intracellular loop (FIG. 1), which is known to be critical for G-protein binding.[6,7] Hence, the difference in the amino acid sequence of the rabbit α_{2A}-adrenoceptor (which has recently been published[8]) compared with the human orthologue, in particular the introduction of a proline-rich sequence that is not present in any other species, may lead to a modified conformation. This modified conformation probably affects receptor activation by

TABLE 1. α_{2A}-Adrenoceptor homology among various species

	Human	Pig	Rabbit	Mouse	Rat	Guinea pig	Cattle	*Takifugu rubripes*
Human	—	94	80	92	90	92	89	63
Pig	90	—	79	92	91	92	91	65
Rabbit	89	85	—	78	77	77	76	60
Mouse	86	86	83	—	97	87	84	64
Rat	88	86	84	95	—	90	87	64
Guinea pig	90	88	87	87	87	—	90	62
Cattle	90	91	72	84	86	87	—	63
Takifugu rubripes	47	46	44	45	45	48	45	—

Values in the upper right portion represent overall percentage amino acid sequence identity; those in the lower left portion demonstrate nucleotide sequence identity.

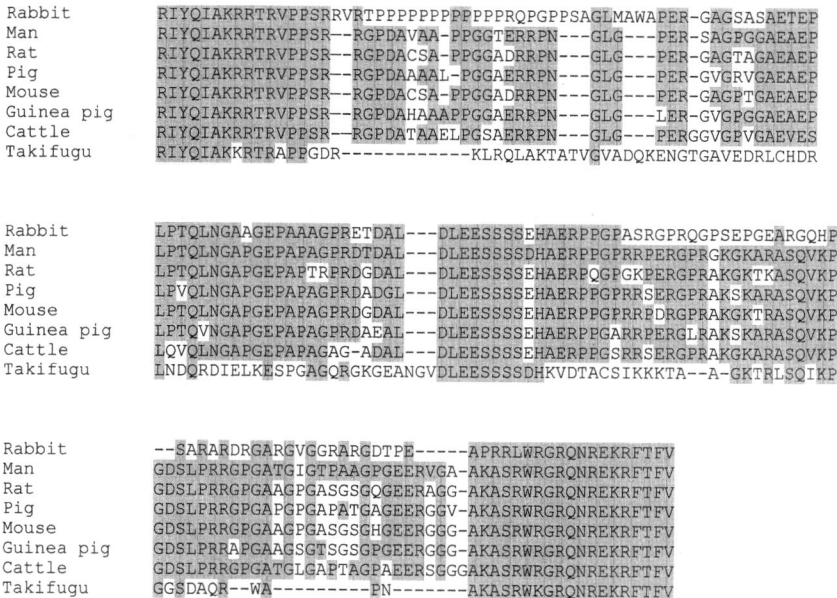

FIGURE 1. Alignment of α_{2A}-adrenoceptor amino acid sequences of the third intracellular loop from eight species.

some of the α_{2A}-adrenoceptor ligands such as rilmenidine and oxymetazoline that act as antagonists (very low efficacy partial agonists) at the human α_{2A}-adrenoceptor, whereas they behave as full agonists at the rabbit α_{2A}-adrenoceptor.

Furthermore, the amino acid sequences of the transmembrane domains also substantially influence the pharmacologic characteristics of the α_{2A}-adrenoceptor.[9–13] Compared with the sequence of the human α_{2A}-adrenoceptor, there are substantial changes of seven amino acids and three deletions of two amino acids each, in the highly conserved transmembrane domains 3, 4, and 5 that may also play an important role for the pharmacologic character of the rabbit α_{2A}-adrenoceptor (for details, see[5,8]).

Implications for the Use of the Rabbit α_{2A}-Adrenoceptor as a Model for the Human α_{2A}-Adrenoceptor

The observation that the pharmacological properties of rilmenidine, clonidine, and oxymetazoline at α_{2A}-adrenoceptors differ substantially between various species[3,5,14] in concert with the present molecular data suggests that the rabbit α_{2A}-adrenoceptor is no reliable predictive model for the action of ligands at the human α_{2A}-adrenoceptor. It is of interest to note that rilmenidine acts as an antagonist not only at human, but also at the pig α_{2A}-adrenoceptor,[14] and that the pig and human α_{2A}-adrenoceptor are structurally most similar among mammals in the amino acid sequence (TABLE 1).[5] Hence, the action of ligands at central α_{2A}-adrenoceptors in humans can be predicted most reliably from experiments performed in pig preparations.

ACKNOWLEDGMENTS

The technical assistance of Mrs. M. Hartwig, Mrs. B. Wenzel, and Mrs. P. Breiden is gratefully acknowledged. The study was supported by a grant from the Deutsche Forschungsgemeinschaft.

REFERENCES

1. SZABO, B. 2002. Imidazoline antihypertensive drugs: a critical review on their mechanism of action. Pharmacol. Ther. **93:** 1–35.
2. BRUBAN, V., J. FELDMAN, H. GRENEY, *et al.* 2001. Respective contributions of α-adrenergic and non-adrenergic mechanisms in the hypotensive effect of imidazoline-like drugs. Br. J. Pharmacol. **133:** 261–266.
3. JASPER, J.R., J.D. LESNICK, L.K. CHANG, *et al.* 1998. Ligand efficacy and potency at recombinant α_2 adrenergic receptors. Biochem. Pharmacol. **55:** 1035–1043.
4. MOLDERINGS, G.J. & M. GÖTHERT. 1995. Subtype determination of presynaptic α_2-autoreceptors in the rabbit pulmonary artery and human saphenous vein. Naunyn Schmiedeberg's Arch. Pharmacol. **352:** 483–490.
5. MOLDERINGS, G.J., H. BÖNISCH, M. BRÜSS, *et al.* 2000. Species-specific pharmacological properties of human α_{2A}-adrenoceptors. Hypertension **36:** 405–410.
6. EASON, M.G. & S.B. LIGGETT. 1996. Chimeric mutagenesis of putative G-protein coupling domains of the α_{2A}-adrenergic receptor. J. Biol. Chem. **271:** 12826–12832.
7. WADE, S.M., M.K. SCRIBNER, H.M. DALMAN, *et al.* 1996. Structural requirements for G(o) activation by receptor-derived peptides: activation and modulation domains of the alpha$_2$-adrenergic receptor i3c region. Mol. Pharmacol. **50:** 351–358.
8. BRÜSS, M., H. BÖNISCH, M. GÖTHERT & G.J. MOLDERINGS. 2003. Molecular structure of the rabbit α_{2A}-adrenoceptor: a contribution to the α_{2A}-adrenoceptor versus I1 imidazoline receptor controversy. Naunyn Schmiedeberg's Arch. Pharmacol. **367:** 328–331.
9. SURYANARAYANA, S., D.A. DAUNT, M. VON ZASTROW & B.K. KOBILKA. 1991. A point mutation in the seventh hydrophobic domain of the α_2-adrenergic receptor increases its affinity for a family of β receptor antagonists. J. Biol. Chem. **266:** 15488–15492.
10. BLAXALL, H.S., D.A. HECK & D.B. BYLUND. 1993. Molecular determinants of the alpha$_{2D}$ adrenergic receptor subtype. Life Sci. **53:** 255–259.
11. CERESA, B.P. & L.E. LIMBIRD. 1994. Mutation of an aspartate residue highly conserved among G-protein-coupled receptors results in nonreciprocal disruption of α_2-adrenergic receptor-G-protein interactions. J. Biol. Chem. **269:** 29557–29564.
12. SALMINEN, T., M. VARIS, T. NYRÖNEN, *et al.* 1999. Three-dimensional models of α_{2A}-adrenergic receptor complexes provide a structural explanation for ligand binding. J. Biol. Chem. **274:** 23405–23413.
13. PAUWELS, P.J. & F.C. COLPAERT. 2000. Heterogenous ligand-mediated Ca^{++} responses at wt and mutant α_{2A}-adrenoceptors suggest multiple ligand activation binding sites at the α_{2A}-adrenoceptor. Neuropharmacology **39:** 2101–2111.
14. ALI, A., H.Y. CHENG, K.N. TING & V.G. WILSON. 1998. Rilmenidine reveals differences in the pharmacological characteristics of prejunctional α_2-adrenoceptors in the guinea-pig, rat and pig. Br. J. Pharmacol. **125:** 127–135.

BU98008, a Highly Selective Imidazoline$_1$-Receptor Ligand

E.S.J. ROBINSON, R.E. PRICE, D.J. NUTT, AND A.L. HUDSON

Psychopharmacology Unit, School of Medical Sciences, Bristol BS8 1TD, UK

ABSTRACT: BU98008 (1-(4, 5-dihydro-1H-imidazol-2-yl)isoquinoline) is a novel isoquinoline derivative. Radioligand binding studies revealed it had high affinity for the I_1 receptor in rat kidney membranes but low affinity for the I_2 binding site and α_2-adrenoceptor in rat brain membranes. Further evaluation of BU98008 in vivo revealed no effect on blood pressure following peripheral administration. These preliminary data suggest BU98008 may be an antagonist at I_1 receptors. Further evaluation following central administration must be performed before a hypotensive action can be excluded.

KEYWORDS: I_1-receptor; blood pressure; radioligand binding

INTRODUCTION

Increased blood pressure in hypertension has been shown to be associated with increased sympathetic tone, and many drugs used to treat hypertension target either sympathetic outflow or adrenoceptors located on cardiovascular tissue. Clonidine and related antihypertensive drugs lower sympathetic tone and reduce blood pressure as well as potentially displaying beneficial effects in cardiac failure. Although these drugs have been used for many years, the exact mechanism by which they decrease sympathetic tone is not clear. The original hypothesis was based on the fact that clonidine is an α_2-adrenoceptor agonist. Clonidine, however, was shown to bind to a non-catecholamine site or imidazoline binding site (I-BS) as well as to α_2-adrenoceptors in the medulla oblongata.[1] Later, the sympathoinhibitory effects of clonidine and the new antihypertensive agents rilmenidine and moxonidine were attributed to activation of these I-BSs. This binding site is now termed the I_1-receptor based on its affinity selectivity for clonidine and related compounds and its functional role in regulating blood pressure.[2] Interest in I_1-receptors as targets for novel, nonsedating antihypertensive agents has led to the synthesis of new ligands with improved selectivity for I_1 receptors compared with α_2-adrenoceptors. The present study has evaluated the relative affinities and functional properties of BU98008 (1-(4, 5-dihydro-1H-imidazol-2-yl)isoquinoline), a novel isoquinoline derivative.

Address for correspondence: A.L. Hudson, Psychopharmacology Unit, School of Medical Sciences, University Walk, Bristol BS81TD, UK. Voice: (+44) 117 928 8608; fax: (+44) 117 928 9700.
e-mail: a.l.Hudson@bristol.ac.uk

METHODS

Radioligand Binding

Radioligand binding studies were carried out as previously described.[3,4] Membranes from whole rat brain (I_2 or α_2-adrenoceptors) or rat kidney (I_1) were incubated with [^{3}H]2-BFI, [^{3}H]RX821002 or [^{3}H]clonidine + 10 µM rauwolscine to label I_2-, α_2-adrenoceptors, or I_1-receptors respectively. Results from the competition experiments were analyzed using iterative nonlinear regression analysis, and IC_{50} values calculated. Where an appropriate K_D was available, the K_i was calculated using the Cheng-Prussoff equation.[5]

Radio Telemetry

Male spontaneously hypertensive rats were surgically implanted with a telemetry device for the measurement of arterial blood pressure, heart rate, body temperature, and an index of locomotor activity. This work was carried out at Quintiles Scotland Ltd (Edinburgh, UK). Animals were dosed with BU98008 (0.1, 1.0, and 10 mg kg^{-1} intraperitoneally) or clonidine (0.1mg kg^{-1} orally) as a positive control. Data were recorded from −0.5 to 9 hours after treatment and analyzed using a one-way ANOVA with repeated measures followed by Dunnett's post hoc. A value of $P < 0.05$ was considered significant, and all data were obtained from eight animals per group.

RESULTS

Radioligand Binding Studies

BU98008 displays nanomolar affinity for I_1 receptors in rat kidney membranes (IC_{50} = 82.48 nM) and has low affinity for I_2-BS (2.5 µM) and α_2-adrenoceptors (27.6 µM). Relative to the α_2-adrenoceptor, BU98008 has a lower affinity than that previously reported for rilmenidine and is some 300-fold more selective for I_1 receptors than for α_2-adrenoceptors.

Radio Telemetry

Functional evaluation of BU98008 in spontaneously hypertensive rats failed to show any significant, dose-dependent effects of blood pressure (FIG. 1). The positive control, clonidine, induced a reduction in both systolic and diastolic blood pressure (FIG. 1). BU98008 (10 mg/kg^{-1}) and clonidine both reduced heart rate and body temperature (FIG. 2). Clonidine significantly reduced locomotor counts, and BU98008 at the highest dose reduced activity only a single time point (FIG. 2).

DISCUSSION

BU98008 is a highly selective, high-affinity I_1 receptor ligand. The radioligand binding studies have shown that BU98008 binds with nanomolar affinity at the rat

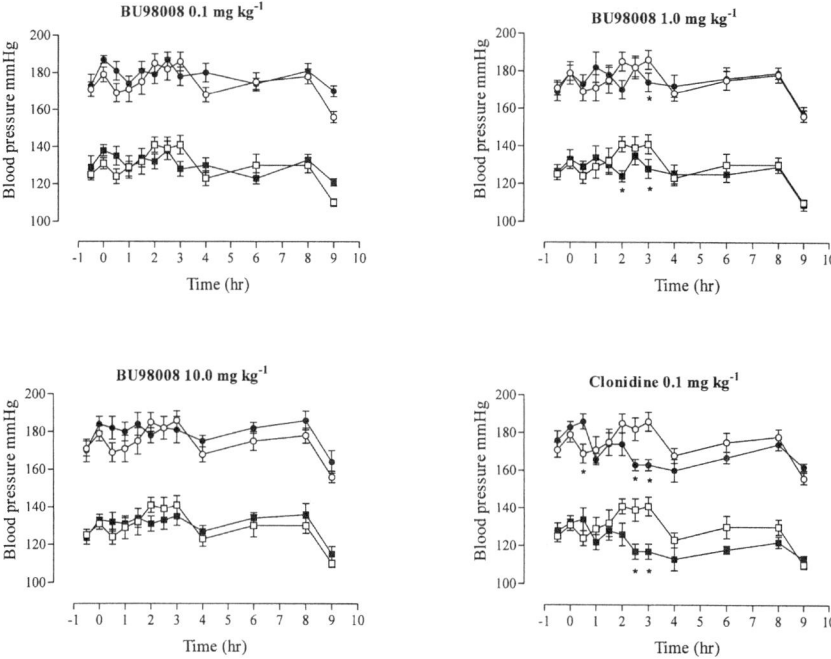

FIGURE 1. Effects of BU98008 and clonidine on systolic and diastolic blood pressure in SHR. The results are shown as mean ± SEM for drug treatment (*closed symbol*) or vehicle (*open symbol*). * $P < 0.05$ versus saline.

kidney I_1 receptor but has micromolar affinity for α_2-adrenoceptors and I_2 binding sites. Given its affinity and selectivity for I_1 receptors, BU98008 was tested in spontaneously hypertensive rats for its ability to decrease blood pressure. Systemic administration of 0.1, 1.0, and 10 mg/kg^{-1} BU98008 failed to induce any significant dose-dependent effects on either systolic or diastolic blood pressure suggesting this compound lacked efficacy at I_1 receptors. Considerable variability was observed using this method of quantification, however, and the positive control, clonidine, also failed to produce the dramatic decrease in blood pressure that would be predicted for the dose given. One explanation for the lack of effect on blood pressure seen with BU98008 is that it is an I_1 receptor antagonist. This hypothesis could be further evaluated further by comparing the ability of BU98008 to attenuate clonidine-induced hypotension with the known I_1-receptor antagonist, efaroxan.

In terms of the other parameters monitored, BU98008 at 0.1 and 1.0 mg/kg^{-1} did not affect heart rate, body temperature, or locomotor function. At 10mg kg^{-1} a small but significant decrease in heart rate was observed, and a significant reduction in body temperature was apparent up to 4 hours after drug administration. It is possible that at the highest dose tested the effects of BU98008 are mediated through α_2-adrenoceptors, although very little effect on locomotor activity was observed. Further

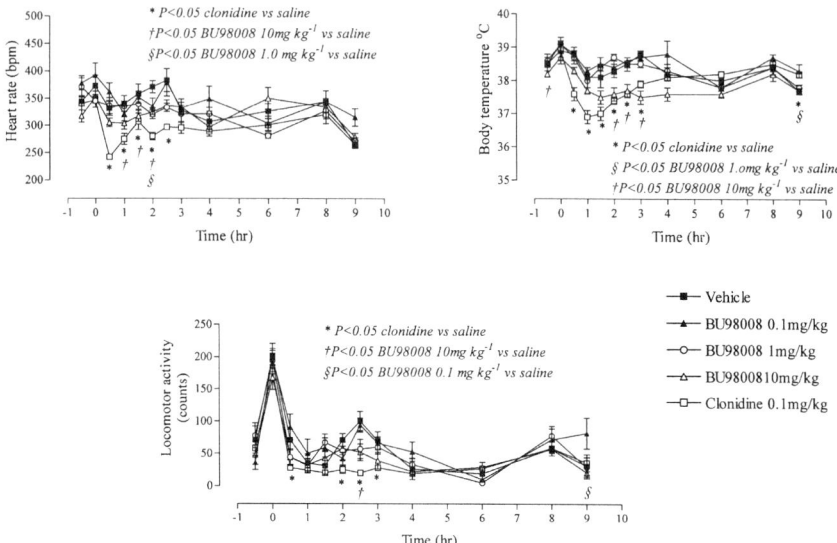

FIGURE 2. Effects of BU98008 and clonidine on heart rate and body temperature in spontaneously hypertensive rats. The results are shown as mean ± SEM.

evaluation using selective α_2-adrenoceptor antagonists will enable determine the mechanisms underlying the hypothermic response and tachycardia.

In a previous study using a highly selective I_1-receptor ligand, AGN192403, Munk and coworkers[6] also failed to observe a hypotensive effect. At present no information on the bioavailability of either of these compounds is available, and therefore, their ability to cross the blood–brain barrier and activate I_1 receptors in the rostral ventrolateral medulla (RVLM) is not known. It has also been shown, using $\alpha_{2A/D}$-adrenoceptor mutant mice, that peripheral administration of clonidine, rilmenidine, and moxonidine in conscious animals failed to induce a reduction in blood pressure.[7] Microinjection of moxonidine into the RVLM of anesthetized mice of the same mutant mouse strain resulted in a reduction in blood pressure.[8] The difference between these results remains to be explained. These data suggest the hypotensive effects of peripherally administered moxonidine are dependent on α_2-adrenoceptors with the I_1-mediated effects on blood pressure only apparent following central administration. Given the results from these experiments, it would be interesting to test both AGN192403 and BU98008 in anesthetized animals following central administration. This approach would also address the question of bioavailability.

In conclusion, BU98008 seems to lack intrinsic activity at I_1 receptors. These data are similar to those reported for the highly selective I_1-receptor ligand AGN 192403. This compound has a high affinity and selectivity for I_1 receptors relative to α_2-adrenoceptors and, like BU98008, failed to reduce blood pressure when tested in vivo. Further studies will investigate the interaction of BU98008 with clonidine and characterize the effect of BU98008 following central administration.

ACKNOWLEDGMENTS

BU98008 was kindly synthesized by Dr. Stephen Husbands, Department of Pharmacy and Pharmacology, University of Bath, Bath, UK. The Sulis Seedcorn Foundation provided funding for these studies.

REFERENCES

1. ERNSBERGER, P., et al. 1987. Clonidine binds to imidazole binding sites as well as α_2-adrenoceptors in ventrolateral medulla. Eur. J. Pharmacol. **134:** 1–13.
2. EGLEN, R.M., et al. 1998. "Seeing through a glass darkly": casting light on imidazoline "I" sites. Trends Pharmacol. Sci. **19:** 381–390.
3. PARKER, C.A., et al. 1998. [^{3}H]Clonidine binding sites in rat kidney: a model for putative central imidazoline1-sites. Br. J. Pharmacol. **125:** 76P.
4. MALLARD, N.J., et al. 1992. Characterisation and autoradiographical localisation of non-adrenoceptor idazoxan binding sites in rat brain. Br. J. Pharmacol. **106:** 1019–1027.
5. CHENG, Y.C. & W.H. PRUSOFF. 1973. Relationship between the inhibition constant (K_i) and the concentration of inhibitor which causes 50% inhibition (IC_{50}) of an enzymatic reaction. Biochem. Pharmacol. **22:** 3099–3108.
6. MUNK, S.A., et al. 1996. Synthesis and pharmacologic evaluation of 2-endo-amino-3-exo-isopropylbicyclo[2.2.1]heptane: a potent imidazoline$_1$ receptor specific agent. J. Med. Chem. **39:** 1193–1195.
7. ZHU, Q.-M. 1999. Cardiovascular effects of rilmenidine, moxonidine and clonidine in conscious wild-type and D79N α_2-adrenoceptor transgenic mice. Br. J. Pharmacol. **126:** 1522–1530.
8. TOLENTINO-SILVA, F.P. 2000. α_2-adrenergic receptors are not required for central antihypertensive action of moxonidine in mice. Brain Res. **862:** 26–35.

Apparent Absence of Direct Renal Effect of Imidazoline Receptor Agonists

D.D. SMYTH,[a,b] D. PIRNAT,[a] B. FORZLEY,[a] AND S.B. PENNER[a,b]

[a]*Department of Pharmacology & Therapeutics, University of Manitoba, Winnipeg, Manitoba, Canada*

[b]*Department of Internal Medicine, University of Manitoba, Winnipeg, Manitoba, Canada*

ABSTRACT: Imidazoline receptor agonists such as moxonidine and rilmenidine increase sodium excretion whether administered within the central nervous system, intravenously, or directly into the renal artery. To determine if this natriuresis was mediated by a direct renal effect and was independent of the renal sympathetic nerves, we used two different preparations in the pentobarbital-anesthetized rat. In the first series of studies, rats were unilaterally nephrectomized 7 to 10 days before the experiment. On the day of the experiment, the remaining kidney was denervated (surgical and 10% phenol/95% ethyl alcohol) or sham treated. The effect of an intravenous infusion of rilmenidine was determined. Rilmenidine (10 nmol/kg/minute) decreased blood pressure and increased urine flow rate and sodium excretion in the sham- but not the denervation-treated rats. The response to furosemide (5.05 nmol/kg/minute) remained intact following denervation. We then used a two-kidney rat model that allowed for separate urine collection from each ureter. We used low infusion rates of moxonidine directly into the left renal artery. An increase in urine flow rate from the left but not the right kidney would suggest a direct renal action. Low infusion rates of moxonidine (10, 30 nmol/kg/minute) increased urine flow rate similarly from both ureters. A low infusion rate of furosemide (9.1 nmol/kg/minute) into the left renal artery increased urine flow rate only from the left ureter. The failure of moxonidine to increase urine flow rate selectively only in the left kidney indicated the agonist acts at an extrarenal site to increase urine flow rate from both kidneys equally. The complete attenuation of the response to rilmenidine indicates the importance of the renal nerves and suggests that the extrarenal site is most probably the central nervous system. Collectively, these studies do not support a direct renal action of imidazoline agonists in producing natriuresis.

KEYWORDS: kidney; denervation; imidazoline receptor

INTRODUCTION

A number of laboratories have observed natriuresis following administration of an imidazoline agonist into the central nervous system,[1–3] into a peripheral vein,[4–6] or directly into the renal artery.[7] These studies failed to determine whether these

Address for correspondence: D.D. Smyth, Department of Pharmacology and Therapeutics, University of Manitoba, 753 McDermot Avenue, Winnipeg, Manitoba, Canada R3E OW3. Voice: (204) 789-3356; fax: (204) 789-3932.
e-mail: dsmyth@ms.umanitoba.ca

Ann. N.Y. Acad. Sci. 1009: 288–295 (2003). © 2003 New York Academy of Sciences.
doi: 10.1196/annals.1304.059

effects were mediated by a direct renal effect (tubular or vascular), a secondary change in natriuretic hormone levels, or an indirect effect such as altering renal sympathetic nerve activity.

Although Kline and Cechetto[8] initially proposed a major role of the central nervous system and the renal sympathetic nerves in natriuresis, our laboratory and others suggested additional mechanisms might be involved. For example, natriuresis observed following imidazoline receptor activation has been closely correlated with an increased release of atrial natriuretic factor and increased urinary excretion of cyclic guanosine monophosphate (cGMP).[6,9] This finding indicated an effect independent of the renal nerves. Studies in our laboratory have also indicated that imidazoline receptor agonists may be acting at two unique sites, within the central nervous system and within the kidney, to increase sodium excretion.[3,10]

In the present study we attempted to demonstrate a direct renal effect of imidazoline receptor agonists. First we determined if acute renal denervation would selectively alter the response to intravenous administration of rilmenidine. Second, we attempted to demonstrate a direct renal action of moxonidine by infusion at low rates directly into the left renal artery such that natriuresis would be observed only in the left kidney.

METHODS

Experimental Preparation

The general experimental protocol has been previously described.[11] Male Sprague-Dawley rats (17–225 g) were obtained from the University of Manitoba (Charles River Breeding Stock), and care was provided according to guidelines of the Canadian Council on Animal Care. The animals were kept in cages (two or three rats per cage) at 22°C with a 12-hour light/dark cycle and fed a standard Purina rat chow diet with free access to tap water.

Renal Denervation Studies

Seven to 10 days before the experimental day, under ether anesthesia, the right kidney was removed through a flank incision. On the day of the experiment the rats (280–340 g) were anesthetized (50 mg/kg Nembutal [BDH Chemical Ltd., Poole, England] administered intraperitoneally). A thermostatically controlled heating blanket maintained body temperature at 37°C. A tracheostomy was performed (PE-240), and the animal was allowed to breathe spontaneously. The left carotid artery was cannulated (PE-50) for monitoring blood pressure and heart rate. The left jugular vein was cannulated (PE-160) for the continuous infusion of saline (0.9% NaCl) at 97 µL/minute to produce moderate diuresis. A second catheter was inserted into the first line with a 21-gauge needle for the administration of saline (3.4 µL/minute), rilmenidine (30 nmol/kg/minute), or furosemide (5.05 nmol/kg/minute). The remaining kidney was exposed by a left flank incision, and the ureter was cannulated (PE-10) for timed urine collections into preweighted vials. The kidney was denervated surgically by cutting and stripping all visible nerves from the renal artery and by painting the renal artery and vein with 10% phenol in 95% ethyl alcohol. In the sham-operated animals, the nerves were exposed but were not cut or painted with the phenol/ethanol mixture. The preparation was allowed to stabilize for 45 minutes.

After the first 30-minute control urine collection, an infusion of rilmenidine (10 nmol/kg/minute), saline (0.9% NaCl), or furosemide (5.05 nmol/kg/minute) was started and maintained at 3.4 µL/minute for the second and third collection, each of 30 minutes' duration.

Left Renal Artery Infusion Studies

Left renal artery infusion studies were performed in two-kidney rats. On the day of the study Sprague-Dawley rats (280–300 g) were anesthetized. The trachea, carotid artery, and jugular vein were cannulated, as described previously, for measurement of heart rate, blood pressure, and the administration of saline. Both ureters were cannulated for timed collection of urine. The left ureter was cannulated through a flank incision (PE-10). A 31-gauge needle was inserted into the left renal artery for the direct infusion of the saline vehicle (3.4 µL/minute), moxonidine (10 and 30 nmol/kg/minute), or furosemide (9.1 nmol/kg/minute). The right ureter was cannulated through an abdominal incision (PE-10). Urine volume was measured gravimetrically. Following a 45-minute stabilization period, a 30-minute baseline urine collection was obtained. Immediately following this first collection, a constant infusion (3.4 µL/minute) of vehicle, moxonidine, or furosemide was started and maintained for the duration of the experiment. Two further 30-minute collections were obtained during this infusion from the ipsilateral (left) and contralateral (right) kidney.

Analysis

Sodium concentrations in the urine were measured with a Nova Electrolyte Analyzer (13+) (Nova Biochemical Canada, Mississaugua). The data points presented represent the difference between the third and the first collection periods. All data have been presented as the mean ± standard error with at least five animals per group and analyzed by ANOVA followed by multiple comparison tests to identify significant differences.

RESULTS

Renal Denervation Studies

In the sham-denervated rats, rilmenidine increased urine flow rate and sodium excretion as compared with the control saline group (FIG. 1). In the sham-treated animals, as compared with the saline control group, rilmenidine decreased blood pressure (0.8 ± 1.4 versus −12.5 ± 4.8 mm Hg) and heart rate (3.3 ± 3.0 versus −36.7 ± 3.0 beats per minute [bpm]). In the animals that underwent renal denervation, rilmenidine failed to increase urine flow rate and sodium excretion as compared with the saline control infusion (FIG. 1). Similar to the sham-treated animals, rilmenidine decreased heart rate (6.7 ± 3.9 versus −40.0 ± 6.7 bpm) but failed to decrease blood pressure (8.3 ± 3.0 versus 1.7 ± 3.7 mm Hg) as compared with the animals receiving saline vehicle alone.

Unlike rilmenidine, furosemide (5.05 nmol/kg/minute) increased urine flow rate in the sham-treated as well as the denervated rats (FIG. 2). Furosemide failed to alter blood pressure or heart rate in the sham-treated and denervated rats.

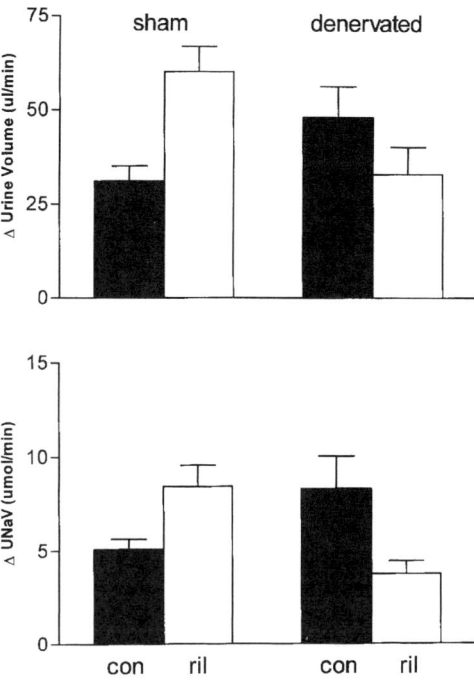

FIGURE 1. Effects of intravenous infusion of 0.9% saline vehicle control (*solid bars*) or rilmenidine (*open bars*) at 10 nmol/kg/minute on urine flow rate and sodium excretion in sham-operated and renal denervated rats. Con, control; ril, rilmenidine.

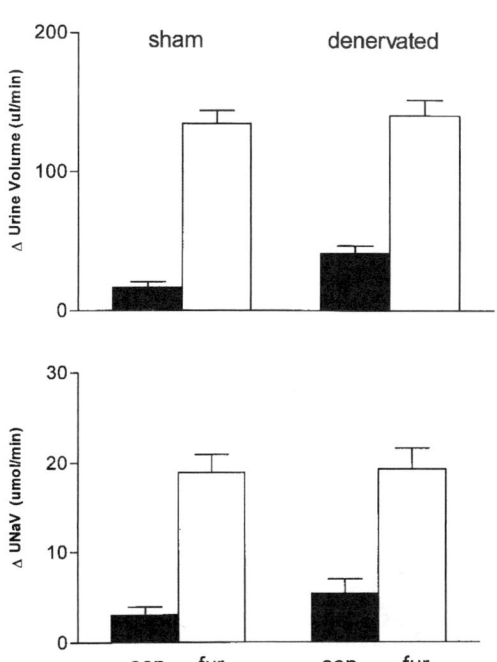

FIGURE 2. Effects of intravenous infusion of 0.9% saline vehicle control (*solid bars*) or furosemide at 5.05 nmol/kg/minute (*open bars*) on urine flow rate and sodium excretion in sham-operated and renal denervated rats. Con, control; fur, furosemide.

FIGURE 3. Effects of infusion of 0.9% saline vehicle control or moxonidine (3.0 and 10.0 nmol kg/minute) directly into the left renal artery on urine flow rate and sodium excretion from the left (*open bars*) and right kidney (*solid bars*). Con, control.

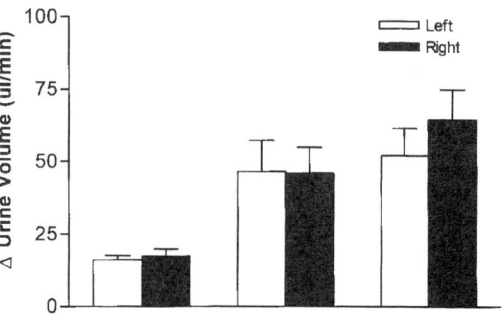
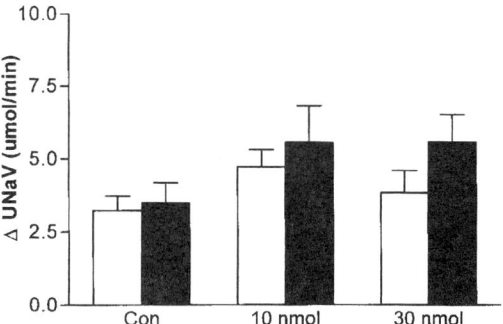

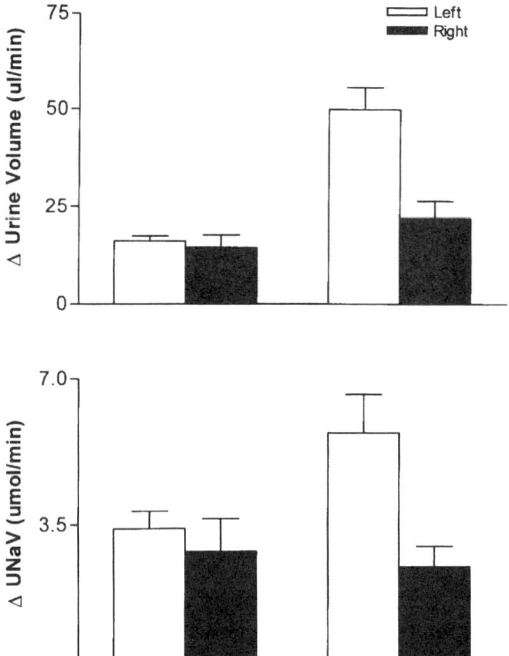

FIGURE 4. Effects of infusion of 0.9% saline vehicle control or furosemide (9.1 nmol/kg/minute) directly into the left renal artery on urine flow rate and sodium excretion from the left (*open bars*) and right kidney (*solid bars*). Con, control.

Left Renal Artery Infusion Studies

As compared with the group receiving saline, moxonidine (10 and 30 nmol/kg/minute) infused into the left renal artery failed to alter blood pressure but decreased heart rate at both doses (-12.0 ± 9.1 versus -60.0 ± 12.1 versus -68.6 ± 12.7 bpm). The infusion of saline or moxonidine (10 and 30 nmol/kg/minutes) directly into the left renal artery resulted in similar levels of urine flow and sodium excretion from the ipsilateral (left) and contralateral (right) kidney (FIG. 3).

Furosemide infusion (9.1 nmol/kg/minute) into the left renal artery increased urine flow rate and sodium excretion from the left (ipsilateral) but not from the right (contralateral) kidney (FIG. 4). Furosemide failed to alter blood pressure and heart rate.

DISCUSSION

The mechanism(s) by which imidazoline receptor agonists increase urine flow rate and sodium excretion have not been clarified. Imidazoline receptors have been identified within the central nervous system at sites known to regulate sympathetic nerve activity,[12,13] within the right and left atria,[9] and on tubules in the kidney.[14,15] Conceivably, stimulation of these receptors at any one of these sites could potentially alter sodium excretion.

Renal sympathetic nerve denervation has been reported to attenuate completely the response to rilmenidine, an I_1 imidazoline receptor agonist.[8] These studies were consistent with others that have demonstrated the ability of imidazoline receptor agonists to alter renal sympathetic nerve activity.[13] Although these findings seemed to demonstrate a major, if not exclusive, role for the renal sympathetic nerves, they were at odds with other studies that indicated that mechanisms not directly involving the renal nerves may also mediate the natriuresis. Mukaddam-Daher and colleagues[9] provided convincing evidence that atrial natriuretic factor has a role in natriuresis. In vitro studies found that imidazoline receptor agonists produced a dose-related release of atrial natriuretic factor from isolated atria. Studies in whole animals found that the natriuresis was associated with an increase in plasma atrial natriuretic factor and increased cGMP excretion in the urine.[6,16] Previous studies from our laboratory had also suggested another mechanism for the natriuresis that did not involve the central nervous system and changes in renal sympathetic nerve activity. A number of separate studies had demonstrated that the response to central administration of an imidazoline receptor agonist was not the same as that seen following peripheral administration.[1,3,7,10,17] For example, intracerebroventricular (i.c.v.) administration of the imidazoline receptor antagonist idazoxan completely blocked the natriuretic effect of i.c.v.-administered moxonidine[10] but only partially blocked the effect of moxonidine administered directly into the renal artery.[7] Similarly, pretreatment with intravenous idazoxan resulted in a complete attenuation of the response to intrarenal moxonidine, whereas the response to i.c.v. moxonidine remained unaltered.[3] Another series of studies found that pretreatment with intravenous prazosin completely attenuated the response to i.c.v. moxonidine[18] but failed to alter the response to an intrarenal infusion of moxonidine.[10] Collectively these studies indicated two unique sites where imidazoline receptor agonists seemed to increase sodium excretion, one within the central nervous system and one peripheral. These studies, however, failed to demonstrate a direct renal effect of imidazoline receptor agonists.

As shown in a preliminary report from our laboratory,[19] renal denervation attenuated the response to an imidazoline receptor agonist indicating the importance of these nerves in the response to these agonists.[8] The maintained response to furosemide in these denervated rats, however, indicted that this finding was not a general, nonspecific loss in responsiveness to all natriuretic substances. The second series of studies investigated whether a direct renal effect was present. It was thought that if a direct renal effect were present, it should be possible to find a dose of moxonidine that would alter sodium handling to a greater extent in the kidney receiving the direct infusion, because this kidney would be the site of highest drug concentration. If a direct effect were not present, the drug would overflow into the systemic circulation and thereby result in changes (possibly increases in atrial natriuretic factor or altered sympathetic nerve activity) that would alter sodium excretion similarly from both kidneys. The doses of moxonidine selected were the lowest that produced a consistent increase in urine flow rate. At both doses, the increases in urine flow rate and sodium excretion were similar from both ureters. Furosemide, on the other hand, increased urine flow rate and sodium excretion selectively from the kidney receiving the direct infusion. This finding indicated that it was possible to increase urine flow rate selectively with this model.

In a previous study from our laboratory,[17] we had reported that renal denervation attenuated the blood pressure–lowering effect of rilmenidine administered by i.c.v. injection. In the present study, renal denervation also attenuated the blood pressure–lowering effect of rilmenidine following intravenous infusion. The kidney has been documented to play a significant role in the long-term regulation of blood pressure. The ability of renal denervation to attenuate the acute blood pressure response to rilmenidine was not anticipated. The mechanism by which this attenuation occurred will require further study.

Collectively, these results confirm the importance of the renal nerves in the mediation of the natriuretic response to imidazoline receptor agonists. As well, it seems that these agents do not act directly on the kidney to alter sodium excretion.

REFERENCES

1. PENNER, S.B. & D.D. SMYTH. 1994. Sodium excretion following central administration of an I1 imidazoline preferring agonist, moxonidine. Br. J. Pharmacol. **112:** 1089–1094.
2. PENNER, S.B. & D.D. SMYTH. 1995. The role of the peripheral sympathetic nervous system in natriuresis following central administration of an I1 imidazoline agonist moxonidine. Br. J. Pharmacol. **116:** 2631–2636.
3. SMYTH, D.D. & S.B. PENNER. 1998. Imidazoline receptor mediated natriuresis: central and/or peripheral effect? J. Auton. Nerv. Sys. **72:** 155–162.
4. KLINE, R.L., J. VAN DER MARK & D.F. CECHETTO. 1994. Natriuretic effect of rilmenidine in anesthetized rats. Am. J. Cardiol. **74:** 20A–24A.
5. HOHAGE, H., E. SCHLATTER & J. GREVEN. 1997. Effect of moxonidine and clonidine on renal function and blood pressure in anesthetized rats. Clin. Nephrol. **47:** 316–324.
6. MUKADDAM-DAHER, S. & J. GUTKOWSKA. 2000. Atrial natriuretic peptide is involved in the renal actions of moxonidine. Hypertension **35:** 1215–1220.
7. ALLAN, D., S.B. PENNER & D.D. SMYTH. 1993. Renal imidazoline preferring receptors and solute excretion in the rat. Br. J. Pharmacol. **108:** 870–875.

8. KLINE, R.L. & D.F. CECHETTO. 1993. Renal effects of rilmenidine in anesthetized rats: importance of renal nerves. J. Pharmacol. Exp. Ther. **266:** 1556–1562.
9. MUKADDAM-DAHER, S., C. LAMBERT & J. GUTKOWSKA. 1997. Clonidine and ST-91 may activate imidazoline binding sites in the heart to release atrial natriuretic peptide. Hypertension **30:** 83–87.
10. PENNER, S.B. & D.D. SMYTH. 1994. Central and renal I_1 imidazoline preferring receptors: two unique sites mediating natriuresis in the rat. Cardiovasc. Drugs Ther. **8:** 43–48.
11. BLANDFORD, D.E. & D.D. SMYTH. 1988. Dose selective dissociation of water and solute excretion after renal α_2-adrenoceptor stimulation. J. Pharmacol. Exp. Ther. **247:** 1181–1186.
12. ERNSBERGER, P., T.H. DAMON, L.M. GRAFF, et al. 1993. Moxonidine, a centrally acting agent, is a selective ligand for I1 imidazoline site. J. Pharmacol. Exp. Ther. **264:** 172–182.
13. HEAD, G.A. & S.L. BURKE. 2000. Comparison of renal sympathetic baroreflex effects of rilmenidine and alpha-methylnoradrenaline in ventrolateral medulla of the rabbit. J. Hypertension **18:** 1263–1276.
14. ERNSBERGER, P., W.L. WESTBROOKS, M.O. CHRISTEN & S.G. SCHAFER. 1992. A second generation of centrally acting antihypertensive agents on putative I1 imidazoline receptors. J. Cardiovasc. Pharmacol. **20:** S1–S10.
15. ZAKEIL, N., P. ERNSBERGER & J.G. DOUGLAS. 1993. Distribution of I1 imidazoline and α2-adrenergic binding sites in renal tubule epithelial cells. [Abstract 837] FASEB J. **7** (Part I): A145.
16. GUTKOWSKA, J., S. MUKADDAM-DAHER & J. TREMBLAY. 1997. The peripheral action of clonidine analog ST-91: involvement of atrial natriuretic factor. J. Pharmacol. Exp. Ther. **281:** 670–676.
17. PENNER, S.B. & D.D. SMYTH. 1997. Renal denervation altered the hemodynamic and renal effects following intracerebroventricular administration of the I1 imidazoline agonist, rilmenidine, in pentobarbital anesthetized rats. Neurochem. Int. **30:** 55–62.
18. PENNER, S.B. & D.D. SMYTH. 1995. Rilmenidine alters renal function when administered intracerebroventricular (ICV) or intrarenal. Ann. N. Y. Acad. Sci. **763:** 353–356.
19. PIRNAT, D., S.B. PENNER & D.D. SMYTH. 2002. Effects of rilmenidine and guanfacine in acute renal denervated rats. Proc. West. Pharmacol. Soc. **45:** 15–17.

Atypical [³H]Clonidine Binding Sites in Human Caudate and Platelets on Cryostat-cut Sections

H. ZHU, A. HALARIS, AND J.E. PILETZ

University of Mississippi Medical Center, Jackson, Mississippi 39216, USA

ABSTRACT: Pharmacological characterization is described for a human imidazoline binding site (I-site) labeled by [³H]clonidine using standard autoradiographic method. Under conditions that mask α_2-adrenergic sites, only a single high affinity site was observed in human caudate and blood platelet sections. Affinity constants (K_i) were highly correlated between the two tissues ($r = 0.90$, $P = 0.0003$). This site is dissimilar to classical I_1 and I_2 sites, even though both tissues possess abundant I_1 and I_2 sites by filtration binding methods. It is suggested that the isotonic buffer conditions inherent to the procedure alter drug affinities to the classical I_1 site.

KEYWORDS: clonidine; human brain; platelets; imidazoline receptors

INTRODUCTION

Clonidine was originally developed as a high affinity agonist for α_2-adrenoceptors (α_2AR), but it also binds with only slightly lower affinity to non-adrenergic I_1-imidazoline receptors (IR_1).[1] Filtration binding methods have been developed whereby [³H]clonidine binding to α_2AR is masked.[2] The additional [³H]clonidine binding sites have been characterized in human brain and platelet membrane fractions.[2] The I_1 site possesses preferential affinity for clonidine, is enriched in plasma membrane fractions,[3] and is distributed in brain differently than α_2AR or the other major subtype of imidazoline binding site, I_2.[4,5] By comparison, I_2 sites possess preferential affinity for idazoxan-like compounds, are co-localized with brain monoamine oxidase B (MAO-B) in rat and human brain,[6] and some I_2 sites are physically linked to MAO-A and MAO-B on mitochondria membranes.[7]

In addition to the two major classes of clonidine binding sites (I_1 and α_2AR sites), an atypical [³H]clonidine binding site has been described in brain by autoradiographic methods.[5] Unfortunately, standard autoradiographic techniques have proven insufficient to regionalize classical I_1 sites. A well-documented key to detecting classical I_1 sites by filtration binding has been the use of extremely hypotonic (5 mmol/L) buffers.[2] By contrast, previous studies with [³H]clonidine autoradiography have utilized at least 50 mmol/L buffers, because 5 mmol/L hypotonic buffers are disruptive to tissue sections. It has been speculated that I_1 sites differ in their pharmacological properties depending on buffer and assay conditions.[2]

Address for correspondence: He Zhu, M.D., Department of Psychiatry, University of Mississippi Medical Center, 2500 North State Street, Jackson, MS 39216-4505, USA. Voice: 601-984-5798; fax: 601-984-5899.
e-mail: hzhu@psychiatry.umsmed.edu

In our study, competition curves of [^{3}H]clonidine binding using autoradiographic conditions are described for cryostat-cut human caudate and compacted platelets. The results have revealed a unique cirazoline-sensitive site in the absence of I_1 or I_2 sites. To our knowledge, a cirazoline-selective I-site has never been reported to exist in platelets. This atypical [^{3}H]clonidine binding site possesses pharmacological properties in common with a [^{3}H]cirazoline-labeled site in rat brain and kidney described using filtration binding studies by Angel and coworkers.[8] It is suggested that classical I_1 pharmacology in hypotonic buffer may convert to an atypical cirazoline-preferring rank-ordered potency in more isotonic buffer.

MATERIALS AND METHODS

Brain tissues from deceased subjects (three males and two females) were obtained at the Cuyahoga County Coroner's Office, Ohio, in accordance with an approved Institutional Review Board protocol. Four subjects died of cardiovascular failure and one died of asphyxiation secondary to smoke inhalation. The average age at death was 52 ± 10 years (age range 24–80 years). Death ensued within 4 hours of injury. Shortly thereafter, the cadavers were transported to the coroner's facility and refrigerated prior to autopsy. The average postmortem interval (from death to freezing of brain tissue) was 16 ± 3 hours (range 6–21 hours). Toxicological screening was performed for 50 compounds in blood, bile, urine, and/or vitreous fluids of cadavers. Four of the subjects showed no detectable drugs in the toxicological screen. One subject had evidence of a small amount of lidocaine in the blood. Postmortem psychological autopsies with next-of-kin revealed no neurological or psychiatric histories. A block of brain tissue containing caudate was dissected and processed as previously described.[5] Frozen blocks of brain tissue were mounted on a specimen chuck of a cryostat microtome (Cryocut 1800; Leica, Reicher-Jung, Deerfield, IL), and sections from the head of the caudate (20 µm thick) were cut at –16°C and thaw-mounted onto gelatin-coated microscope slides. Sections were dried under refrigeration and stored at –82°C until use.

Intact platelets were obtained from concentrates (1-day outdated) from the Mississippi Blood Services (Jackson, MS). The platelets were adjusted to pH 6.5 with a citric acid solution made isotonic with saline and centrifuged at 7,500 ×g for 10 minutes. Pellets were resuspended and transferred into conical microcentrifuge tubes and centrifuged at 11,000 rpm for 10 minutes at 4°C. After being frozen at –80°C for at least 24 hours, the platelet plug was mounted on a specimen chuck of a cryostat microtome. Platelet sections (8 mm in diameter) were prepared exactly as for brain caudate.

The autoradiographic technique was identical to our earlier report.[5] [^{3}H]Clonidine (70.5 Ci/mmol) was purchased from NEN Life Science Products (Boston, MA). Moxonidine and BDF6143 were gifts of Lilly Forschung GmbH Company (Hamburg, Germany). Tizanidine was a gift of Sandoz Pharmaceuticals (Tokyo, Japan). Cirazoline and RX 821002 (methoxyidazoxan) were from the former Research Biochemicals International (Natick, MA). Agmatine, harmane, norepinephrine (NE), oxymetazoline and idazoxan were from Sigma Chemical Company (St. Louis, MO). Drug stock solutions were prepared fresh before each experiment (0.01 mol/L) in either distilled water, ethanol, or 10 mmol/L acetic acid, depending on solubilities; they were then serially diluted with reaction buffer (50 mmol/L Tris-HCl, 2 mmol/L

MgCl$_2$, 252 µmol/L ascorbic acid, pH 7.4) containing [^{3}H]clonidine. A drop of solution covered each tissue slice on the slides. After incubation and washing, each slice was wiped from its slide using glass fiber filters and then radioactivity was determined on the wipes by liquid scintillation counting. Competition experiments were performed at the near-K$_D$ concentration of 50 nmol/L radioligand.[5] Total I-site binding was defined in the presence of 12.5 µmol/L RX821002 to mask α$_2$AR. Specific binding to I-sites was determined by subtracting the binding of [^{3}H]clonidine in the presence of 12.5 µmol/L RX 821002 plus 100 µmol/L cirazoline (to displace I-sites) from binding of [^{3}H]clonidine in the presence of only 12.5 µmol/L RX 821002. The preferred affinity (K$_D$ and K$_i$) and density (B$_{max}$) constants were chosen by statistical F test using LIGAND, whereas actual values reported (expressed as mean ± SEM) came from Prism to be consistent with our plotting program, InPlot (GraphPad, San Diego, CA). We masked α$_2$AR with RX821002, which behaves as a selective antagonist of α$_2$AR. A very useful feature of this compound is its lack of binding at I$_1$ and I$_2$ sites (IC$_{50}$ at I sites ≥ 60 µmol/L).[9,10]

In a previous study, we also proved that with 12.5 µmol/L RX821002 mask, the specific binding to I-sites was only fractionally lower compared to the results with NE mask (60 µmol/L).[5] Therefore, I$_1$ and I$_2$ may, if present, be unaffected by 12.5 µmol/L RX821002 to block α$_2$AR.

RESULTS

Competition curves of 50 nmol/L [^{3}H]clonidine binding with 10^{-10} to 10^{-4} mol/L concentrations of inhibitors were generated under co-incubation with 12.5 µmol/L of RX821002 (α$_2$-masked). On caudate sections the total non-adrenergic binding of

TABLE 1. Affinity (K$_i$) values for I-sites in human caudate and platelet sections labeled with 50 nmol/L [^{3}H]clonidine

Competitors	Caudate (nmol/L)	Platelets (nmol/L)
Cirazoline	88.3 ± 2.1	1.7 ± 0.07 (34%)
		5,460 ± 224 (56%)
Tizanidine	175 ± 6.7	100 ± 3.1
Rilmenidine	349 ± 9.8	690 ± 30.1
Harmane	521 ± 12	2,330 ± 111
BDF6143	693 ± 19	493 ± 12.1
Idazoxan	1,330 ± 32	818 ± 27.0
Oxymetazoline	≈36,000[a]	5,180 ± 170
Norepinephrine	≈50,400[a]	≈253,700[a]
Moxonidine	≈55,600[a]	≈59,300[a]
Agmatine	≈100,000[a]	≈236,400[a]

[a] In these cases the non-linear regression fits were forced through y = 0.

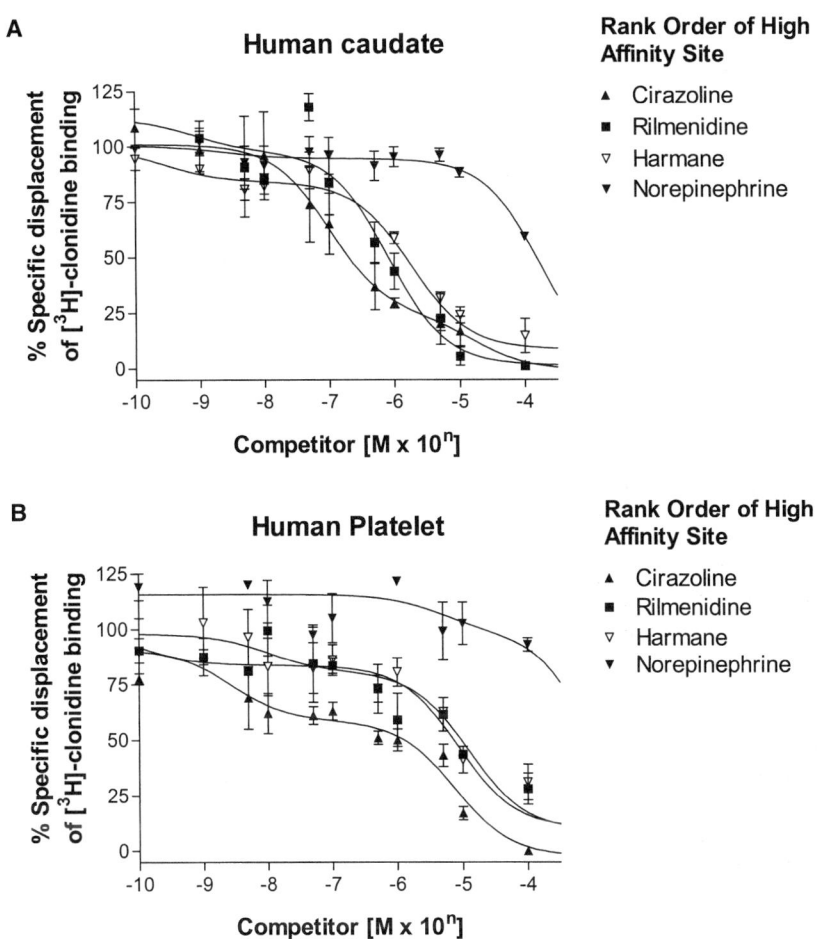

FIGURE 1. Inhibition of binding of [^{3}H]clonidine (50 nmol/L) to I-sites in human (**A**) caudate and (**B**) platelets sections by cirazoline, rilmenidine, harmane, and norepinephrine. In all cases, the binding of [^{3}H]clonidine to α_2-adrenoceptors was masked by adding 12.5 µmol/L RX 81002. Each point represents the mean ± SEM of values generated from two to three separate experiments.

[^{3}H]clonidine amounted to 1,503 ± 222 cpm, whereas non-specific binding in the presence of additional 100 µmol/L cirazoline amounted to 433 ± 28 cpm (i.e., 71.2% I-site specific binding). On platelet plug sections the total non-adrenergic binding amounted to 1,112 ± 171 cpm, whereas non-specific binding amounted to 551 ± 81 cpm (i.e., 50.4% I-site specific binding). Saturation binding experiments confirmed a single class of I-sites on slide-mounted platelet sections; the [^{3}H]clonidine B_{max} was 12.2 ± 4.5 fmol/mg protein and the K_D was 86.8 ± 40.6 nmol/L ($n = 3$).

As shown in TABLE 1 and FIGURE 1, six compounds fully displaced [^{3}H]clonidine binding from both caudate and platelet I-sites on tissue sections. However, 100 µmol/L NE and agmatine displaced no binding. Moxonidine and oxymetazoline could only displace about 50% of [^{3}H]clonidine binding on either tissue. The rank order of IC$_{50}$ values for the six compounds that completely displaced I-sites (generated using a single site model) on human caudate was thus as follows: cirazoline > tizanidine > rilmenidine > harmane > BDF6143 > idazoxan. The rank order of IC$_{50}$ values for I-sites on human platelets was similar: cirazoline > tizanidine > BDF6143 > rilmenidine > idazoxan > harmane. Similar K$_i$ values were also identified by [^{3}H]clonidine for both caudate and platelet I-sites on tissue sections (TABLE 1). Linear analysis showed that the affinity constants (pK$_i$) for the I-sites labeled in human caudate and platelets were highly correlated ($r = 0.90$, $P = 0.0003$).

DISCUSSION

Imidazoline receptors bind clonidine, idazoxan, and other imidazoline-related compounds.[1] All known imidazoline receptors exhibit low affinity for NE and other biogenic amines (K$_i$ values ≥ 100 µmol/L).[1] The two major subclasses, I$_1$ and I$_2$, have been identified based on differential affinities for various imidazoline compounds.[1,3] The I$_1$ receptor, which has preferential affinity for clonidine, is expressed on the platelet cell surface.[3] I$_2$ receptors preferentially bind idazoxan and are localized to the mitochondrial membranes of many cells, including platelets.[3]

The results in TABLE 1 indicate that the I-site labeled autoradiographically by [^{3}H]clonidine in human caudate and platelets lacks identity with the classical I-sites. First, the I$_1$-sensitive ligands, moxonidine and oxymetazoline, possessed very low affinity. This contradicts the rank-order of compounds published[3] for human I$_1$ sites by filtration binding assays, which is moxonidine ≥ oxymetazoline > tizanidine ≥ agmatine ≥ efaroxan = clonidine > cirazoline > BDF6143 >> idazoxan >> NE. Second, the established rank-order for I$_2$ sites in filtration binding assays was also inconsistent with our results: cirazoline > idazoxan >> oxymetzoline > moxonidine ≥ efaroxan > clonidine.[3] Third, the monophasic nature of most of our competition curves tends to dismiss the possibility that a true I$_1$ or I$_2$ site was present in our data, but merely obscured. Instead, our data match closely with a [^{3}H]-cirazoline-labeled I-site described in rat brain and kidney membranes.[8] In our hands, cirazoline was the only competitor with a preferred two-site fit. A previous filtration binding study using [^{125}I]p-iodoclonidine also revealed a biphasic competition curve for cirazoline at platelet I$_1$ sites, but monophasic competition curves for cirazoline at α_{2A}, α_{2B} and α_{2C} binding sites.[11]

The endogenous β-carboline, harmane, displayed moderate affinity in human caudate and platelets (K$_i$ = 521 nmol/L and 2,330 nmol/L, respectively) for I-sites labeled autoradiographically by [^{3}H]clonidine (TABLE 1 and FIG. 1). This supports the candidacy of harmane as an endogenous I-site ligand.[12] Harmane has been reported[12] to have high affinity for I$_1$ and I$_2$ sites and to be active in modulating blood pressure in the central nervous system.

Human caudate and platelets have thus been shown to possess I-sites that have their highest affinity for cirazoline. Because there was no evidence of classical I-sites even though these tissues are known to possess I$_1$ and I$_2$ sites, it is suggested that something about the autoradiographic technique may have converted classical I-sites into atypical I-sites. The buffer may be the main variable, since a filtration procedure with 50 mmol/L buffer has been reported to yield [^{3}H]-cirazoline competition curves which are highly compatible with our data.[8]

ACKNOWLEDGMENTS

We appreciate Gregory Ordway and Craig Stockmeier for providing the human brain tissues, and Sharonda Swilley and Hilary Flint (University of Mississippi Medical Center) for help with tissue sectioning. This research was supported by federal grants MH49248 and MH57601.

REFERENCES

1. ERNSBERGER, P., M.E. GRAVES, L.M. GRAFF, et al. 1995. I$_1$-Imidazoline receptors: definition, characterization, distribution and transmembrane signalling. Ann. N. Y. Acad. Sci. **763:** 22–42.
2. ERNSBERGER, P., J.E. PILETZ, L.M. GRAFF & M.E. GRAVES. 1995. Optimization of radioligand binding assays for I$_1$-imidazoline sites. Ann. N. Y. Acad. Sci. **763:** 163–168.
3. PILETZ, J.E. & K. SLETTEN. 1993. Nonadrenergic imidazoline binding sites on human platelets. J. Pharmacol. Exp. Ther. **267:** 1493–1502.
4. KAMISAKI, Y., T. ISHIKAWA, Y. TAKAO, et al. 1990. Binding of [^{3}H]p-aminoclonidine to two sites, α_2-adrenoceptors and imidazoline binding sites: distribution of imidazoline binding sites in rat brain. Brain Res. **514:** 15–21.
5. PILETZ, J.E., G.A. ORDWAY, H. ZHU, et al. 2000. Autoradiographic comparison of [^{3}H]clonidine binding to non-adrenergic sitres and α_2-adrenergic receptors in human brain. Neuropsychopharmacology **23:** 697–708.
6. GARCIA-SEVILLA, J.A., A. MIRALLES, M. SASTRE, et al. 1995. I$_2$-imidazoline receptors in the healthy and pathologic human brain. Ann. N. Y. Acad. Sci. **763:** 178–193.
7. RADDATZ, R., A. PARINI & S.M. LANIER. 1997. Localization of the imidazoline binding domain on monoamine oxidase B. Mol. Pharmacol. **52:** 549–553.
8. ANGEL, I., M. LE ROUZIC, C. PIMOULE, et al. 1995. [^{3}H]Cirazoline as a tool for the characterization of imidazoline sites. Ann. N. Y. Acad. Sci. **763:** 112–124.
9. CLARKE, R.W. & J. HARRIS. 2002. Rx 821002 as a tool for physiological investigation of alpha (2)-adrenoceptors. CNS Drug Rev. **8:** 177–192.
10. DE VOS, H., G. BRICCA, J. DEKEYSER, et al. 1994. Imidazoline receptors, non-adrenergic idazoxan binding sites, and α_2 adrenoceptors in the human central nervous system. Neuroscience **59:** 589–598.
11. PILETZ, J.E., H. ZHU & D.N. CHIKKALA. 1996. Comparison of ligand binding affinities at human I$_1$-imidazoline binding sites and the high affinity state of α_2-adrenoceptor subtypes. J. Pharmacol. Exp. Ther. **279:** 694–702.
12. HUDSON, A., R. PRICE, R.J. TYACKE, et al. 1999. Harmane, norharmane and tetrahydro beta-carboline have high affinity for rat imidazoline binding sites. Br. J. Pharmacol. **126:** 2P.

Novel Ligands for the Investigation of Imidazoline Receptors and Their Binding Proteins

A.L. HUDSON,[a] R.J. TYACKE,[a] M.D. LALIES,[a] N. DAVIES,[a] D.P. FINN,[a] O. MARTÍ,[b] E. ROBINSON,[a] S. HUSBANDS,[c] M.C.W. MINCHIN,[d] A. KIMURA,[a] AND D.J. NUTT[a]

[a]*Psychopharmacology Unit, School of Medical Sciences, University of Bristol, Bristol BS8 1TD, UK*

[b]*Department de Biologia Cellular de Fisiologia I d'Immunologia, Unitat de Fisiologia Animal, Universitat Autonoma de Barcelona, Barcelona, Spain*

[c]*Department of Pharmacy and Pharmacology, University of Bath, Bath, UK*

[d]*Yamanouchi Research UK, Byfleet, Surrey KT14 6RA, UK*

ABSTRACT: New ligands for imidazoline receptors are described so that these receptors can be more fully explored and understood. BU224, (2-(4,5-dihydroimidaz-2-yl)-quinoline, shows high affinity and is selective for the imidazoline-2 (I_2) class of receptors. BU224 was tested in the rat Porsolt forced swim paradigm where it was found to decrease time spent immobile and increase the time spent swimming, consistent with an antidepressant profile. BU224 was tritiated and, in radioligand binding studies, was found to label a single population of saturable sites with high affinity. In vitro brain autoradiography with [^{3}H]BU224 also showed a pattern of distribution similar to the known labeling of I_2 receptors. A new series of four 2BFI (2-(benzofuranyl)-2-imidazoline) derivatives were investigated as potential ligands for imaging brain I_2 receptors using positron emission tomography (PET). At least two, BU20012 and BU20013, retained high affinity and moderate selectivity and penetrated the brain when administered peripherally in the mouse. 2BFI has undergone the Mannich reaction to immobilized diaminodipropyl amine to fabricate an affinity column, which was used to isolate a protein from rabbit brain; this protein was sequenced and identified as the enzyme creatine kinase.

KEYWORDS: imidazoline receptors; BU224; 2BFI; imidazoline binding sites; creatine kinase

INTRODUCTION

Imidazoline (I) receptors are a heterogeneous group of proteins, which are broadly divided into I_1, I_2, and I_3 sites based on physiologic functions and pharmacologic tools available.[1] There is need for new and novel ligands to explore the func-

Address for correspondence: Dr. Alan L. Hudson, Head of Preclinical Research, Psychopharmacology Unit, School of Medical Sciences, University of Bristol, Bristol BS8 1TD, UK. Voice: (+44) 0 117 928 8608; fax: (+44) 0 117 928 9700.
e-mail: a.l.hudson@bristol.ac.uk

tions and potential therapeutic roles of these proteins in disease states. Much work centers around the I_2 receptor because compounds acting at this site are able to elevate extracellular brain monoamines and may therefore play a role in mood disorders.[2] Previously, we reported that [^{3}H]2-(2-benzofuranyl)-2-imidazoline (2BFI) is a selective ligand for I_2 receptors, and its use in tissue binding studies has revealed the distribution of these receptors in brain using the technique of quantitative autoradiography.[3] 2BFI, in its unlabelled form, has been shown to be active in the Porsolt forced swim paradigm, indicative of antidepressant activity (see Hudson, Nutt, & Husbands[4]). A quinoline-based series of compounds were synthesized, and one of these, BU224 (2-(4,5-dihydroimidaz-2-yl)-quinoline, was found to have high affinity ($K_i = 2.1$ nM) and high selectivity for I_2 receptors in brain membranes.[2] BU224 was able to penetrate the brain following peripheral administration and, typical of I_2 site–selective compounds, BU224 was shown, using in vivo brain dialysis, to elevate extracellular noradrenaline in rat frontal cortex.[2] In view of the biologic profile demonstrated by BU224, further studies were performed with this compound.

CHARACTERIZATION OF BU224

BU224 was investigated in a modified force swim test to see if it could mimic the antidepressant profile of 2BFI. The test was based on a single swim in a cylindrical plastic tank (height 22 cm) filled with warm water (25°C), because these conditions have been shown to produce reliable and dose-dependant effects.[5] Male Sprague-Dawley rats (300–350 g) were injected three times with either sterile saline or BU224 (10 mg/kg) intraperitoneally at 24, 18, and 1 hour before testing. The rats' swimming behavior was recorded on videotape for the first 5 minutes and then analyzed for swimming behavior versus time spent immobile. FIGURE 1A shows that the rats treated with BU224 spent significantly ($P < 0.001$) less time immobile compared with the saline-treated animals. The animals spent significantly ($P < 0.001$) more time mildly swimming (FIG. 1B). This result indicates antidepressant-like activity for BU224 and, taken together with our previous work with 2BFI, suggests that this class of I_2 ligands could possess therapeutic potential for the treatment of depression. It is unknown what mechanism of action is responsible for this profile, but one might speculate that the ability of these compounds to elevate extracellular monoamines in the brain, as demonstrated by in vivo brain dialysis, could be responsible for the antidepressant profile. How 2BFI and BU224 are able to increase extrasynaptic levels of noradrenaline is unknown at present although inhibition of monoamine oxidase remains a possibility.[6,7]

CHARACTERIZATION OF [^{3}H]BU224

A dibrominated form of BU224 was prepared with substitution on the aromatic ring and then catalytic tritium exchange was performed by Dupont NEN (Boston, MA, USA) to yield a ligand of high specific activity. Initial experiments showed that [^{3}H]BU224 bound to rat brain membranes in a specific and saturable manner (B_{max} 119.5 + 45 fmol/mg protein^{-1}) with high affinity ($K_D = 3.2 + 1.7$ nM) and low nonspecific binding.[8] Subsequent experiments demonstrated [^{3}H]BU224 to be a suitable

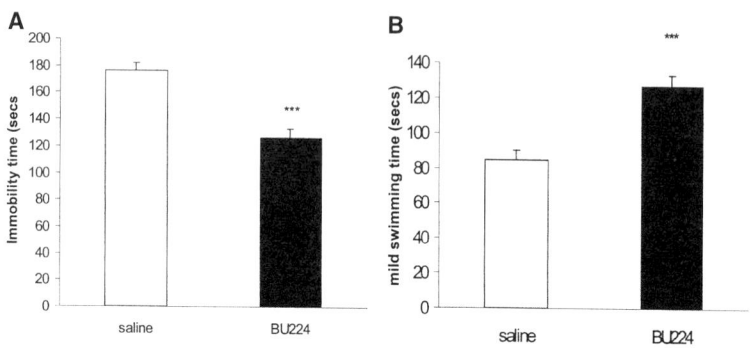

FIGURE 1. The effect of BU224 in the rat Porsolt forced swim test. (**A**) Immobility time. (**B**) Mild swimming time. Mean ± SE mean, N = 8. *** $P < 0.001$. (From Finn et al.,[5] with permission.)

ligand for in vitro autoradiography of I_2 receptors in rat brain. Sections of tissue were incubated with 1 nM of [^{3}H]BU224 alone or with 10 µM 2BFI to define specific binding, apposed to tritium sensitive film for 4 to 6 weeks, and then analyzed on a computerized densitometer. The resulting images showed [^{3}H]BU224 binding to be high in those brain areas known to be dense in I_2 receptors, notably the arcuate nucleus, interpeduncular nucleus, area postrema, pineal gland, and the ependyma (FIG. 2). Subsequent comparisons with the published values of densities obtained using [^{3}H]2BFI and [^{3}H]idazoxan (in the presence of rauwolscine to block α_2-adrenocep-

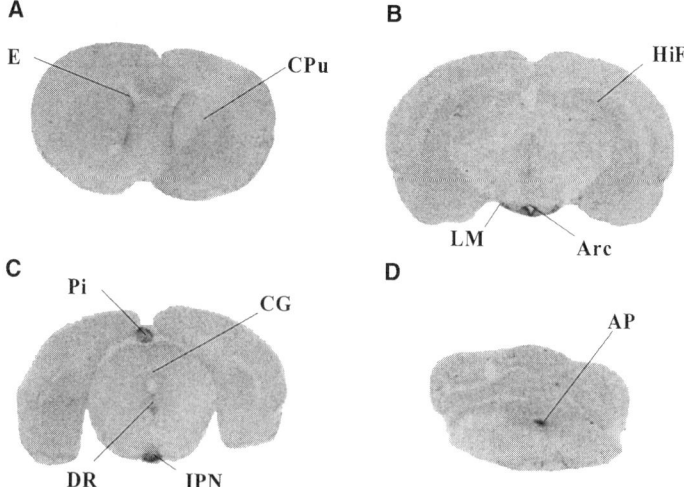

FIGURE 2. Autoradiograms showing the distribution of [3H]BU224 in rat brain. Sections taken from (**A**) bregma 0.26 mm; (**B**) bregma 3.3 mm; (**C**) bregma 7.06 mm; (**D**) bregma 13.8 mm. AP, area postrema; Arc, arcuate nucleus; CG, central grey; CPu, caudate putamen; DR, dorsal raphe; E, ependyma; HiF, hippocampal fissure; IPN, interpeduncular nucleus; LM, Later mammilary body; Pi, pineal gland. (From Robinson et al.,[8] with permission.)

tors) showed a positive correlation for all brain areas analyzed.[8] Overall, these results demonstrated [^{3}H]BU224 to be a useful ligand for the study of I$_2$ receptors.

POTENTIAL PET LIGANDS FOR I$_2$ RECEPTORS

Studies have demonstrated that the density of central I$_2$ receptors changes in a number of disease states (TABLE 1). These changes in density may be a direct or indirect consequence of a particular disease. Monitoring a change in the brain density of I$_2$ receptors may provide a diagnostic tool or an insight into these diseases. Positron emission tomography (PET) is a relatively noninvasive technique in which a suitable positron-emitting moiety such as carbon-11 or fluorine-18 is incorporated into the molecule of interest. A tracer amount of the ligand is then administered to the patient. A PET scanner is used to monitor the gamma emissions and determine a three-dimensional map of the receptor or binding protein in the patient's brain. As an interim step in the development of potential PET ligands to image I$_2$ receptors, we have synthesized and tested four new derivatives of 2BFI for affinity and bioavailability (FIG. 3).

In radioligand binding assays, BU99017 and BU99018, the ethyl and fluoroethyl derivatives of 2BFI, were found to displace [^{3}H]2BFI (1 nM) binding to rat whole-brain membranes in a biphasic manner demonstrating high affinity (nM) for at least 50% of the sites labeled (TABLE 2). BU99017 and BU99018 proved of low affinity for α$_2$-adrenoceptors labeled with the selective ligand [^{3}H]RX821002. The corresponding propyl and fluoropropyl derivatives, BU20012 and BU20013, were of slightly lower affinity for rat brain I$_2$ sites but still showed nM affinity for around 50% of the sites labeled (TABLE 2). Again both compounds demonstrated low affinity for rat brain α$_2$-adrenoceptors, indicating that these ligands are selective for I$_2$ receptors over α$_2$-adrenoceptors. Overall, BU99018 maintained the best affinity and selectivity as compared with the parent compound 2BFI. BU99018 and BU99017 are

TABLE 1. I$_2$ imidazoline receptors identified by radioligand binding in human brain in various pathologic states

Disorder	I$_2$-Imidazoline Receptor	
	[^{3}H]-Idazoxan	[^{3}H]-2BFI
Aging (4–89 yr)	↑(r = 0.59)	
Suicide/depression	↓(40%)	
Opioid addiction	↓(39%)	
Alcohol dependence	No change	No change
Alzheimer's disease	↑(63%)	
Parkinson's disease	No change	No change
Huntington's disease		↓(56%)
Glial tumor	↑(184%)	↑(203%)

Modified from García-Sevilla et al.,[10] 1999.

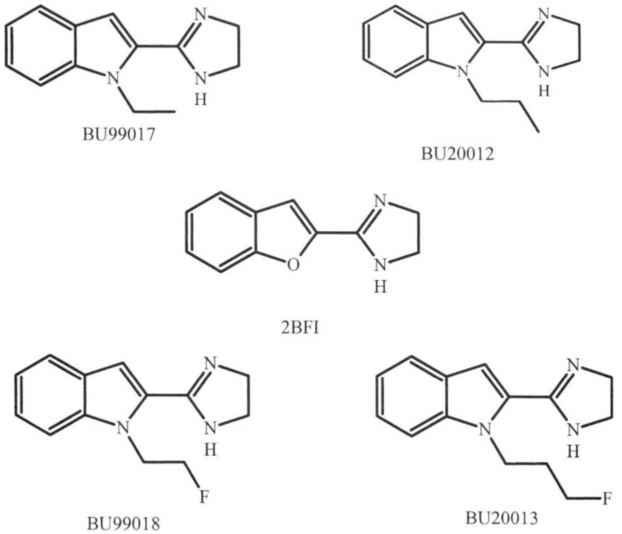

FIGURE 3. The structures of the potential PET ligands BU99017, BU99018, BU20012, and BU20013, which are derivatives of the I_2 receptor–selective ligand 2BFI.

thought to be unstable, however, and therefore further work has been performed with BU20012 and BU20013. Subsequent in vivo experiments in mice (male Swiss, 26–34 g) showed that tail vein administration of BU20012 (0.3, 1.0, 3.0, 10 mg/kg or vehicle) resulted in its subsequent detection in the brain. For this procedure animals were humanely killed 30 minutes after injection. Brains were removed, homogenized in 1 mL of assay buffer, centrifuged, and the resulting supernatant assayed versus [^{3}H]2BFI (1 nM) binding to rat brain membranes to give an estimation of brain concentration of the test compounds. The result of this crude bioassay showed dose-

TABLE 2. Calculated equilibrium dissociation constants (K_i) and selectivity for the test compounds at the I_2-BS and the α_2-adrenoceptor in rat whole-brain membranes

Compound	I_2-BS K_i (nM) ± SD		α_2-adrenoceptor		Selectivity α_2/I_2 high
	High	Low	K_i (nM) ± SD	nH ± SD	
2BFI	1.7 ± 0.2[a]	242 ± 106[a]	3736 ± 147[b]	NA	2198
BU99017	1.8 ± 0.6	403 ± 28	370 ± 31	−0.95 ± 0.03	205
BU99018	3.6 ± 1.9	1964 ± 1458	2584 ± 997	−1.11 ± 0.11	717
BU20012	3.1 ± 1.6	573 ± 83	210 ± 60	−0.98 ± 0.11	68
BU20013	6.0 ± 2.4	1528 ± 571	722 ± 182	−1.00 ± 0.07	120

Data represent the mean of three experiments performed in triplicate ± SD.
[a] From Lione et al.[3]
[b] From Nutt et al.[11]

dependent brain entry of BU20012 indicating good bioavailablity. For example, increasing the dose of BU20012 given intravenously resulted in brain levels reaching µM levels at a dose of 10 mg/kg. These results showed that BU20012 could have good potential as a PET ligand for brain I_2 receptors in future imaging studies in humans

IDENTIFICATION OF AN I_2 BINDING PROTEIN

2-BFI has, with the aid of Pharmalink gel (Pierce Chemical, Rockford, IL, USA), undergone the Mannich reaction to immobilized diaminodipropyl amine, which was then used as the resin for an affinity column. Rabbit (New Zealand white, 2.5–4.0 kg, either sex) whole-brain P_2 membranes were solubilized in the detergent CHAPS (0.5% w/v), centrifuged to remove insoluble matter, and the supernatant loaded onto the 2BFI-affinity column. Following a salt wash to remove nonspecifically bound proteins, idazoxan (20 mM) was used to elute proteins. These proteins were subjected to SDS-polyacrylamide gel electrophoresis, which revealed a strong band with a mass of around 45 kD which was subjected to N-terminal sequencing by Edman degradation. The sequence was found to match the 43-kD protein, creatine kinase (EC 2.7.3.2). Further studies have shown this enzyme to be an I_2 binding protein, and it is now the subject of further experiments (see Kimura *et al.*, this volume).

CONCLUSIONS

This study provides evidence on the usefulness of I_2 site-selective compounds as tools with which to study these receptors. The I_2-selective compound BU224 showed efficacy in the rat Porsolt forced swim paradigm in an antidepressant manner similar to 2BFI. A tritiated form of BU224 has also demonstrated usefulness as a new radioligand for the characterization and visualization of I_2 receptors in rat brain. Several new derivatives of 2BFI with the potential to be labeled with ^{11}C or ^{18}F have shown access to the brain with high affinity and selectivity for I_2 receptors. In their labeled forms, these derivatives could be used to image I_2 sites in human brain using PET. 2BFI has been immobilized to form an affinity column that has retained a protein from solubilized rabbit-brain membranes which was subsequently identified as creatine kinase. Given that I_2 receptors are a family of proteins, it may be possible to design and synthesize subtype selective ligands in the future and increase our understanding of the functions of these receptors.

ACKNOWLEDGMENT

We thank the Wellcome Trust for their generous financial support.

REFERENCES

1. EGLEN, R.M., A.L. HUDSON, D.A. KENDALL, *et al.* 1998. "Seeing through a glass darkly": casting light on imidazoline "I" sites. Trends Pharmacol. Sci. **19:** 381–390.
2. HUDSON, A.L., R. GOUGH, R. TYACKE, *et al.* 1999. Novel selective compounds for the investigation of imidazoline receptors. Ann. N.Y. Acad. Sci. **881:** 81–91.

3. LIONE, L.A., D.J. NUTT & A.L. HUDSON. 1998. Characterisation and localisation of [^{3}H]2-(2-benzofuranyl)-2-imidazoline binding in rat brain: a selective ligand for imidazoline I$_2$ receptors. Eur. J. Pharmacol. **353:** 123–135.
4. HUDSON, A., D. NUTT & S. HUSBANDS. 2001. Imidazoline receptors and their role in depression. Pharmaceutical News **8**(3): 18–24.
5. FINN, D.P., O. MARTÍ, M.S. HARBUZ, et al. 2003. Behavioral, neuroendocrine and neurochemical effects of the imidazoline I$_2$ receptor selective ligand BU224 in naive rats and rats exposed to the stress of the forced swim test. Psychopharmacology **167:** 195–202.
6. LALIES, M.D., A. HIBELL, A.L. HUDSON, et al. 1999. Inhibition of central monoamine oxidase by imidazoline2 site-selective ligands. Ann. N. Y. Acad. Sci. **881:** 114–117.
7. PATERSON, L.M., R.J. TYACKE, D.J. NUTT, et al. 2003. Relationship between imidazoline$_2$ sites and monoamine oxidase. Ann. N. Y. Acad. Sci. This volume.
8. ROBINSON, E.S.J., R.J. TYACKE, D.J. NUTT, et al. 2002. Distribution of [^{3}H]BU224, a selective imidazoline I$_2$ binding site ligand, in rat brain. Eur. J. Pharmacol. **450:** 55–60.
9. KIMURA A., R.J. TYACKE, M.C.W. MINCHIN, D.J. NUTT, et al. 2003. Identification of an I$_2$ binding protein from rabbit brain. Ann. N. Y. Acad. Sci. This volume.
10. GARCÍA-SEVILLA, J.A., P.V. ESCRIBÁ & J. GUIMÓN. 1999. Imidazoline receptors and human brain disorders. Ann. N. Y. Acad. Sci. **881:** 392–409.
11. NUTT, D.J., N. FRENCH, S. HANDLEY, et al. 1995. Functional studies of specific imidazoline-2 receptor ligands. Ann. N. Y. Acad. Sci. **763:** 125–139.

The Effects of Chronic Administration of Inhibitors of Flavin and Quinone Amine Oxidases on Imidazoline I_1 Receptor Density in Rat Whole Brain

ANDREW HOLT, KATHRYN G. TODD, AND GLEN B. BAKER

Neurochemical Research Unit, Department of Psychiatry, 1E7.44 Walter C. Mackenzie Health Sciences Centre, University of Alberta, Edmonton, Alberta, Canada T6G 2B7

ABSTRACT: Many imidazoline ligands have been shown to bind to the active sites of several amine oxidases, and endogenous ligands such as agmatine and tryptamine are amine oxidase substrates. In order to ascertain whether concentrations of endogenous imidazoline receptor agonists might be regulated by amine oxidase activities, rats were administered saline, clorgyline, deprenyl, MDL 72274A, aminoguanidine, or a combination of clorgyline, deprenyl, and aminoguanidine, for 14 days, and then binding parameters for [^{3}H]clonidine at imidazoline I_1 receptors were determined in whole brain. Several EC 1.4.3.4, 1.4.3.6, and 1.5.3.11 amine oxidase activities were also measured ex vivo in tissues from treated animals. Results showed that drug treatments did not alter the affinity of clonidine for imidazoline I_1 receptors. There was a tendency toward a reduction in receptor density when monoamine oxidase (MAO)-A + MAO-B, MAO-B + semicarbazide-sensitive amine oxidase (SSAO), or SSAO + diamine oxidase (DAO) were inhibited, and a marked reduction in density when MAO-A + MAO-B + SSAO were inhibited. These data suggest that amines that are substrates both for MAO and for SSAO, such as tryptamine and other trace amines, may act as endogenous imidazoline I_1 receptor agonists, at which they may have neuromodulatory efficacy. A role for β-carbolines, which can form endogenously from tryptamine, is also supported by the present findings.

KEYWORDS: imidazoline I_1 receptor; I_1 agonists; rat brain; clonidine; monoamine oxidase; MAO; semicarbazide-sensitive amine oxidase; SSAO; clorgyline; deprenyl; aminoguanidine; MDL 72274A; agmatine; tryptamine; trace amines; β-carbolines

INTRODUCTION

The contention that a physical link exists between amine oxidase enzymes and imidazoline binding sites is beyond argument. The presence of a high affinity site on

---

Address for correspondence: Andrew Holt, AL*viva* Biopharmaceuticals Inc., 218-111 Research Drive, Saskatoon, Saskatchewan, Canada S7N 3R2. Voice: 306-956-6884; fax: 306-956-6877.
e-mail: aholt@alviva.ca

monoamine oxidase (EC 1.4.3.4; MAO) that binds a variety of imidazoline receptor site (IR) ligands has been clearly established,[1,2] while inhibition of MAO as a result of secondary interactions of such ligands with the enzyme active site has also been confirmed.[2–4] However, the failure of researchers to demonstrate any effects of IR ligands on MAO activity through binding to the high affinity site, as well as the inconsequential nature of the low affinity active site-directed inhibition, support the view that while physical links between MAO and IR certainly exist, functional links may not.

In contrast, evidence appears outwardly supportive of the existence of both physical and functional relations between IR and EC 1.4.3.6 amine oxidase enzymes. This nebulous group of copper-containing glycoproteins, which share trihydroxyphenylalanine quinone as a redox-active cofactor,[5,6] remain largely unaffected by classical MAO inhibitors but are sensitive to inhibition by semicarbazide and other carbonyl reagents.[7] Accordingly, the somewhat unsatisfactory term "semicarbazide-sensitive amine oxidase" (SSAO) is most often used to identify these enzymes, although its use is usually restricted to specify only those tissue-bound SSAO enzymes found predominantly in the vasculature and on adipocytes. Soluble SSAO enzymes are rather referred to as plasma amine oxidases (PAO), or as diamine oxidase (DAO) for those cytoplasmic SSAO enzymes found, for example, in kidney and intestinal tissue. In addition to observations of low affinity inhibition of bovine PAO by several imidazoline ligands,[3] an endogenous imidazoline receptor ligand, agmatine,[8] is a reasonably good substrate for porcine[9] and rat[10] kidney DAO activities. However, the idea that DAO might regulate the availability of agmatine to act as an agonist at imidazoline receptors is questionable, exemplified by the preponderance of agmatine and imidazoline receptors, and the paucity of DAO activity, in the brain. Thus, the nature of any functional interplay between amine oxidases and imidazoline receptors or binding sites remains unclear.

A review of literature covering these areas brings to light a remarkable pattern of apparent coincidences, in that many ligands acting with some selectivity at the active sites of several EC 1.4.3.4 or 1.4.3.6 amine oxidases, or at I_1 receptors or I_2 binding sites, exhibit a consistent ability to cross-react with most or all of the other enzymes or receptors in this group. Although these are too numerous to list here, the notable exception in this regard is the failure of recognized amine oxidase inhibitors to bind to imidazoline I_1 receptors. Nevertheless, what can be deduced from these observations of cross-compatibility is that some degree of structural similarity, both steric and electronic, must exist between the active sites of several amine oxidases and imidazoline receptors or binding sites. Perhaps the most obvious explanation for the existence of this structural similarity is that the enzymes share with the receptors one or more common endogenous ligands. However, in the absence of further evidence, trying to predict the identity of these ligands would be a somewhat baseless exercise.

Most endogenous receptor ligands are agonists, and many receptors respond to a prolonged increase in agonist concentration with a shift in equilibrium favoring intracellular receptor localization followed by uncoupling from second messenger mechanisms, internalization, and eventually receptor down-regulation.[11] Based on the assumption that one or more substrates for one or more amine oxidases act as agonists at imidazoline receptors, we attempted to exploit this response by administering selective amine oxidase inhibitors to rats for two weeks and determining the effects of treatments on imidazoline receptor density. In the event that receptor down-regulation was observed, a detailed analysis of amine oxidase inhibition in the same animals should provide information regarding the relative contributions of different amine oxidases to turnover of the proposed agonist, and thus information on possible candidates that might fulfill this role.

METHODS

Animal Treatment Regimens

Male Sprague-Dawley rats (230–280 g), obtained from Ellerslie Biosciences (Edmonton, Canada), were housed in pairs in an environmentally-controlled room, with a 12 hour light-dark cycle and with access to standard rat chow and water ad libitum. Animals were randomized and divided into six treatment groups of eight rats. Drugs were administered by IP injection in a volume of 1 mL/kg, once daily for 14 days, as indicated in TABLE 1. While single drug treatment with phenelzine would have achieved substantial inhibition of MAO, SSAO, and DAO, the use of a combination of more selective amine oxidase inhibitors was preferred, since phenelzine would also inhibit pyridoxal-dependent enzymes, including decarboxylases involved in the synthesis of a variety of amines such as agmatine. In this regard, while aminoguanidine can be thought of as selective in terms of amine oxidase inhibition, it is nevertheless recognized that enzymes such as nitric oxide synthase (NOS) are targets for this inhibitor.[17] However, in the present experiments, we considered that inhibition of NOS would be unlikely to influence imidazoline receptor density, whereas inhibition of decarboxylases might be expected to have an effect in this respect.

Twenty-four hours after the last injection, animals were killed by decapitation, and brains, livers, lungs, and a 5 cm section of small intestine were removed, washed rapidly in ice-cold saline and frozen on solid CO_2 prior to storage at $-70°C$ until required.

TABLE 1. Amine oxidase inhibitors used, with abbreviations (column 2), intended targets, and references supporting the choice of inhibitor and dose with respect to the intended targets

Drug Treatment		Intended Enzyme Target(s)	References
Vehicle (saline)	VEH	—	—
Clorgyline (2 mg/kg)	CLRG	MAO-A	12
(-)-Deprenyl (1 mg/kg)	DEP	MAO-B	13
MDL-72274A (2 mg/kg)	MDL	SSAO (+ PAO)	14
Aminoguanidine (10 mg/kg)	AG	DAO + SSAO	15, 16
Clorgyline + Deprenyl + Aminoguanidine	COMB	MAO-A + -B + SSAO + DAO	—

Analysis of [^{3}H]clonidine Binding to Rat Whole Brain Membranes

A decision was made to examine the effects of amine oxidase inhibitors on the density of I_1, rather than I_2 or I_3, receptors, for two main reasons: the evidence that I_1 binding sites corresponded to true receptors was far more compelling than for I_2 or I_3 sites, and little evidence existed for direct binding of amine oxidase inhibitors to I_1 receptors, reducing the likelihood of effects on receptor density occurring through a mechanism unrelated to enzyme inhibition.

The procedure used to determine binding constants for [^{3}H]clonidine to rat brain I_1 receptors was based on that described by Ernsberger et al.[18] Whole brains were homogenized gently in 20 volumes of 0.32 mol/L sucrose containing phenylmethylsulphonyl fluoride (50 µmol/L) and buffered to pH 7.5 at 25°C with Tris base. Homogenates were centrifuged at $1000 \times g$ and 4°C for 5 minutes. The supernatants were further centrifuged at $50,000 \times g$ and 4°C for 20 minutes. The P2 (plasma membrane) pellets were resuspended in approximately 10 volumes of Tris (50 mmol/L, pH 8.0 at 25°C) containing ethylenediaminetetraacetic acid (EDTA; 5 mmol/L). In order to reduce background interference, membranes were washed by centrifugation ($50,000 \times g$, 4°C, 20 minutes), pellets were resuspended in Tris containing NaCl (25 mmol/L) and preincubated at 25°C for 30 minutes. Homogenates were subjected to further centifugation ($50,000 \times g$, 4°C, 20 minutes), pellets were resuspended in Tris and centrifuged once more, as described above. Pellets were frozen rapidly on isopentane/solid CO_2 and were stored at –70°C for no more than 7 days.

Prior to binding analyses, pellets were thawed gently and resuspended in binding buffer (HEPES [5 mmol/L, pH 7.8] containing EDTA [500 µmol/L], egtazic acid [EGTA; 500 µmol/L], $MgCl_2$ [500 µmol/L], and ascorbic acid [100 µmol/L], to a final protein concentration of approximately 0.5 mg/mL. The use of a KCl pH electrode was avoided during binding buffer preparation.

Eight-point binding curves were determined in triplicate for both total and nonspecific binding, in washed glass tubes. Assays, in a volume of 500 µL, contained brain homogenate (200 µL), [^{3}H]clonidine (100 µL, assay concentrations 1.25 nmol/L [67 Ci/mmol] to 24 nmol/L [3.6 Ci/mmol]), noradrenaline (100 µL, assay concentration 100 µmol/L, to mask α2-adrenergic receptors), and either incubation buffer (100 µL, in total binding assays) or cirazoline (100 µL, assay concentration 10 µmol/L, in non-specific binding assays). Assays were initiated by addition of homogenate, and after vortex-mixing, samples were incubated at 22°C for 30 minutes. Cell membranes were collected on Whatman GF/B paper pre-treated with polyethyleneimine (0.3% vol/vol, 4°C, 4 hours) and were washed rapidly four times with 3 mL of icecold Tris buffer (pH 8.07 at 5°C). Filters were counted for tritium in Ready-Safe scintillation cocktail for 3 minutes.

Determination of Amine Oxidase Activities Ex Vivo

MAO-A and MAO-B activities in liver homogenates, and SSAO activity in lung homogenates, were determined radiochemically as described previously,[19,20] with [^{14}C]5-HT (250 µmol/L, 1 µCi/µmol), [^{14}C]β-phenylethylamine (50 µmol/L, 1 µCi/µmol), and [^{14}C]benzylamine (5 µmol/L, 10 µCi/µmol) as respective substrates. Lung homogenates were preincubated with deprenyl (1 µmol/L, 37°C, 30 min) to inhibit any MAO-B present that may contribute to metabolism of benzylamine.

DAO in intestinal homogenates was measured by a peroxidase-linked absorbance assay, modified from that described by Holt et al.[21] Intestines were homogenized in 10 volumes of potassium phosphate buffer (50 mmol/L, pH 7.4), endogenous amines were oxidized by adding approximately 10 mg of MnO_2, and samples were centrifuged at $1800 \times g$ for 10 minutes. Supernatants were retained, with care taken to ensure that no MnO_2 was transferred with the supernatants. Assays, done in triplicate, contained homogenate (100 μL) and a mixture of chromogen and substrate (200 μL). The chromogenic portion of the mixture, prepared in phosphate buffer, was composed of 4-aminoantipyrine (600 μmol/L), 2,4-dichlorophenol (600 μmol/L), and horseradish peroxidase (type II; 4 IU/mL), while the substrate was putrescine (150 μmol/L). Assay concentrations of these constituents were thus two-thirds of initial concentrations. Blanks contained phosphate buffer in place of homogenate. The change in absorbance in each well was monitored continuously at 498 nm in a Molecular Devices SPECTRAmax Plus platereader, and DAO activities were determined by linear regression analyses of data to yield initial rates.

Polyamine oxidase (EC 1.5.3.11) was also measured in intestinal homogenates. Drug treatments were not expected to affect this enzyme. However, since any perturbations to polyamine cycling might indirectly affect agmatine levels through a feedback mechanism, it was felt prudent to ensure that this enzyme system had remained unaltered by drug administration. Polyamine oxidase was measured in a manner identical to that used for DAO measurements, except that N^1-acetylspermine (150 μmol/L) replaced putrescine in the chromogen/substrate mixture. In addition, homogenates were preincubated with aminoguanidine (100 nmol/L, 37°C, 10 minutes) to inhibit intestinal DAO; the product of polyamine oxidase-mediated N^1-acetylspermine metabolism is putrescine, which would be further metabolized by DAO, resulting in anomalously high rates of change in absorbance.

Data Analysis

The coefficients of variation (CV) of triplicate values obtained in binding experiments were examined and either single outlying dpm values, or mean triplicate values, were discarded in those cases where CV was greater than 12%. The dpm values were then corrected for protein content[22] and were converted to fmol/mg protein following determination of specific activities of the clonidine solutions used. One site hyperbolic binding curves were fitted to specific binding data with the nonlinear regression facility of GraphPad Prism 3.03 (GraphPad Software, San Diego, CA) and K_D and B_{max} data were obtained. Application of a two-site equation did not improve the fits obtained.

Statistical comparisons between groups in binding and enzyme assays were made by one-way ANOVA followed by Tukey's post hoc test (GraphPad Prism 3.03).

Materials

[Benzene ring-^{3}H]clonidine hydrochloride, 5-[2-^{14}C]hydroxytryptamine binoxalate, and β-[ethyl-1-^{14}C]phenylethylamine hydrochloride were purchased from New England Nuclear (Boston, MA). [7-^{14}C]Benzylamine hydrochloride was obtained from Amersham (UK). Clorgyline, clonidine, aminoguanidine, benzylamine, 5-hydroxytryptamine, β-phenylethylamine, putrescine, and N^1-acetylspermine were obtained as their hydrochloride salts from Sigma (St. Louis, MO). (−)Deprenyl hydrochloride was purchased from RBI (Natick, MA). MDL-72274A was a gift

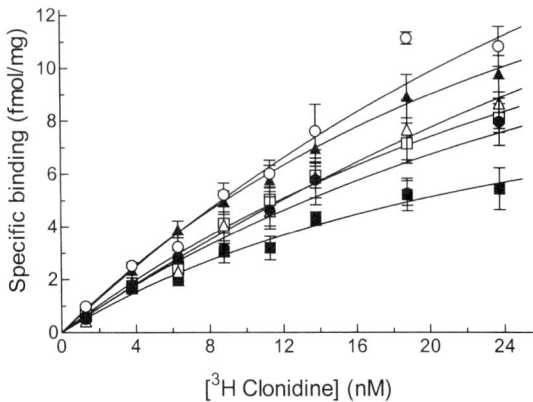

FIGURE 1. Effects of chronic amine oxidase inhibitor administration on specific binding of clonidine (1.25-24 nmol/L) to imidazoline I_1 sites in rat whole brain. Treatment groups were VEH (*open circles*), CLRG (*closed circles*), DEP (*open triangles*), AG (*closed triangles*), MDL (*open squares*) and COMB (*closed squares*). Abbreviations are as listed on Table 1.

from Dr. R. Knippenberg (Hoescht Marion Roussel Inc., Bridgewater, NJ), and cirazoline was a gift from Dr. V. Rovei (Synthelabo Recherche, Bagneux, France). All other assay constituents were of research grade.

RESULTS

FIGURE 1 shows specific binding curves obtained for each of the treatment groups, and TABLE 2 lists binding constants obtained from these data. While we expected K_D values to lie in the low nanomolar range,[18] those measured were rather higher, with the result that the highest concentration of radioligand used (24 nmol/L) was rather lower than the mean K_D value. Consequently, it was not possible to establish B_{max} values, and thus K_D values, with any degree of confidence.

Since differences in K_D values observed did not approach statistical significance, this problem was circumvented by comparing specific binding at individual radio-

TABLE 2. Effects of chronic amine oxidase inhibitor administration on single-site binding parameters for clonidine binding to rat brain I_1 receptors

Group	VEH	CLRG	DEP	MDL	AG	COMB
K_D (nmol/L)	57.0 ± 26.0	43.7 ± 22.8	84.1 ± 77.2	43.3 ± 16.4	34.8 ± 11.5	28.9 ± 12.9
B_{max} (fmol/mg)	37.9 ± 13.4	21.4 ± 8.1	40.2 ± 30.9	23.4 ± 6.4	24.6 ± 5.7	12.5 ± 3.7

Data obtained from nonlinear regression analyses of the specific binding data presented in Figure 1.

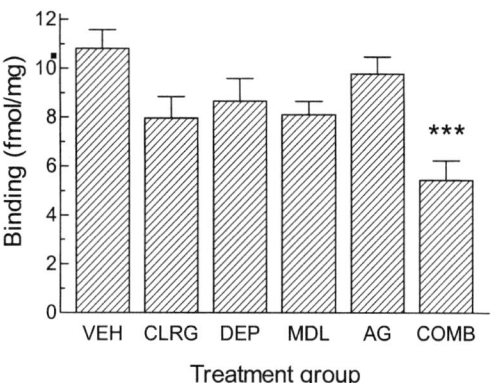

FIGURE 2. Effects of chronic amine oxidase inhibitor administration on single point clonidine binding (24 nmol/L) to rat brain I_1 receptors. Abbreviations are as listed in Table 1. *** $P < 0.001$, compared with VEH group (one-way ANOVA followed by Tukey's Multiple Comparison post hoc test).

ligand concentrations (single point binding). FIGURE 2 shows how binding of clonidine at 24 nmol/L varied between treatment groups; this pattern of variation was similar at the other (lower) clonidine concentrations (not shown). A substantial (50%) and highly significant ($P < 0.001$) reduction in clonidine binding was evident in the combination treatment group, while moderate but not significant reductions were observed in clorgyline and MDL-72274A groups.

The effects of inhibitor treatments on amine oxidase activities ex vivo are shown in FIGURE 3. Polyamine oxidase activities were unaltered by any of the drug treatments, and results are not shown. MAO-A was inhibited substantially by clorgyline, although chronic deprenyl also caused a significant degree of inhibition. A similar observation was made for MAO-B, against which deprenyl was relatively effective, but clorgyline also had significant potency. Furthermore, MDL-72274A, which is a potent and selective SSAO inhibitor in vitro, failed to maintain these attributes in vivo, causing moderate inhibition of both SSAO and MAO-B. SSAO was also inhibited effectively by aminoguanidine, which showed no potency versus either MAO isozyme. All three enzymes were inhibited effectively by combination drug treatment. Interestingly, while aminoguanidine was a potent inhibitor of DAO, this enzyme appeared to be resistant to inhibition when other amine oxidases had been inhibited by combination drug treatment. This was not due to loss, or chemical instability or reactivity, of aminoguanidine in the presence of other inhibitors, since it maintained its effectiveness versus SSAO in the combination group. It is possible that DAO may become resistant in order to compensate for lost MAO and SSAO activities; SSAO may play such a role under conditions of compromised MAO activities.[23]

TABLE 3 provides an overview of data from single point binding and enzyme inhibition assessments. The greatest reduction in receptor density was observed following substantial inhibition of MAO-A, MAO-B, and SSAO. If both MAO isozymes were inhibited to some degree, without a substantial effect on SSAO, with either clorgyline or deprenyl, effects on receptor density were minor and just failed to reach statistical significance. The individual contributions of MAO-A and MAO-B could not be estimated from the available data, although similar reductions in receptor density in the clorgyline group (MAO-A and -B inhibited) and in the MDL-72274A group (MAO-B and SSAO inhibited), coupled with the failure of substantial inhibition of SSAO with aminoguanidine to alter receptor density, certainly indicates that

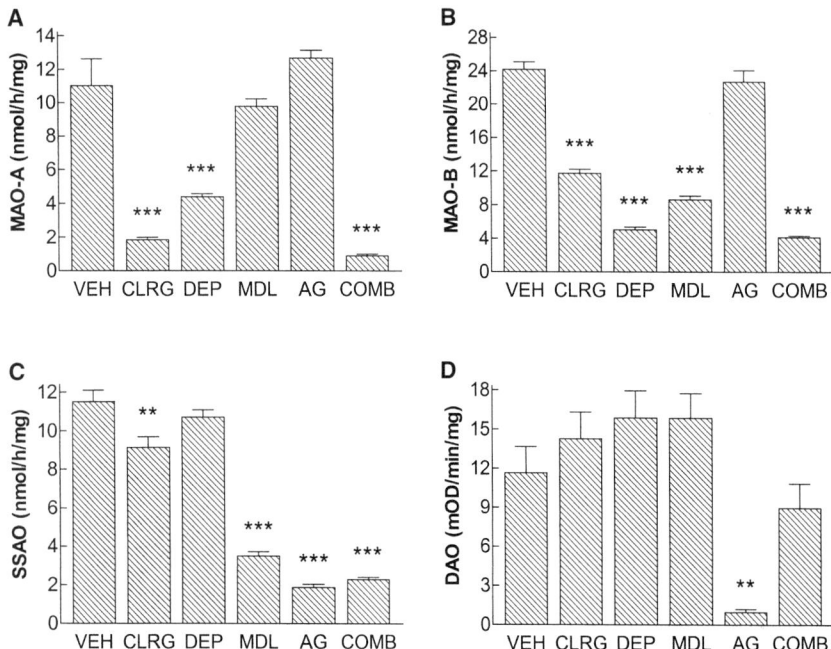

FIGURE 3. Ex vivo effects of chronic amine oxidase inhibitor administration on (**A**) liver MAO-A, (**B**) liver MAO-B, (**C**) lung SSAO, and (**D**) intestinal DAO activities in the rat. Abbreviations are as listed in Table 1. ** $P < 0.01$, *** $P < 0.001$, compared with VEH group (one-way ANOVA followed by Tukey's Multiple Comparison post hoc test).

TABLE 3. Summary of the effects of amine oxidase inhibitor treatments on clonidine binding (single point data from Figure 2) and amine oxidase activities ex vivo (data from Figure 3)

	MAO-A	MAO-B	SSAO	DAO	Binding
CLRG	↓↓↓↓***	↓↓***	↓**	—	↓
DEP	↓↓***	↓↓↓***	—	—	↓
MDL	—	↓↓↓***	↓↓↓***	—	↓
AG	—	—	↓↓↓↓***	↓↓↓↓**	—
COMB	↓↓↓↓***	↓↓↓↓***	↓↓↓↓***	↓	↓↓***

A dash indicates a drug-induced reduction in enzyme activity or clonidine binding of less than 20%, while one, two, three, or four downward arrows indicate reductions in enzyme activity or binding by 20–40%, 40–60%, 60–80%, and greater than 80%, respectively.

** $P < 0.01$.
*** $P < 0.001$.

both forms of MAO, as well as SSAO, play a role. Results from the aminoguanidine group also suggested that any contribution of DAO to turnover of an endogenous I_1 agonist would be insubstantial.

The available data thus suggest that the most likely candidate for an endogenous I_1 agonist is a substrate for both forms of MAO, as well as for SSAO, but probably not for DAO.

DISCUSSION

Currently, the most popular candidate for an endogenous imidazoline receptor agonist is agmatine,[8,24–26] although this polyamine does not mimic the effects of synthetic imidazoline receptor agonists in many respects (for example,[27–29]). Agmatine is a good DAO substrate[9,10] although DAO activity in brain is extremely low. It is also metabolized by tissue-bound SSAO from porcine aorta (A. Holt, unpublished observation), this enzyme being present in brain microvasculature.[30] It has been presumed that the involvement of MAO in agmatine oxidation is most unlikely, given that agmatine is a polyamine with two primary amine groups,[25] and we have been unable to detect agmatine turnover by MAO in rat brain homogenates in a peroxidase-coupled assay at concentrations of the amine up to 4 mmol/L (A. Holt, unpublished observation). However, tissue-bound SSAO enzymes are also, in general, thought not to use diamines or polyamines as substrates (although histamine is a substrate in some tissues), and the involvement of MAO in other tissues or species thus should not be precluded entirely at this time. Indeed, Raasch et al.[31] described loss of agmatine in rat liver homogenates, which could have been due to oxidation by MAO, as well as what appeared to be a biphasic inhibition of kynuramine deaminating activity in rat liver mitochondria, perhaps indicating selectivity of agmatine for one form of MAO over the other. The higher affinity component had an IC_{50} of less than 10 µmol/L, some 500-fold lower than the K_m for agmatine metabolism by rat brain mitochondrial agmatinase,[32] and while the concentration of agmatine in whole rat brain (2.4 ng/g, or approximately 18 nmol/L)[33] is very much lower than these values, the possibility of micromolar, or even millimolar, concentrations of agmatine in intracellular compartments in distinct brain regions is very real.[25] Since endogenous enzyme substrates often exist at concentrations at or a little below the K_m values for the enzymes responsible for their degradation, which allows those enzymes to respond immediately to changes in substrate concentration with changes in activity, then any demonstration of agmatine metabolism by MAO with a micromolar K_m value suggests that MAO may be more important than agmatinase with respect to regulation of brain agmatine concentrations.

In the present study, the possibility certainly exists that agmatinase might have been inhibited by one or more of the amine oxidase inhibitors used. The most likely candidate to have had such an effect would have been aminoguanidine, since bacterial agmatinase, at least, is inhibited by agmatine analogues.[34] However, the failure of aminoguanidine alone to alter receptor density suggests that any such interaction would likely be of secondary importance.

Besides agmatine, other amine oxidase substrates have been reported to bind to IR. Tryptamine, 5-HT, and histamine had higher affinities for I_2 sites in rat and rabbit brain than did agmatine.[35] Of these, tryptamine had the highest affinity (26.7 µmol/L in rat, 3.0 µmol/L in rabbit) and is the only one metabolized by both forms of MAO, as well as SSAO.[36] Other substrates shared by MAO and SSAO include β-phenylethylamine, *m*- and *p*-tyramine, and dopamine,[7,36] although high affinity of these amines for I_1 or I_2 sites has not been demonstrated. Nevertheless, tryptamine, β-phenylethylamine, and *m*- and *p*-tyramine are of particular interest as novel endogenous agonists. These amines belong to a small group of ligands known as the trace amines,[37] the other member of which is octopamine, a substrate for MAO but not SSAO. While the existence of specific receptors for trace amines has been known for several years,[38,39] these have come to prominence recently following the cloning of a family of human trace amine receptors[40] at which trace amines appear to act as agonists.[41] Interestingly, human trace amine receptors have been implicated in the etiology of affective disorders,[40] and administration of the antidepressant amine oxidase inhibitor, tranylcypromine, at doses that might be expected to inhibit MAO and SSAO, resulted in a down-regulation of tryptamine receptors in much the same way as occurred with I_1 receptors in the present study.[42] Similarly, chronic phenelzine administration, which would inhibit MAO and SSAO, resulted in a more substantial down-regulation of tryptamine receptors than did treatment with the MAO-A-selective antidepressant, moclobemide.[43] In addition, functional studies have suggested that trace amine agonists act as neuromodulators, rather than neurotransmitters,[44,45] and some of the synergistic interactions observed between central imidazolinergic and adrenergic systems in blood pressure control[26,46] are consistent with a neuromodulatory role for imidazoline agonists. Thus, some trace amine receptors share with some imidazoline receptors common ligands, common pathophysiologic implications[47] and responses to drug administration, and a common proposed neuromodulatory action.[26,48] It is an intriguing possibility that some of the imidazoline receptor subtypes described thus far might represent subtypes, perhaps as yet uncharacterized, of trace amine receptors.

While tryptamine, on the basis of the evidence presented here, might seem to be a reasonable candidate as an endogenous I_1 agonist, its micromolar affinity for IR (albeit for I_2 sites)[35] has been used as an argument against this likelihood, particularly when compared with the nanomolar affinities attainable with synthetic compounds. However, the affinities of numerous endogenous neurotransmitters for their receptors lie in the low micromolar range[49] and if tryptamine or other trace amines are to be discounted as potential endogenous I_1 agonists, it should instead be because of a lack of efficacy in functional studies, if such a lack exists. That said, endogenous ligands have been described for I_1 receptors which do indeed bind with nanomolar affinites. The β-carbolines can be formed chemically through a Pictet-Spengler condensation reaction between indolealkylamines, such as tryptamine, and an aldehyde,[50] a reaction that would be expected to yield higher concentrations of product in the presence of elevated concentrations of reactants. Nanomolar affinities have been demonstrated for several β-carbolines, as well as dihydro- and tetrahydro-β-carbolines, at both I_1 receptors and I_2 binding sites.[51] Furthermore, observations by Musgrave and Badoer[52] suggest that the β-carboline harmane acts as an agonist at I_1 receptors to produce hypotension when injected into the rostral ventrolateral medulla of the rat.

While β-carbolines are not themselves amine oxidase substrates, they are formed endogenously from such compounds, and thus might be expected to increase in concentration following administration of appropriate amine oxidase inhibitors. Intriguingly, it has recently been demonstrated that the product of agmatine oxidation by a plant copper amine oxidase from *Pisum sativum* is N-amidino-2-hydroxypyrrolidine.[53] This compound forms as a result of an internal cyclization of 4-guanidinbutyraldehyde, the oxidation product of agmatine metabolism presumed to be released by diamine oxidase.[9,54] However, no agmatine aldehyde could be detected in bulk solvent during incubation of agmatine with the *Pisum sativum* enzyme; rather, only the cyclic pyrrolidine was present, and the authors suggested that cyclisation may even take place within the active site of the enzyme.[53] Remarkably, the pyrrolidine was shown to inhibit NOS enzymes rather more potently than did agmatine, while it was equipotent with agmatine in displacing clonidine from rat heart I_1 receptors. If this pyrrolidine product of agmatine oxidation by amine oxidases can also act as an agonist at I_1 receptors, then a response of down-regulation following amine oxidase inhibition, as was observed in the present study, would be unexpected. It is thus possible that N-amidino-2-hydroxypyrrolidine is devoid of efficacy and might thus act to antagonize the effects of agmatine, and the concentration ratios of agmatine to N-amidino-2-hydroxypyrrolidine in different tissues would then assume some degree of functional importance. Alternatively, such a cyclization reaction might be specific to the plant enzyme. It is thought that pyrrolines, formed by cyclization of aldehydes of diamines and polyamines, play important roles in plant physiology.[55] However, while substrates and products may be shared between plant and mammalian copper amine oxidases, catalytic mechanisms may be different, and it should not be assumed that N-amidino-2-hydroxypyrrolidine would indeed be formed following oxidation of agmatine by mammalian SSAO (and DAO) enzymes.[56,57]

In summary, we have shown that substantial inhibition of MAO-A and/or MAO-B, in combination with inhibition of SSAO, results in a substantial and significant down-regulation of rat brain I_1 sites. The effects on receptor density of inhibition of MAO isoforms in the absence of SSAO inhibition were less marked, suggesting that the endogenous agonist increased in concentration by amine oxidase inhibition and responsible for receptor down-regulation is a substrate for both MAO and SSAO. While agmatine should not be precluded as a candidate, the involvement of tryptamine and/or other trace amines as well as β-carbolines that can form endogenously from tryptamine and that are thought to act as agonists at I_1 receptors, seem to be supported by the present findings.

REFERENCES

1. REMAURY, A., R. RADDATZ, C. ORDENER, *et al.* 2000. Analysis of the pharmacological and molecular heterogeneity of I(2)-imidazoline-binding proteins using monoamine oxidase-deficient mouse models. Mol. Pharmacol. **58:** 1085–1090.
2. RADDATZ, R., S.L. SAVIC, V. BAKTHAVACHALAM, *et al.* 2000. Imidazoline-binding domains on monoamine oxidase B and subpopulations of enzyme. J. Pharmacol. Exp. Ther. **292:** 1135–1145.
3. CARPÉNÉ, C., P. COLLON, A. REMAURY, *et al.* 1995. Inhibition of amine oxidase activity by derivatives that recognize imidazoline I_2 sites. J. Pharmacol. Exp. Ther. **272:** 681–688.
4. OZAITA, A., G. OLMOS, M.A. BORONAT, *et al.* 1997. Inhibition of monoamine oxidase A and B activities by imidazol(ine)/guanidine drugs, nature of the interaction and distinction from I_2-imidazoline receptors in rat liver. Br. J. Pharmacol. **121:** 901–912.
5. JANES, S.M., M.M. PALCIC, C.H. SCAMAN, *et al.* 1992. Identification of topaquinone and its consensus sequence in copper amine oxidases. Biochemistry **31:** 12147–12154.

6. HOLT, A., G. ALTON, C. SCAMAN, et al. 1998. Identification of the quinone cofactor in mammalian semicarbazide-sensitive amine oxidase. Biochemistry **37:** 4946–4957.
7. LYLES, G.A. 1996. Mammalian plasma and tissue-bound semicarbazide-sensitive amine oxidases: biological, pharmacological and toxicological aspects. Int. J. Biochem. Cell Biol. **28:** 259–274.
8. LI, G., S. REGUNATHAN, C.J. BARROW, et al. 1994. Agmatine: an endogenous clonidine-displacing substance in the brain. Science **263:** 966–969.
9. HOLT, A. & G.B. BAKER. 1995. Metabolism of agmatine (clonidine-displacing substance) by diamine oxidase and the possible implications for studies of imidazoline receptors. Prog. Brain Res. **106:** 187–197.
10. LORTIE, M.J., W.F. NOVOTNY, O.W. PETERSON, et al. 1996. Agmatine, a bioactive metabolite of arginine. Production, degradation, and functional effects in the kidney of the rat. J. Clin. Invest. **97:** 413–420.
11. KOENIG, J.A. & J.M. EDWARDSON. 1997. Endocytosis and recycling of G protein-coupled receptors. Trends Pharmacol. Sci. **18:** 276–287.
12. CAMPBELL, I.C., D.S. ROBINSON, W. LOVENBERG & D.L. MURPHY. 1979. The effects of chronic regimens of clorgyline and pargyline on monoamine metabolism in the rat brain. J. Neurochem. **32:** 49–55.
13. MURPHY, M.P., P.H. WU, N.W. MILGRAM & G.O. IVY. 1993. Monoamine oxidase inhibition by L-deprenyl depends on both sex and route of administration in the rat. Neurochem. Res. **18:** 1299–1304.
14. PALFREYMAN, M.G., I.A. MCDONALD, P. BEY, et al. 1986. The rational design of suicide substrates of amine oxidases. Biochem. Soc. Trans. **14:** 410–413.
15. YU, P.H. & D.-M. ZUO. 1997. Aminoguanidine inhibits semicarbazide-sensitive amine oxidase activity: implications for advanced glycation and diabetic complications. Diabetologia **40:** 1243–1250.
16. SHORE, P.A. & V.H.J. COHN. 1960. Comparative effects of monoamine oxidase inhibitors on monoamine oxidase and diamine oxidase. Biochem. Pharmacol. **5:** 91–95.
17. BRYK, R. & D.J. WOLFF. 1998. Mechanism of inducible nitric oxide synthase inactivation by aminoguanidine and L-N^6-(1-iminoethyl)lysine. Biochemistry **37:** 4844–4852.
18. ERNSBERGER, P., J.E. PILETZ, L.M. GRAFF & M.E. GRAVES. 1995. Optimization of radioligand binding assays for I1-imidazoline sites. Ann. N. Y. Acad. Sci. **763:** 163–168.
19. LYLES, G.A. & B.A. CALLINGHAM. 1982. *In vitro* and *in vivo* inhibition by benserazide of clorgyline-resistant amine oxidases in rat cardiovascular tissues. Biochem. Pharmacol. **31:** 1417–1424.
20. HOLT, A. & B.A. CALLINGHAM. 1995. Further studies on the ex-vivo effects of procarbazine and monomethylhydrazine on rat semicarbazide-sensitive amine and monoamine oxidase activities. J. Pharm. Pharmacol. **47:** 837–845.
21. HOLT, A., D. SHARMAN, G. BAKER & M. PALCIC. 1997. A continuous spectrophotometric assay for monoamine oxidase and related enzymes in tissue homogenates. Anal. Biochem. **244:** 384–392.
22. LOWRY, O.H., N.J. ROSEBROUGH, A.L. FARR & J. RANDALL. 1951. Protein measurement with the Folin phenol reagent. J. Biol. Chem. **193:** 265–275.
23. MURPHY, D.L., K.B. SIMS, F. KAROUM, et al. 1991. Plasma amine oxidase activities in Norrie disease patients with an X-chromosomal deletion affecting monoamine oxidase. J. Neural. Transm. Gen. Sect. **83:** 1–12.
24. REIS, D.J. & S. REGUNATHAN. 2000. Is agmatine a novel neurotransmitter in brain? Trends Pharmacol. Sci. **21:** 187–193.
25. RAASCH, W., U. SCHAFER, J. CHUN & P. DOMINIAK. 2001. Biological significance of agmatine, an endogenous ligand at imidazoline binding sites. Br. J. Pharmacol. **133:** 755–780.
26. RAASCH, W., B. JUNGBLUTH, U. SCHAFER, et al. 2003. Modification of noradrenaline release in pithed spontaneously hypertensive rats by I1-binding sites in addition to alpha2-adrenoceptors. J. Pharmacol. Exp. Ther. **304:** 1063–1071.
27. BERDEU, D., R. PUECH, M.M. LOUBATIÈRES-MARIANI & G. BERTRAND. 1996. Agmatine is not a good candidate as endogenous ligand for imidazoline sites of pancreatic β cells and vascular bed. Eur. J. Pharmacol. **308:** 301–304.

28. HEAD, G.A., C.K. CHAN & S.J. GODWIN. 1997. Central cardiovascular actions of agmatine, a putative clonidine-displacing substance, in conscious rabbits. Neurochem. Int. **30:** 37–45.
29. RAASCH, W., U. SCHAFER, F. QADRI & P. DOMINIAK. 2002. Agmatine, an endogenous ligand at imidazoline binding sites, does not antagonize the clonidine-mediated blood pressure reaction. Br. J. Pharmacol. **135:** 663–672.
30. ZUO, D.-M. & P.H. YU. 1994. Semicarbazide-sensitive amine oxidase and monoamine oxidase in rat brain microvessels, meninges, retina and eye sclera. Brain Res. Bull. **33:** 307–311.
31. RAASCH, W., H. MUHLE & P. DOMINIAK. 1999. Modulation of MAO activity by imidazoline and guanidine derivatives. Ann. N. Y. Acad. Sci. **881:** 313–331.
32. SASTRE, M., S. REGUNATHAN, E. GALEA & D.J. REIS. 1996. Agmatinase activity in rat brain: a metabolic pathway for the degradation of agmatine. J. Neurochem. **67:** 1761–1765.
33. RAASCH, W., S. REGUNATHAN, G. LI & D.J. REIS. 1995. Agmatine is widely and unequally distributed in rat organs. Ann. N. Y. Acad. Sci. **763:** 330–334.
34. KHRAMOV, V.A. 1976. [Inhibition of bacterial agmatinase by substrate analogs.] Vopr. Med. Khim. **22:** 804–808.
35. HUDSON, A.L., S. LUSCOMBE, R.E. GOUCH, et al. 1999. Endogenous indoleamines demonstrate moderate affinity for I_2 binding sites. Ann. N. Y. Acad. Sci. **881:** 212–216.
36. ELLIOTT, J., B.A. CALLINGHAM & D. SHARMAN. 1989. Semicarbazide-sensitive amine oxidase (SSAO) of the rat aorta. Interactions with some naturally occurring amines and their structural analogues. Biochem. Pharmacol. **38:** 1507–1515.
37. DAVIS, B.A. & A.A. BOULTON. 1994. The trace amines and their acidic metabolites in depression—an overview. Prog. Neuro-Psychopharmacol. & Biol. Psychiat. **18:** 17–45.
38. MOUSSEAU, D.D. & R.F. BUTTERWORTH. 1994. The [^{3}H]tryptamine receptor in human brain: kinetics, distribution, and pharmacologic profile. J. Neurochem. **63:** 1052–1059.
39. ROBB, S., T.R. CHEEK, F.L. HANNAN, et al. 1994. Agonist-specific coupling of a cloned *Drosophila* octopamine/tyramine receptor to multiple second messenger systems. EMBO J. **13:** 1325–1330.
40. BOROWSKY, B., N. ADHAM, K.A. JONES, et al. 2001. Trace amines: Identification of a family of mammalian G protein-coupled receptors. PNAS **98:** 8966–8971.
41. BUNZOW, J.R., M.S. SONDERS, S. ARTTAMANGKUL, et al. 2001. Amphetamine, 3,4-Methylenedioxymethamphetamine, Lysergic acid diethylamide, and metabolites of the catecholamine neurotransmitters are agonists of a rat trace amine receptor. Mol. Pharmacol. **60:** 1181–1188.
42. GOODNOUGH, D.B., G.B. BAKER, D.D. MOUSSEAU, et al. 1994. Effects of low- and high-dose tranylcypromine on [^{3}H]tryptamine binding sites in the rat hippocampus and striatum. Neurochem. Res. **19:** 5–8.
43. URICHUK, L.J., K. ALLISON, A. HOLT, et al. 2000. Comparison of neurochemical effects of the monoamine oxidase inhibitors phenelzine, moclobemide and brofaromine in the rat after short- and long-term administration. J. Affect. Disorders **58:** 135–144.
44. BOULTON, A.A., A.V. JUORIO & I.A. PATERSON. 1990. Phenylethylamine in the CNS: effects of monoamine oxidase inhibiting drugs, deuterium substitution and lesions and its role in the neuromodulation of catecholaminergic neurotransmission. J. Neural Transm. Suppl. **29:** 119–129.
45. ISHITANI, R., M. KIMURA, M. TAKEICHI & D.M. CHUANG. 1994. Tryptamine induces phosphoinositide turnover and modulates adrenergic and muscarinic cholinergic receptor function in cultured cerebellar granule cells. J. Neurochem. **63:** 2080–2085.
46. BRUBAN, V., J. FELDMAN, H. GRENEY, et al. 2001. Respective contributions of alpha-adrenergic and non-adrenergic mechanisms in the hypotensive effect of imidazoline-like drugs. Br. J. Pharmacol. **133:** 261–266.
47. HALARIS, A. & J.E. PILETZ. 2001. Imidazoline receptors: possible involvement in the pathophysiology and treatment of depression. Hum. Psychopharmacol. **16:** 65–69.
48. REIS, D.J. & S. REGUNATHAN. 1999. Agmatine: an endogenous ligand at imidazoline receptors is a novel neurotransmitter. Ann. N. Y. Acad. Sci. **881:** 65–80.
49. BOWMAN, W.C. & M.J. RAND. 1980. Textbook of Pharmacology, 2nd ed. Blackwell Scientific Publications. Oxford, U.K. p 39.38.

50. YU, A.M., J.R. IDLE, K.W. KRAUSZ, et al. 2003. Contribution of individual cytochrome P450 isozymes to the O-demethylation of the psychotropic beta-carboline alkaloids harmaline and harmine. J. Pharmacol. Exp. Ther. **305:** 315–322.
51. HUSBANDS, S.M., R.A. GLENNON, S. GORGERAT, et al. 2001. β-carboline binding to imidazoline receptors. Drug Alcohol Depend. **64:** 203–208.
52. MUSGRAVE, I.F. & E. BADOER. 2000. Harmane produces hypotension following microinjection into the RVLM: possible role of I_1-imidazoline receptors. Br. J. Pharmacol. **129:** 1057–1059.
53. ASCENZI, P., M. FASANO, M. MARINO, et al. 2002. Agmatine oxidation by copper amine oxidase. Eur. J. Biochem. **269:** 884–892.
54. SATRIANO, J., D. SCHWARTZ, S. ISHIZUKA, et al. 2001. Suppression of inducible nitric oxide generation by agmatine aldehyde: beneficial effects in sepsis. J. Cell Physiol. **188:** 313–320.
55. ŠEBELA, M., A. RADOVÁ, R. ANGELINI, et al. 2001. FAD-containing polyamine oxidases: a timely challenge for researchers in biochemistry and physiology of plants. Plant Sci. **160:** 197–207.
56. ŠEBELA, M., Z. LAMPLOT, M. PETŘIVALSKÝ, et al. 2003. Recent news related to substrates and inhibitors of plant amine oxidases. Biochim. Biophys. Acta **1647:** 355–360.
57. PIETRANGELI, P., S. NOCERA, MONDOVI & L. MORPURGO. 2003. Is the catalytic mechanism of bacteria, plant, and mammal copper-TPQ amine oxidases identical? Biochim. Biophys. Acta **1647:** 152–156.

In Vivo Effects of the I_2-Alkylating Agent BU99006 on the Immunodensity of Imidazoline Receptor Proteins in the Mouse Brain

JESUS A. GARCIA-SEVILLA[a,b] AND MARCEL FERRER-ALCON[b]

[a]*Laboratory of Neuropharmacology, Associate Unit of the Institute of Neurobiology Ramón y Cajal (CSIC), Department of Biology, University of the Balearic Islands, E-07122 Palma de Mallorca, Spain*

[b]*Clinical Research Unit, Department of Psychiatry, Medical School, University of Geneva, CH-1225 Chêne-Bourg/GE, Switzerland*

ABSTRACT: The binding sites for imidazol(ine)/guanidine drugs (identified inter alia with [^{3}H]-clonidine and [^{3}H]-idazoxan) are heterogeneous in nature, and various pharmacologic types of imidazoline receptors (IRs) have been characterized ($I_1R, I_{2A}R, I_{2B}R$, and I_3R). IR-receptor proteins have also been immunodetected using an antibody raised against an ≈70-kD idazoxan/clonidine binding protein, which probably recognizes all types of IRs. In this study, the in vivo effects of the selective I_2-alkylating agent BU99006 (5-isothiocyanato-2-benzofuranyl-2-imidazoline) on immunoreactive IR proteins were assessed in the mouse brain to unravel the molecular nature of the I_2R subtypes. In mouse tissues (cerebral cortex, liver, testis, and kidney) this antibody revealed the presence of 30-, 43-, 45-, 66-, and/or 85-kD IR proteins. Treatment with BU99006 (20 mg/kg, intraperitoneally, for 4 hours) significantly decreased the immunodensity of specific IR proteins in the brain (30 kD: −49%; 45 kD: −37%; 66 kD: −18%). In contrast, the immunoreactivities of 43-kD and 85-kD IR proteins were not altered after I_2R alkylation. Prolonged treatment with BU99006 (20 mg/kg, intraperitoneally. for 8 hours) resulted in modest but significant increases in the expression of all the immunodetected IR proteins in the mouse brain (20%–36%), suggesting compensatory increases in IR protein synthesis after alkylation of I_2 sites. The results indicate that the 30-kD and 45-kD proteins, but not the 43-kD and 85-kD proteins, immunodetected in the mouse brain are related to the I_2R.

KEYWORDS: imidazoline receptor proteins; I_2-receptor alkylation; BU99006 (5-isothiocyanato-2-benzofuranyl-2-imidazoline); mouse brain

INTRODUCTION

Historically and based on the rank order of affinity for different ligands, imidazoline receptors (IRs) have been classified into three main types: a clonidine-preferring

Address for correspondence: Jesus A. Garcia-Sevilla, Clinical Research Unit, Department of Psychiatry, Medical School, University of Geneva, HUG Belle-Idée, CH-1225 Chêne-Bourg/GE, Switzerland. Voice: (+41) 22-305 57 56; fax: (+41) 22-305 57 99.
e-mail: jesus.a.garcia-sevilla@hcuge.ch

Ann. N.Y. Acad. Sci. 1009: 323–331 (2003). © 2003 New York Academy of Sciences.
doi: 10.1196/annals.1304.041

receptor (I_1R, involved in the control of blood pressure), an idazoxan-preferring receptor (I_2R, modulated in various psychiatric disorders), and an atypical imidazoline site found on pancreatic β cells (I_3R, involved in insulin secretion).[1,2] Moreover, I_2R has been further subclassified into the I_{2A}-subtype of binding site (high affinity for the guanidide amiloride) and the I_{2B}-subtype of binding site (low affinity for amiloride).[3] The I_{2A}-subtype is expressed in rabbit tissues and in human placenta, whereas the I_{2B}-subtype predominates in the rat and human brain.[3,4] Some of these sites represent binding domains on monoamine oxidases (MAOs), which are proteins of 50- to 55-Kd size.[2] In addition, various IR proteins between 27 and 85 Kd in size have been visualized or purified from various tissues and cells,[5] but their possible association with particular pharmacologic subtypes of IR is not precisely known. Thus, the I_2-IR labeled by [^{3}H]-idazoxan in the rat brain was shown to be heterogeneous in nature because its pharmacologic modulation was related to several proteins (≈66, ≈45, and ≈30 Kd).[6]

Irreversible blockers of neurotransmitter receptors have been widely used as specific tools to elucidate the functional and structural properties of their binding sites.[7] The lack of selective alkylating agents for IRs has been a major obstacle. Therefore effort has been spent in looking for alkylating agents for I_2R.[8] Initial studies indicated that in the rat brain the potent peptide-coupling agent EEDQ[7] was unable to alkylate in vitro I_2R,[9] and it acted through an indirect mechanism to reduce in vivo the density of these sites ([^{3}H]-idazoxan binding) and of various related IR proteins (≈66, ≈45, and ≈30 Kd).[6,9] Later, the 4′-NCS analogue of tolazoline, isothiocyanatobenzyl imidazoline (IBI), was shown to alkylate a portion of I_2R both in vitro and in vivo.[8] Recently, another isothiocyanate-containing selective irreversible ligand, BU99006 (5-isothiocyanato-2-benzofuranyl-2-imidazoline), has been developed for the I_2R.[10] This new alkylating agent, like its parent ligand (2BFI), displayed higher affinity, selectivity, and potency for I_2 sites compared with IBI.[11] In vivo, BU99006 (15 mg/kg) was shown to induce an almost complete loss of I_2 sites ([^{3}H]-2BFI) in rat brain.[11] Therefore, the present study was designed to assess whether BU99006 is able in vivo to reduce the immunodensity of any IR protein expressed in the mouse brain (≈85, ≈66, ≈43/45, and ≈30 Kd) and in this way to unravel further the molecular nature of the I_2R.

METHODS

BU99006 Treatment of Mice and Tissue Samples

Male brown mice (20–25 g) were used (SV129 strain). The irreversible I_2 ligand BU99006 (20 mg/kg) was injected intraperitoneally in a volume of 0.1 mL per 10 g of body weight. Control animals received saline on the same injection schedule. The mice were decapitated after 4 to 8 hours of treatment, and the brains were removed and frozen at –80°C. Other mouse tissues were taken from control animals. These experiments in mice were performed according to standard ethical guidelines.

Gel Electrophoresis and Immunoblot Assays

Mouse brain samples (total homogenates from the cerebral cortex, hippocampus, and corpus striatum), other mouse tissues, and various cell samples were prepared as described.[12] Briefly, the tissues were homogenized (50 mM Tris-HCl buffer, pH 6.8, 1 mM EDTA, 2% sodium dodecyl sulfate, SDS) in the presence or absence of various protease inhibitors (1.3 mM pefabloc, 10 µg/mL leupeptin, 5 µg/mL E64, 10 µg/mL antipain, and 10 µg/mL pepstatin A),[12] and aliquots of the mixtures were combined with solubilization buffer (50 mM Tris-HCl [pH 6.8], 2% SDS, 10% glycerol, 2.5% β-mercaptoethanol and 0.1% bromophenol blue) to reach a final protein concentration of about 3 µg/µL The samples were boiled and stored at −20°C. In routine experiments, 40 µg of protein from each mouse tissue or cell sample was subjected to electrophoresis on 15-well, 12% polyacrylamide minigels (SDS-PAGE type). Resolved proteins were electrophoretically transferred to nitrocellulose membranes that were incubated in phosphate-buffered saline solution containing 5% nonfat dry milk, 0.2% Tween 20 (Sigma Chemie, Buchs, Switzerland), and 0.5% bovine serum albumin (blocking solution). The membranes were incubated overnight at 4°C in blocking solution containing the appropriate primary antibody: a polyclonal rabbit antibody against IR proteins[6,13,14] (dilution 1:3000), a polyclonal rabbit antibody against Bcl-2 oncoprotein (dilution 1:1000; Santa Cruz Biotechnology, Santa Cruz, CA), or a monoclonal anti-dynamin antibody (dilution 1:3000; Transduction Laboratories, Lexington, KY). The secondary antibody, horseradish peroxidase–linked donkey anti-rabbit IgG or sheep anti-mouse IgG, was incubated at 1:5000 dilution in blocking solution at room temperature for 2 hours. Immunoreactivity was detected with an Enhanced Chemiluminescence (ECL) system, followed by exposure to Hyperfilm ECL (Amersham, Bucks, UK) for 5 to 15 minutes (autoradiograms).

Quantification of Target Proteins

The autoradiograms were quantitated by densitometric scanning by measuring the integrated optical density (IOD) units. For a direct comparison, tissues from two groups of five mice (i.e., saline-treated versus BU99006-treated) were run together in the same gel to assess differences in the effects of the I_2–alkylating agent; 40 µg of protein (known to be within the linear range for immunolabeling of the target proteins) were loaded in each lane for the different blots. Comparison of IOD units for the two groups of mice in the same gel were assessed 2 or 3 times in different gels with similar results. Mean ± SEM values of representative immunoblots are shown. Student's two-tailed *t* test was used for the statistical evaluations. The level of significance was chosen as $P = 0.05$.

Drugs

BU99006 hydrochloride synthesized by Stephen M. Husbands was kindly provided by Alan L. Hudson, Psychopharmacology Unit, University of Bristol, UK.

RESULTS

Immunodetection of IR Proteins and Effects of Proteases

The immunologic detection of IR proteins in various mouse tissues and cell lines was performed using antiserum against a ≈70-Kd idazoxan/clonidine-binding protein purified from bovine chromaffin cells.[13,14] In the mouse cerebral cortex, this antibody allowed the detection of ≈85-, ≈66-, ≈45-, and ≈30-Kd IR proteins (FIG. 1). The prominent ≈66-Kd IR protein in the mouse brain roughly corresponds to the ≈70-Kd IR protein originally identified in bovine chromaffin cells.[13,14] A similar set

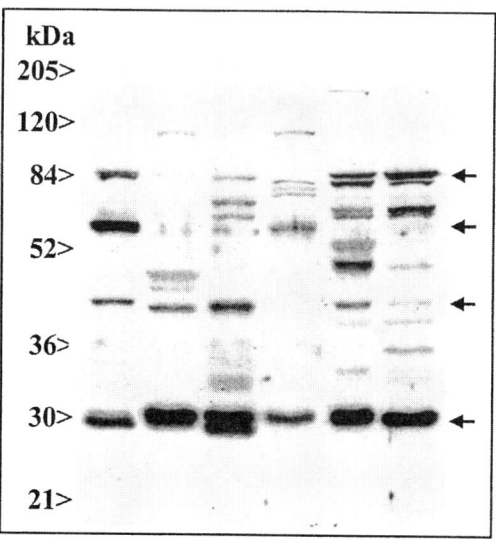

FIGURE 1. Representative autoradiograph of a Western blot depicting immunodetectable imidazoline receptor proteins (≈85 Kd, ≈66 Kd, ≈43/45 Kd, and ≈30 Kd, *arrows*) in mouse tissues and cells using anti-imidazoline receptor antiserum. The apparent molecular masses of the various proteins were determined by calibrating the blot with prestained molecular weight markers. AS, human astrocytoma U-373 cells; MB, mouse brain (cerebral cortex); MK, mouse kidney; ML, mouse liver; MT, mouse testis; SH, human SH-SY5Y neuroblastoma cells (40 μg protein for each sample prepared with protease inhibitors).

of peptides were immunodetected in SH-SY5Y neuroblastoma cells and in astrocytoma U-373 cells (FIG. 1), indicating that these IR proteins are expressed in neurons and glial cells. Similar IR proteins were also visualized in the mouse liver (except the 66-Kd band), testis, and kidney (except the 45-Kd band) (FIG. 1).

Membranes prepared from mouse brains without protease inhibitors resulted in lowered immunodensities of 85-Kd ($-46\% \pm 3\%, P < 0.01$), 66-Kd ($-19\% \pm 8\%, P > 0.05$), and 45-Kd ($-28\% \pm 4\%, P < 0.01$) IR proteins but not of 43- and 30-Kd IR proteins (FIG. 2). Similar results have previously been used to suggest that various IR proteins of low molecular mass are degradation products from an 85-Kd IR protein and that the use of a protease-inhibitor cocktail avoids its proteolytic breakage.[15] In our hands the 85-Kd IR was susceptible to degradation, but previous data[5] and the current results (FIG. 2) do not suggest that the 43-Kd and 30-Kd IR proteins are degradation products of the 85-Kd IR protein. A previous study[16] also showed that protease inhibitors block the process of protein degradation after receptor alkylation. Therefore, it was decided that the effects of the I_2–alkylating agent BU99006 on IR proteins should be assessed in samples prepared without protease inhibitors.

In Vivo Effects of BU99006 on the Immunodensity of Brain IR Proteins

FIGURE 3 shows a representative immunoblot from in vivo treatments with the I_2– alkylating agent BU99006 (20 mg/kg, intraperitoneally for 4 hours). BU99006 sig-

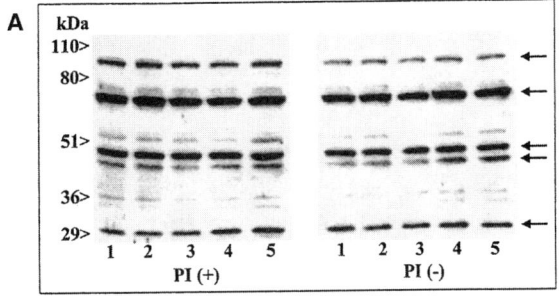

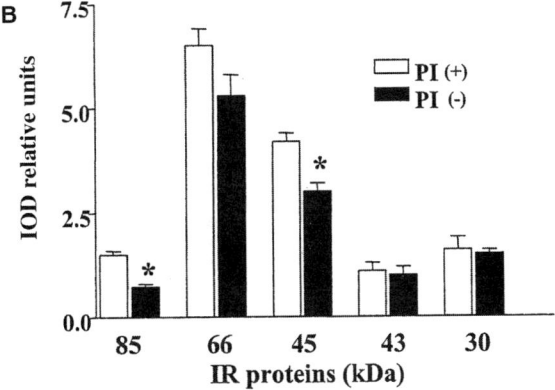

FIGURE 2. Immunodetection of IR proteins (≈85 Kd, ≈66 Kd, ≈45 Kd, ≈43 Kd, and ≈30 Kd, *arrows*) in mouse brain (pool of cerebral cortex, hippocampus, and corpus striatum) using anti-imidazoline receptor antiserum. A total homogenate was divided into two aliquots and incubated in the presence or absence of protease inhibitors (PI) for 2 hours. (**A**) Representative immunoblot (40 μg protein) for samples prepared with (PI+) or without (PI−) protease inhibitors (1.3 mM pefabloc, 10 μg/L leupeptin, 5 μg/mL E64, 10 μg/mL antipain, and 10 μg/mL pepstatin A). The comparison is five different samples PI+ versus five different samples PI−. The apparent molecular masses of the various IR proteins were determined by calibrating the blot with prestained molecular weight markers. (**B**) The columns are mean ± SEM values (integrated optical density units, IOD) of the corresponding bands shown in the above immunoblot (n = 5 for each protein band). * $P < 0.01$ when compared with the corresponding control PI+ (Student's two-tailed *t*-test).

nificantly decreased the immunodensity of specific IR proteins in the mouse brain (30 Kd: −49% ± 8%, $P < 0.001$; 45 Kd: −37% ± 7%, $P < 0.01$; 66 Kd: −18 % ± 4%, $P < 0.05$) (FIG. 3). In contrast, the immunoreactivities of 43-Kd and 85-Kd IR proteins were not altered by BU99006 treatment (FIG. 3). This experiment was repeated with similar results, and the 43-Kd and 85-Kd IR proteins were found unaltered by BU99006 treatment. In other brain samples prepared with protease inhibitors, BU99006 (20 mg/kg, intraperitoneally for 4 hours) did not decrease the immunodensity of IR proteins, except slightly that of 30-Kd protein (−11%, $P = 0.07$) (data not shown).

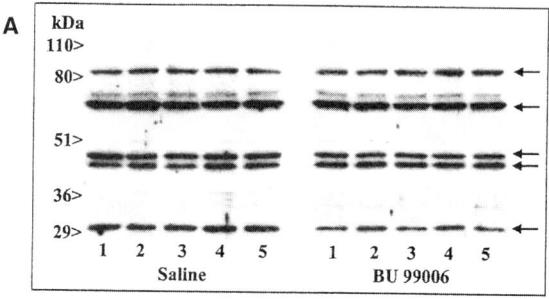

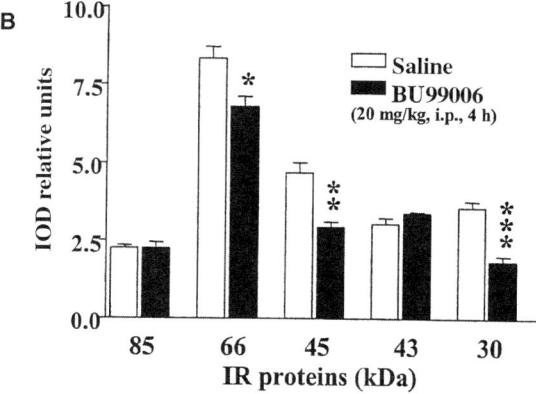

FIGURE 3. Four-hour treatment with the I_2–alkylating agent BU99006 (20 mg/kg, intraperitoneally) affects the immunodensity of IR proteins ($\approx$85 Kd, $\approx$66 Kd, $\approx$45 Kd, $\approx$43 Kd, and $\approx$30 Kd, *arrows*) in mouse brain (pool of cerebral cortex, hippocampus, and corpus striatum) detected by anti-imidazoline receptor antiserum. (**A**) Representative immunoblot (40 μg protein; samples prepared without protease inhibitors) for the effects of saline and BU99006 (five saline-treated mice versus five BU99006-treated mice). The apparent molecular masses of the various IR proteins were determined by calibrating the blot with prestained molecular weight markers. (**B**) The columns are mean ± SEM values (IOD) of the corresponding IR band shown in the above immunoblot (n = 5 for each protein band). * $P < 0.05$; ** $P < 0.01$; *** $P < 0.001$ when compared with the corresponding saline group (Student's two-tailed *t*-test).

Longer treatment with BU99006 (20 mg/kg, intraperitoneally for 8 hours) resulted in modest but significant increases in the expression of all the immunodetected IR proteins in the mouse brain (+20%–36%, $P < 0.05$) (FIG. 4). This finding suggests a compensatory mechanism for IR protein synthesis after alkylation of I_2 sites. The time courses for complete alkylation (1 hour) and global recovery ($t_{1/2}$ = 2–4 hours) of I_2 sites ([^{3}H]-2BFI binding) in the rodent brain after BU99006 have also been shown to be rapid (see Paterson *et al.*, this volume).[11]

None of the treatments with BU99006 (20 mg/kg, intraperitoneally for 4 hours and 8 hours) modified significantly the immunodensities of dynamin (a cytoskeletal

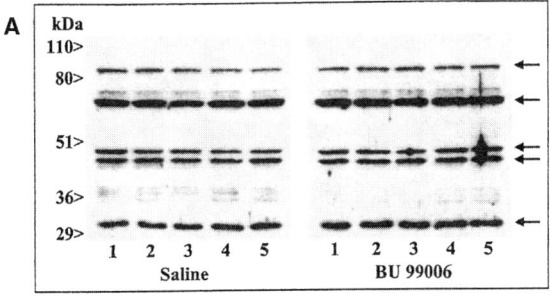

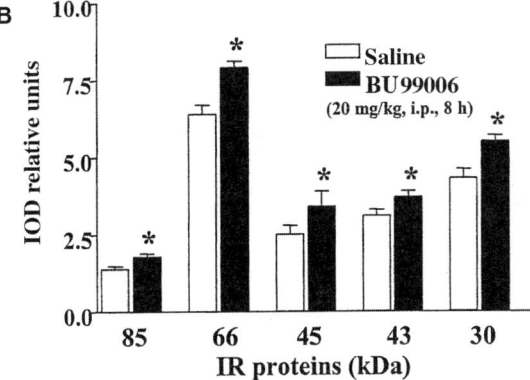

FIGURE 4. Eight-hour treatment with the I_2–alkylating agent BU99006 (20 mg/kg, intraperitoneally.) affects the immunodensity of IR proteins (≈85 Kd, ≈66 Kd, ≈45 Kd, ≈43 Kd, and ≈30 Kd, *arrows*) in the mouse brain (pool of cerebral cortex, hippocampus, and corpus striatum) detected with anti-imidazoline receptor antiserum. (**A**) Representative immunoblot (40 μg protein; samples prepared without protease inhibitors) for the effects of saline and BU99006 (5 saline-treated mice versus 5 BU99006-treated mice). The apparent molecular masses of the various IR proteins were determined by calibrating the blot with prestained molecular weight markers. (**B**) The columns are mean ± SEM values (IOD) of the corresponding IR band shown in the above immunoblot (n = 5 for each protein band). * At least $P < 0.05$ when compared with the corresponding saline group (Student's two-tailed *t*-test).

protein associated with receptor endocytosis) or Bcl-2 (a mitochondrial anti-apoptotic protein) used as negative controls in the same mouse brains (data not shown).

DISCUSSION

The in vivo study with the I_2–alkylating agent BU99006 provides evidence that 30-Kd and 45-Kd (and perhaps 66-Kd) proteins, but not 43-Kd and 85-Kd proteins, are probably related to the I_2R. This conclusion is based on the high affinity and selectivity of BU99006 for I_2 sites in the brain.[10,11] The data are also in agreement with previous studies indicating the existence of a close association between I_2 sites and the 30-, 45-, and/or 66-Kd IR proteins in the brain.[5,6,17]

Some I_2 sites labeled by [^{3}H]-idazoxan were shown to be heterogeneous in nature and related to various IR proteins that are not MAOs.[6] Notably, drug-induced changes in the immunodensity of the 30-Kd IR protein and the density of I_2 sites were strongly correlated in the rat brain.[6] Moreover, the I_2–alkylating agent BU99006 markedly decreased the immunodensity of the 30-Kd IR protein, providing evidence that this protein is clearly related to the I_2R. In 1995, the isolation and molecular characterization of a 45-Kd IR protein from the rat brain was reported,[18] and its pharmacologic profile was shown to correspond to an I_2 site.[18] Cirazoline, an I_2-ligand, is a unique drug in modulating the 45-Kd protein but not other, IR proteins.[6] Recently, a 45-Kd IR protein was isolated from the rabbit brain and, through N-terminal amino acid sequencing, was identified as the brain creatine kinase (Kimura *et al.*, in this volume).[19] Although this finding suggests that the 45-Kd peptide (immunoreactivity reduced by BU99006) is not a transmembrane I_2R protein, it remains to be demonstrated whether the anti-imidazoline receptor antiserum used for its identification is also able to recognize the enzyme creatine kinase. Direct evidence for the possible association of the 66-Kd IR protein (not related to MAO) with I_2R[5,6] is weak because BU99006 treatment did not strongly decrease its immunodensity.

The I_2–alkylating agent BU99006 did not alter the expression of 43-Kd and 85-Kd IR proteins in the mouse brain, perhaps because these proteins are of the I_1R subtype. A 43-Kd protein has previously been related to an I_1R,[20] and the immunodensity of an 85-Kd IR protein was shown to correlate with the density of I_1-binding sites[15] (see also Menaouar *et al.*, in this volume).

In conclusion, the effects of BU99006 on IR proteins described here provide new insights into the molecular nature of IR, and particularly of the 45-Kd and 30-Kd I_2R.

ACKNOWLEDGMENTS

This study was supported by grants BFI 2000-0306 from the Ministerio de Ciencia y Tecnologia (MCT, Madrid, Spain) and 32-57066.99 from the Fond National Suisse pour la Recherche Scientifique (FNSRS, Bern, Switzerland) J.A.G.-S. is a member of the Institut d'Estudis Catalans (Barcelona, Spain).

REFERENCES

1. REGUNATHAN, S. & D.J. REIS. 1996. Imidazoline receptors and their endogenous ligands. Annu. Rev. Pharmacol. **36:** 511–544.
2. EGLEN, R.M., A.L. HUDSON, D.A. KENDALL, *et al.* 1998. "Seeing through a glass darkly": casting light on imidazoline "I" sites. Trends Pharmacol. Sci. **19:** 381–390.
3. MIRALLES, A., G. OLMOS, M. SASTRE, *et al.* 1993. Discrimination and pharmacological characterization of I_2-imidazoline sites with [^{3}H]-idaxozan and alpha-2 adrenoceptors with [^{3}H]-RX821002 (2-methoxy idaxozan) in the human and rat brains. J. Pharmacol. Exp. Ther. **264:** 1187–1197.
4. OLMOS, G., R. ALEMANY & J.A. GARCÍA-SEVILLA. 1996. Pharmacological and molecular discrimination of brain I_2-imidazoline receptor subtypes. Naunyn-Schmiedeberg's Arch. Pharmacol. **354:** 709–716.

5. ESCRIBÁ, P.V., A. OZAITA & J.A. GARCÍA-SEVILLA. 1999. Pharmacologic characterization of imidazoline receptor proteins identified by immunologic techniques and other methods. Ann. N. Y. Acad. Sci. **881:** 8–25.
6. ESCRIBÁ, P.V., R. ALEMANY, M. SASTRE, et al. 1996. Pharmacological modulation of immunoreactive imidazoline receptor proteins in rat brain: relationship with non-adrenoceptor [^{3}H]-idaxozan binding sites. Br. J. Pharmacol. **118:** 2029–2036.
7. MELLER, E., M. GOLDSTEIN, A.J. FRIEDHORFF, et al. 1988. N-Ethoxycarbonyl-2-ethoxy-1,2-dihydroquinoline (EEDQ): a new tool to probe CNS receptor function. Adv. Exp. Med. Biol. **235:** 121–136.
8. BORONAT, M.A., G. OLMOS, D.D. MILLER, et al. 1998. Isothiocyanato benzyl imidazoline is an alkylating agent for I_2-imidazoline binding sites in rat and rabbit tissues. Naunyn-Schmiedeberg's Arch. Pharmacol. **357:** 351–355.
9. MIRALLES, A., C. RIBAS, G. OLMOS, et al. 1993. Differential effects of the alkylating agent N-ethoxycarbonyl-2-ethoxy-1,2-dihydroquinoline on brain α_2-adrenoceptors and I_2-imidazoline sites in vitro and in vivo. J. Neurochem. **61:** 1602–1610.
10. COATES, P.A., P. GRUNDT, E.S.J. ROBINSON, et al. 2000. Probes for imidazoline binding sites: synthesis and evaluation of a selective, irreversible I_2 ligand. Bioorg. Med. Chem. Lett. **10:** 605–607.
11. TYACKE, R.J., E.S.J. ROBINSON, D.J. NUTT, et al. 2002. 5-Isothiocyanato-2-benzofuranyl-2-imidazoline (BU99006) an irreversible imidazoline$_2$ binding site ligand: in vitro and in vivo characterisation in rat brain. Neuropharmacology **43:** 75–83.
12. FERRER-ALCÓN, M., J.A. GARCÍA-SEVILLA, P.H. JAQUET, et al. 2000. Regulation of nonphosphorylated and phosphorylated forms of neurofilament proteins in the prefrontal cortex of human opioid addicts. J. Neurosci. Res. **61:** 338–349.
13. WANG, H., S. REGUNATHAN, M.P. MEELEY, et al. 1992. Isolation and characterization of imidazoline receptor protein from bovine adrenal chromaffin cell. Mol. Pharmacol. **42:** 792–801.
14. WANG, H., S. REGUNATHAN, D.A. RUGGIERO, et al. 1993. Production and characterization of antibodies specific for the imidazoline receptor protein. Mol. Pharmacol. **43:** 509–515.
15. IVANOV, T.R., H. ZHU, S. REGUNATHAN, et al. 1998. Co-detection by two imidazoline receptor protein antisera of a novel 85 kilodalton protein. Biochem. Pharmacol. **55:** 649–655.
16. OZAITA, A., P.V. ESCRIBÁ & J.A. GARCÍA-SEVILLA. 1999. The alkylating agent EEDQ facilitates protease-mediated degradation of the human brain α_{2A}-adrenoceptor as revealed by a sequence-specific antibody. Neurosci. Lett. **263:** 105–108.
17. GARCÍA-SEVILLA, J.A., P.V. ESCRIBÁ & J. GUIMÓN. 1999. Imidazoline receptors and human brain disorders. Ann. N. Y. Acad. Sci. **881:** 392–409.
18. ESCRIBÁ, P.V., A. OZAITA, A. MIRALLES, et al. 1995. Molecular characterization and isolation of a 45-kilodalton imidazoline receptor protein from the rat brain. Mol. Brain Res. **32:** 187–196.
19. KIMURA, A., R.J. TYACKE, M.C.W. MINCHIN, et al. 2003. Identification of a putative imidazoline-2 binding protein. Br. J. Pharmacol. **138:** 173P.
20. DONTENWILL, M., C. VONTHRON, H. GRENEY, et al. 1999. Identification of human I_1 eceptors and their relationship to α_2-adrenoceptors. Ann. N. Y. Acad. Sci. **881:** 123–134.

Restoration of First-Phase Insulin Secretion by the Imidazoline Compound LY374284 in Pancreatic Islets of Diabetic db/db Mice

M.B. BRENNER, J. GROMADA, A.M. EFANOV, K. BOKVIST, AND H.-J. MEST

Lilly Research Laboratories, Hamburg, Germany

ABSTRACT: The effect of the imidazoline compound LY374284 has been studied in pancreatic islets of db/db mice, a progressive model of diabetes. In perifusion experiments, pancreatic islets of db/db mice showed a progressive deterioration of glucose-induced insulin release with increasing age, whereby the first phase of insulin secretion was almost completely abolished and the second phase was substantially decreased by 15 weeks of age. LY374284 restored the first phase of glucose-induced insulin secretion in islets of 16-week-old db/db mice to 70% of that observed in islets isolated from age-matched nondiabetic db/+ mice. LY374284 did not affect insulin secretion at a low glucose concentration (3.3 mmol/L). A similar restoration of first phase insulin secretion was observed after application of glucagon-like peptide-1, whereas a sulfonylurea agent, tolbutamide, was inactive. LY374284 did not affect cytosolic Ca^{2+} concentration or cellular ATP content. Furthermore, LY374284 strongly enhanced insulin secretion in islets of db/db and db/+ mice maximally depolarized by 30 mmol/L K^+ and 250 μmol/L diazoxide. The present data suggest that the imidazoline compound LY374284 restores biphasic insulin secretion in islets of diabetic db/db mice by amplifying glucose-induced insulin secretion at a site distal to Ca^{2+}-influx.

KEYWORDS: imidazoline; GLP-1; sulfonylureas; db/db mice; insulin secretion

INTRODUCTION

One characteristic of type 2 diabetes is the loss of first-phase insulin secretion which is associated with a marked impairment of glycemic control.[1] It has been shown that a selective restoration of the early phase of insulin release improves postprandial glucose homeostasis more effectively than normalization of the second-phase secretion.[2,3] Sulfonylureas, the traditional treatment of type 2 diabetes, block ATP-sensitive K^+ (K_{ATP}) channels in the β-cell plasma membrane and stimulate insulin release independently of ambient glucose concentration.[4] The strong insulinotropic effect of these compounds at low glucose concentrations is often accompanied by hypoglycemic episodes in diabetic patients.[5] Compounds with a 2-aryl-imidazoline moiety are known as potent stimulators of insulin secretion in pancreatic β cells and attract substantial interest because of their possible use in the treatment of type 2 diabetes.[6] The insulinotropic action of imidazolines was first thought to be caused

---

Address for correspondence: Dr. Martin Brenner, Lilly Research Laboratories, Essener Strasse 93, D-22419 Hamburg, Germany. Voice: (+49) 40-52724-494; fax: (+49) 40-52724-617.
e-mail: brenner_martin@lilly.com

exclusively by the closure of K_{ATP} channels and the subsequent increase in cytosolic Ca^{2+} concentration ($[Ca^{2+}]_i$).[7] Recently, it has been shown in rat pancreatic islets that the imidazoline compound BL 11282 (LY374284) stimulates glucose-dependent insulin secretion without modulation of K_{ATP} channel activity.[8] The same is true for the intestinally derived peptide hormone glucagon-like peptide-1 (GLP-1), which stimulates insulin secretion by binding to a specific G-protein–coupled receptor, activation of adenylate cyclase, and generation of cAMP.[9,10] Therefore, orally available agents that restore the first phase of insulin secretion and act only at elevated glucose levels could provide a therapeutic alternative to sulfonylureas. The purpose of the present study was to investigate the influence of the imidazoline compound, LY374284, on the impaired insulin secretion in islets of diabetic db/db mice.

METHODS

Diazoxide, Hank's buffer (HBSS), Krebs-Ringer buffer (KRB), phosphate buffered saline (PBS), Histopaque-1077®, and tolbutamide were obtained from Sigma (Taufkirchen, Germany), glucagon like peptide-1 (7-36) amide (GLP-1) was from Bachem (Heidelberg, Germany) and fura-2 from Molecular Probes (Eugene, OR, USA). Collagenase was from Serva (Heidelberg, Germany) and LY374284 was from Lilly Research Laboratories (Hamburg, Germany). RPMI-1640 medium, penicillin/streptomycin and fetal bovine serum were obtained from Invitrogen (Karlsruhe, Germany). Bovine serum albumine was from Applichem (Darmstadt, Germany).

Isolation and Culture of Pancreatic Islets

Male C57Bl/KS db/+ (16 weeks old) and C57Bl/KS db/db mice (13–20 weeks old) were from our own colony. Animals were housed with a 12-hour daylight cycle and had free access to standard chow and water. Islet isolation was based on standard methods.[11,12] Mice were killed by cervical dislocation (approved by local authorities). The common bile duct was cannulated with a 27-gauge needle, and the pancreas was distended with 3 mL of Hank's buffer, containing 2% bovine serum albumin and 1 mg/mL collagenase. Subsequently, the pancreas was removed and digested in Hank's buffer at 37°C. Islets were purified on a Histopaque-1077 gradient (Sigma, Taufkirchen, Germany) for 15 minutes at 750 × gravity. The islets were cultured overnight in RPMI-1640 medium (Invitrogen, Karlsruhe, Germany) containing 10% fetal bovine serum (FBS) and 100 U/mL penicillin as well as 100 μg/mL streptomycin.

Insulin Secretion

Perifusion experiments were carried out using a 12-channel perifusion system.[13] Each reaction chamber was loaded with 25 islets and perifused with 500 μL/minute Krebs-Ringer buffer. After perifusing islets with Krebs-Ringer buffer containing 3.3 mmol/L glucose for 40 minutes, the glucose concentration was increased to 16.7 mmol/L in the absence and presence of test compounds. The perifusate was collected in 5-minute to 30-second intervals and stored at −20°C until assayed for insulin by radioimmunoassay as described before.[14] In static incubation experiments, islets were starved for 30 minutes in Krebs-Ringer buffer containing 3.3 mmol/L glucose. Subsequently, groups of five islets were picked up and incubated in 0.25 mL Krebs-Ringer buffer containing 16.7 mmol/L glucose, 30 mmol/L K^+, and 250 µmol/L diazoxide.

ATP Measurement

ATP content was determined in batches of 30 size-matched islets using a luminescent cell viability kit (Promega, Manheim, Germany).

Measurement of $[Ca^{2+}]_i$

Islets of 16-week-old db/+ and db/db mice were dissociated into cell clusters in Ca^{2+}-free phosphate buffered saline (PBS) and seeded on glass cover slips. The clusters were loaded with 0.5 µmol/L fura-2/AM for 25 minutes before superfusion with Krebs-Ringer buffer, containing either 3.3 mmol/L or 16.7 mmol/L glucose. $[Ca^{2+}]_i$ measurements (sample rate, 0.5 Hz) were made using an Axiovert 200 inverted microscope with a Plan-Neofluar 25× objective (Carl Zeiss, Göttingen, Germany) and an Ionoptix (Milton, MA) fluorescence imaging software. The excitation wavelengths were 340 nm and 380 nm. The emitted light was recorded at 510 nm with a video camera.

Statistical Analysis

Data are expressed as means ± SE for the indicated number of observations. The difference of means was assessed with Student's t-test using the statistical software package SigmaStat 2.0 (Jandel, San Rafael, CA, USA).

RESULTS

Insulin Secretion in db/db Islets Deteriorates Between 13 and 20 Weeks of Age

FIGURE 1A shows the dynamics of insulin secretion from db/db islets evoked by a glucose stimulus of 16.7 mmol/L. Although islets of 13-week-old db/db mice have an insulin secretion pattern comparable to that of their nondiabetic counterparts (db/+), islets of 15-, 16-, and 20-week-old animals show a substantial decrease, especially in the first phase of insulin secretion. The areas under the curves (AUCs) from FIGURE 1A were calculated to quantify the progression of the insulin secretory defect (FIG. 1B). Glucose-induced insulin secretion from db/+ islets of 16-week-old animals was used as control and set to 100%. There was no significant difference in insulin secretion between islets of 13-week-old db/db animals and control animals. In contrast, first-phase glucose-induced insulin secretion was dramatically reduced by 80% at 16 weeks of age. Likewise, second-phase insulin secretion was significantly reduced by 50% (FIG. 1B). In all subsequent experiments, islets of 16-week-old mice were used.

LY374284 Improves First-phase Insulin Secretion in Islets of Db/db Mice

FIGURE 2 shows the effects of several compounds on the kinetics of insulin secretion from islets of 16-week-old db/db mice. No effect of the imidazoline compound

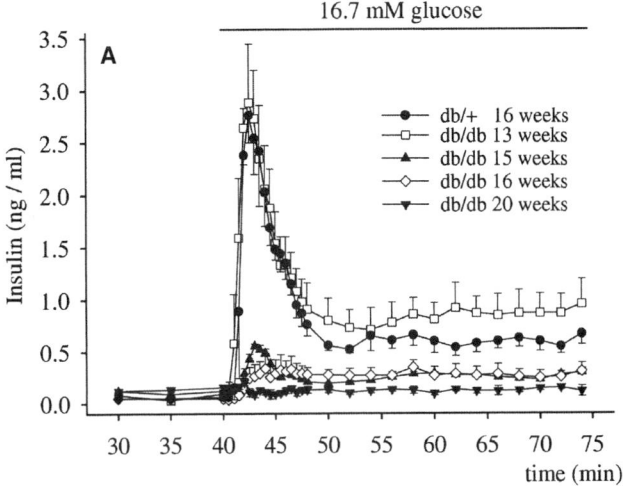
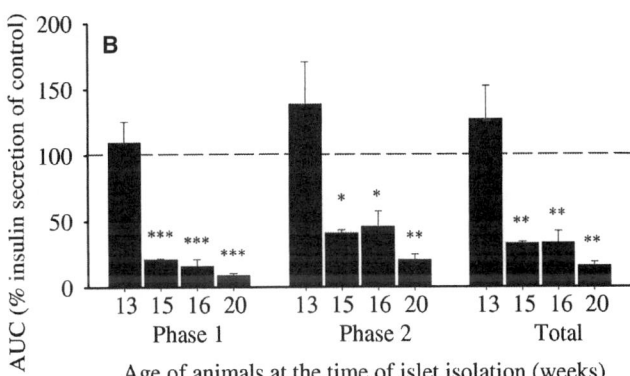

FIGURE 1. Progressive deterioration of glucose-induced insulin secretion in perifused db/db islets. (**A**) Secretion patterns of perifused islets of 16-week-old db/+ and 15-, 16- as well as 20-week-old db/db mice. Islets were perifused for 40 minutes with Krebs-Ringer buffer containing 3.3 mmol/L glucose before glucose concentration was raised to 16.7 mmol/L. (**B**) AUCs calculated from the secretion patterns in FIGURE 1A. AUCs of insulin secretion in db/db islets are expressed as percentage of insulin secretion in db/+ islets. Data are means ± SE from three independent experiments. *$P < 0.05$, **$P < 0.01$, ***$P < 0.001$ versus insulin secretion in db/+ islets.

LY374284 on insulin secretion was observed at a low prestimulatory glucose concentration (3.3 mmol/L). LY374284 significantly increased first-phase insulin secretion and even increased second-phase secretion as compared with controls (FIG. 2C). On average, glucose-induced insulin release in the presence of LY374284 was restored to 68% ± 12% (first phase) and 159% ± 22% (second phase) of control (FIG. 2D). The strong insulinotropic action of LY374284 was not mimicked by 100 μmol/L tolbutamide (FIG. 2A). It is noteworthy that tolbutamide significantly increased insulin secretion at 3.3 mmol/L glucose to 369% ± 68% of control ($P < 0.05$) (FIG. 2A).

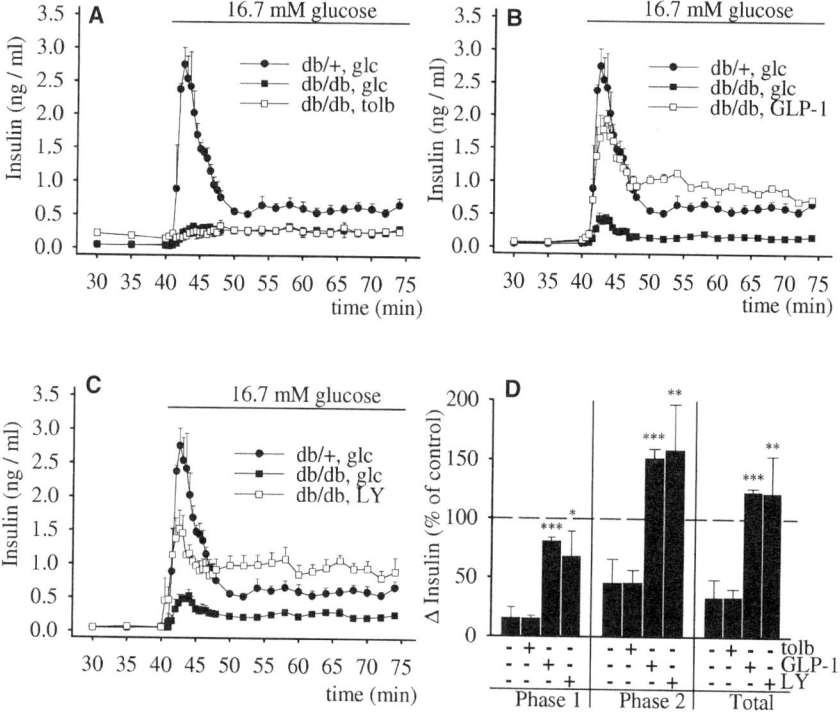

FIGURE 2. Restoration of the biphasic insulin secretion pattern in islets of db/db mice. Islets of 16-week-old db/+ and db/db mice were perifused for 40 minutes with Krebs-Ringer buffer containing 3.3 mmol/L glucose before glucose concentration was raised to 16.7 mmol/L (glc). Compounds were added throughout the whole experiment as depicted. (**A**) Stimulation of insulin secretion in db/db islets by 100 μmol/L tolbutamide (tolb). (**B**) Potentiation of insulin secretion in db/db islets by 30 nmol/L GLP-1. (**C**) Potentiation of insulin secretion in db/db islets by 10 μmol/L LY374284 (LY). (**D**) AUCs of insulin secretion calculated from the secretion patterns in FIGURE 2A, 2B, and 2C. AUCs of insulin secretion in db/db islets is expressed as percentage of insulin secretion in db/+ islets induced by 16.7 mmol/L glucose. Data are means ± SE from three independent experiments. * $P < 0.05$, ** $P < 0.01$, *** $P < 0.001$ versus insulin secretion in db/db islets induced by 16.7 mmol/L glucose.

On the other hand, GLP-1 significantly enhanced both first and second phase of insulin secretion in db/db islets in a manner similar to that observed with LY374284 (FIG. 2B).

Effects of Glucose and LY374284 on $[Ca^{2+}]_i$

FIGURE 3 shows the effects of high glucose concentration (16.7 mmol/L) and 10 μM LY374284 on $[Ca^{2+}]_i$ in clusters of β cells from db/db and db/+ mice. In β cells from 16-week-old db/+ mice, glucose produced a small initial decrease in $[Ca^{2+}]_i$ after a delay of 89 ± 7 seconds (n = 11) followed by a robust oscillatory (FIG. 3A) or steady

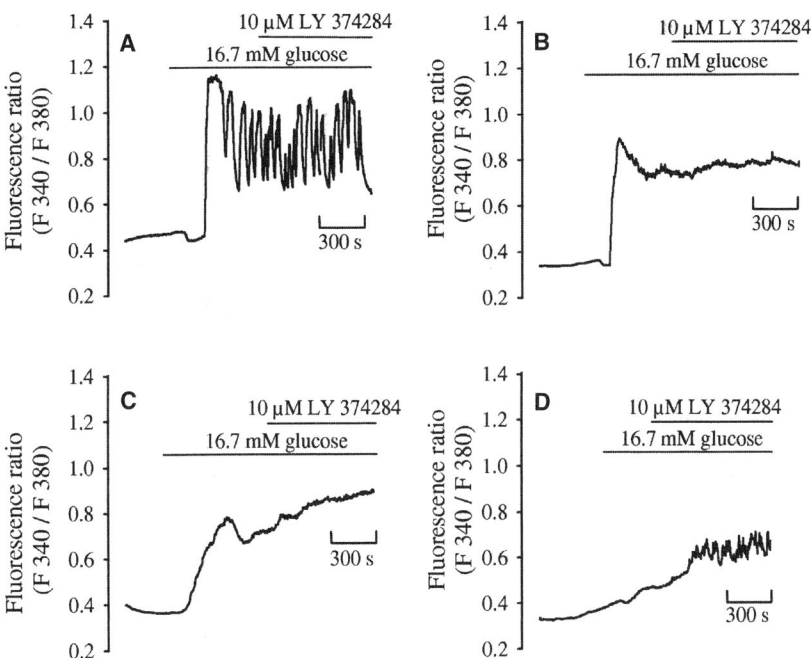

FIGURE 3. Two types of effects of 16.7 mmol/L glucose and 10 μmol/L LY374284 on fura-2 fluorescence ratio F_{340}/F_{380} reflecting $[Ca^{2+}]_i$ in db/+ (**A, B**) and db/db (**C, D**) β-cell clusters. Traces are representative of 11 experiments.

(FIG. 3B) rise in $[Ca^{2+}]_i$. This pattern of increase in $[Ca^{2+}]_i$ was in sharp contrast to that observed in clusters of β cells from db/db mice, as illustrated by a lack of the initial transient decrease and a delayed onset (165 ± 10 seconds; n = 11) and slower rate of increase in $[Ca^{2+}]_i$ (FIG. 3C, D).

LY374284 Does Not Increase Cellular ATP Content in Islets of Db/db Mice

FIGURE 4B shows cellular ATP content in islets of 16-week-old db/db mice. It is evident that glucose stimulation produced a small but not significant increase in cellular ATP, which did not change following application of LY374284. Much stronger increases in cellular ATP content were observed in islets from db/+ mice following glucose stimulation (FIG. 4A). Again, LY374284 was without effect.

LY374284 Stimulates Insulin Secretion in Maximally Depolarized Islets

We have previously demonstrated that imidazoline compounds stimulate Ca^{2+}-dependent exocytosis in pancreatic β cells.[15] To explore the possibility that LY374284 potentiates insulin secretion at a level distal to an elevation of $[Ca^{2+}]_i$,

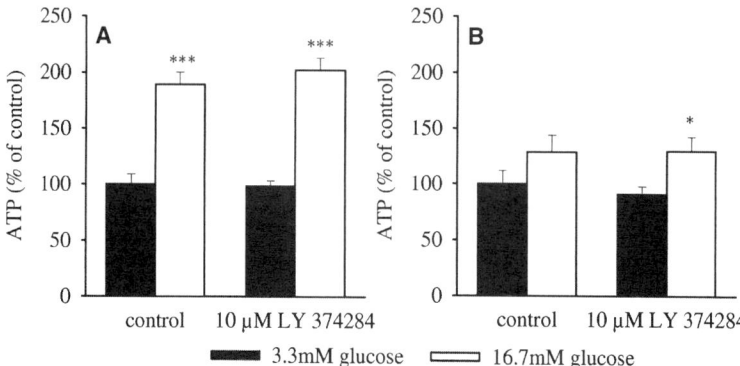

FIGURE 4. Effects of 16.7 mmol/L glucose and 10 µmol/L LY374284 on ATP content in islets of 16-week-old db/+ (**A**) and db/db (**B**) mice. ATP levels are expressed as percentage of the ATP level at 3.3 mmol/L glucose. Data are means ± SE for 9 to 12 observations from three to four independent experiments. * $P < 0.05$, *** $P < 0.001$ versus ATP levels at either 3.3 mmol/L glucose or 3.3 mmol/L glucose plus 10 µmol/L LY374284.

islets of db/db and db/+ mice were clamped at a depolarized stage using 30 mmol/L K^+, 16.7 mmol/L glucose, and 250 µmol/L diazoxide.[16] Under these maximally depolarized conditions, LY374284 (50 µM) strongly increased insulin secretion in islets of both diabetic and control mice (FIG. 5). This finding suggests that LY374284 directly stimulates insulin exocytosis.

DISCUSSION

One of the major signs of human type 2 diabetes is the gradual loss of biphasic insulin secretion.[1] The present data demonstrate a gradual deterioration of glucose-induced insulin secretion in islets of db/db mice that was characterized by both a reduced first- and second-phase response. Sulfonylureas have been widely used in the

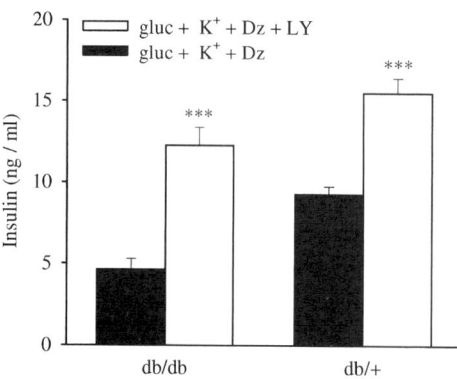

FIGURE 5. Effect of LY374284 on insulin secretion in maximally depolarized db/+ and db/db islets. Islets were starved for 30 minutes in Krebs-Ringer buffer containing 3.3 mmol/L glucose. Subsequently five islets were grouped and stimulated with Krebs-Ringer buffer containing 30 mmol/L K^+ (K^+), 250 µmol/L diazoxide (Dz), and 16.7 mmol/L glucose (gluc). Data are means ± SE for six observations from two independent experiments. *** $P < 0.001$ versus control.

treatment of type 2 diabetes. A major criticism of this group of compounds is that they induce insulin secretion by closure of K_{ATP} channels independently of the ambient glucose concentration.[4] Therefore, treatment of diabetic patients with sulfonylureas involves the risk of hypoglycemic episodes.[5] Our data revealed that tolbutamide enhanced insulin secretion at a low glucose concentration in perifused islets of db/db mice but was unable to increase glucose-induced insulin secretion. This finding clearly contrasts with the marked enhancement of glucose-stimulated insulin secretion in islets of db/db mice exposed to the imidazoline compound LY374284 or the peptide GLP-1. The latter two compounds did not affect insulin secretion at nonstimulatory glucose concentrations.

Recent attention was focused on imidazoline compounds for the potential treatment of type 2 diabetes,[6] because some of these compounds selectively potentiate insulin secretion at elevated glucose levels without interfering with the activity of K_{ATP} channels.[8,14,17] The present study extends these observations by showing no effect of LY374284 on cellular ATP content or $[Ca^{2+}]_i$ in islets isolated from diabetic db/db mice. A change in $[Ca^{2+}]_i$ is a good indicator of K_{ATP} channel activity because closure of the channels leads to membrane depolarization, activation of voltage-gated Ca^{2+} channels, and Ca^{2+} influx. Instead our data showed that LY374284 directly stimulates insulin exocytosis as illustrated by the strong enhancement of insulin secretion in maximally depolarized islets. This finding is consistent with other data showing that imidazoline compounds directly stimulate Ca^{2+}-dependent exocytosis in pancreatic β cells.[15]

In conclusion, we have described a progressive insulin secretion defect in islets of diabetic db/db mice. The imidazoline compound LY374284 partly restored first-phase and completely normalized second-phase insulin secretion in those islets. These observations may be of therapeutic relevance because the importance of early-phase insulin secretion in the control of postprandial hyperglycemia in type 2 diabetes.

ACKNOWLEDGMENTS

The technical assistance of Eva-Marie Azizi, Claudia Schöber, and Clemens Borkenstein is highly appreciated.

REFERENCES

1. PFEIFER, M.A., *et al.* 1981. Insulin secretion in diabetes mellitus. Am. J. Med. **70:** 579–588.
2. STEINER, K.E., *et al.* 1982. The relative importance of first- and second-phase insulin secretion in countering the action of glucagon on glucose turnover in the conscious dog. Diabetes **31:** 964–972.
3. MITRAKOU, A., *et al.* 1992. Role of reduced suppression of glucose production and diminished early insulin release in impaired glucose tolerance. N. Engl. J. Med. **326:** 22–29.
4. ASHCROFT, F.M. 1996. Mechanisms of the glycaemic effects of sulfonylureas. Horm. Metab. Res. **28:** 456–463.
5. PFEIFFER, E.F., *et al.* 1976. Hypoglycemia in diabetics. Horm. Metab. Res. Suppl. **6:** 112–126.
6. SCHULZ, A. & A. HASSELBLATT. 1989. An insulin-releasing property of imidazoline derivatives is not limited to compounds that block alpha-adrenoceptors. Naunyn Schmiedebergs Arch. Pharmacol. **340:** 321–327.

7. PLANT, T.D. & J.C. HENQUIN. 1990. Phentolamine and yohimbine inhibit ATP-sensitive K+ channels in mouse pancreatic beta-cells. Br. J. Pharmacol. **101:** 115–120.
8. EFANOV, A.M., *et al.* 2001. The novel imidazoline compound BL11282 potentiates glucose-induced insulin secretion in pancreatic beta-cells in the absence of modulation of K(ATP) channel activity. Diabetes **50:** 797–802.
9. THORENS, B. 1992. Expression cloning of the pancreatic beta cell receptor for the gluco-incretin hormone glucagon-like peptide 1. Proc. Natl. Acad. Sci. U. S. A. **89:** 8641–8645.
10. GROMADA, J., *et al.* 1995. Stimulation of cloned human glucagon-like peptide 1 receptor expressed in HEK 293 cells induces cAMP-dependent activation of calcium-induced calcium release. FEBS Lett. **373:** 182–186.
11. LACY, P.E. & M. KOSTIANOVSKY. 1967. Method for the isolation of intact islets of Langerhans from the rat pancreas. Diabetes **16:** 35–39.
12. PERDRIZET, G.A., *et al.* 1995. Albumin improves islet isolation: specific versus nonspecific effects. Transplant. Proc. **27:** 3400–3402.
13. BRENNER, M. & H.J. MEST. 2003. Comparison of the insulin secretory kinetics from MIN6-pseudoislets and mouse islets. Naunyn Schmiedebergs Arch. Pharmacol. **367**(Suppl 1): R73.
14. MEST, H.J., *et al.* 2001. Glucose-induced insulin secretion is potentiated by a new imidazoline compound. Naunyn Schmiedebergs Arch. Pharmacol. **364:** 47–52.
15. HOY, M., *et al.* 2003. Imidazoline NNC77–0074 stimulates insulin secretion and inhibits glucagon release by control of Ca(2+)-dependent exocytosis in pancreatic alpha- and beta-cells. Eur. J. Pharmacol. **466:** 213–221.
16. GEMBAL, M., *et al.* 1992. Evidence that glucose can control insulin release independently from its action on ATP-sensitive K+ channels in mouse B cells. J. Clin. Invest. **89:** 1288–1295.
17. EFANOV, A.M., *et al.* 2002. Insulinotropic activity of the imidazoline derivative RX871024 in the diabetic GK rat. Am. J. Physiol. Endocrinol. Metab. **282:** E117–E124.

Effect of Postmortem Delay on Imidazoline Receptor-Binding Proteins in Human and Mouse Brain

JOHN K. MA,[a] HE ZHU,[a] AND JOHN E. PILETZ[a,b]

[a]*Department of Psychiatry, University of Mississippi Medical Center, Jackson, Mississippi 39216, USA*

[b]*Department of Biology, Jackson State University, Jackson, Mississippi, USA*

ABSTRACT: Immunoreactive proteins of 45-kD and 29/30-kD doublet bands are candidate imidazoline receptor binding proteins (IRBP) based on associations with I_1 or I_2 binding sites, respectively. It was reported that the density of cortical membrane 29/30-kD I_2 protein is diminished whereas a 45-kD I_1 protein is increased in depressed suicide victims versus controls. IRBP immunoreactive bands of similar size have been suggested to be breakdown products of the 170-kD protein known as IRAS (putative full-length I_1 receptor). This study compares nonpathologic human brains collected and frozen after postmortem delays of 13.4 hours ± 1.7 (SEM) with brains of longer postmortem delays (26.1 hours ± 1.2). The fresher human brains possessed more full-length IRAS ($P = 0.05$). In another study, the postmortem decay of IRBP bands in mouse brain was shown to be linear over time. The results are relevant to previous studies of IRBP bands in postmortem brains of depressed suicide victims.

KEYWORDS: imidazoline receptor; postmortem; antiserum; IRAS

INTRODUCTION

Microinjection studies into the brainstem have linked an I_1-imidazoline receptor subtype to sympathetic drive and the control of blood pressure.[1] Aberrations in sympathetic drive are also known to occur in depressed patients.[2] The I_1-selective agonist moxonidine has also been reported[3] to induce calming behavior in mice. Another class of imidazoline binding sites, designated I_{2A} and I_{2B}, has been associated with monoamine oxidases A (MAO-A) and B (MAO-B).[4] Because MAO inhibition was the first discovered mechanism of antidepressant drug action, imidazoline receptors may play a role in depression.

The isolation of an imidazoline receptor binding protein (IRBP) was first performed with bovine adrenomedullary plasma membranes.[5] Surprisingly, this protein was shown to possess both I_1 and I_2 binding properties based on affinity chromatography resins.[5] The fact that imidazoline receptors and α_2-adrenoreceptors possessed

---

Address for correspondence: He Zhu, M.D., Department of Psychiatry, University of Mississippi Medical Center, 2500 North State Street, Jackson, MS 39216-4505, USA. Voice: 601-984-5798; fax: 601-984-5899.
e-mail: HZhu@psychiatry.umsmed.edu

Ann. N.Y. Acad. Sci. 1009: 341–346 (2003). © 2003 New York Academy of Sciences.
doi: 10.1196/annals.1304.043

almost equal affinities for most imidazoline compounds[6] led to the use of immunologic techniques, rather than radioligand binding, for ease of quantification. Therefore, bovine IRBP was used to produce a polyclonal antiserum, designated IRBP antiserum.[7] IRBP antiserum was in turn used to isolate a human cDNA clone that encodes an imidazoline binding protein named IRAS.[8] From these studies, a large number of polypeptides are now known to react with IRBP antiserum on Western blots. Sizes are (1) 70 kD for the original IRBP isolated from bovine adrenomedulla; (2) 170–210 kD for the various species forms of IRAS; (3) 85 kD for a major immunoreactive protein found in fresh rat brain membranes; and (4) 45, 35, and 29 kD for various peptides that are enriched in tissue membranes prepared in the absence of protease inhibitors.[9] Associational studies have also suggested that an I_2 site is encoded by 29/30-kD doublet IRBP in cortical membranes, and an I_1 site is encoded by a 45-kD peptide in brain.[10]

Literature reports exist of both increased[11] and decreased[12] densities of IRBPs in brains of depressed suicide victims versus normal controls. Unfortunately, the studies are difficult to compare. One problem is the inaccessibility of human brain tissue until after death. This problem has led to inevitable questions of postmortem decay. The objective of the present study was to investigate the effect of postmortem delay (PMD) on IRBP levels in brain.

MATERIALS AND METHODS

Human Cortex

Human brain tissues were obtained in accordance with approved Institutional Review Board protocols (supplied by Dr. Gregory Ordway, University of Mississippi). All subjects died of sudden natural or accidental causes within 4 hours of injury, and the brains were collected at the time of autopsy at the Cuyahoga County Coroner's Office, Ohio (collected by Dr. Craig Stockmeier, University of Mississippi). Subjects were divided into two groups according to long and short PMD. Eight subjects in each group were paired closely for age, sex, cause of death, and evidence of alcohol consumption. Ages were 39.3 years ± 5.5 (SEM) in the longer-PMD group and 39.4 years ± 5.6 in the shorter-PMD group. Six pairs were males, and two pairs were females. Race and smoking history were identical in five of the eight pairs. Toxicologic screening was performed at the coroner's office for 50 compounds in the blood, bile, urine, and/or vitreous fluids; only one subject had evidence of a small amount of lidocaine in the blood. Thus, the main difference was PMD: 26.1 hours ± 1.2 (SEM) in the longer-PMD group versus 13.4 hours ± 1.7 in the shorter-PMD group ($P < 0.001$).

Following the dissection on ice, blocks of cortex were placed on dry ice for 10 minutes and stored at −80°C. The frozen blocks of cortex were subsequently mounted on a specimen chuck of a cryostat microtome (Cryocut 1800, Leica, Reicher-Jung, Deerfield, IL, USA). Two 20-μm slices of Brodmann's area 9 from each subject were cut at −16°C and placed in microcentrifuge tubes. The slices were sonicated for 6 seconds in 200 μL of ice-cold Tris-sucrose buffer containing eight protease inhibitors.[9] Aliquots (2×10 μg) were assayed for total protein concentration using Lowry-Biuret reagent kit from Sigma (St. Louis, MO, USA), and the remaining homogenates were flash-frozen and stored at −80°C until Western blotting.

Mouse Cortex

Male C57Bl/6 mice (Jackson Labs, Bar Harbor, ME), weighing 24 to 30 g, were housed five per cage under a 12-hour light/dark cycle with free access to food and water. Acclimatization to the new environment lasted at least 1 week before experimentation. Thirty-three mice were divided into six groups of five or six. All were killed by decapitation. One group was immediately dissected on ice. Other decapitated heads were kept at room temperature for up to 6 hours, and some were then placed at 4°C to simulate the procedure of human brain collection at the coroner's office. For mice, the six PMD times were 0, 3, 6, 12, 24, and 30 total hours. A single left cortical hemisphere was obtained and immediately frozen in liquid nitrogen. This solid brain hemisphere was pulverized with a stainless steel mortar and pestle set in dry ice. From this, approximately 0.2 mg of powder was immediately processed, as described previously.

Western Blotting

Each sample consisted of 10 µg protein/10 µL buffer, which was denatured and electrophoresed through 13.7% polyacrylamide gels (SDS-PAGE). A batch preparation of standard mouse-brain homogenate was also run on each slab gel at 4, 7, 10, 13, and 16 µg, which served as a standard curve. Our use of nitrocellulose membranes (Hybond ECL, Amersham, Arlington Heights, IL, USA) and IRBP antiserum (1:3,000 dilution in TBST/10% milk as primary antibody) followed by anti-rabbit Ig G antibody (1:3,000 dilution in TBST/10% milk as secondary antibody) has been previously described.[12] Bands were detected with Amersham's Enhanced Chemiluminesence (ECL) detection system by film exposure (ECL Hyperfilm) for 3 to 10 minutes. Each sample was duplicated on different gels. To detect β-actin as a standard, the same blots were stripped and incubated with a 1:9,000 dilution of β-actin antiserum (Chemicon International, Temecula, CA, USA). Detection was by ECL using 1:3,000 dilution of anti-mouse IgG antibody (Amersham). Films were scanned using a Molecular Dynamics personal densitometer and analyzed with the Image Quant program (Molecular Dynamics, Sunnyvale, CA, USA). The main human IRBP brain bands were 200 kD, 48 kD, 45 kD, and 40 kD in size. Mouse brain IRBP bands of 85 kD, 70 kD, and 35 kD were singled out from each postmortem category (0, 3, 6, 12, 24, and 30 hours). Standard curves gave assurance that optical densities (OD) were within a linear response range for the film and allowed for normalizing between films. IRBP OD values of each sample were compared with the amount of β-actin in each sample to ensure equal loading in each lane. Statistical analyses and regression lines were obtained from GraphPad Prism (San Diego, CA, USA). Results are expressed as mean ± SEM, and Student's two-tailed t-tests were performed.

RESULTS

The only statistically significant finding among our human samples was that the immunodensity of a 200-kD IRBP band was 33% higher in the shorter-PMD group than in the longer-PMD group ($P = 0.05$, unpaired). The size of this band is consistent with full-length IRAS. No other differences were detected in 48-kD, 45-kD, or

40-kD IRBP bands in the human samples between the short- and long-PMD groups. Likewise, no difference in β-actin was detected between human PMD groups in the same samples ($P = 0.51$, unpaired).

Compared with the bands in human brain, the prominent IRBP bands of mouse cortex were of smaller size (85 kD, 70 kD, and 35 kD). No immunostaining was detectable above the 85-kD size in fresh mouse brains, and therefore full-length IRAS was not detected. Because we used eight protease inhibitors, this absence of the 200-kD IRAS band in mouse brain seems unlikely to be an artifact of tissue processing.

The rates of decay of mouse cortical IRBP bands are shown in FIGURE 1. The 85-kD IRBP band decreased more rapidly than the other IRBP bands and was almost completely absent after 30 hours of PMD. This decay was statistically significant for the 85-kD band after 24 hours and 30 hours of PMD ($P < 0.05$). Likewise, the 70-kD IRBP band showed a statistically significant decline after 24 hours and 30 hours of PMD ($P < 0.05$). The slight decline in the 35 kD IRBP band did not reach statistical significance at any time point, however (FIG. 1). In fact, the level of 35-kD peptide at 3 hours and 6 hours postmortem seemed higher than at baseline (NS [not statistically significant]). Overall, the 35-kD band paralleled levels of β-actin, which also did not change after 30 hours of PMD. Thus, murine IRBP bands degraded in the following order: 85 kD > 70 kD > 35 kD (FIG. 1).

DISCUSSION

The present human study shows that longer PMDs, from 13 hours to 26 hours, are associated with a significant reduction in amount of a 200-kD IRBP band in Brod-

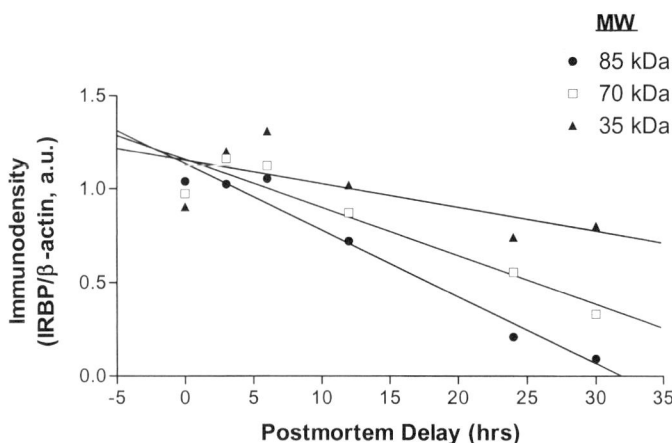

FIGURE 1. Rates of postmortem decay of IRBPs of different molecular weights expressed in ratio to the reference β-actin antigen. Thirty-three mouse brains were studied with different postmortem delays (0, 3, 6, 12, 24, and 30 hours). The correlation coefficients and P values for these correlations were as follow: 85 kD ($r = -0.98$, $P = 0.0004$); 70 kD ($r = -0.94$, $P = 0.0045$); 35 kD ($r = -0.68$, $P = 0.139$).

man's area 9 of human cortex. Based on its size and immunoreactivity, this band is almost surely full-length human IRAS, which encodes the I_1 imidazoline receptor.[8] For unknown reasons, the size is slightly larger than cloned IRAS (167 kD). Also, IRBP antiserum did not detect a similar 200-kD band in mouse brain, but murine IRBP bands of 85 kD and 70 kD were identified and found to be diminished by approximately 96% and approximately ≈85%, respectively, after 30 hours of PMD (FIG. 1). Because β-actin levels were unchanged in the same samples, the IRBP bands seem to be selectively more sensitive to proteolysis.

The present findings add to previous studies that suggest that an 85-kD band is a proteolytic product of full-length IRAS[13] and that the human 85-kD IRBP band is particularly susceptible to proteolysis, depending on method of tissue preparation.[9,14] From a techniques standpoint, the good news is that no significant decay was apparent in mouse brain during the first 6 hours of PMD, and thereafter the postmortem decay occurred in a linear, predictable fashion (FIG. 1).

Despite an obvious loss of 85-kD and 70-kD IRBP bands in mouse brain, no significant changes were observed in the 35-kD IRBP at any time of PMD (FIG. 1). In fact, the 35-kD band tended towards higher levels after only 3 hours or 6 hours of PMD (FIG. 1). One explanation may be that the 35-kD IRBP derives from the 85-kD or 70-kD IRBP. This possibility would explain a slight increase in the 35-kD band during short PMDs up to 6 hours (FIG. 1). Thereafter, a slower rate of degradation of the 35-kD band (FIG. 1) might also be expected because of its simultaneous formation from the 85-kD and/or 70-kD peptides, along with its own steady decay. In any case, PMD should be carefully documented and controlled in future studies of IRBP with human brain tissues.

ACKNOWLEDGMENTS

We gratefully acknowledge Drs. Greg Ordway and Craig Stockmeier for obtaining and providing the human brain samples. This research was supported by federal grants MH49248 and MH57601.

REFERENCES

1. BOUSQUET, P., J. FELDMAN & J. SCHWARTZ. 1984. Central cardiovascular effects of alpha adrenergic drugs: differences between catecholamines and imidazolines. J. Pharmacol. Exp. Ther. **230:** 232–236.
2. MANJI, H.K., M.V. RUDORFER & W.Z. POTTER. 1994. Affective disorders and adrenergic function. *In* Adrenergic Dysfunction and Psychobiology. O.G. Cameron, Ed.: 365–401. American Psychiatric Press Inc. Washington, DC.
3. ZHU, H., I.A. PAUL, D.E. STEC, *et al.* 2003. Non-adrenergic exploratory behavior induced by moxonidine at mildly hypotensive doses. Brain Res. **964:** 9–20.
4. TESSON, F., I. LIMON-BOULEZ, P. URBAN, *et al.* 1995. Localization of I2-imidazoline binding sites on monoamine oxidases. J. Biol. Chem. **270:** 9856–9861.
5. WANG, H., S. REGUNATHAN, M.P. MEELEY, *et al.* 1992. Isolation and characterization of imidazoline receptor protein from bovine adrenal chromaffin cells. Mol. Pharmacol. **42:** 792–801.
6. ERNSBERGER, P., M.E. GRAVES, L.M. GRAFF, *et al.* 1995. I1-Imidazoline receptors: definition, characterization, distribution and transmembrane signalling. Ann. N. Y. Acad. Sci. **763:** 22–42.
7. WANG, H., S. REGUNATHAN, D.A. RUGGIERO, *et al.* 1993. Production and characterization of antibodies specific for the imidazoline receptor protein. Mol. Pharmacol. **43:** 509–515.

8. PILETZ, J.E., T.R. IVANOV, J.D. SHARP, et al. 2000. Imidazoline receptor antisera-selected (IRAS) cDNA: cloning and characterization. DNA Cell Biol. **19:** 319–329.
9. IVANOV, T.R., H. ZHU, S. REGUNATHAN, et al. 1998. Co-detection by two imidazoline receptor protein antisera of a novel 85 kilodalton protein. Biochem. Pharmacol. **55:** 649–655.
10. ESCRIBA, P.V., A. OZAITA & J.A. GARCIA-SEVILLA. 1999. Pharmacologic characterization of imidazoline receptor proteins identified by immunologic techniques and other methods. Ann. N. Y. Acad. Sci. **881:** 8–25.
11. GARCIA-SEVILLA, J.A., P.V. ESCRIBA, M. SASTRE, et al. 1996. Immunodetection and quantitation of imidazoline receptor proteins in platelets of patients with major depression and in brains of suicide victims. Arch. Gen. Psychiatry **53:** 803–810.
12. PILETZ, J.E., H. ZHU, G. ORDWAY, et al. 2000. Imidazoline receptor proteins are decreased in the hippocampus of individuals with major depression. Biol. Psychiatry **48:** 910–919.
13. PILETZ, J.E., J.C. JONES, H. ZHU, et al. 1999. Imidazoline receptor antisera-selected cDNA clone and mRNA distribution. Ann. N. Y. Acad Sci. **881:** 1–7.
14. IVANOV, T.R., Y. FENG, H. WANG, et al. 1998. Imidazoline receptor proteins are regulated in platelet-precursor MEG-01 cells by agonists and antagonists. J. Psychiatr. Res. **32:** 65–79.

Association Between I_2 Binding Sites and Monoamine Oxidase-B Activity in Platelets

H. ZHU[a] AND J.E. PILETZ[a,b]

[a]*University of Mississippi Medical Center, Jackson, Mississippi 39216, USA*

[b]*Jackson State University, Jackson, Mississippi 39217, USA*

ABSTRACT: An I_2 imidazoline binding site on monoamine oxidase-B (MAO-B) is known to be encoded by a noncatalytic part of the enzyme, different from that which recognizes mechanism-based inhibitors. Herein, the relationship between I_2-imidazoline binding sites and MAO-B activity has been assessed using a semi-purified source of MAO-B: platelet mitochondrial membranes. A positive correlation between I_2 sites and MAO-B activity was observed (r = 0.61, P = 0.0016) among 24 human subjects. Nevertheless, the variance in MAO-B activity cannot be completely accounted for in relation to I_2 sites. Therefore, I_2 density and MAO-B activity are only weakly correlated in platelets.

KEYWORDS: monoamine oxidase; MAO-B; imidazoline receptors; platelets

INTRODUCTION

Two major subtypes of imidazoline binding sites are known (I_1 and I_2). I_1 sites possess high affinity for clonidine relative to idazoxan and are associated with plasma membranes.[1] I_2 sites possess high affinity for idazoxan relative to clonidine and are associated with mitochondria membranes.[2]

Some I_2 sites are encoded by monoamine oxidases (MAOs).[3,4] MAOs catalyze the oxidative deamination of amine neurotransmitters such as norepinephrine and dopamine as well as various xenobiotics. Inhibition of the two subtypes of this enzyme (MAO-A and MAO-B) has therapeutic value for treating depression and Parkinson's disease. The I_2 site on MAO-B is distinct from the amino acid sequence, which recognizes mechanism-based enzyme inhibitors such as pargyline and deprenyl,[5] but some I_2-selective ligands inhibit enzyme activity.[6] Paradoxically, I_2 sites exist within only a subset of MAO-A and MAO-B molecules.[7] Of particular relevance, Raddatz and coworkers reported[3] that the platelet I_2 site is less accessible to radioligand binding than MAO-B molecules in other tissues.

The aim of the present study was to explore the relationship between I_2 sites and MAO-B enzyme activity in different human platelet samples. For this purpose a purified source of MAO-B was used: purified internal membranes from human platelets. A previous report[8] showed that [^{3}H]idazoxan binding to I_2 sites correlates

---

Address for correspondence: He Zhu, M.D., Department of Psychiatry, University of Mississippi Medical Center, 2500 North State Street, Jackson, MS 39216-4505, USA. Voice: 601-984-5798; fax: 601-984-5899.

e-mail: HZhu@psychiatry.umsmed.edu

positively with monoamine oxidase (r = 0.960) and negatively with the inner mitochondrial membrane marker, cytochrome oxidase (r = −0.950) activities. Therefore, a robust correlation between I_2 sites and MAO-B activity was expected if the platelet enzyme is the same as the liver enzyme.

MATERIALS AND METHODS

Twenty-four adult subjects were recruited through local advertisements. They consisted of 17 females and 7 males (average age: 38.6 years ± 10.1 SD). Each subject signed a consent form before the morning blood collection. All were physically healthy on examination, unmedicated, and not using chemical substances of any kind. Subjects followed precise exercise and dietary restrictions before the blood drawing to avoid platelet activation.[9] Platelets were prepared as previously described[10,11] from fresh blood samples (100 mL) or from recently outdated platelet concentrates from Mississippi Blood Services (called Red Cross standards). The platelets were resuspended in isotonic-buffer solution containing 100 µM phenylmethylsulfonyl fluoride, homogenized on ice, and subjected to two cycles of snap freezing and thawing on ice. The lysates were then layered over a discontinuous 14.5% and 34% sucrose gradient which was centrifuged at 105,000 × gravity for 90 minutes at 4°C.[10] The pellet from the sucrose gradient was dissolved in 1.5 mL ice-cold membrane buffer optimized for imidazoline binding assays.[12] The pellet is called "internal membranes" because it is enriched in mitochondrial and endoplasmic-reticulum markers.[11]

MAO-B assays were conducted with platelet internal membranes (25 µg protein/tube) in 0.05 M phosphate buffer, pH 7.4, plus substrates in a total volume of 1.0 mL for 20 minutes at 37°C. The MAO-B radioactive substrate, β-[ethyl-1-^{14}C]phenylethylamine hydrochloride (PEA 44 mCi/mmol), was purchased from NEN Life Science Products (Boston, MA, USA). Substrates were [^{14}C]-labeled and unlabeled PEA in an overall concentration of 10 µM (radioactivity about 50,000 cpm). The selective MAO-B inhibitor, Ro16-6491 (100 µM), was used to define specific activity. After incubation, 0.2 mL of 3 M HCl was added and vigorously shaken for 15 minutes with 3 mL toluene. One mL of the organic phase was collected after low-speed centrifugation (10 minutes), and radioactivity was determined in a liquid scintillation counter. Total and nonspecific activities were determined in duplicate. Results are given in terms of specific nmol min^{-1} mg^{-1} protein from duplicate assays of each sample.

A cirazoline derivative, 2-(3-amino-4-iodophenoxy)methylimidazoline (AMIPI) was synthesized, radio-iodinated, and converted into the photolabile azide ([^{125}I]AZIPI) for use as the photoaffinity I_2 ligand (2000 Ci/mmol).[3] This kind gift came from Rita Raddatz and Steve Lanier (Medical University of South Carolina, Charleston, SC, USA). Platelet internal membrane (60 µg protein/tube) was then incubated in the dark with 2 nM [^{125}I]AZIPI for 30 minutes at room temperature (total volume, 80 µL), followed by cooling on ice for 5 minutes. Just before photolysis (5 minutes at 254-nm wavelength), samples were diluted with 0.8 mL of ice-cold membrane buffer containing 2 mM dithiothreitol. Photolabeled membranes were then pelleted at 4°C, washed with 1 mL membrane buffer, and repelleted. Samples (25 µg protein/lane) were dissolved in denaturing buffer, boiled briefly, and then subjected to 10% SDS-polyacrylamide gel electrophoresis (SDS-PAGE) according to previously described methods.[9] After electrotransfer onto nitrocellulose membranes, the blots were dried at room temperature for 1 hour and exposed to Hyperfilm MP (Amersham Life Science, Arlington Heights, IL, USA) at −80°C for 10–14 days. Afterwards, to detect β-actin as a protein loading standard, the blots were incubated with a 1:10,000 dilution of β-actin antiserum (Chemicon International, Temecula, CA, USA) as the primary antibody, followed by the secondary antibody (horseradish peroxidase-linked sheep anti-mouse Ig G at 1:3,000 dilution), and finally detected by an Enhanced Chemiluminescent system (Amersham, Piscataway, NJ).[9] Films were scanned using a densitometer and analyzed with the Image Quant program (Molecular Dynamics, Sunnyvale, CA, USA). Samples on different blots were normalized by optical density (OD) in comparison with Red Cross standards (n = 3 concentrations on each slab gel). OD values were obtained twice for each sample, averaged from different blots, and results were expressed as the ratio of [^{125}I]AZIPI band:β-actin band.

RESULTS

The photoaffinity ligand, [^{125}I]AZIPI, was used to label I_2 sites covalently in human platelet internal membranes. [^{125}I]AZIPI incorporated into a single protein band on SDS-PAGE with the molecular weight expected of MAO-B (approximately 59 kD). In FIGURE 1, the 59-kD MAO-B bands (*upper panel*) are shown juxtaposed above the 43-kD β-actin reference bands (*lower panel*). FIGURE 1 displays bands labeled in platelet internal membranes from six representative subjects. Over all, it was calculated that I_2 sites averaged 5.01 ± 3.43 (SD)-fold higher intensity than β-actin intensity in the same fractions (n = 24 subjects). Two control experiments are also particularly noteworthy: (1) the extent of the [^{125}I]AZIPI labeling varied in a protein-dependent manner; (2) labeling of the 59-kD MAO-B band was totally blocked by addition of 100 μM cirazoline, an imidazoline agent (data not shown).

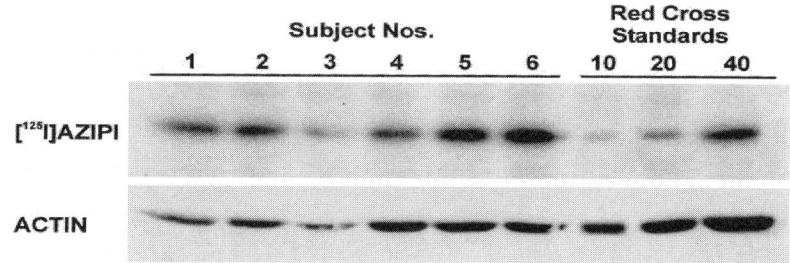

FIGURE 1. (*Upper panel*) [^{125}I]AZIPI photo-labeling of a 59-kD band from the internal membrane fraction of platelets from six healthy adult subjects (lanes 1–6). Samples (25 μg protein per lane) were run on SDS-polyacrylamide gels, transferred to nitrocellulose blots, and the blots exposed to X-ray film. (*Lower panel*) Western blot of a 43-kD band revealed by probing the same blot with anti-β-actin antibody (1:10,000 dilution) and developing the film by enhanced chemiluminescence. Red Cross standards were platelet internal membrane protein (10, 20, and 40 μg/lane) prepared from a bag of platelet concentrates from the blood bank.

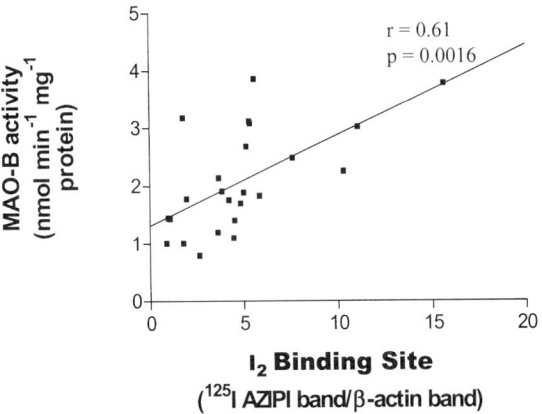

FIGURE 2. Linear correlation between [^{125}I]AZIPI photo-labeling of I_2 sites and MAO-B enzyme activity across 24 samples of human platelet internal membranes (r = 0.61, P = 0.0016). Points are individual values from different subjects.

MAO-B enzyme activity was next measured in aliquots of the same platelet internal membranes as used for [^{125}I]AZIPI binding. [^{14}C]-PEA was used as substrate, and Ro16-6491 (100 µM) was included as a blank. Neither agent has any known interaction with imidazoline binding sites. Overall, the activity of MAO-B averaged 2.078 ± 0.889 nmol min^{-1} mg^{-1} protein in the subjects' internal membrane fractions (n = 24).

Next, the relationship between I_2 sites and MAO-B activity in platelet internal membrane was investigated. Using linear regression analysis, a significant positive correlation was established between [^{125}I]AZIPI-labeling of I_2 sites and MAO-B catalytic activity across platelet internal membrane fractions from different subjects (r = 0.61, P = 0.0016, n = 24) (FIG. 2). Many samples deviated from the expected 1:1 correspondence, and thus not all the variance in I_2 sites could be accounted for by MAO-B activity.

DISCUSSION

An I_2 site is known to be encoded by a domain within MAO-B.[3,4] It is therefore not surprising that I_2 sites have been correlated with the number of MAO-B molecules in the brain.[8,13] Such correlations were found to be significant across eight human brain regions (r = 0.84) and in the frontal cortex of 11 postmortem control human brains (r = 0.70) by using [^{3}H]idazoxan to label I_2 sites and [^{3}H]lazabemide to label MAO-B active sites.[14] Another report[8] found [^{3}H]idazoxan binding to I_2 sites was highly positively correlated with MAO (r = 0.960) and negatively with the inner mitochondrial membrane marker cytochrome oxidase (r = −0.950) activities in human and rabbit liver subcellular fractions. Furthermore, some I_2-selective ligands inhibit MAO-A and MAO-B enzyme activity.[6] One would therefore expect a positive correlation to exist between platelet I_2 sites and MAO-B enzyme activity in platelets, especially when using membrane-enriched subcellular fractions. On the other hand, Lanier and coworkers[7] have shown that only a subset of MAO-A and MAO-B molecules actually express I_2 sites. Furthermore, platelet I_2 sites have been reported[3] to be disproportionately low compared with the high level of MAO-B expressed in platelets.

In the present study, the levels of MAO-B catalytic activity and I_2 sites were positively correlated among samples from 24 subjects (FIG. 2). The strength of the correlation (r = 0.61, FIG. 2) was substantially lower than that expected from earlier studies reported in brain and liver, however.[8,14] Therefore, it seems that factors in addition to the number of platelet MAO-B molecules should be involved in determining the level of I_2 sites in platelets. This study adds weight to the previous findings that platelet I_2 sites are not found on every MAO-B molecule.[3]

ACKNOWLEDGMENTS

We thank Dr. Angleos Halaris for providing resources to recruit subjects. We also thank Dr. Stephen Lanier and Dr. Rita Raddatz for providing the [^{125}I]AZIPI (while based at the University of South Carolina, Charleston). This research was supported by federal grants MH49248 and MH57601.

REFERENCES

1. ERNSBERGER, P., M.E. GRAVES, L.M. GRAFF, et al. 1995. I_1-Imidazoline receptors: definition, characterization, distribution and transmembrane signalling. Ann. N. Y. Acad. Sci. **763:** 22–42.
2. TESSON, F. & A. PARINI. 1991. Identification of an imidazoline-guanidinium receptive site in mitochondria from rabbit cerebral cortex. Eur. J. Pharmacol. **208:** 81–83.
3. RADDATZ, R., A. PARINI & S.M. LANIER. 1995. Imidazoline/guanidinium binding domains on monoamine oxidases. Relationship to subtypes of imidazoline-binding proteins and tissue-specific interaction of imidazoline ligands with monoamine oxidase B. J. Biol. Chem. **270:** 27961–27968.
4. TESSON, F., I. LIMON-BOULEZ, P. URBAN, et al. 1995. Localization of I_2-imidazoline binding sites on monoamine oxidases. J. Biol. Chem. **270:** 9856–9861.
5. RADDATZ, R., A. PARINI & S.M. LANIER. 1997. Localization of the imidazoline binding domain on monoamine oxidase B. Mol. Pharmacol. **52:** 549–553.
6. LALIES, M., A. HIBELL, A. HUDSON, et al. 1999. Inhibition of central monoamine oxidase by imidazoline-2 site-selective ligands. Ann. N. Y. Acad. Sci. **881:** 114–117.
7. LANIER, S.M., R. RADDATZ & A. PARINI. 1998. Relationship between alpha 2-adrenergic receptors and imidazoline/guanidinium receptive sites. Adv. Pharmacol. **42:** 474–477.
8. TESSON, F., C. PRIP-BUUS, A. LEMOINE, et al. 1991. Subcellular distribution of imidazoline-guanidinium-receptive sites in human and rabbit liver. Major localization to the mitochondrial outer membrane. J. Biol. Chem. **266:** 155–160.
9. ZHU, H., A. HALARIS, S. MADAKASIRA, et al. 1999. Effect of bupropion on immunodensity of putative imidazoline receptors on platelets of depressed patients. J. Psychiatr. Res. **33:** 323–333.
10. PILETZ, J., A. HALARIS, A. SARAN, et al. 1990. Elevated [^{3}H]para-aminoclonidine binding to platelet purified plasma membranes from depressed patients. Neuropsychopharmacology. **3:** 201–210.
11. PILETZ, J.E. & K. SLETTEN. 1993. Nonadrenergic imidazoline binding sites on human platelets. J. Pharmacol. Exp. Ther. **267:** 1493–1502.

12. ERNSBERGER, P., J.E. PILETZ, L.M. GRAFF, et al. 1995. Optimization of radioligand binding assays for I-1 imidazoline sites. Ann. N. Y. Acad. Sci. **763**:163–168.
13. SASTRE, M. & J.A. GARCIA-SEVILLA. 1993. Opposite age-dependent changes of alpha-2A adrenoceptors and nonadrenoceptor [^{3}H]idazoxan binding sites (I_2-imidazoline sites) in the human brain: strong correlation of I_2 with monoamine oxidase-B sites. J. Neurochem. **61:** 881–889.
14. GARCIA-SEVILLA, J.A., A. MIRALLES, M. SASTRE, et al. 1995. I_2-imidazoline receptors in the healthy and pathologic human brain. Ann. N. Y. Acad. Sci. **763:** 178–193.

Relationship Between Imidazoline$_2$ Sites and Monoamine Oxidase

L.M. PATERSON, R.J. TYACKE, D.J. NUTT, AND A.L. HUDSON

Psychopharmacology Unit, School of Medical Sciences, University of Bristol, Bristol BS8 1TD, UK

ABSTRACT: I_2 site–selective compounds are known to interact with and inhibit monoamine oxidase (MAO), but it remains unclear as to whether this interaction occurs through an allosteric or competitive interaction. This study used the new selective, irreversible I_2 ligand BU99006, to clarify the relationship between MAO and the I_2 binding sites (I_2-BS). Results demonstrate that irreversible binding of BU99006 to rat brain membranes does not inhibit the enzyme or interfere with its interaction with other imidazoline enzyme inhibitors. This finding suggests that the I_2 sites that react with BU99006 are not those implicated in MAO inhibition and points to the existence of at least two distinct I_2 binding proteins.

KEYWORDS: imidazoline$_2$ binding sites; BU99006; 2BFI; monoamine oxidase

INTRODUCTION

Selective imidazoline$_2$ (I_2) ligands, such as 2BFI and BU224, exert several effects in vivo such as elevation of brain monoamines, efficacy in the Porsolt swim test,[1] and increased feeding behavior in rats.[2] The precise mechanism is unknown; however, these compounds are known to bind and inhibit monoamine oxidase (MAO).[3] Inhibition of this enzyme would offer a possible explanation for monoamine modulation by imidazolines but would not explain their effects on feeding, because MAO inhibitors decrease food intake. Although MAO inhibition by these ligands is well documented,[3,4,5] the exact mechanism of inhibition is not clear. It has been proposed to occur though an allosteric interaction of the imidazoline ligands with the enzyme.[6] Other data, however, suggest a more competitive form of inhibition.[5] Alternatively, a mechanism independent of MAO may be employed to cause the in vivo effects of I_2 ligands.

This study aimed to clarify the interaction of I_2-selective ligands with MAO using a new I_2-selective irreversible ligand, BU99006,[7,8,9] and other selective MAO and I_2 compounds. BU99006 has previously been shown to significantly reduce specific I_2 binding in rat brain.[8] Determination of the effects of BU99006 on MAO activity will allow a better assessment of the relationship between I_2 binding sites and MAO.

Address for correspondence: Dr. Alan L. Hudson, Head of Preclinical Science, Psychopharmacology Unit, School of Medical Sciences, University of Bristol, Bristol BS8 1TD, UK. Voice: (+44) 0 117 928; fax: (+44) 0 117 928 9700.
e-mail: a.l.hudson@bristol.ac.uk

MATERIALS AND METHODS

Rat whole brain pellets were prepared and pretreated as previously described.[8] Aliquots of homogenates were preincubated with 10 μM BU99006, 100 nM clorgyline, 100 nM deprenyl, or vehicle at 37°C for 20 minutes. Samples were then diluted with excess buffer (50 mM sodium orthophosphate, 1m M $MgCl_2$, pH 7.4) and centrifuged (32,000 gravity, 4°C for 20 minutes). Supernatants were discarded, and the pellet was washed twice to remove any unbound ligand. Samples were assayed either for their ability to bind specifically the I_2 selective ligand [^{3}H]2BFI (5 nM; NSB defined with 10 μM BU224)[10] or for MAO activity using a modified radiochemical assay as previously described.[5] Selective substrates for MAO-A and MAO-B were 200 μM [^{3}H]-serotonin and 20 μM [^{3}H]PEA, respectively. Data were analyzed using software supplied with GraphPad Prism version 3.03 for Windows (San Diego, California, USA). Significance was determined using one-way ANOVA with Dunnett's post hoc test.

RESULTS

BU99006 pretreatment caused a significant reduction in I_2 binding in rat brain membranes, as defined with specific [^{3}H]2BFI binding, which is similar to that previously shown.[8] This reduction did not occur with either clorgyline or deprenyl pretreatment (FIG. 1A).

Pretreatment with clorgyline or deprenyl resulted in a complete loss of MAO-A and MAO-B enzyme activities, respectively, as would be expected from selective irreversible inhibitors (FIG. 1B). On the other hand, BU99006 pretreatment had no effect on MAO activity (FIG.1B). Furthermore, the IC_{50} for inhibition of MAO-A by BU224 in control membranes was (in accordance with previously published data[3]) a value unaltered in BU99006 pretreated membranes (FIG. 2), as was the case with 2BFI in both MAO-A and MAO-B assays (data not shown). Overall, the results suggested that the I_2 sites that irreversibly react with BU99006 are not those implicated in the inhibition of MAO by imidazolines.

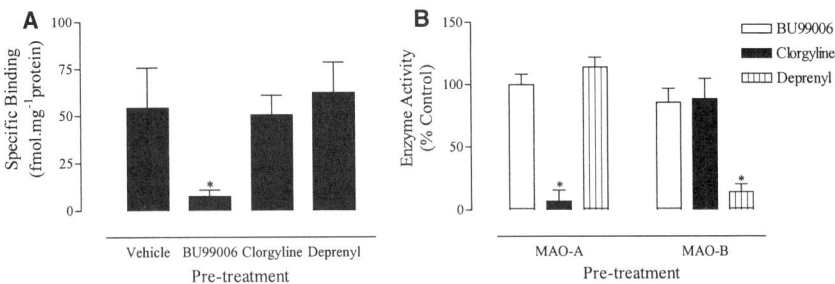

FIGURE 1. (**A**) Specific [^{3}H]2BFI binding in rat brain membranes, following pretreatment with vehicle, 10 μM BU99006, 100 nM clorgyline, or 100 nM deprenyl. (**B**) The effect of the same pretreatment on MAO-A and MAO-B activities. Bars represent mean ± S.D. * Indicates a significant difference from control, $P < 0.01$.

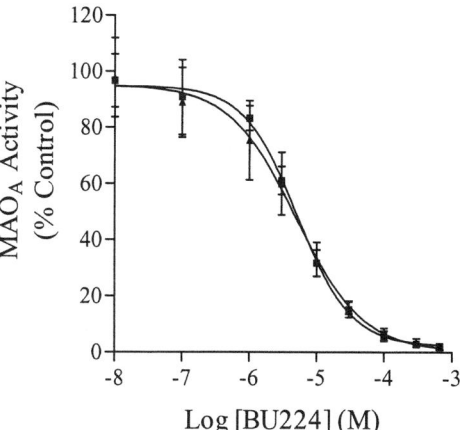

FIGURE 2. Inhibition of MAO-A by BU224 in vehicle and BU99006 (10 µM) pretreated rat whole brain membranes. Points represent mean, and vertical bars represent the SD. Legend shows IC_{50} values for inhibition.

DISCUSSION AND CONCLUSIONS

It seems that the irreversible binding of I_2 binding sites by BU99006 does not compromise the activity of MAO. The exact mechanism of interaction is not entirely obvious, but the evidence suggests that an allosteric modulation is unlikely, because 2BFI and BU224 are still able to inhibit MAO even though the I_2 site is irreversibly occupied by BU99006. Furthermore, 2BFI and BU224 are structurally similar to classical MAO substrates and inhibitors, making a competitive mechanism of inhibition seem more likely. This evidence points to the existence of other I_2 proteins, which are irreversibly bound by BU99006. The half-life of one of these proteins was estimated at 4.3 hours in rat brain.[9] Candidate proteins have been isolated, including creatine kinase[11] and imidazoline receptor antisera-selected (IRAS) protein.[12] Further work will determine which, if any, of these proteins are responsible for the reported in vivo I_2 binding site function.

ACKNOWLEDGMENT

This work was kindly funded by the Medical Research Council.

REFERENCES

1. HUDSON, A.L., D.J. NUTT & S.M. HUSBANDS. 2001. Imidazoline receptors and their role in depression. Pharmaceutical News **8:** 18–24.
2. EDWARDS, M.M., *et al.* 2002. Investigation of the acute administration of imidazoline ligands on food intake. Br. J. Pharmacol. **135:** 110P.

3. LALIES, M.D., et al. 1999. Inhibition of central monoamine oxidase by imidazoline2 site-selective ligands. Ann. N.Y. Acad. Sci. **881:** 114–117.
4. CARPENE, C., et al. 1995. Inhibition of amine oxidase activity by derivatives that recognize imidazoline I_2 sites. J. Pharmacol. Exp. Ther. **272:** 681–688.
5. OZAITA, A., et al. 1997. Inhibition of monoamine oxidase A and B activities by imidazol(ine)/guanidine drugs, nature of the interaction and distinction from I_2-imidazoline receptors in rat liver. Br. J. Pharmacol. **121:** 901–912.
6. RADDATZ, R., A. PARINI & S.M. LANIER. 1997. Localization of the imidazoline binding domain on monoamine oxidase B. Mol. Pharmacol. **52:** 549–553.
7. COATES, P.A., et al. 2000. Probes for imidazoline binding sites: synthesis and evaluation of a selective, irreversible I_2 ligand. Bioorg. Med. Chem. Lett. **10:** 605–607.
8. TYACKE, R.J., et al. 2002. 5-Isothiocyanato-2-benzofuranyl-2-imidazoline (BU99006) an irreversible imidazoline-2 binding site ligand: in vitro and in vivo characterisation in rat brain. Neuropharmacology **43:** 75–83.
9. PATERSON, L.M., et al. 2003. In vivo estimation of imadazoline$_2$ binding site turnover. Ann. N.Y. Acad. Sci. This volume.
10. LIONE, L.A., D.J. NUTT & A.L. HUDSON. 1998. Characterisation and localisation of [^{3}H]2-(2-benzofuranyl)-2-imidazoline binding in rat brain: a selective ligand for imidazoline I_2 receptors. Eur. J. Pharmacol. **353:** 123–135.
11. KIMURA, A., et al. 2003. Identification of a putative imidazoline-2 binding protein from rabbit brain. Br. J. Pharmacol. **138**(Suppl): 173P.
12. PILETZ, J.E., et al. 2000. Imidazoline receptor antisera-selected (IRAS) cDNA: cloning and characterization. DNA Cell Biol. **19:** 319–329.

Initial Evaluation of Novel Selective Ligands for Imidazoline$_2$ Receptors in Rat Whole Brain

R.J. TYACKE,[a] F. SĄCZEWSKI,[b] P. TABIN,[b] J. SĄCZEWSKI,[b] D.J. NUTT,[a] AND A.L. HUDSON[a]

[a]*Psychopharmacology Unit, School of Medical Sciences, University of Bristol, Bristol BS8 1TD, UK*

[b]*Department of Chemical Technology of Drugs, Medical University of Gdańsk, 80-416 Gdańsk, Poland*

ABSTRACT: Indazim, the indazole analogue of 2BFI, and four methyl-substituted analogues were tested for their affinity at the imidazoline$_2$ binding site (I$_2$-BS), and this affinity was compared with their affinity at the α_2-adrenoceptor to determine their structure, affinity relationship, and selectivity at the I$_2$-BS. These studies showed that these ligands were highly selective for the I$_2$-BS compared with 2BFI and that substitution at the 4 and 7 positions increased affinity without affecting selectivity.

KEYWORDS: imidazoline$_2$ binding site; indazim; 2BFI; α_2-adrenoceptor

INTRODUCTION

Since their discovery and identification imidazoline binding sites (I-BSs) have been found throughout the body and brain of a number of different species. Further research has led to their subsequent subdivision into I$_1$-BS and I$_2$-BS based on their relative affinities for clonidine and idazoxan, respectively. Also a third pharmacologically distinct subtype, I$_3$-BS, has been identified. The functions of these binding sites have been studied, and the I$_1$- and I$_3$-BSs have been implicated in hypertension and insulin regulation, respectively (for review see Eglen et al.[1]).

A functional role for the I$_2$-BS has also been investigated, and it has been implicated in various mood disorders. I$_2$ ligands demonstrate antidepressant properties in animal models.[2] One hindrance in determining the actual function of the I$_2$-BS is that the high-affinity ligands available still retain some affinity for the α_2-adrenoceptor (α_2AR). Because many of these functions are also thought to be mediated through α_2AR, questions still remain. In this study, we have investigated the affinity and selectivity of a series of novel imidazoline ligands at the I$_2$-BS and the α_2AR. These ligands are based on indazim (2-(4,5-dihydro-1*H*-imidazol-2-yl)-2*H*-indazole), the indazole analogue of the selective I$_2$-BS ligand 2BFI (2-(1-benzofuran-2-yl)-4,5-dihydro-1*H*-imidazole) (TABLE 1).

Address for correspondence: Dr. Alan L. Hudson, Head of Preclinical Science, Psychopharmacology Unit, School of Medical Sciences, University of Bristol, Bristol BS8 1TD, UK. Voice: (+44) 0 117 925 3066; fax: (+44) 0 117 928 9500.
e-mail: a.l.hudson@bristol.ac.uk

Ann. N.Y. Acad. Sci. 1009: 357–360 (2003). © 2003 New York Academy of Sciences.
doi: 10.1196/annals.1304.046

TABLE 1. Summary of the calculated equilibrium dissociation constants (Ki) for the test compounds at the I2-BS and the a2AR in rat whole-brain membranes

Compound	K_i I_2-BS (nM) Mean ± SD	Ki α_2AR (nM) Mean ± SD
Indazim	213.3 ± 102.4	>10 000
4-Me-Indazim	39.5 ± 19.0	>10 000
5-Me-Indazim	201.6 ± 59.2	>10 000
6-Me-Indazim	138.2 ± 60.3	>10 000
7-Me-Indazim	52.5 ± 31.5	>10 000
2BFI	2.9 ± 1.2	2688.7 ± 174.0

METHODS

Crude P_2 membranes from male Wistar rats (approximately 250 g) whole brains were prepared as previously described.[3] Membrane aliquots (400 µL, approximately 0.2 mg protein) were incubated (RT, 45 minutes) with 10 concentrations of the test compounds over the range 0.03 nM to 10 µM in the presence of 1 nM [^{3}H]2BFI (I_2-BS), or 1 nM [^{3}H]RX821002 (α_2AR) to a final volume of 500 µL. Nonspecific binding was determined using 10 µM BU224 (I_2-BS) or rauwolscine (α_2AR). Bound ligand was separated from free by rapid filtration and determined by liquid scintillation counting. The resulting data were analyzed individually using GraphPad Prism version 3.02 for Windows (San Diego, CA, USA), and the determined IC_{50} values were used to calculate the equilibrium dissociation constants (K_i) by the method of Cheng & Prusoff.[4]

RESULTS AND DISCUSSION

The data for the displacement of [^{3}H]2BFI by the test ligands were best fit to a single-site model with Hill slopes close to unity (FIG. 1), and the K_i values calculated were all found to be in the nanomolar range (TABLE 1). Indazim, 5-Me-indazim, and 6-Me-indazim showed moderate affinity for the I_2-BS, whereas 4-Me-indazim and 7-Me-indazim demonstrated the highest affinity. The affinity of the indazims at the α_2AR as determined using [^{3}H]RX821002 was found to be very poor, with none of them showing more than 10% displacement at the highest concentration tested. Only 2BFI had any measurable affinity for the α_2AR, and these data (not shown) were also best fit to a single-site model.

Indazim and its derivatives, such as 2BFI, are planar molecules, and this configuration has previously been shown to improve affinity for the I_2-BS.[5] Substitution on

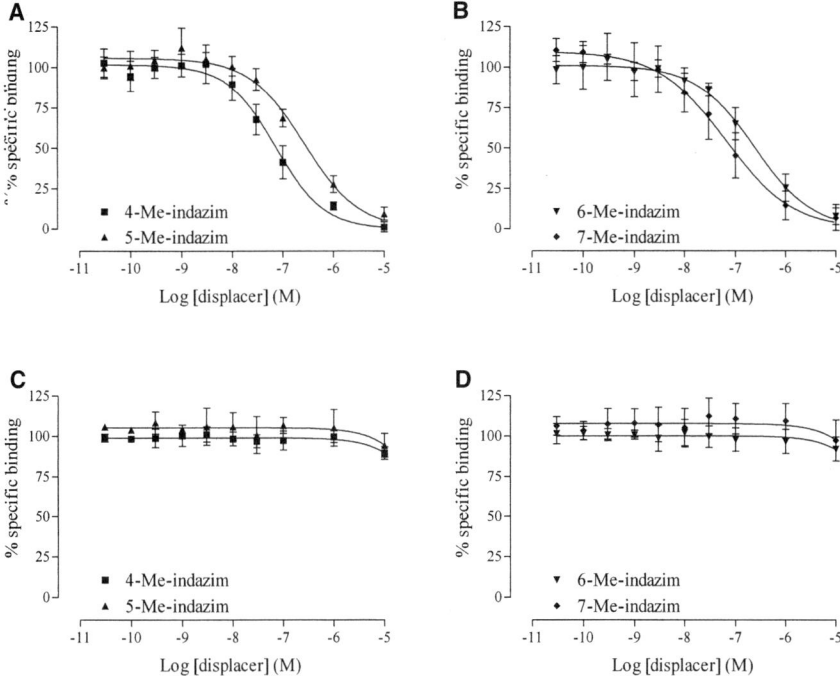

FIGURE 1. Displacement of [^{3}H]2BFI (**A**, **B**) and [^{3}H]RX821002 (**C**, **D**) by the test compounds in rat whole brain membranes. Data were analyzed as described in the text and are the mean ± S.D. for three or four separate experiments performed in triplicate.

the indazole ring at positions 4 and 7 would seem also to favor binding to the I_2-BS, at least in this class of molecule. It is clear from the methyl substitutions that relatively large hydrophobic groups are very well tolerated. However, the best chemical characteristic of the substituted group is unclear. For this reason further investigations with different substituents at these positions are required to understand fully the structure affinity relationship between these compounds and the I_2-BS.

In conclusion, all these indazim compounds represent highly selective ligands for the I_2-BS compared with the α_2AR and should prove to be useful tools in determining the contribution, if any, that α_2ARs play in the function of I_2-BS. Compared with 2BFI, these new compounds are much more selective for the I_2-BS than for the α_2AR but demonstrate reduced affinity.

ACKNOWLEDGMENTS

F. Sączewski acknowledges the Polish State Committee for Scientific Research for Grant No. 6 P05F 03821.

REFERENCES

1. EGLEN, R.M., et al. 1998. "Seeing through a glass darkly": casting light on imidazoline "I" sites. Trends Pharmacol. Sci. **19**: 381–390.
2. HUDSON, A.L., D.J. NUTT & S.M. HUSBANDS. 2001. Imidazoline receptors and their role in depression. Pharmaceutical News **8**: 26–32.
3. LIONE, L.A., D.J. NUTT & A.L. HUDSON. 1998. Characterisation and localisation of [^{3}H]2-(2-benzofuranyl)-2-imidazoline binding in rat brain: a selective ligand for imidazoline I_2 receptors. Eur. J. Pharmacol. **353**: 123–135.
4. CHENG, Y.C. & W.H. PRUSOFF. 1973. Relationship between the inhibition constant (K_i) and the concentration of inhibitor which causes 50% inhibition (IC_{50}) of an enzymatic reaction. Biochem. Pharmacol. **22**: 3099–3108.
5. HUSBANDS, S.M., et al. 2001. β-carboline binding to imidazoline receptors. Drug Alcohol Depend. **64**: 203–208.

Investigation of the Affinities of Two New β-Carbolines for Rat Brain Imidazoline$_2$ Receptors

R.J. TYACKE,[a] A. LAU,[a] B. GRELLA,[b] R.A. GLENNON,[b] D.J. NUTT,[a] AND A.L. HUDSON[a]

[a]*Psychopharmacology Unit, School of Medical Sciences, University of Bristol, Bristol BS8 1TD, UK*

[b]*Medicinal Chemistry, Virginia Commonwealth University, Richmond, Virginia 23298, USA*

> ABSTRACT: The β-carbolines are possible endogenous ligands and modulators of the imidazoline binding sites (I-BSs). Relatively little is known about this class of compound and its interaction with the I-BS. Presented here are the binding data for two aryl ring substituted dihydro-β-carbolines at the imidazoline$_2$ binding site (I$_2$-BS) and α$_2$-adrenoceptor: BG-326 (5-bromo-4,9-dihydro-3*H*-β-carboline) and BG-350 (5-methoxy-4,9-dihydro-3*H*-β-carboline). Both compounds show good affinity and selectivity for the I$_2$-BS.
>
> KEYWORDS: imidazoline$_2$ binding site; β-carboline; 2BFI; α$_2$-adrenoceptor

INTRODUCTION

The ability of the α$_2$-adrenoceptor (α$_2$AR) agonist clonidine and the antagonist idazoxan to label a subpopulation of binding sites that were not displaceable by the endogenous ligand noradrenaline led to the discovery of imidazoline binding sites (I-BSs). They have been subdivided into three types: I$_1$-, I$_2$-, and I$_3$-BS. Functions have been shown for two of these subtypes: I$_1$-BS is involved in the central control of blood pressure, and I$_3$-BS modulates insulin release (for review see Eglen *et al.*[1]). As yet there is no clear function attributable to I$_2$-BSs although they have been linked to monoamine oxidase, appetite and feeding, and a number of disease states such as depression and Huntington's disease.[2]

Much study has been devoted to finding the endogenous ligand for these sites, and a number of possible candidates have been suggested. The β-carbolines are a group of psychoactive indoles (e.g., harmane[3] and norharmane[4]) that have been found endogenously in animals. They have been found to bind with high affinity to I$_1$-BS and I$_2$-BS,[5] and harmane has been shown to modulate blood pressure following microinjection into the rostral ventrolateral medulla through the I$_1$-BS.[6] Therefore, it has

---

Address for correspondence: Dr. Alan L. Hudson, Head of Preclinical Science, Psychopharmacology Unit, School of Medical Sciences, University of Bristol, Bristol BS8 1TD, UK. Voice: (+44) 0 117 925 3066; fax: (+44) 0 117 928 9500.

e-mail: hudson@bristol.ac.uk

been proposed that the β-carbolines may be one of the endogenous ligands for I-BS. In this study binding data for two novel dihydro-β-carbolines at the I_2-BS and α_2AR are presented. These analogues bear either an electron-withdrawing bromo group (i.e., BG-326; 5-bromo-4,9-dihydro-3H-β-carboline) or an electron-donating methoxy group (i.e., BG-350; 5-methoxy-4,9-dihydro-3H-β-carboline) at the 5 position of the aryl ring and were meant to explore the electronic effects of this region of the dihydro-β-carboline nucleus on binding.

METHODS

Crude P_2 membranes from rat (male, Wistar, approximately 250 g) whole brains were prepared as previously described.[7] Membrane aliquots (400 μL, approximately 0.2 mg protein) were incubated (45 minutes RT) with seven concentrations of the test compounds over the range 0.1 nM to 100 μM in the presence of 1 nM [^{3}H]2BFI (I_2-BS), or 1 nM [^{3}H]RX821002 (α_2AR) to a final volume of 500 μL. Nonspecific binding was determined using 10 μM BU224 (I_2-BS) or rauwolscine (α_2AR). Bound ligand was separated from free by rapid filtration and determined by liquid scintillation counting. The resulting data were analyzed individually using GraphPad Prism version 3.02 for Windows (San Diego, CA, USA), and the determined IC_{50} values were used to calculate the equilibrium dissociation constants (K_i) by the method of Cheng and Prusoff.[8]

RESULTS AND DISCUSSION

For the α_2AR site, the data were best fit to a single-site model of binding (TABLE 1), and the Hill slopes for the displacement of [^{3}H]RX821002 were close to unity. However, the Hill slopes for the displacement of [^{3}H]2BFI from I_2-BS were not close to unity. Further analysis showed that they fitted well to a two-site model, but this was

TABLE 1. Calculated equilibrium dissociation constants (K_i) and Hill slopes (n_H) for the test compounds at the I_2-BS and the α_2AR in rat whole brain membranes

Compound	K_i I_2-BS (nM)	n_H	K_i α_2AR (nM)	n_H
BG326 R = Br	76.6 ± 25.9	0.59 ± 0.02	3808.3 ± 1347.0	1.18 ± 0.08
BG350 R = OCH$_3$	80.5 ± 30.4	0.71 ± 0.17	1026.7 ± 358.1	1.02 ± 0.11

The data presented are the mean ± SD.

not found to be statistically significant on using the F test. Both BG-326 and BG-350 showed good affinity for the I_2-BS and poor affinity for the α_2AR, but BG-350 had an approximately threefold higher affinity for the α_2AR compared with BG-326.

Dihydro-β-carbolines have been shown to have good affinity for the I_2-BS. This affinity has been attributed to the increased planarity of the molecule produced by the double bond between the carbon and nitrogen in the third ring. Also, substitution on the aryl ring has been shown to be beneficial for binding at the I_2-BS in other β-carbolines.[9] These data agree with these findings.

The substitutions used in these two molecules, bromine and methoxyl, are similar in size but differ in their electronic and lipophilic properties. Although neither of the substitutions used here had any apparent affect on the affinity at the I_2-BS, the bromine (BG-326) was less well tolerated in the ligand's binding to the α_2AR, thereby conferring greater selectivity. Hence, whereas the electronic nature of the dihydro-β-carboline 5-position might have little influence on binding at I_2-BS, an electron-withdrawing substituent adversely affects binding at α_2AR. It is clear that aryl ring–substituted dihydro-β-carbolines bind with high affinity and selectivity to the I_2-BS. Further investigations are required to understand fully the β-carbolines' binding to both the I-BS and the α_2AR.

REFERENCES

1. EGLEN, R.M., et al. 1998. "Seeing through a glass darkly": casting light on imidazoline "I" sites. Trends Pharmacol. Sci. **19:** 381–390.
2. HUDSON, A.L., D.J. NUTT & S.M. HUSBANDS. 2001. Imidazoline receptors and their role in depression. Pharmaceutical News **8:** 26–32.
3. ADELL, A., T.A. BIGGS & R.D. MYERS. 1996. Action of harman (1-methyl-beta-carboline) on the brain: body temperature and in vivo efflux of 5-HT from hippocampus of the rat. Neuropharmacology **35:** 1101–1107.
4. FEKKES, D., et al. 1992. Norharman, a normal body constituent. Lancet **339:** 506.
5. HUDSON, A.L., et al. 1999. Harmane, norharman and tetrahydro-β-carboline have high affinity for rat imidazoline binding sites. Br. J. Pharmacol. **126:** 2P.
6. MUSGRAVE, I.F. & E. BADOER. 2000. Harmane produces hypotension following microinjection into the RVLM: possible role of I1-imidazoline receptors. Br. J. Pharmacol. **129:** 1057–1059.
7. LIONE, L.A., D.J. NUTT & A.L. HUDSON. 1998. Characterisation and localisation of [^{3}H]2-(2-benzofuranyl)-2-imidazoline binding in rat brain: a selective ligand for imidazoline I_2 receptors. Eur. J. Pharmacol. **353:** 123–135.
8. CHENG, Y.C. & W.H. PRUSOFF. 1973. Relationship between the inhibition constant (K_i) and the concentration of inhibitor which causes 50% inhibition (IC_{50}) of an enzymatic reaction. Biochem. Pharmacol. **22:** 3099–3108.
9. HUSBANDS, S.M., et al. 2001. β-carboline binding to imidazoline receptors. Drug Alcohol Depend. **64:** 203–208.

Identification of an I_2 Binding Protein From Rabbit Brain

A. KIMURA,[a] R.J. TYACKE,[a] M.C.W. MINCHIN,[b] D.J. NUTT,[a] AND A.L. HUDSON[a]

[a]*Psychopharmacology Unit, School of Medical Sciences, University Walk, University of Bristol, Bristol BS8 1TD, UK*

[b]*Yamanouchi UK Ltd., Pyrford Road, West Byfleet, Surrey KT14 6RA, UK*

> ABSTRACT: Imidazoline-2 binding proteins exist as a heterogeneous population. The aim of this study was to isolate and identify I_2 binding proteins from rabbit brain using an affinity column synthesized with a highly selective I_2 ligand, 2-(2-benzofuranyl)2-imidazoline (2BFI). The results revealed an approximately 45-kD protein to be brain creatine kinase (EC 2.7.3.2). [^{3}H]-2BFI (5nM) was able to bind specifically to the purified enzyme. This study has identified brain creatine kinase as a novel I_2 binding protein.
>
> KEYWORDS: I_2 binding proteins; rabbit brain; 2BFI; creatine kinase

INTRODUCTION

Imidazoline-2 binding proteins (I_2BPs) are found throughout the brain and are known to be involved in feeding and various other brain conditions such as depression (for reviews, see references 1, 2). Despite advances in understanding the effects of imidazoline ligands, the identities of most I_2BPs remain unknown. Imidazoline binding proteins exist as a heterogeneous population that includes the two subtypes (A and B) of monoamine oxidase (for review, see reference 3). The aim of this study was to isolate and identify I_2BPs other than monoamine oxidase from rabbit brain using a highly selective I_2 ligand, 2-(2-benzofuranyl)2-imidazoline (2BFI).

METHODS

The methods for isolation and identification of I_2 binding proteins were used as previously described[4] and modified from other methods.[5,6] For radioligand binding studies, either pure creatine kinase (Sigma Chemicals, Poole, UK) or rabbit whole-brain P_2 membranes were incubated with [^{3}H]-2BFI (5 nM) and bovine serum albumin (0.8 g/mL) for 30 minutes, and the reactions were terminated by addition of polyethylene glycol (15% final) followed by centrifugation at 11,000 gravity for 10 minutes at 4°C. The resulting pellets were washed twice with ice-cold Tris-HCl (50 mM Tris, 1 mM $MgCl_2$, pH 7.4), and the radioactivity was counted.

Address for correspondence: Dr. Alan L. Hudson, Head of Preclinical Science, Psychopharmacology Unit, School of Medical Sciences, University of Bristol, Bristol BS8 1TD, UK. Voice: (+44) 0 117 928 8608; fax: (+44) 0 117 928 9700.

e-mail: a.l.hudson@bristol.ac.uk

RESULTS AND DISCUSSION

Proteins eluted off the 2BFI affinity column by idazoxan (20 mM) were subjected to SDS-polyacrylamide gel electrophoresis, which revealed a strong band around 45 kD as well as weaker bands (FIG. 1). Following N-terminal sequencing and searching in a protein sequence database (Protein Information Resources[7]), the identity of this 45-kD protein was determined to be rabbit brain creatine kinase (EC 2.7.3.2; 43 kD). Creatine kinase is a key enzyme of the cellular energy metabolism, and it catalyses a reversible phosphoryl transfer reaction from phosphocreatine to ADP to produce ATP. This enzyme exists in two cytosolic isoforms, brain creatine kinase (B-CK) and muscle creatine kinase (M-CK), and two mitochondrial isoforms, ubiquitous Mi_a-CK and sarcomeric Mi_b-CK (for review, see Wallimann & Hemmer[8]). We have identified the brain isoform that was used in radioligand binding studies. Pure rabbit brain creatine kinase (Sigma Chemicals) was able to bind [^{3}H]-2BFI (5 nM). This binding was displaceable by a selective I_2 site ligand 2-(4, 5-dihydroimidaz-2-yl)-quinoline (BU224, 10 µM) establishing specific binding to I_2 sites (FIG. 2). This specific binding was abolished in the presence of an I_2 irreversible ligand, BU99006 (10 µM),[9] further supporting the existence of an I_2 binding domain on this enzyme.

An I_2 BP with a molecular weight of approximately 45 kD has previously been observed in rat brain,[6] but its identity remains unknown. In this study we have identified an I_2BP of molecular weight at approximately 45 kD in rabbit brain to be brain creatine kinase.

Further studies are required to clarify how this enzyme functionally interacts with I_2 ligands. Also, the identities of other proteins isolated in this study need to be determined and the roles they play in various brain disorders need to be examined.

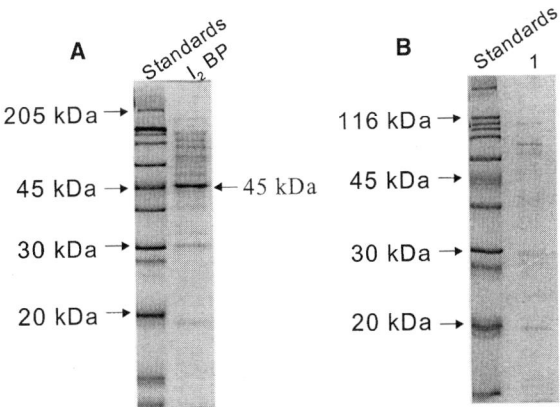

FIGURE 1. (**A**) I_2BPs isolated by a 2BFI affinity column. There is a strong band at approximately 45 kD. (**B**) Proteins nonspecifically bound to the blank 2BFI affinity column (*Lane 1*). There was no band at approximately 45 kD.

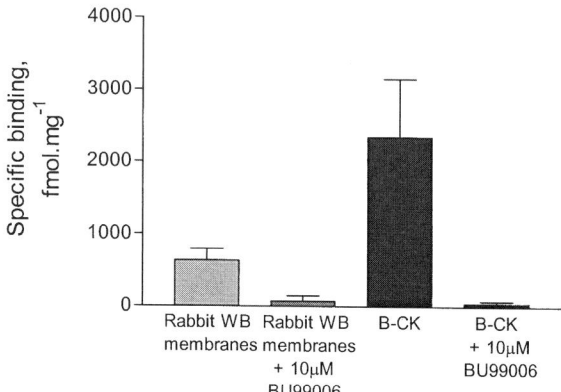

FIGURE 2. Specific binding of [^{3}H]-2BFI to purified rabbit brain creatine kinase and rabbit whole-brain membranes with and without pretreatment with BU99006 (10 μM). Data show mean ± SEM; N = 5. B-CK, purified brain creatine kinase; WB, whole brain.

ACKNOWLEDGMENTS

This study was supported by Yamanouchi UK Ltd. We thank Dr. Graham Kemp at University of St. Andrews, UK, for his assistance with protein sequencing.

REFERENCES

1. GARCÍA-SEVILLA, J.A., P.V. ESCRIBA & J. GUIMON. 1999. Imidazoline receptors and human brain disorders. Ann. N. Y. Acad. Sci. **881:** 392–409.
2. HUDSON, A.L., D.J. NUTT & S.M. HUSBANDS. 2001. Imidazoline receptors and their role in depression. Pharmaceutical News **8:** 26–32.
3. EGLEN, R.M., A.L. HUDSON, D.A. KENDALL, et al. 1998. "Seeing through a glass darkly": casting light on imidazoline "I" sites. Trends Pharmacol. Sci. **19:** 381–390.
4. KIMURA, A., R.J. TYACKE, M.C.W. MINCHIN, et al. 2003. Identification of a putative imidazoline-2 binding protein. Br. J. Pharmacol. **138**(Suppl): 173.
5. WANG, H., S. REGUNATHAN, M.P. MEELEY, et al. 1992. Isolation and characterization of imidazoline receptor protein from bovine adrenal chromaffin cells. Mol. Pharmacol. **42:** 792–801.
6. ESCRIBA, P.V., A. OZAITA, A. MIRALLES, et al. 1995. Molecular characterization and isolation of a 45-kilodalton imidazoline receptor protein from rat brain. Mol. Brain Res. **32:** 187–196.
7. WU, C.H., H. HUANG, L. ARMINSKI, et al. 2002. The Protein Information Resources: an integrated public resource of functional annotation of protein. Nucleic Acids Res. **30:** 35–37.
8. WALLIMANN, T. & W. HEMMER. 1994. Creatine kinase in non-muscle tissues and cells. Mol. Cell. Biochem. **133/134:** 193–220.
9. TYACKE, R.J., E.S.J. ROBINSON, D.J. NUTT, et al. 2002. 5-Isothiocyanato-2-benzofuranyl-2-imidazoline (BU99006) an irreversible imidazoline-2 binding site ligand: in vitro and in vivo characterisation in rat brain. Neuropharmacology **43:** 75–83.

In Vivo Estimation of Imidazoline$_2$ Binding Site Turnover

L.M. PATERSON, E.S.J. ROBINSON, D.J. NUTT, AND A.L. HUDSON

Psychopharmacology Unit, School of Medical Sciences, University of Bristol, Bristol BS8 1TD, UK

ABSTRACT: Turnover of imidazoline$_2$ (I$_2$) binding sites in the mouse and rat brain has been measured following an acute intravenous dose of BU99006. This ligand selectively and irreversibly knocks out I$_2$ sites, as defined by [^{3}H]2BFI binding. Recovery was measured using radioligand binding and autoradiography to determine global and regional changes in I$_2$ density. The density of I$_2$ sites in brain recovered from BU99006 treatment with a half-life of 2.1 hours in mice and 4.3 hours in rats. Monoamine oxidase (MAO) activity and MAO binding density were unaltered in the brains of BU99006-treated animals. These data suggest that the I$_2$ site that reacts with BU99006 recovers rapidly and is independent of MAO.

KEYWORDS: imidazoline$_2$ binding site; BU99006; 2BFI; half-life; autoradiography

INTRODUCTION

The nature of the imidazoline$_2$ (I$_2$) binding site is not well defined. A number of I$_2$ binding proteins seem to exist, a proportion of which are located on monoamine oxidases (MAO), but this interaction is little understood. I$_2$ ligands exert several effects in vivo, for example, the elevation of monoamines in rat brain[1] and hyperphagic effects.[2] The latter effects are contrary to the effects of MAO inhibitors on food intake. Research into the identity of I$_2$ proteins has in part been hampered by the lack of selective ligands. A new chemical tool, BU99006, has been developed within our laboratory to aid their study.[3] This ligand is the isothiocyanate derivative of 2BFI and as such will selectively and irreversibly knock out the I$_2$ binding site, as defined by [^{3}H]2BFI binding, both in vitro and in vivo in rat brain.[4] The irreversible nature of BU99006 makes it an ideal ligand with which to study I$_2$ function. The present study aimed to determine the turnover of I$_2$ binding proteins in vivo following intravenous injection of BU99006 at 5 mg/kg. This dose of BU99006 is known to remove permanently the protein's ability to bind [^{3}H]2BFI.[4] Only when new protein is synthesized do sites become available for [^{3}H]2BFI binding. Therefore, the recovery of I$_2$ binding sites is an estimate of the half-life of the protein. A pilot study was first carried out in mice to give a preliminary value for the half-life. A further, more comprehensive study was then performed in rats, in which MAO activity and binding were also assayed.

Address for correspondence: Dr Alan L. Hudson, Head of Preclinical Science, Psychopharmacology Unit, School of Medical Sciences, University of Bristol, Bristol BS8 1TD, UK. Voice: (+44) 0 117 928 8608; fax: (+44) 0 117 928 9700.
e-mail: a.l.hudson@bristol.ac.uk

MATERIALS AND METHODS

Male Ca/CBA mice (25–35 g) or Wistar rats (200–225 g) were intravenously injected at t = 0 with 5mg kg^{-1} BU99006 or 0.9% saline vehicle (controls), through the tail vein. This method ensured swift delivery of a maximal drug concentration, with minimal first-pass metabolism. Animals were killed at various time points after injection. The brains were removed and either sectioned for autoradiography or homogenized.[5] Radioligand binding assays were carried out as previously described.[5] Briefly, either whole brain homogenates or parasagittal brain sections were incubated (40 minutes RT) with 5 or 1 nM [^{3}H]2BFI, respectively, with or without 10 μM BU224, to determine the I_2-specific binding component. MAO binding density was determined in rat brain using the radioligands [^{3}H]Ro 41-1049 (MAO-A selective) and [^{3}H]Lazabemide (MAO-B selective) at 10-nM concentration. The MAO inhibitors, 1 μM clorgyline or 100 μM deprenyl, were added to determine MAO-A and MAO-B specific binding, respectively.[6] MAO activity was determined using a radiochemical assay as previously described.[7] Selective substrates for MAO-A and MAO-B were 200 μM [^{3}H]serotonin and 20 μM [^{3}H]PEA, respectively. Incubations were performed over a 10-minute period, over which time enzyme reaction rates were linear. All data analysis was performed using statistical tests available in GraphPad Prism, version 3.03 for Windows (San Diego, CA, USA).

RESULTS

An acute dose of 5 mg kg^{-1} BU99006 resulted in a significant loss in I_2 binding sites as defined with [^{3}H]2BFI within 1 hour following intravenous injection in both mouse and rat brain. This loss occurred in all areas studied by autoradiography of the mouse brain (data not shown). The result reflected previous data indicating that a global reduction in I_2 binding sites occurs 20 minutes after injection of a 15-mg kg^{-1} dose of BU99006 in rat brain.[4]

Analysis of the recovery of the I_2 binding site revealed its turnover rate to be relatively rapid. In brains of both rats and mice, the specific binding of [^{3}H]2BFI returned from 15% to 100% of controls within 8 hours after injection of BU99006. Half-lives of 2.1 hours in mouse brain and 4.3 hours in rat brain were calculated (FIG. 1). The recovery rates seemed relatively uniform throughout all areas of the brain with measurable levels of I_2 binding (data not shown).

Determination of MAO binding density using the selective ligands [^{3}H]Ro 41-1049 and [^{3}H]Lazabemide for MAO-A and MAO-B, respectively, revealed no significant changes after BU99006 administration in rat brain. Furthermore, no significant changes in the activity of either isozyme were observed by the radiochemical enzyme assay.

DISCUSSION AND CONCLUSIONS

A previous study has shown that the ligand BU99006 can irreversibly bind to the I_2 site labeled by the classical I_2 ligand 2BFI, and this ligand rapidly enters the brain within 20 minutes following intravenous injection.[4] Our present study reveals that I_2

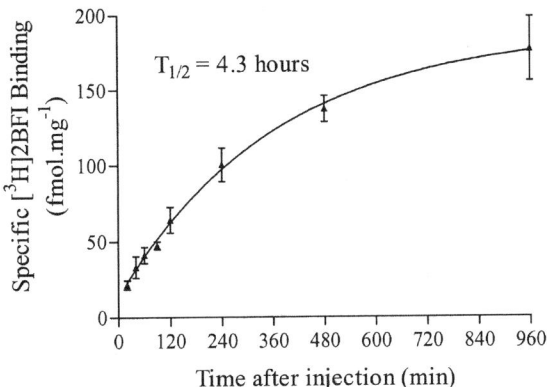

FIGURE 1. Estimation of half-life of the I_2 binding protein. The graph shows the recovery of 5nM [^{3}H]2BFI binding, over time, following a single intravenous dose of 5 mg kg^{-1} BU99006 in rat brain. Specific binding was defined using 10 μM BU224. Data were fitted using iterative nonlinear regression curve analysis, and a half-life of 4.3 hours was calculated. Each point represents mean ± S.D., N = 4.

binding proteins have a half-life of 4.3 hours in rat brain. The I_2 site irreversibly bound by BU99006 is therefore not likely to be one associated with MAO, because this protein has a turnover of approximately 11 days.[8] Furthermore, BU99006 did not affect the binding or activity of either isozyme of MAO in this study (data not shown). The data support the existence of an I_2 binding protein independent from MAO[9] that has a more rapid turnover rate, as described herein.

It would seem there are at least two distinct I_2 binding proteins. One I_2 site is likely to be responsible for the inhibition of MAO, the other (bound by BU99006) is located elsewhere. Several possible candidates have been isolated from rabbit brain including the enzyme creatine kinase.[10] Further work will determine which of these sites is responsible for the reported in vivo function of the I_2-selective ligands, and it seems likely that BU99006 will play an important role in this research.

ACKNOWLEDGMENTS

This work was funded by grants from the Medical Research Council and Wellcome Trust. We would also like to thank Dr. Borroni at Hoffmann La Roche for the kind gift of the ligands [^{3}H]Ro 41-1049 and [^{3}H]Lazabemide.

REFERENCES

1. HUDSON, A.L., D.J. NUTT & S.M. HUSBANDS. 2001. Imidazoline receptors and their role in depression. Pharmaceutical News **8**: 18–24.
2. EDWARDS, M.M., *et al.* 2002. Investigation of the acute administration of imidazoline ligands on food intake. Br. J. Pharmacol. **135**: 110P.

3. COATES, P.A., et al. 2000. Probes for imidazoline binding sites: synthesis and evaluation of a selective, irreversible I_2 ligand. Bioorg. Med. Chem. Lett. **10:** 605–607.
4. TYACKE, R.J., et al. 2002. 5-Isothiocyanato-2-benzofuranyl-2-imidazoline (BU99006) an irreversible imidazoline$_2$ binding site ligand: in vitro and in vivo characterisation in rat brain. Neuropharmacology **43:** 75–83.
5. LIONE, L.A., D.J. NUTT & A.L. HUDSON. 1998. Characterisation and localisation of [^{3}H]2-(2-benzofuranyl)-2-imidazoline binding in rat brain: a selective ligand for imidazoline I_2 receptors. Eur. J. Pharmacol. **353:** 123–135.
6. SAURA, J., et al. 1992. Quantitative enzyme radioautography with [^{3}H]Ro 41–1049 and [^{3}H]Ro 19–6327 in vitro: localization and abundance of MAO_A and MAO_B in rat CNS, peripheral organs, and human brain. J. Neurosci. **12:** 1977–1999.
7. OZAITA, A., et al. 1997. Inhibition of monoamine oxidase A and B activities by imidazol(ine)/guanidine drugs, nature of the interaction and distinction from I_2-imidazoline receptors in rat liver. Br. J. Pharmacol. **121:** 901–912.
8. GORIDIS, C. & N.H. NEFF. 1971. Monoamine oxidase: an approximation of turnover rates. J. Neurochem. **18:** 1673–1682.
9. PATERSON, L.M., et al. 2002. The irreversible I_2 ligand BU99006 abolished [^{3}H]-2BFI binding without effect on monoamine oxidase activity. J. Pyschopharm. **16:** A63.
10. KIMURA, A., et al. 2003. Identification of a putative imidazoline-2 binding protein. Br. J. Pharmacol. **138**(Suppl.): 173P.

Specificity of Nonadrenergic Imidazoline Binding Sites in Insulin-Secreting Cells and Relation to the Block of ATP-Sensitive K⁺ Channels

TIMM GROSSE-LACKMANN,[a] BERND J. ZÜNKLER,[b] AND INGO RUSTENBECK[a]

[a]*Institute of Pharmacology and Toxicology, Technical University of Braunschweig, D-30106 Braunschweig, Germany*

[b]*Federal Institute for Drugs and Medical Devices, D-53113 Bonn, Germany*

ABSTRACT: To characterize the specificity of nonadrenergic imidazoline binding sites of insulin-secreting HIT cells, competitive binding of insulinotropic imidazolines and quinine was measured and compared with the effect of these compounds on native K_{ATP} channels and with a heterologously expressed variant of the pore-forming subunit (Kir6.2 ΔC26). There were two nonadrenergic imidazoline binding sites for [^{3}H]clonidine with K_d values of 61 nM and 4.5 μM, respectively. Quinine reduced specific binding incompletely (73%) with K_i values of 75 nM and 133 μM. Clonidine, N-allyl-clonidine (alinidine), and quinine inhibited native K_{ATP} channels as well as Kir6.2ΔC26 channels. Co-expression of Kir6.2ΔC26 and SUR1 (the regulatory subunit of K_{ATP}) did not increase the potency of quinine. There are nonadrenergic imidazoline binding sites in insulin-secreting HIT cells which also recognize quinine. One of these sites is Kir6.2, the pore-forming subunit of the K_{ATP} channel.

KEYWORDS: K_{ATP} channel; quinine; imidazoline compounds; nonadrenergic imidazoline binding sites; insulin secretion

INTRODUCTION

A number of imidazoline compounds stimulate insulin secretion with characteristics that make them interesting as potential oral antidiabetic agents. Nonadrenergic imidazoline binding sites have been shown to exist on insulin-secreting RINm5F[1] and HIT cells.[2] When [^{3}H]clonidine was used as an imidazoline radioligand, the competition binding curves were biphasic, indicating the presence of at least two imidazoline binding sites on HIT cell membranes.[2] The implication was that these imidazoline binding sites might be related to the inhibition of the ATP-sensitive potassium (K_{ATP}) channels reported with imidazoline compounds such as phentolamine.[3] Taking advantage of a C-terminally truncated variant of the pore-forming subunit of the K_{ATP} channels, Kir6.2, which expresses independently of sulphonylurea receptor-1 (SUR1), it was shown that phentolamine blocks K_{ATP} channels by

Address for correspondence: I. Rustenbeck, Institute of Pharmacology and Toxicology, Technical University of Braunschweig, Mendelssohnstr. 1, D-38106, Braunschweig, Germany. Voice: (+49) 531-5670; fax: (+49) 531-8287.
e-mail: i.rustenbeck@tu-bs.de

Ann. N.Y. Acad. Sci. 1009: 371–377 (2003). © 2003 New York Academy of Sciences.
doi: 10.1196/annals.1304.050

interaction with the pore-forming subunit.[3] In the same line, affinity chromatography showed that the imidazoline efaroxan interacted with the pore-forming subunit.[4] Thus the question arose whether the pore-forming subunit corresponds to one of the nonadrenergic imidazoline binding sites characterized in HIT cells.[5]

In the present experiments we used the antimalarial agent quinine as an experimental tool because of three properties: (1) it induces insulin secretion, (2) it blocks K_{ATP} channels in pancreatic B-cells and insulin-secreting HIT cells, and (3) it directly affects Kir6.2.[6–9] We tested whether quinine was able to displace [^{3}H]clonidine from nonadrenergic binding sites at HIT cell membranes and compared its blocking action on K_{ATP} channels and Kir6.2 with that of clonidine.

MATERIALS AND METHODS

Cell Culture and Transfection

HIT T15 cells were cultured in RPMI 1640 and HEK 293 cells in M199. Both media were supplemented with 10% fetal calf serum. For transient expression studies, the cDNA of Kir6.2ΔC26 was subcloned in a pADtrack CMV vector containing the cDNA of the green fluorescent protein (GFP). HEK cells were plated on glass cover slips at a density of 3×10^5 per 35-mm dish. After 24 hours, the cells were transiently transfected by incubation with 1 μg plasmid DNA and 5 μg lipofectamine in 1 mL serum-free M199 medium for 6 hours. For the coexpression of Kir6.2ΔC26 and SUR1, Kir6.2ΔC26 (in pcDNA3) was stably expressed in HEK 293 cells which were then used for transient transfection with SUR1 (using pADtrack CMV). The cDNA of Kir6.2ΔC26 was kindly provided by F. Ashcroft (University of Oxford), and the cDNA of SUR1 was provided by J. Bryan (Baylor College of Medicine, Houston, TX).

Electrophysiologic Recordings

The cell-attached configuration of the patch-clamp technique was used to measure channel currents. Pipettes were pulled from borosilicate glass and had resistances between 3 and 8 MOhm when filled with solution. Currents were recorded by an EPC 7 patch-clamp amplifier (HEKA, Lambrecht, Germany), low pass-filtered and stored on videotape. The pipette holding potential was 0 mV. All experiments were performed at room temperature. Data were analyzed off-line using pClamp (Axon Instruments, Foster City, CA, USA) and TAC software (Bruxton Corporation, Seattle, WA, USA). The channel activity ($N * P_O$) was measured before, during and after the presence of each test agent. It was calculated as $1/T * \Sigma n_i * t_i$, where N is the number of channels, P_O the open probability of a single channel, t_i the time spent at each current level n_i and T the total recording time, which was 50 seconds. The duration of one experiment was 20 to 30 minutes because of the slow onset and offset of the quinine effect. The concentration-dependent block of channel activity by the test agents was fitted to the equation $P/P_c = 1 - [ligand]^{nH}/([ligand]^{nH} + IC_{50}^{nH})$.

Receptor Binding Assay

Membranes from HIT T15 cells were prepared, and competition binding experiments were performed as described previously.[2] [^{3}H]clonidine (5 nM) was used as radioligand, and binding to α-adrenoceptors was prevented by masking with 100 μM noradrenaline. All binding isotherms were determined from three independent experiments, each performed in triplicate. Binding was analyzed by nonlinear least-squares curve fitting using Prism software (GraphPad Software, San Diego, CA, USA). The IC_{50} values were converted into inhibitory constants (K_i) by use of the Cheng-Prusoff equation ($K_i = IC_{50}/(1 + [ligand]/K_d)$. B_{max} and K_d values for [^{3}H]clonidine binding were derived from competition with unlabelled clonidine according to the equations $B_{max} = B_0*IC_{50}/[ligand]$ and $K_d = IC_{50} - [ligand]$, where B_0 is the difference between the upper and the lower plateau values of the binding site.

RESULTS

The homologous displacement of [^{3}H]clonidine by unlabelled clonidine from HIT cell membranes gave a biphasic curve with K_d values of 61 nM for the high-affinity site and 4.5 μM for the low-affinity site. The corresponding binding capacities (B_{max}) were 41.3 fmol/mg and 20.1 pmol/mg (FIG. 1). Quinine also displaced [^{3}H]clonidine from two nonadrenergic imidazoline binding sites with K_i values of 75 nM and 133 μM (FIG. 1). The binding capacities of these sites corresponded to 17% and 83%, respectively, of the displaced label. The displacement by quinine was not complete, however, in that the lower plateau of the competition curve was significantly different from zero: about 27% of the specific activity remained bound (95% confidence interval 15.6%–38.6%).

In other studies, clonidine and quinine were observed to inhibit the activity of native K_{ATP} channels in intact HIT cells in a concentration-dependent manner. The cell-attached configuration was chosen to minimize the influence of channel rundown, because the effect of quinine was only slowly reversible. Only one concentration was tested per patch. There was no change in the single channel amplitude within the tested concentration range. The IC_{50} values were 44.2 ± 14.6 μM for clonidine and 5.3 ± 1.2 μM for quinine. The corresponding values of the Hill coefficient were 1.0 and 1.7 (FIG. 2).

When the truncated variant of the pore-forming subunit, Kir6.2ΔC26, was transiently expressed in HEK293 cells, channel activity could be consistently observed in green fluorescent cells. These channels had about the same current amplitude as

FIGURE 1. Displacement of [^{3}H]-clonidine from HIT cell membranes by unlabelled clonidine and quinine.

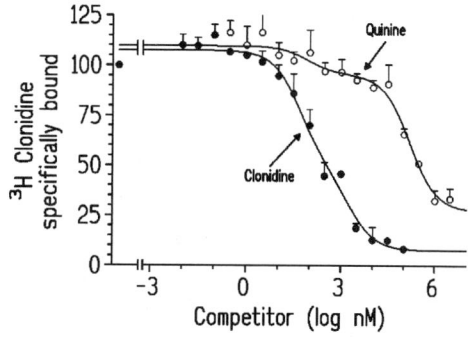

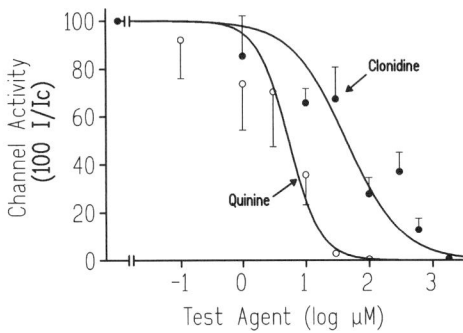

FIGURE 2. Concentration-dependent inhibition of native K_{ATP} channels in HIT cells by clonidine and quinine.

native K_{ATP} channels but had much shorter open times and proved to be susceptible to inhibition by quinine (FIG. 3). At concentrations that were maximally effective to block native K_{ATP} channels, phentolamine (100 μM) and clonidine (100 μM), but not glibenclamide (1 μM), strongly reduced Kir6.2ΔC26 channel activity. Both clonidine and quinine were able to induce a virtually complete block of channel activity (FIG. 4, *top*). The IC_{50} for clonidine-induced block was 40.1 ± 13.7 μM (Hill coefficient 0.7); the IC_{50} for quinine was 14.6 ± 2.1 μM (Hill coefficient 1.4). Alinidine (N-allyl-clonidine), which has a low affinity to α-adrenoceptors, was a more efficient blocker of these channels than clonidine, with an IC_{50} of 0.38 ± 0.05 μM (Hill coefficient 0.93) (FIG. 4, *middle*). Channels consisting of coexpressed Kir6.2ΔC26/SUR1 subunits also showed the same fast kinetics of channel openings as Kir6.2ΔC26 channels: (0.67 ± 0.08 milliseconds versus 0.74 ± 0.08 milliseconds intraburst open time). Here, the IC_{50} for quinine-induced block was 29.8 ± 5.7 μM (Hill coefficient 1.3) (FIG. 4, *bottom*).

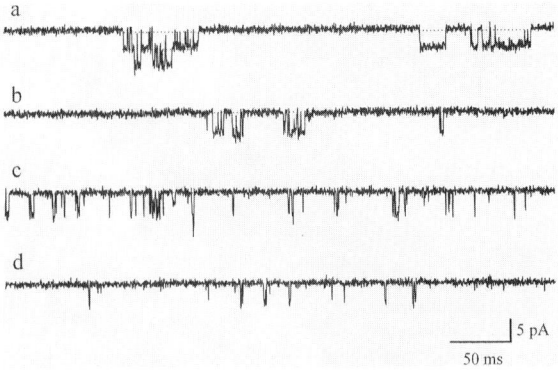

FIGURE 3. Comparison of the kinetics of channel openings of native K_{ATP} channels (*traces a and b*) and of Kir6.2ΔC26 channels (*traces c and d*). In traces b and d, 10 μM quinine is continuously present, leading to a marked reduction in channel activity.

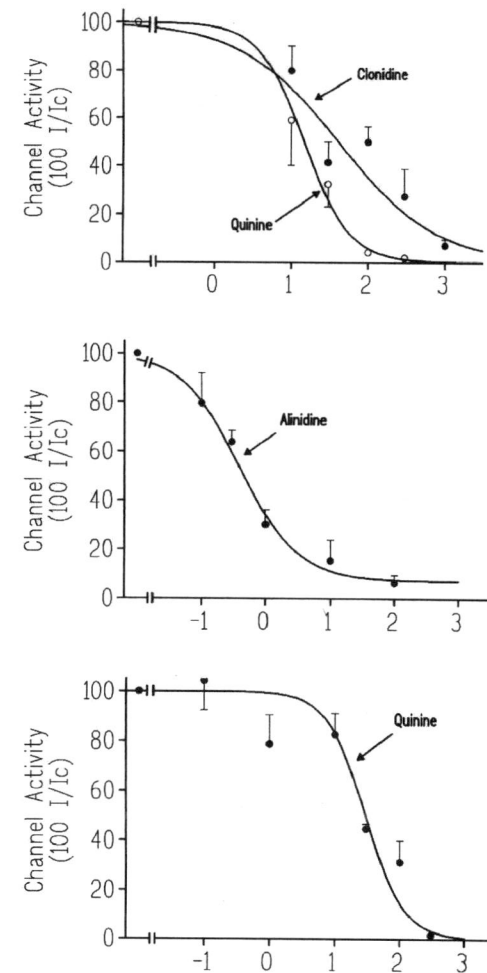

FIGURE 4. (*Top*) Concentration-dependent inhibition of Kir6.2ΔC26 channels by clonidine and quinine. (*Middle*) Concentration-dependent inhibition of Kir6.2ΔC26 channels by alinidine. (*Bottom*) Concentration-dependent inhibition of Kir6.2ΔC26/SUR1 channels by quinine.

DISCUSSION

Clonidine was chosen for these studies because it is an established ligand for imidazoline I_1 receptors provided α-adrenoceptors are masked. Furthermore, clonidine stimulates insulin secretion from pancreatic B cells when $α_2$-adrenoceptors are blocked.[10] Thus, clonidine can be expected to label the functionally relevant imidazoline binding sites in insulin-secreting cells. Both affinity and capacity of clonidine binding as determined in the present experiments were in good agreement with earlier data.[2] Similarly, the electrophysiologic characteristics of the Kir6.2ΔC26 and the Kir6.2ΔC26/SUR1 channels corresponded with published data.[3,11]

Quinine displaced [^{3}H]clonidine from at least two nonadrenergic binding sites at

HIT cell membranes. In contrast to all imidazolines tested earlier,[2] however, quinine did not displace [^{3}H]clonidine completely. Probably, there is more than one low-affinity site for imidazolines, which could not be resolved in the competition binding and one of which was not recognized by quinine. Alternatively, clonidine and quinine do not compete for the same site, in which case displacement of clonidine could be caused by an allosteric mechanism. This lack of competition may explain the lack of direct correlation between the potency to close K_{ATP} or Kir6.2 channels and the ability to displace [^{3}H]clonidine. In addition, methodologic differences may play a role. Binding was indirectly measured by competition binding in isolated membranes, whereas the potency was determined using intact cells. Nevertheless, it seems obvious that Kir6.2 forms a low-affinity imidazoline binding site. The additional presence of SUR1 does not seem to affect the channel-blocking potency of quinine, in contrast to the channel block by ATP^{4-}, which is also exerted at Kir6.2.[11]

The observation that quinine displaced [^{3}H]clonidine not only with low-affinity sites (83% of sites) but also with high-affinity sites (17% of sites) was unexpected and shows that even this classic nonadrenergic imidazoline site is not exclusively specific for ligands with an imidazoline moiety. Although it seems unlikely that the high-affinity site is involved in the insulinotropic effect of the imidazolines, which usually requires micromolar concentrations, it is conceivable that occupation of this site may modulate the signalling initiated by closure of the K_{ATP} channels.

ACKNOWLEDGMENTS

The skillful technical assistance of Ute Sommerfeld and Corinna Dickel is gratefully acknowledged. This work was supported by a grant from the Deutsche Forschungsgemeinschaft (Ru 368/3-1).

REFERENCES

1. CHAN, S.L.F., K.E. SCARPELLO & N.G. MORGAN. 1997. Identification and characterization of non-adrenergic binding sites in insulin-secreting cells with the imidazoline RX821002. Adv. Exp. Med. Biol. **426:** 159–163.
2. RUSTENBECK, I., C. HERRMANN, P. RATZKA, et al. 1997. Imidazoline/guanidinium binding sites and their relation to inhibition of K_{ATP} channels in pancreatic B-cells. Naunyn-Schmiedeberg's Arch. Pharmacol. **356:** 410–417.
3. PROKS, P. & F.M. ASHCROFT. 1997. Phentolamine block of K_{ATP} channels is mediated by Kir6.2. Proc. Natl. Acad. Sci. U. S. A. **94:** 11716–11720.
4. MONKS, L.K., K.E. COSGROVE, M. DUNNE, et al. 1999. Affinity isolation of imidazoline binding proteins from rat brain using 5-amino-efaroxan as a ligand. FEBS Lett. **447:** 61–64.
5. RUSTENBECK, I., M. KÖPP, P. RATZKA, et al. 1999. Imidazolines and the pancreatic B-cell: actions and binding sites. Ann. N. Y. Acad. Sci. **881:** 229–240.
6. HENQUIN, J.C. 1982. Quinine and the stimulus-secretion coupling in pancreatic β-cells: glucose-like effects on potassium permeability and insulin release. Endocrinology **110:** 1325–1332.
7. BOKVIST, K., P. RORSMAN & P.A. SMITH. 1990. Block of ATP-regulated and Ca^{2+}-activated K^+ channels in mouse pancreatic β-cells by external tetraethylammonium and quinine. J. Physiol. **423:** 327–342.
8. GROSSE-LACKMANN, T., & I. RUSTENBECK. 2000. Quinine blocks K_{ATP} channels by binding to the imidazoline site at the pore-forming subunit [abstract]. Naunyn-Schmiedeberg's Arch. Pharmacol. **361:** R78.

9. GRIBBLE, F., T.M.E. DAVIS, C. HIGHAM, *et al.* 2000. The antimalarial agent mefloquine inhibits ATP-sensitive K-channels. Br. J. Pharmacol. **131:** 756–760.
10. SCHULZ, A. & A. HASSELBLATT. 1989. Dual action of clonidine on insulin release: suppression, but stimulation when α-receptors are blocked. Naunyn-Schmiedeberg's Arch. Pharmacol. **340:** 712–714.
11. TUCKER, S.J., F. GRIBBLE, C. ZHAO, *et al.* 1997. Truncation of Kir6.2 produces ATP-sensitive K^+ channels in the absence of the sulfonylurea receptor. Nature **387:** 179–183.

Moxonidine, a Mixed α_2-Adrenergic and Imidazoline Receptor Agonist, Identifies a Novel Adrenergic Target for Spinal Analgesia

LAURA S. STONE,[a] CAROLYN A. FAIRBANKS,[a,b,c] AND GEORGE L. WILCOX[a,b]

[a]*Department of Neuroscience, University of Minnesota, Minneapolis, Minnesota 55455, USA*

[b]*Department of Pharmacology, University of Minnesota, Minneapolis, Minnesota 55455, USA*

[c]*Department of Pharmaceutics, University of Minnesota, Minneapolis, Minnesota 55455, USA*

> ABSTRACT: Moxonidine is a mixed α_2-adrenergic and imidazoline receptor agonist with an improved side effect profile compared to clonidine. Intrathecal (i.t.) moxonidine has been found to possess analgesic activity that, in contrast to the majority of α_2-adrenoceptor (α_2AR) agonists, does not require activation of the α_{2A}AR subtype, which mediates many of the side effects associated with α_2AR use. In addition, moxonidine (i.t.) interacts in a synergistic manner with opioid agonists and this synergy is retained in neuropathic pain states. Moxonidine may therefore be clinically useful in the treatment of chronic neuropathic pain, either alone or as a coadjuvant with opioids.
>
> KEYWORDS: intrathecal; α_{2C} adrenergic receptor; synergy; pain

INTRODUCTION

Moxonidine, a mixed imidazoline-1 receptor (I_1R) and α_2-adrenergic receptor (α_2AR) agonist, was developed as a centrally acting antihypertensive agent with an improved side effect profile over clonidine.[1] Clinical trials have indicated that it is well tolerated and several studies have reported that patients experience a reduction in the side effects of sedation and dry mouth compared to clonidine.[2–5]

Binding studies have shown that moxonidine binds to the I_1R site on human platelets with 13-fold higher affinity than clonidine ($K_i = 4.2 \pm 3.2$ nmol/L and $K_i = 55 \pm 10$ nmol/L, respectively).[6] However, both clonidine and moxonidine also bind with relatively high affinity to α_2ARs. Examination of human α_2ARs stably expressed in transfected Chinese Hamster Ovary cells revealed that the affinity of moxonidine was comparable between the α_2AR subtypes (K_i: α_{2A}AR = 13.0 ± 4.2; α_{2B}AR = 9.5 ± 4.1 nmol/L; and α_{2C}AR = 15.6 ± 9.8 nmol/L). In the same study the affinity of clonidine was found to be comparable between the α_{2A}AR and α_{2C}AR subtypes while slightly lower at α_{2B}ARs (K_i: α_{2A}AR = 8.7 ± 2.0; α_{2B}AR = 31 ± 6.0 nmol/L; α_{2C}AR = 9.4 ± 2.3 nmol/L).[2] Overall these data demonstrate that moxonidine has

Address correspondence to: George L. Wilcox, Department of Neuroscience, 6-145 Jackson Hall, 321 Church Street SE, University of Minnesota, Minneapolis, MN 55455, USA. Voice: 612-625-1474; fax: 612-624-7910.

e-mail: george@umn.edu

Ann. N.Y. Acad. Sci. 1009: 378–385 (2003). © 2003 New York Academy of Sciences.
doi: 10.1196/annals.1304.051

improved affinity for I_1Rs compared to clonidine, yet the two agonists share similar affinities for the α_2AR subtypes.

SPINAL α_2-ADRENERGIC ANALGESIA

Agonists acting at α_2ARs have analgesic properties following both systemic[7] and spinal[8–10] administration in multiple species including humans.[11–18] Development of the use of clonidine for the treatment of pain has been particularly important for the management of patients who are under-responsive to conventional opioid therapy.[12,14,17–18] In addition, α_2AR agonists interact synergistically when co-administered with opioids spinally[19–27] and systemically.[21] By taking advantage of this property, effective analgesia can be achieved at lower doses of drug, a strategy that may lead to a reduction in the side effects associated with both adrenergic and opioid therapies.

In addition to combination therapies, untoward side effects can sometimes be minimized through the development of more selective agents. It is therefore important to understand the relative contributions of the I_1R and α_2AR subtypes in mediating the effects of these compounds. Although pharmacologic studies have largely excluded I_1R activation as the mechanism underlying the analgesic action of these agents,[28–29] the question remains as to which of the α_2AR subtypes(s) is(are) necessary and sufficient to produce α_2AR agonist-mediated analgesia.

Differential localization of the α_2AR subtypes suggests differential involvement in spinal analgesia. The $\alpha_{2A}AR$ and $\alpha_{2C}AR$ subtypes have been localized to primary sensory neurons and/or spinal cord by several investigators at both the RNA and protein level.[30–39] More specifically, the $\alpha_{2A}AR$ has been shown to be expressed by substance P–containing, capsaicin-sensitive primary afferent neurons, the majority of which are thought to be nociceptors. These neurons synthesize $\alpha_{2A}ARs$ and transport them into the spinal cord on their central terminals.[30] Activation of α_2ARs on the terminals of sensory neurons results in decreased glutamate release and attenuation of nociceptive neurotransmission,[40] and α_2AR agonist-mediated reductions in glutamate release have been attributed to the activation of $\alpha_{2A}ARs$ on capsaicin-sensitive terminals in the spinal cord.[41] In contrast to the $\alpha_{2A}AR$ subtype, the majority of $\alpha_{2C}AR$-immunoreactivity can be attributed to expression by neurons intrinsic to the spinal cord.[42–44] Although there is one report suggesting expression of $\alpha_{2B}AR$ in adult dorsal root ganglia or spinal cord neurons,[34] these findings have not been confirmed in other studies.[31,37–39]

Several lines of evidence implicate the $\alpha_{2A}AR$ subtype as the primary mediator of spinal α_2AR agonist-mediated analgesia. The first, based on pharmacologic data, implicated the $\alpha_{2A}AR$ subtype based on the relative potencies of several α_2AR agonists in comparison to their relative affinities at each subtype.[45,46] Subsequently, the use of mice in which the $\alpha_{2A}AR$ had been rendered dysfunctional illustrated more substantively that the $\alpha_{2A}AR$ subtype is required for full analgesic potency and efficacy of spinally delivered NE, clonidine, UK-14,304, and dexmedetomidine[47,48] as well as that of systemically administered dexmedetomidine.[49,50] Furthermore, the synergistic interactions between spinally delivered opioid agonists deltorphin II and DAMGO and the α_2AR agonist UK-14,304 were also shown to depend on the presence of a functional $\alpha_{2A}AR$.[47] Finally, applying antisense oligonucleotides to selectively reduce expression of the $\alpha_{2A}AR$, Wang et al.[51] demonstrated a reduction in the potency of spinally delivered clonidine in a model of acute pain whereas knockdown of the $\alpha_{2C}AR$ had no effect.

In addition to its analgesic effects, converging lines of evidence suggest that the $\alpha_{2A}AR$ subtype mediates additional effects associated with α_2AR agonists including sedation,[49,50,52] epileptogenesis,[53] anesthetic sparing,[50] hypothermia,[49] and hypotension.[54] Thus, the development of $\alpha_{2A}AR$-selective agonists as analgesics is unlikely to result in an improved side effect profile and may therefore have limited therapeutic utility.

A role for the $\alpha_{2B}AR$ and $\alpha_{2C}AR$ subtypes is also indicated based on pharmacologic studies. Takano et al. have suggested that, whereas clonidine and dexmedetomidine analgesia is meditated by $\alpha_{2A}AR$, the analgesic efficacy of the α_2AR agonist ST-91 may involve activation of non-$\alpha_{2A}ARs$ when delivered intrathecally.[55,56] Interestingly, dexmedetomidine and ST-91 will synergize when co-administered in the spinal cord, an interaction that strongly supports different sites of action for each compound.[57] Furthermore, studies using genetically engineered mice have revealed that the antinociceptive response to nitrous oxide is also mediated by activation of the $\alpha_{2B}AR$ and/or $\alpha_{2C}AR$.[58,59]

MOXONIDINE-INDUCED SPINAL ANALGESIA IN ACUTE PAIN ASSAYS

The spinal analgesic properties of moxonidine were first reported by Fairbanks and Wilcox.[48] In that and subsequent studies the following observations have been reported: (1) moxonidine produces dose-dependent analgesia in multiple acute pain assays; (2) these effects are mediated by an action at α_2ARs; (3) the $\alpha_{2A}AR$ is not required for moxonidine analgesia; (4) the site of action is not the terminals of descending NE-containing terminals; (5) moxonidine acts synergistically with spinal morphine as well as the δ-opioid receptor agonist deltorphin II, but does not synergize with the μ-selective agonist DAMGO; (6) moxonidine analgesia has an $\alpha_{2C}AR$-dependent component; and (7) unlike the α_2AR agonist UK-14,304, the $\alpha_{2A}AR$ was neither necessary nor sufficient for moxonidine to synergize with deltorpin II—only the $\alpha_{2C}AR$ is required for that interaction.[60,61] Interestingly, antagonist studies in both the $\alpha_{2A}AR$-dysfunctional and $\alpha_{2C}AR$-KO mice indicated that moxonidine's residual analgesia observed in both cases was mediated by α_2AR and not I_1Rs. The presence of an $\alpha_{2C}AR$-dependent component in moxonidine's analgesic profile was validated by the observation that treating animals with $\alpha_{2C}AR$-selective antisense oligonucleotides significantly decreased (6-fold) moxonidine's potency compared to mismatch-control mice.

These data suggest that moxonidine, in its ability to elicit analgesia through a non-$\alpha_{2A}AR$-dependent mechanism, may provide an improved therapeutic window over clonidine and other $\alpha_{2A}AR$-requiring analgesics. Implicit in that hypothesis is the assumption that the non-$\alpha_{2A}AR$-dependent nature of moxonidine-induced analgesia allows for the prediction that moxonidine will have reduced activity in other $\alpha_{2A}AR$-mediated effects such as sedation. It is not clear why clonidine and moxonidine, which are non-selective among the α_2AR subtypes in binding assays in vitro, should have differential functional selectivity in vivo. It may therefore be premature to assume that an improved side effect profile will necessarily correlate with a non-

α_{2A}AR analgesic action in cases where the compound has non-subtype-selective binding properties. Nonetheless, the results of the clinical hypotension trials, in which moxonidine treatment resulted in less sedation and dry mouth than clonidine, support the notion that moxonidine may represent a significant improvement over clonidine or other α_{2A}AR-dependent analgesic agents.

MOXONIDINE IN CHRONIC NEUROPATHIC PAIN

Chronic neuropathic pain is characterized by spontaneous persistent pain and hypersensitivity to thermal and mechanical stimuli. Neuropathic pain is thought to be under-responsive to conventional opioid regimens,[62] although the degree of this under-responsiveness is controversial.[63] In contrast, adrenergic agonists have been shown to be highly effective against neuropathic pain in humans[14,17,64] and animals,[65,66] although to a limited degree following systemic administration,[67] and their analgesic activity may be enhanced in neuropathic pain conditions.[68,69] In addition, several studies have demonstrated that adrenergic-opioid synergy persists in neuropathic pain.[70,71] Accordingly, intrathecal moxonidine dose-dependently reverses nerve injury-induced hypersensitivity[71] and systemically administered moxonidine attenuates formalin-induced nocifensive behaviors, a common model for chronic, on-going pain.[72] Importantly, the analgesic synergy between moxonidine and morphine are retained in the neuropathic state.[71] A combination of moxonidine with an opioid may therefore represent a powerful approach to the treatment of chronic neuropathic pain.

Anatomical studies have demonstrated that, while expression of α_{2A}AR is down-regulated in the dorsal horn of the spinal cord, the α_{2C}AR is either up-regulated or unchanged.[73] Thus, increases in α_2AR agonist potency in neuropathic conditions may be mediated by an increase in the analgesic contribution of α_{2C}ARs. This hypothesis is consistent with the study by Duflo *et al.*,[74] in which the α_{2A}AR-dependent component of clonidine analgesia was lost following nerve injury, leaving only a non-α_{2A}AR-mediated action. This shift in pharmacology away from α_{2A}AR and toward α_{2C}AR suggests that selective or α_{2C}AR-preferring agonists such as moxonidine may be particularly advantageous in the treatment of chronic neuropathic pain free of the many side effects associated with α_{2A}AR activation.

CONCLUSIONS

Despite moxonidine's mixed I_1R/α_2AR profile, both moxonidine and clonidine produce analgesia following spinal delivery via activation of α_2ARs. However, the α_2AR subtype mediating the action of these agents differs between the two compounds. Clonidine analgesia in acute pain models has an absolute requirement for α_{2A}AR activation. Several other commonly used α_2AR agonists (UK-14,304, dexmedetomidine) share this dependency on α_{2A}AR. Moxonidine analgesia and synergy with opioids are non-α_{2A}AR-dependent and have an α_{2C}AR component. The importance of moxonidine's non-α_{2A}AR mechanism of action is underscored by the observations linking many α_2AR side effects to activation of the α_{2A}AR subtype. It is not clear why agonists such as clonidine and moxonidine, which share similar affinity across subtypes, might show subtype-selectivity in their analgesic activity in vivo. The observation that moxonidine may function as a partial agonist at the $\alpha_{2A}AR$ in some assays may explain its ability to "unmask" analgesic properties of non-$\alpha_{2A}ARs$.[75] Moxonidine's improved side effect profile may therefore be explained as a consequence of its partial efficacy at the side-effect mediating $\alpha_{2A}ARs$. It should be noted, however, that moxonidine displays full agonist efficacy at $\alpha_{2A}AR$ in many functional assays.[76,77]

In summary, the $\alpha_{2C}AR$-mediated site of action of moxonidine, the anatomic and pharmacologic shift toward $\alpha_{2C}ARs$ in neuropathic conditions and the retention of moxonidine/morphine synergy following nerve injury highlight moxonidine's potential as a therapeutic agent, either alone or in combination with an opioid, in the treatment of chronic neuropathic pain.

REFERENCES

1. ARMAH, I.B. & W. STENZEL. 1981. BE-5895, a new clonidine-type antihypertensive aminopyrimidine derivative. Naunyn Schmiedebergs Arch. Pharmacol. **316**(Suppl): R–42.
2. PLÄNITZ, V. 1984. Crossover comparison of moxonidine and clonidine in mild to moderate hypertension. Eur. J. Clin. Pharmacol. **27:** 147–152.
3. OLLIVIER, J.P. & M.O. CHRISTEN. 1994. I1-imidazoline-receptor agonists in the treatment of hypertension: an appraisal of clinical experience. J. Cardiovasc. Pharmacol. **24:** S39–48.
4. KRAFT, K. & H. VETTER. 1994. Twenty-four-hour blood pressure profiles in patients with mild-to-moderate hypertension: moxonidine versus captopril. J. Cardiovasc. Pharmacol. **24:** S29–33.
5. KÜPPERS, H.E., B.A. JAGER, J.H. LUSZICK, et al. 1997. Placebo-controlled comparison of the efficacy and tolerability of once-daily moxonidine and enalapril in mild-to-moderate essential hypertension. J. Hypertension **15:** 93–97.
6. PILETZ, J.E., H. ZHU & D.N. CHIKKALA. 1996. Comparison of ligand binding affinities at human I-1-Imidazoline binding sites and the high affinity state of alpha-2 adrenoceptor subtypes. J. Pharmacol. Exp. Ther. **279:** 694–702.
7. PAALZOW, L. 1974. Analgesia produced by clonidine in mice and rats. J. Pharm. Pharmacol. **26:** 361–363.
8. REDDY, S.V.R., J.L. MADERDRUT & T.L. YAKSH. 1980. Spinal cord pharmacology of adrenergic agonist-mediated antinociception. J. Pharmacol. Exp. Ther. **213:** 525–533.
9. REDDY, S.V. & T.L. YAKSH. 1980. Spinal noradrenergic terminal system mediates antinociception. Brain Res. **189:** 391–401.
10. YAKSH, T.L. & S.V. REDDY. 1981. Studies in the primate on the analgesic effects associated with intrathecal actions of opiates, alpha-adrenergic agonists and baclofen. Anesthesiology **54:** 451–454.
11. EISENACH, J.C., S.Z. LYSAK & C.M. VISCOMI. 1989. Epidural clonidine analgesia following surgery: phase I. Anesthesiology **71:** 640–646.
12. EISENACH, J.C., R.L. RAUCK, C. BUZZANELL, et al. 1989. Epidural clonidine analgesia for intractable cancer pain: phase I. Anesthesiology **71:** 647–652.
13. MENDEZ, R., J.C. EISENACH & K. KASHTAN. 1990. Epidural clonidine analgesia after cesarean section. Anesthesiology **73:** 848–852.
14. RAUCK, R.L., J.C. EISENACH, K. JACKSON, et al. 1993. Epidural clonidine treatment for refractory reflex sympathetic dystrophy. Anesthesiology **79:** 1163–1169.
15. EISENACH, J.C., R. D'ANGELO, C. TAYLOR, et al. 1994. An isobolographic study of epidural clonidine and fentanyl after cesarean section. Anesth. Analg. **79:** 285–290.
16. EISENACH, J.C., S. DUPEN, M. DUBIOS, et al. 1995. Epidural clonidine analgesia for intractable cancer pain. Pain **61:** 391–399.

17. SIDDALL, P.J., M. GRAY, S. RUTKOWSKI, et al. 1994. Intrathecal morphine and clonidine in the management of spinal cord injury pain: a case report. Pain **59:** 147–148.
18. COOMBS, D.W., R.L. SAUNDERS, J.D. FRATKIN, et al. 1986. Continuous intrathecal hydromorphone and clonidine for intractable cancer pain. J. Neurosurg. **64:** 890–894.
19. PLUMMER, J.L., P.L. CMIELEWSKI, G.K. GOURLAY, et al. 1992. Antinociceptive and motor effects of intrathecal morphine combined with intrathecal clonidine, noradrenaline, carbachol or midazolam. Pain **49:** 145–152.
20. WILCOX, G.L., K.H. CARLSSON, A. JOCHIM, et al. 1987. Mutual potentiation of antinociceptive effects of morphine and clonidine on motor and sensory responses in rat spinal cord. Brain Res. **405:** 84–93.
21. OSSIPOV, M., S. HARRIS, P. LLOYD, et al. 1990. An isobolographic analysis of the antinociceptive effect of systemically and intrathecally administered combinations of clonidine and opiates. J. Pharmacol. Exp. Ther. **255:** 1107–1116.
22. OSSIPOV, M., R. LOZITO, E. MESSINEO, et al. 1990. Spinal antinociceptive synergy between clonidine and morphine, U69593, and DPDPE: isobolographic analysis. Life Sci. **47:** PL71–PL76.
23. OSSIPOV, M., S. HARRIS, P. LLOYD, et al. 1990. Antinociceptive interaction between opioids and medetomidine: systemic additivity and spinal synergy. Anesthesiology **73:** 1227–1235.
24. SULLIVAN, A.F., M.R. DASHWOOD & A.H. DICKENSON. 1987. α2 adrenoceptor modulation of nociception in rat spinal cord: location, effects and interactions with morphine. Eur. J. Pharmacol. **138:** 169–177.
25. DRASNER, K. & H.L. FIELDS. 1988. Synergy between the antinociceptive effects of intrathecal clonidine and systemic morphine in the rat. Pain **32:** 309–312.
26. MONASKY, M.S., A.R. ZINSMEISTER, C.W. STEVENS, et al. 1990. Interaction of intrathecal morphine and ST-91 on antinociception in the rat: dose-response analysis, antagonism and clearance. J. Pharmacol. Exp. Ther. **254:** 383–392.
27. YAKSH, T.L. 1985. Pharmacology of spinal adrenergic systems which modulate spinal nociceptive processing. Pharmacol. Biochem. Behav. **22:** 845–858.
28. MONROE, P.J., D.L. SMITH, H.R. KIRK, et al. 1995. Spinal nonadrenergic imidazoline receptors do not mediate the antinociceptive action of intrathecal clonidine in the rat. J. Pharmacol. Exp. Ther. **273:** 1057–1062.
29. TAKANO, Y. & T.L. YAKSH. 1992. Characterization of the pharmacology of intrathecally administered alpha-2 agonists and antagonists in rats. J. Pharmacol. Exp. Ther. **261:** 764–772.
30. STONE, L.S., C. BROBERGER, L. VULCHANOVA, et al. 1998. Differential distribution of alpha$_{2A}$ and alpha$_{2C}$ adrenergic receptor immunoreactivity in the rat spinal cord. J. Neurosci. **18:** 5928–5937.
31. NICHOLAS, A.P., V. PIERIBONE & T. HOKFELT. 1993. Distributions of mRNAs for alpha-2 adrenergic receptor subtypes in rat brain: an in situ hybridization study. J. Comp. Neurol. **328:** 575–594.
32. SHI, T.J.S., U. WINZER-SERHAN, F. LESLIE, et al. 1999. Distribution of alpha(2)-adrenoceptor mRNAs in the rat lumbar spinal cord in normal and axotomized rats. Neuroreport. **10:** 2835–2839.
33. SHI, T.J.S., U. WINZER-SERHAN, F. LESLIE, et al. 2000. Distribution and regulation of alpha(2)-adrenoceptors in rat dorsal root ganglia. Pain **84:** 319–330.
34. GOLD, M.S., S. DASTMALCHI & J.D. LEVINE. 1997. Alpha 2 adrenergic receptor subtypes in rat dorsal root and superior cervical ganglion neurons. Pain **69:** 179–190.
35. ROSIN, D.L., E.M. TALLEY, A. LEE, et al. 1996. Distribution of alpha 2C-adrenergic receptor-like immunoreactivity in the rat central nervous system. J. Comp. Neurol. **372:** 135–165.
36. TALLEY, E.M., D.L. ROSIN, A. LEE, et al. 1996. Distribution of alpha 2A-adrenergic receptor-like immunoreactivity in the rat central nervous system. J. Comp. Neurol. **372:** 111–134.
37. SCHEININ, M., J.W. LOMASNEY, H.D. HAYDEN, et al. 1994. Distribution of alpha 2-adrenergic receptor subtype gene expression in rat brain. Brain Res. Mol. Brain Res. **21:** 133–149.

38. ZENG, D.W. & K.R. LYNCH. 1991. Distribution of alpha 2-adrenergic receptor mRNAs in the rat CNS. Brain Res. Mol. Brain Res. **10:** 219–225.
39. BLAXALL, H.S., N.A. HASS & D.B. BYLUND. 1994. Expression of alpha 2-adrenergic receptor genes in rat tissues. Receptor **4:** 191–199.
40. PAN, Y.Z., D.P. LI & H.L. PAN. 2002. Inhibition of glutamatergic synaptic input to spinal lamina II_O neurons by presynaptic alpha-2-adrenergic receptors. J. Neurophysiol. **87:** 1938–1947.
41. LI, X.H. & J.C. EISENACH. 2001. α_{2A}-adrenoceptor stimulation reduces capsaicin-induced glutamate release from spinal cord synaptosomes. J. Pharmacol. Exp. Ther. **299:** 939–944.
42. OLAVE, M.J. & D.J. MAXWELL. 2002. An investigation of neurones that possess the alpha 2C-adrenergic receptor in the rat dorsal horn. Neuroscience **115:** 31–40.
43. OLAVE, M.J. & D.J. MAXWELL. 2003. Axon terminals possessing the alpha 2c-adrenergic receptor in the rat dorsal horn are predominantly excitatory. Brain Res. **965:** 269–273.
44. OLAVE, M.J. & D.J. MAXWELL. 2003. Neurokinin-1 projection cells in the rat dorsal horn receive synaptic contacts from axons that possess $alpha_{2C}$-adrenergic receptors. J. Neurosci. **23:** 6837–6846.
45. MILLAN, M.J. 1992. Evidence that an $alpha_{2A}$-adrenoceptor subtype mediates antinociception in mice. Eur. J. Pharmacol. **215:** 355–356.
46. MILLAN, M.J., K. BERVOETS, J.M. RIVET, et al. 1994. Multiple alpha-2 adrenergic receptor subtypes. II. Evidence for a role of rat R alpha-2A adrenergic receptors in the control of nociception, motor behavior and hippocampal synthesis of noradrenaline. J. Pharmacol. Exp. Ther. **270:** 958–972.
47. STONE, L.S., L. MACMILLAN, K.F. KITTO, et al. 1997. The α_{2a}-adrenergic receptor subtype mediates spinal analgesia evoked by α2 agonists and is necessary for spinal adrenergic/opioid synergy. J. Neurosci. **17:** 7157–7165.
48. Fairbanks, C.A. & G.L. Wilcox. 1999. Moxonidine, an α_2 adrenergic and imidazoline receptor agonist, produces spinal antinociception in mice. J. Pharmacol. Exp. Ther. **290:** 403–412.
49. HUNTER, J.C., D.J. FONTANA, L.R. HEDLEY, et al. 1997. Assessment of the role of alpha2-adrenoceptor subtypes in the antinociceptive, sedative and hypothermic action of dexmedetomidine in transgenic mice. Br. J. Pharmacol. **122:** 1339–1344.
50. LAKHLANI, P.P., L.B. MACMILLAN, T.Z. GUO, et al. 1997. Substitution of a mutant alpha(2a)-adrenergic receptor via hit and run gene targeting reveals the role of this subtype in sedative, analgesic, and anesthetic-sparing responses in vivo. PNAS **94:** 9950–9955.
51. WANG, X.M., Z.J. ZHANG, R. BAINS, et al. 2002. Effect of antisense knock-down of alpha(2a)- and alpha(2c)-adrenoceptors on the antinociceptive action of clonidine on trigeminal nociception in the rat. Pain **98:** 27–35.
52. MIZOBE, T., K. MAGHSOUDI, K. SITWALA, et al. 1996. Antisense technology reveals the alpha2A adrenoceptor to be the subtype mediating the hypnotic response to the highly selective agonist, dexmedetomidine, in the locus coeruleus of the rat. J. Clin. Invest. **98:** 1076–1080.
53. JANUMPALLI, S., L.S. BUTLER, L.B. MACMILLAN, et al. 1998. A point mutation (D79N) of the α2A adrenergic receptor abolishes the antiepileptogenic action of endogenous norepinephrine. J. Neurosci. **18:** 2004–2008.
54. MACMILLAN, L.B., L. HEIN, M.S. SMITH, et al. 1996. Central hypotensive effects of the $alpha_{2a}$-adrenergic receptor subtype. Science **273:** 801–803.
55. TAKANO, Y., M. TAKANO & T.L. YAKSH. 1992. The effect of intrathecally administered imiloxan and WB4101: possible role of α2-adrenoceptor subtypes in the spinal cord. Eur. J. Pharmacol. **219:** 465–468.
56. TAKANO, Y. & T.L. YAKSH. 1993. Chronic spinal infusion of dexmedetomidine, ST-91 and clonidine: spinal alpha2 adrenoceptor subtypes and intrinsic activity. J. Pharmacol. Exp. Ther. **264:** 327–335.
57. GRAHAM, B.A., D.L. HAMMOND & H.K. PROUDFIT. 2000. Synergistic interactions between two alpha(2)-adrenoceptor agonists, dexmedetomidine and ST-91, in two substrains of Sprague-Dawley rats. Pain **85:** 135–143.

58. GUO, T.Z., M.F. DAVIES, W.S. KINGERY, et al. 1999. Nitrous oxide produces antinociceptive response via alpha2B and/or alpha2C adrenoceptor subtypes in mice. Anesthesiology **90:** 470–476.
59. SAWAMURA, S., W.S. KINGERY, M.F. DAVIES, et al. 2000. Antinociceptive Action of nitrous oxide is mediated by stimulation of noradrenergic neurons in the brainstem and activation of α2B adrenoceptors. J. Neurosci. **20:** 9242–9251.
60. FAIRBANKS, C.A., I.J. POSTHUMUS, K.F. KITTO, et al. 2000. Moxonidine, a selective imidazoline/a2 adrenergic receptor agonist, synergizes with morphine and deltorphin II to inhibit substance P-induced behavior in mice. Pain **84:** 13–20.
61. FAIRBANKS, C.A., L.S. STONE, K.F. KITTO, et al. 2002. alpha(2C)-adrenergic receptors mediate spinal analgesia and adrenergic-opioid synergy. J. Pharmacol. Exp. Ther. **300:** 282–290.
62. ARNER, S. & B.A. MEYERSON. 1988. Lack of analgesic effect of opioids on neuropathic and idiopathic forms of pain. Pain **33:** 11–23.
63. PORTENOY, R.K., K.M. FOLEY & C.E. INTURRISI. 1990. The nature of opioid responsiveness and its implications for neuropathic pain: new hypotheses derived from studies of opioid infusions. Pain **43:** 273–286.
64. DAVIS, K.D., R.D. TREEDE, S.N. RAJA, et al. 1991. Topical application of clonidine relieves hyperalgesia in patients with sympathetically maintained pain. Pain **47:** 309–317.
65. YAKSH, T.L., J.W. POGREL, Y.W. LEE, et al. 1995. Reversal of nerve ligation-induced allodynia by spinal alpha-2 adrenoceptor agonists. J. Pharmacol. Exp. Ther. **272:** 207–214.
66. MALMBERG, A.B., L.R. HEDLEY, J.R. JASPER, et al. 2001. Contribution of a2 receptor subtypes to nerve injury-induced pain and its regulation by dexmedetomidine. Br. J. Pharmacol. **132:** 1827–1836.
67. HAO, J.X., W. YU, X.J. XU, et al. 1996. Effects of intrathecal vs. systemic clonidine in treating chronic allodynia-like response in spinally injured rats. Brain Res. **736:** 28–34.
68. XU, X.J., M.J. PUKE & H.Z. WIESENFELD. 1992. The depressive effect of intrathecal clonidine on the spinal flexor reflex is enhanced after sciatic nerve section in rats. Pain **51:** 145–151.
69. POREE, L.R., T.Z. GUO, W.S. KINGERY, et al. 1998. The analgesic potency of dexmedetomidine is enhanced after nerve injury: a possible role for peripheral α2-adrenoceptors. Anesth Analg. **87:** 941–948.
70. OSSIPOV, M.H., Y. LOPEZ, D. BIAN, et al. 1997. Synergistic antinociceptive interactions of morphine and clonidine in rats with nerve-ligation injury. Anesthesiology **86:** 1–9.
71. FAIRBANKS, C.A., H.O. NGUYEN, B.M. GROCHOLSKI, et al. 2000. Moxonidine, a selective imidazoline-a2-adrenergic receptor agonist, produces spinal synergistic antihyperalgesia with morphine in nerve-injured mice. Anesthesiology **93:** 765–773.
72. SHANNON, H.E. & E.A. LUTZ. 2000. Effects of the I-1 imidazoline/alpha(2)-adrenergic receptor agonist moxonidine in comparison with clonidine in the formalin test in rats. Pain **85:** 161–167.
73. STONE, L.S., L. VULCHANOVA, M.S. RIEDL, et al. 1999. Effects of peripheral nerve injury on alpha-2a and alpha-2c adrenergic receptor immunoreactivity in the rat spinal cord. Neuroscience. **93:** 1399–1407.
74. DUFLO, F., X. H. LI, C. BANTEL, et al. 2002. Peripheral nerve injury alters the alpha(2) adrenoceptor subtype activated by clonidine for analgesia. Anesthesiology **97:** 636–641.
75. TAN, C.M., M.H. WILSON, L.B. MACMILLAN, et al. 2002. Heterozygous alpha(2A)-adrenergic receptor mice unveil unique therapeutic benefits of partial agonists. Proc. Natl. Acad. Sci. U. S. A. **99:** 12471–12476.
76. MICHEL, M.C., L.F. BRASS, A. WILLIAMS, et al. 1989. Alpha 2-adrenergic receptor stimulation mobilizes intracellular Ca2+ in human erythroleukemia cells. J. Biol. Chem. **264:** 4986–4891.
77. MOLDERINGS, G.J., H. BONISCH, M. BRUSS, et al. 2000. Species-specific pharmacological properties of human alpha(2A)-adrenoceptors. Hypertension **36:** 405–410.

Evidence for Nonadrenoceptor Responses to Imidazoline Derivatives in the Porcine Isolated Rectal Artery

MINYAN WANG, W.R. DUNN, S.L. CHAN, B. GARFIELD, AND V.G. WILSON

School of Biomedical Sciences, University of Nottingham, Nottingham, UK

ABSTRACT: High concentrations of phentolamine, efaroxan, and idazoxan were found to produce nonadrenoceptor contractions of the porcine isolated rectal artery previously exposed to U46619 and forskolin. These responses were insensitive to the putative imidazoline I_3 receptor antagonist KU-14R, unlike those previously reported in this preparation for oxymetazoline. The pharmacologic nature of this response and the obligate requirement for preconstriction suggests that these imidazoline derivatives modulate ion channel function through a novel nonadrenergic site.

KEYWORDS: phentolamine; idazoxan; imidazolines; non-adrenoceptors; KU-14R

INTRODUCTION

The presence of nonadrenoceptor imidazoline binding sites is well established in the central nervous system,[1,2] various peripheral organs,[3,4] and smooth muscles cells.[5–7] There are, however, surprisingly few functional correlates that exhibit strict pharmacologic identity with the binding sites.[8] Part of the difficulty experienced by various groups has been the paucity of unambiguous nonadrenoceptor responses to the imidazoline derivatives, coupled with the lack of a suitable antagonist that does not also interact with α_2-adrenoceptors. KU-14R (2-(2,3 dihydro-2-benzofuranyl)-2-imidazole) is an imidazoline derivative reported to inhibit selectively the I_3 imidazoline receptor (I_3R) on pancreatic islet cells.[9] This site is thought to mediate the increase in insulin secretion produced by high concentrations of a variety of imidazoline-based agents,[8] including oxymetazoline.[10] We recently showed that oxymetazoline elicited large contractions of the porcine isolated rectal artery following inactivation of α-adrenoceptors by phenoxybenzamine and exposure to a combination of a vasoconstrictor, U46619, and a vasodilator, forskolin.[11] This nonadrenoceptor-mediated response was sensitive to the putative I_3 imidazoline antagonist KU-14R.[11] In the present study, we have examined the effects of various imidazoline derivatives on the porcine isolated rectal artery to determine the pharmacologic characteristics of this nonadrenergic response.

Address for correspondence: V.G. Wilson, School of Biomedical Sciences, University of Nottingham, Queen's Medical Centre, Nottingham NG7 2UH, UK. Voice: 00 44 115 9709472; fax: 00 44 115 9709259.

e-mail: vince.wilson@nottingham.ac.uk

METHODS

Segments of the porcine isolated rectal artery were prepared for isometric tension recording as previously described.[11] All preparations were exposed to 3 µM phenoxybenzamine for 60 minutes to inactivate α-adrenoceptors, followed by repeated washing over a 40-minute period. Each preparation was then exposed to 60 mM KCl, and the response was allowed to reach maximum. Two further responses to 60 mM KCl were elicited until the contractions were reproducible. Following an equilibration period of 30 minutes, each preparation was then stimulated with 5 to 20 nM U-46619 (the thromboxane-mimetic, 9,11 dideoxy-9α, 11α-(epoxymethano)-prosta-5Z,13E-dien-1-oic acid) to produce a contraction equivalent to 50% to 70% of the response to 60 mM KCl. Each preparation was then exposed to increasing concentrations of forskolin (0.1–0.7 µM) to lower the residual vasoconstrictor tone to less than 5% of the final contraction induced by 60 mM KCl. Once a stable contraction was established, the preparations were exposed to cumulatively increasing concentrations of phentolamine, efaroxan, idazoxan, BDF 6143, clonidine, UK-14304, or rilmenidine. Responses to phentolamine and efaroxan were repeated in the presence of 10 µM KU14R (2-(2,3 dihydro-2-benzofuranyl)-2-imidazole).

RESULTS

Following inactivation of all α-adrenoceptors by phenoxybenzamine, the imidazoline-based α-adrenoceptor antagonists phentolamine, idazoxan, efaroxan, BDF 6143, and the α-adrenoceptor agonists, rilmenidine, clonidine, and UK-14304 (all 0.1 µM–100 µM) failed to modify vascular tone in the porcine rectal artery (n = 4–8). In addition, the antagonists failed to elicit a response in phenoxybenazamine-naïve preparations (n = 4). After exposure to U46619 and forskolin, however, the addition of an imidazoline (phentolamine) caused slow-developing, concentration-dependent contractions in all preparations examined (FIG. 1, *upper section*). As shown in FIGURE 1, efaroxan and idazoxan also caused similar contractions in the presence of U46619 and forskolin, with a –log EC_{50} of 5.17 ± 0.12 (n = 10) for phentolamine and a maximum response equivalent to 20% to 30% of the response to 60 mM KCl. An accurate estimate of the –log EC_{50} was not possible for efaroxan because the highest concentration employed (100 µM) was clearly not the maximum response. In contrast to phentolamine and efaroxan, the imidazoline derivative BDF 6143 failed to elicit a response under these conditions in 7 out of 10 preparations; in the remaining 3 preparations the contractions were less than 10% of the response to 60 mM KCl. Under similar conditions, UK-14304 (0.01–10 µM) failed to elicit a response (n = 8), but rilmenidine and clonidine caused small concentration-dependent contractions (<15% of the response to 60 mM KCl).

FIGURE 2 shows that contractions elicited by efaroxan and phentolamine, in the presence of U46619 and forskolin, were not affected by 10 µM KU14R.

DISCUSSION

Investigation of the function of nonadrenergic imidazoline binding sites has proven difficult because of the coexistence of α_2-adrenoceptors in many tissues and the lack

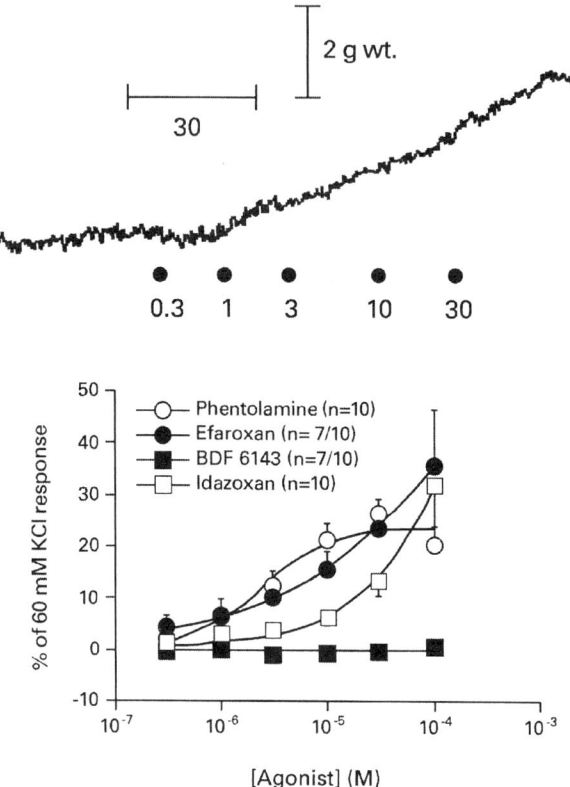

FIGURE 1. (*Upper*) Representative digitized recordings of phentolamine-induced contractions of the porcine isolated rectal artery elicited in the presence of a combination of U46619 and forskolin (following inactivation of α-adrenoceptors by phenoxybenzamine). (*Lower*) The effect of various imidazoline derivatives on the porcine isolated rectal artery (pretreated with phenoxybenzamine) in the presence of forskolin and U46619. Responses have been expressed as percentage of the contraction to 60 mM KCl and are shown as the mean ± SEM of 7 to 10 observations conducted in 10 different preparations. The time base shown represents 30 minutes.

of selective antagonists.[8] Various approaches have been adopted to circumvent these problems, including the use of preparations largely devoid of α_2-adrenoceptors (e.g., bovine chromaffin cells[12]), investigating only derivatives with known antagonist activity at α_2-adrenoceptors[5,13] or by pharmacologically inactivating α_2-adrenoceptors.[14] In the present study we attempted to use all three approaches to examine nonadrenoceptor vasoactive effects of imidazoline derivatives.

It has previously been established that the porcine isolated rectal artery has a low density of α_2-adrenoceptor binding sites, which accounts for the failure of selective α_2-adrenoceptor agonists under standard in vitro conditions.[15] Functional responses through this receptor to various imidazoline derivatives were only revealed by pharmacologic manipulation with a combination of U46619 and forskolin.[15] Following pretreat-

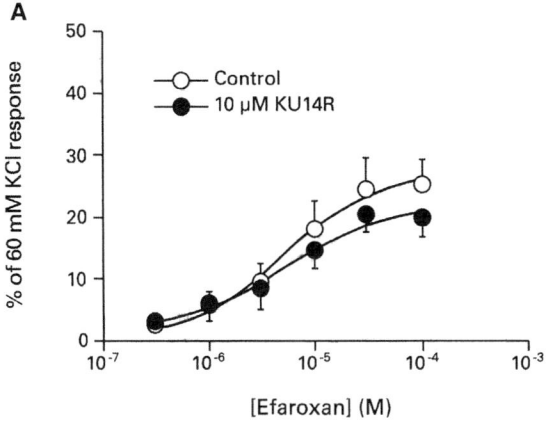

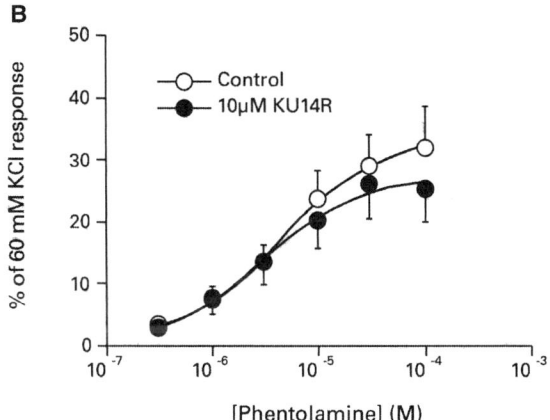

FIGURE 2. The effect of 10 μM KU-14R against (**A**) efaroxan and (**B**) phentolamine-induced contractions of the porcine isolated rectal artery (pretreated with phenoxybenzamine) in the presence of forskolin and U46619. Responses have been expressed as percentage of the contraction to 60 mM KCl and are shown as the mean ± SEM of 8 to 10 observations.

ment with the irreversible α-adrenoceptor antagonist phenoxybenzamine, oxymetazoline was still able to elicit large contractions in the presence of a combination of U46619 and forskolin.[11] This nonadrenoceptor response was sensitive to the putative imidazoline I_3 antagonist KU-14R, suggesting the presence of imidazoline I_3 receptors on vascular smooth muscle.[9] These findings raised the possibility of pharmacologically characterizing the target with different imidazoline derivatives. We have shown that high concentrations of phentolamine, idazoxan, and efaroxan mimicked the action of oxymetazoline in the porcine isolated rectal artery under these conditions. In contrast, UK-14304 did not mimic this response and clonidine, rilmenidine, and BDF-6143 produced weak or inconsistent contractions in only a small proportion of the preparations.

The latter finding with BDF 6143 is particularly important, because it indicates that the pharmacologic characteristics of the nonadrenoceptor response in the rectal artery is different from that reported on peripheral neurons.[14] The effect of phentolamine and efaroxan were examined in greater detail because they produced the most consistent responses. Significantly the contractions to phentolamine and efaroxan were insensitive to KU-14R, indicating that both imidazolines acted through a nonadrenoceptor site different from that previously described for oxymetazoline in this preparation.[11] The small size and inconsistency of the responses to clonidine and rilmenidine precluded us from conducting similar experiments with the antagonist KU14R.

This is the first report of a nonadrenergic response to imidazoline-based α-adrenoceptor antagonists in porcine blood vessels. The contractions were found to be critically dependent on the presence of pre-existing vasoactive tone, produced by the combination of U46619 and forskolin, and in this respect there are parallels with other studies. In the rat isolated portal vein[16] and guinea pig detrusor muscle,[17] high concentrations of phentolamine (>1 µM) have been reported[16,17] to enhance pre-existing spontaneous contractions through a nonadrenoceptor mechanism. In the case of the rat isolated portal vein, the authors proposed that the effect was mediated through ATP-regulated K^+ (K^+_{ATP}) channels.[16] The potential significance of this interaction is underlined by the report of Dunne and colleagues[13] that phentolamine, idazoxan, and efaroxan can also modulate K^+_{ATP} channels in islet cells to increase insulin secretion. These investigators, however, noted greater differences in relative potency between the agents than those reported here.

In conclusion, a series of imidazoline-based derivatives mimicked the nonadrenergic actions of oxymetazoline on the porcine isolated rectal artery. For phentolamine and efaroxan, however, the response does not involve imidazoline I_3R because KU-14R did not inhibit their effect. When taken together, these results fall short of convincing evidence for the presence of functional I_3 imidazoline binding sites in the rectal artery. The potential involvement of K^+_{ATP} channels in the nonadrenoceptor vascular effects of imidazoline derivatives warrants further investigation.

REFERENCES

1. ERNSBERGER, P., M. GRAVES, L. GRAFF, et al. 1995. I_1-imidazoline receptors. Definition, characterization, distribution, and transmembrane signalling. Ann. N. Y. Acad. Sci. **763:** 22–42.
2. MALLARD, N.J., A.L. HUDSON & D.J. NUTT. 1992. Characterization and autoradiographical localization of non-adrenoceptor, idazoxan binding sites in the rat brain. Br. J. Pharmacol. **106:** 1019–1027.
3. MORGAN, N.G., S.L.F. CHAN, C.A. BROWN, et al. 1995. Characterization of the imidazoline binding site involved in regulation of insulin secretion. Ann. N. Y. Acad. Sci. **763:** 361–373.
4. EVANS, R.G. & J. HAYNES. 1995. α_2-adrenoceptor- and imidazoline-preferring binding sites in the dog kidney. Ann. N. Y. Acad. Sci. **763:** 357–360.
5. REGUNATHAN, S., C. YOUNGSON, H. WANG, et al. 1995. Imidazoline receptors in vascular smooth muscle and endothelial cells. Ann. N. Y. Acad. Sci. **763:** 580–590.
6. FELSEN, D., P. ERNSBERGER, P.M. SUTARIA, et al. 1994. Identification, localisation and functional analysis of imidazoline and alpha-adrenergic receptors in canine prostate. J. Pharmacol. Exp. Ther. **268:** 1063–1071.
7. MOLDERINGS, G.J., K. DONECKER & M. GOHERT. 1995. Characterization of non-adrenergic [3H]-clonidine binding sites in rat stomach: high affinity of imidazoline, guanidines and sigma ligands. Naunyn Schmiedeberg's Arch. Pharmacol. **351:** 561–564.

8. EGLEN, R.M., A.L. HUDSON, D.A. KENDALL, *et al.* 1998. "Seeing through a glass darkly": casting light on imidazoline "I" sites. Trends Pharmacol. Sci. **19:** 381–390.
9. CHAN, S.L.F., A.L. PALLETT, J. CLEWS, *et al.* 1998. Characterization of new efaroxan derivatives for use in purification if imidazoline-binding sites. Eur. J. Pharmacol. **355:** 67–76.
10. HIROSE, H., Y. SETO, H. MARUYAMA, *et al.* 1997. Effects of α_2-adrenergic agonism, imidazolines, and G-protein on insulin secretion in β cells. Metabolism **46:** 1146–1149.
11. WANG M., W.R. DUNN, N.A. BLAYLOCK, *et al.* 2001. Evidence for a non-adrenoceptor, imidazoline-mediated contractile response to oxymetazoline in the porcine isolated rectal artery. Br. J. Pharmacol. **132:** 1359–1365.
12. GRENEY, H., P. RONDE, C. MAGNIER, *et al.* 2000. Coupling of I_1 imidazoline receptors to the cAMP pathway: studies with a highly selective ligand, benazoline. Mol. Pharmacol. **57:** 1142–1151.
13. DUNNE, M.J., E.A. HARDING, J.H. JAGGAR, *et al.* 1995. Potassium channels, imidazoline and insulin-secreting cells. Ann. N. Y. Acad. Sci. **763:** 243–261.
14. GÖHERT, M., G.J. MOLDERINGS, K. FINK, *et al.* 1995. α_2-Adrenoceptor-independent inhibition by imidazolines and gaunidines of noradrenaline release from peripheral, but not central noradrenergic neurons. Ann. N. Y. Acad. Sci. **763:** 405–419.
15. BLAYLOCK, N.A., A. SHAH & V.G. WILSON. 2000. Pharmacological evidence for pre- and post-junctional α_2-adrenoceptors in the porcine isolated rectal artery. Br. J. Pharmacol. **131:** 10P.
16. SCHWIETERT, R., D. WILHELM, B. WILLFERT, *et al.* 1992. The effect of some α-adrenoceptor antagonists on spontaneous myogenic activity in the rat portal vein and putative involvement of ATP-sensitive K^+ channels. Eur. J. Pharmacol. **211:** 87–95.
17. SATAKE, N., S. SHIBATA & S. UEDA. 1984. Phentolamine-induced rhythmic contractions in bladder detrusor muscle of guinea-pig. Br. J. Pharmacol. **83:** 965–971.

Cell Signaling by Imidazoline-1 Receptor Candidate, IRAS, and the Nischarin Homologue

J.E. PILETZ,[a,b] G. WANG,[a] AND H. ZHU[a]

[a]*Department of Psychiatry and Human Behavior, University of Mississippi Medical Center, Jackson, Mississippi 39216, USA*

[b]*Department of Biology, Jackson State University, Jackson, Mississippi 39217, USA*

ABSTRACT: IRAS transfection into Chinese hamster ovary (CHO) or pheochromocytoma (PC-12) cell lines leads to the appearance of nonadrenergic binding sites for radiolabeled-clonidine. Nischarin is the mouse homologue of IRAS. IRAS seems to be a cytosolic protein that is anchored to the intracellular side of plasma membranes by a POX domain. Previous studies of IRAS-transfected HEK293 cells, and Nischarin-transfected 3T3 cells have shown this protein can intrinsically mediate cell growth and differentiation independent of imidazoline drugs through binding to insulin receptor substrates (HEK293 cells) and fibronectin receptors (3T3 cells). Herein, a growth-arrested PC-12 cell line stably transfected with IRAS is shown to express lower basal and nerve growth factor-stimulated levels of the activated form of extracellular receptor kinase than found in a vector-only transfected control cell line treated similarly. These findings suggest that IRAS is a membrane-associated mediator of receptor signaling.

KEYWORDS: imidazoline receptors; IRAS; Nischarin; ERK; integrins; PC-12

INTRODUCTION

A few years ago, our laboratory cloned an imidazoline-1 receptor (I_1R) candidate protein named IRAS, the acronym for imidazoline receptor antisera-selected protein.[1] Before our discovery of IRAS, a 70-kD membrane-associated protein had been isolated from bovine adrenal chromaffin (BAC) cell membranes by affinity chromatography with idazoxan-linked and para-aminoclonidine–linked chromatography resins.[2] Reis and colleagues named this protein the imidazoline receptor binding protein (IRBP), because it was selectively eluted from the resins by imidazoline drugs.[2] Using antiserum prepared against BAC IRBP,[3] we were then able to clone a fragment of IRAS cDNA from a human hippocampal lambda phage cDNA expression library.[1] In actuality, four identical copies of this cDNA were isolated out of 500,000 plaques screened with IRBP antiserum, with no false positives. Once our initial cDNA clone had been extended at both ends by amplification methods, its

---

Address for correspondence: He Zhu, M.D., Department of Psychiatry, University of Mississippi Medical Center, 2500 North State Street, Jackson, MS 39216, USA. Voice: 601-984-5798; fax: 601-984-5899.

e-mail: HZhu@psychiatry.umsmed.edu

mRNA was realized to be at least 5,131 base pairs long, not counting the polyA$^+$ tail.[1] Thus, IRAS mRNA was found to encode a 1,504–amino acid protein. Transfection studies further showed that human IRAS-M cDNA (the active splice variant form) yielded a protein size of 167 kD, with apparent fragments of 85 kD and smaller also separated on SDS-polyacrylamide gels (SDS-PAGE).[1] The 167-kD sized protein was bigger than that of the original IRBP, but evidence was found that IRAS is fragmented into peptides in this size range in most native tissues and cell types.[4] The amino acid sequence of IRAS was found to be unique when compared with other protein sequences. In fact, IRAS is structurally unrelated to any known G protein–coupled receptors, including the α_2-adrenoceptors (α_2ARs) which also bind many of the same imidazoline compounds (see the article by Chen *et al.*, in this volume). The amino acid sequence of IRAS is also different from the monoamine and diamine oxidase proteins, which also bind imidazoline compounds.[5] In fact, the amino acid sequence of IRAS is 80% unrelated to any known family of proteins. Nonetheless, IRAS is a highly conserved protein across mammalian species. IRAS is also predicted to possess at least two hydrophobic domains but lacks an expected N-terminal signal sequence for translational insertion through the plasma membrane. At first, the absence of this sequence presented a dilemma. IRAS, however, is probably anchored to the intracellular surface of the plasma membrane by virtue of possessing a phosphoinositide-triphosphate (PI3) binding domain in its N-terminus region, known as a POX domain.[6] This article describes what has been learned in recent years about the imidazoline-binding properties of IRAS and its intracellular signaling functions.

Although IRAS has not yet proven to be a transmembrane protein, much can be said to support IRAS's candidacy as an I_1R. Besides its immunologic connection with the BAC IRBP,[1,3,7] a number of research findings can be mentioned. First, IRAS mRNA was shown by in situ hybridization to be appropriately localized in brain neurons as expected for I_1R binding sites.[7] Second, a positive correlation (r = 0.71) was established between Northern blot estimates of the mRNA for IRAS-M plus IRAS-L (the two main splice variants of the IRAS gene) with radioligand binding density estimates of membranous I_1 sites (B_{max}) over a range of native rat tissues.[4] Further transfection of IRAS cDNA into the Chinese hamster ovary (CHO) cell line resulted in high-affinity I_1-like binding sites without appearance of α_2AR sites or the other major subtype of imidazoline binding sites (I_2).[1] The I_1-like sites encoded by transfected IRAS cDNA were radiolabeled in membrane fractions with [^{125}I]-p-iodoclonidine and were not displaced by adrenergic compounds. In addition, these sites were displaced by two I_1-selective compounds, moxonidine and napthazoline.[1] Thus, the transfection-dependent I_1-like results were consistent with Western blotting data wherein various transfected human IRAS protein forms, the 167-kD band plus breakdown peptides of 85-kD sizes or smaller, were expressed over a background of endogenous IRAS bands in the CHO cells. Concordance was observed between I_1 B_{max} values and IRAS immunoreactivity in the transfected CHO cells, but the overall level of transfection was only twice as high in transfected CHO cells as in nontransfected CHO cells.[1]

More recent evidence in support of IRAS's candidacy as an I_1R is that IRAS cDNA transfection into PC-12 cells results in a rise in I_1 B_{max} in these cells.[8] We found this evidence in three sublines of PC-12 cells overexpressing human IRAS cDNA.[8] An advantage of PC-12 cells is that transfected human IRAS can readily be distinguished on Western blots as a distinctly smaller band than endogenous rat

IRAS (210 kD). As in CHO cells, the level of IRAS transfection by Western blotting corresponded with the level of I_1 sites in the transfected cells (about twofold higher than in controls). A surprise in the transfected PC-12 cell lines was that the rise in human IRAS immunoreactivity as well as I_1 B_{max} values was predominantly localized to cytosol.[8] This finding has led us to hypothesize that the endogenous form of rat IRAS in PC-12 cells might preferentially occupy fully an anchor site in the plasma membrane. In transfected PC-12 cells this preference might leave human IRAS (167-kD form) excluded from the membranes. It is also now realized that IRAS exists in equilibrium between membrane-bound and cytosolic states.[8–10] Finally, when IRAS is overexpressed in PC-12 cells (FIG. 1) or when native PC-12 cells are treated with an I_1 agonist[23], a common effect is attenuation of trophic factor signaling by nerve growth factor (NGF). The details of FIGURE 1 are elaborated later in this article, but the commonality of the effect with that reported[23] for I_1R action reinforces IRAS's candidacy as an I_1R.

Before proceeding to describe the function of IRAS, the I_1-binding site ascribed to IRAS needs mention. A critical examination of the Western blots from IRAS-

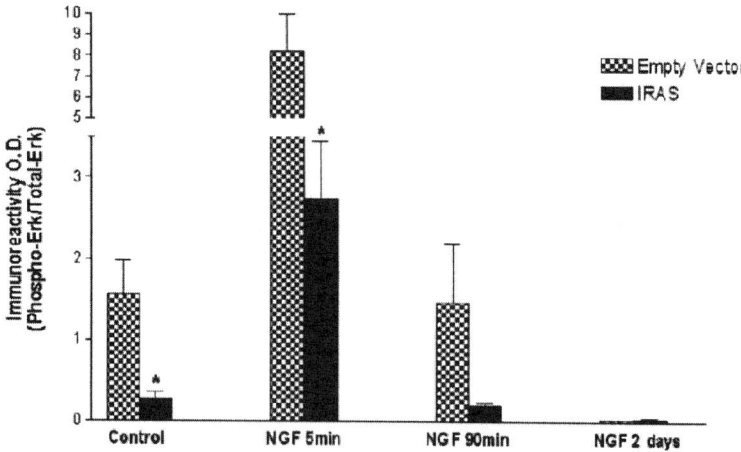

FIGURE 1. Extracellular receptor kinase (ERK) activation by nerve growth factor (NGF) in IRAS-transfected PC-12 cell line. The stable IRAS-transfected PC-12 subline and the vector-only transfected PC-12 subline have been described in reference 8. Equal numbers of cells were plated and grown for 15 hours at 37°C on poly-D-lysine-coated wells in complete medium (standard for PC-12). Both sublines were then exposed to serum reduction (complete DMEM (017)/glutamine/streptomycin/penicillin containing 1% horse serum and no fetal calf serum) for 2 hours. Then, NGF (50 ng/mL) was added along with complete medium (with 10% horse and 5% fetal calf serum) for 5 minutes, 90 minutes, or 2 days. Cells were harvested, lysates were prepared, and denatured supernatants were run onto Western blots by standard procedures. Antiactive ERK and anti-total ERK antiserum (Promega Corp., Madison, WI, USA) were used with enhanced chemiluminescence to detect the bands of interest. Bands were quantified by densitometry with a standard curve of controls on each Western blot. The results are the average ± SE (n = 3 experiments). * $P < 0.05$ versus other cell line.

transfected CHO and PC-12 cells has indicated that the elevation in radioligand binding to I_1 sites is mostly associated with an increase in immunoreactive bands that are only 40 to 70 kD in size.[1,8] In fact, the full-length form of human IRAS (167 kD) seems to be scarce in all native tissues we have examined, a finding which would be consistent with a protein that is normally processed into fragments. This finding raised the intriguing possibility that only certain peptide fragments of IRAS might be causative peptides that behave as I_1 binding sites and could explain why most previous efforts to isolate an I_1 binding protein have resulted in estimates between 40 and 85 kD.[2,11,12] In addition, the possibility of normal processing of IRAS into fragments might explain another paradox, which is the reason for host-cell dependence in transfecting IRAS cDNA to obtain I_1 binding sites.[1] Indeed, transfection of human IRAS cDNA into three cell lines (COS-7, HEK293, and Sf9 cells) has failed to induce I_1 binding sites even though the 167-kD version of the human protein was evidently synthesized in them.[1,10] The evidence remains merely circumstantial, but it is interesting that the same negative host cell lines were distinct in having the transfected form of human IRAS appear mostly in its full-length form. By contrast, IRAS was processed into smaller fragments in CHO and PC-12 cells.[1,8] Thus, one possibility is that fragmentation of full-length IRAS is required to cause a conformational change that leads to high-affinity I_1-binding sites.

The preceding paragraphs have attempted to defend IRAS's candidacy as an I_1R protein. Even though this candidacy still may be debated, a consensus has emerged that IRAS is either the human homologue or closely related to the IRBP originally isolated in BAC cells by Reis and coworkers (see Zhu *et al.*, in this volume). Therefore, IRAS should provide insight into a number of previous studies showing altered levels of IRBP using antiserum made against that BAC protein. Studies with Reis' anti-IRBP antiserum have revealed altered levels of 40- to 45-kD bands in brains of patients with depressive mood disorders.[13,14] Of course, if the connection with IRAS is settled, then another question must arise: how does the function of IRAS relate to changes in the brain as detected with IRBP antiserum? The following section on the function of IRAS addresses this question.

FUNCTIONAL STUDIES OF IRAS

Sano and colleagues were first to report a signaling function for human IRAS.[10] They found that a modest level of overexpression of human IRAS by transfection into the HEK293 kidney cell line led to a twofold rise in the activated (phosphorylated) state of extracellular receptor kinase (ERK). Phosphorylation of ERK is a requirement for cell division. Sano and colleagues[10] found that in HEK293 cells the overexpression of IRAS was specific for phospho-ERK, not enhancing other branches of insulin signaling (e.g., glucose transport). Also, the effect of IRAS transfection was selective to the insulin-ERK pathway because ERK activation by epidermal growth factor was not altered in IRAS-transfected HEK293 cells.[10] Although IRAS was found not to bind to insulin or the insulin receptor, Sano and coworkers[10] demonstrated that IRAS binds to all four isoforms of the insulin receptor substrate proteins (IRSs). Using recombinant DNA methodology these investigators further identified the carboxy-terminal half of IRAS as the domain that binds the IRSs. At first glance, the findings of Sano *et al.*[10] seemed applicable to an I_3R that had been reported to mediate insulinotropic effects,[15] rather than to an I_1R effect. Unpublished results from our laboratory, however, have indicated that tissue culture administration of nanomolar concentrations of the I_1-selective compound, moxonidine, also induces greater ERK activation in PC-12 cells that overexpress human IRAS (permanently transfected PC-12 sublines) than in untransfected controls. Thus, the findings of Sano *et al.*[10] still need to be expanded to include treatments with imidazoline agents.

The discovery[10] of an insulin receptor–signaling pathway for IRAS has led us to speculate that IRAS might function in the absence of an I_1 agonist. To this speculation we now add supportive data (FIG. 1) in the form of ERK activation by NGF, another peptide that activates the tyrosine receptor kinase (*trk*) family of receptors. The effect of NGF treatment to a stable IRAS-transfected PC-12 subline versus to a stable vector-only transfected PC-12 subline is shown. Before NGF addition (50 ng/mL in complete medium), both sublines had been exposed to serum reduction for 2 hours to lower basal phospho-ERK levels and to arrest cell division. NGF administration plus restoration of normal serum levels at time zero was to initiate neurite outgrowth in the absence of ongoing cell division. Controls were treated only with medium or insulin growth factor, because PC-12 cells possess NGF receptors but not IGF receptors. Firstly, basal levels of phospho-ERK were found to be lower before serum reduction in the IRAS-enriched PC-12 subline than in the control PC-12 subline (data not shown). Second, we found that basal levels of phospho-ERK were still lower after 2 hours serum reduction in cells that overexpressed IRAS than in serum reduced control cells (FIG. 1). Third, contrary to expectations arising from insulin's hyperactivation of ERK in IRAS-transfected HEK293 cells,[10] it was found that NGF treatment of IRAS-enriched cells for 5 minutes led to a lower rise in ERK activation than NGF treatment of the control PC-12 subline for 5 minutes (FIG. 1). A similar, although smaller, distinction was also evident after 10 minutes' treatment with NGF (data not shown). Phospho-ERK returned to baseline levels by 90 minutes following NGF treatment and then went to low levels after 2 days of daily NGF treatments (FIG. 1). Neither IGF treatment nor serum repletion alone had any effect on phospho-ERK. Although the finding of lowered phospho-ERK came as a surprise, it was supported by a recent publication on native PC-12 cells.[23] Edwards and Ernsberger[23] reported that stimulation of the I_1R in native PC-12 cells by moxonidine increased ERK activation by more than twofold. Similarly, NGF elicited a fivefold increase in activated ERK in the native PC-12 cells. Similar to the findings shown in FIGURE 1, they reported that moxonidine treatment of NGF-treated PC-12 cells led to a decline in ERK phosphorylation.[23] The moxonidine-induced inhibition of ERK activation in NGF-treated cells was dose-dependent, followed a limited time course, and could be blocked by the I_1R antagonist efaroxan.[23] These authors suggested this inhibition might be result from deactivation of ERK by specific phosphatases induced by moxonidine. Thus, either by overexpressing IRAS or by treating with an I_1-agonist,[23] there seems to be an attenuation of ERK activation by NGF.

Evidence of a second signaling pathway for IRAS comes from studies by Alahari and coworkers[9,16] of IRAS's murine homologue, named Nischarin. Using two-hybrid methodology to identify proteins that bind to the α5 subunit of the fibronectin receptor, Alahari and coworkers[9] identified and cloned Nischarin. When Nischarin cDNA was sequenced, it was found to possess high homology with human IRAS, even though the murine cDNA was truncated at the N-terminal 244 amino acids. The domain of mouse Nischarin that these investigators identified as binding to the α5 subunit protein of the fibronectin receptor was 100% identical to amino acids #684 through 831 in human IRAS.[9] This domain roughly agrees with the "C-terminal domain" as identified in human IRAS by Sano et al.[10] that encodes binding to the insulin receptor substrate protein-4. Like the study of Sano et al.,[10] the investigators of Nischarin have not used imidazoline drugs to explore the function of Nischarin. Instead, with the use of transfected 3T3 fibroblastoid cells grown on extracellular matrix proteins, the overexpression of Nischarin was found to inhibit lamellipodia formation, cell migration, and invasion of epithelial cells.[9,16] Here again, a second messenger signaling role has been revealed for the protein rather than as a classical receptor. Although the specific receptor couplings of the studies are quite different (fibronectin receptor versus insulin receptor mediator), it is intriguing that both signals may converge. In particular, the effects of insulin and fibronectin on neurons are both considered to promote neurite outgrowth.[17] This hypothesis has raised the possibility that IRAS is a protein that binds imidazoline drugs but essentially functions as a neurite outgrowth mediator.

Finally, the most recently discovered system that IRAS mediates is the apoptotic pathway (see Dontenwill et al., in this volume). Dontenwill and coworkers have reported[8] that IRAS-transfected COS and PC-12 cells display prolonged survival against known apoptotic stimuli such as serum starvation, thapsigargin, or staurosporine treatments. The attenuation of apoptosis by IRAS was correlated with a decrease in caspase-3 activity, phosphatidylcholine translocation, and nuclear fragmentation.[8] Conceivably, this promotion of cell survival could also be related to IRAS-mediated ERK activation or to IRAS's action on the fibronectin receptor.[18]

HOW MIGHT THE FUNCTION OF IRAS RELATE TO NEURONAL ACTIVITY?

On one hand, the aforementioned studies have revealed IRAS's intrinsic activity to promote cell growth[10] and survival.[8] On the other hand, in nondividing PC-12 cells treated with NGF, we observed that IRAS transfection caused a reduction in phospho-ERK compared with vector-only transfected controls (FIG. 1). Furthermore, transfection studies with the murine homologue, Nischarin, have reported[9,16] that IRAS overexpression leads to an inhibition of lamellipodia formation in 3T3 cells. Another way of summarizing this information is that IRAS transfections have revealed the intrinsic activity of IRAS on *trk* receptor signaling (although the insulin and NGF receptors responded oppositely with IRAS) and on integrin signaling (the fibronectin receptor). Although these effects of IRAS are diverse, this combination of signals is intriguing because the manner by which signals from *trk*s and integrins integrate is an area of intense research in cell biology.[19] Specifically, there is evidence that the insulin receptor and the α5 subunit of the fibonectin receptor act synergistically to enhance cell adhesion.[20] Furthermore, in model systems of neuronal differentiation, the integration of these two second-messenger signaling pathways is a requirement for neurite outgrowth.[17,21] ERK activation through various *trk*s determines the level and type of gene transcripts produced that commit the neuron either to cell division or to establishment of axonal growth cones.[19] If a neuron is committed to cell division (e.g., by insulin-mediated ERK activation), the fibronectin receptor then should become inhibited, as should its signaling through a pathway known by the acronyms JNK and c-Jun, which would in turn lead to retraction of the cytoskeleton and allowance for cell proliferation. On the other hand, if a neuron is committed to axonal differentiation, as in the case of NGF stimulation (FIG. 1), the opposite should occur. In other words, neurite extension should only appear under a combination of appropriate *trk* inhibition and integrin activation. This requirement is essentially consistent with the IRAS transfection studies of PC-12 cells (FIG. 1). Furthermore, because IRAS overexpression in transfected cell lines modifies the activities of both *trks* and the α5 integrin, IRAS could be pivotal in regulating processes such as neuronal cell division, axonal sprouting, and neuroplasticity. These versatile properties of IRAS provide the basis for much future research.

Finally, it is realized that after neuronal development integrin signaling in the nervous system has commonly been misconstrued as a static system of little importance to neuronal firing and function. It has recently been demonstrated, however, that integrins and their ligands are capable of rapid neuromodulatory actions in mature neurons.[22] Wildering and coworkers[22] showed that ligand for fibronectin can alter neuronal pacemaker properties, intracellular free Ca^{2+} levels, and voltage-gated Ca^{2+} currents in a matter of minutes. Thus, the discovery that the murine form of IRAS, named Nischarin, interacts with the integrin α5 protein[9,16] might be viewed as meditative of rapid neuronal firing. This property of integrins should not be forgotten when trying to determine if the rapid actions of imidazoline compounds on neuronal firing could be mediated by IRAS. If the imidazoline compounds that bind to IRAS also interfere or enhance this presumed activity of IRAS, then this action may explain some of their properties.

ACKNOWLEDGMENTS

We are extremely grateful to Dr. John Naftel (University of Mississippi Medical Center) for freely supplying nerve growth factor. This research was supported by a grant from the National Institute of Mental Health (R01 MH49248).

REFERENCES

1. PILETZ, J.E., T.R. IVANOV, J.D. SHARP, *et al.* 2000. Imidazoline receptor antisera-selected (IRAS) cDNA: cloning and characterization. DNA Cell Biol. **19:** 319–329.
2. WANG, H., S. REGUNATHAN, M.P. MEELEY, *et al.* 1992. Isolation and characterization of imidazoline receptor protein from bovine adrenal chromaffin cells. Mol. Pharmacol. **42:** 792–801.
3. WANG, H., S. REGUNATHAN, D.A. RUGGIERO, *et al.* 1993. Production and characterization of antibodies specific for the imidazoline receptor protein. Mol. Pharmacol. **43:** 509–515.
4. PILETZ, J.E., J.C. JONES, H. ZHU, *et al.* 1999. Imidazoline receptor antisera-selected cDNA clone and mRNA distribution. Ann. N. Y. Acad. Sci. **881:** 1–7.
5. RADDATZ, R., A. PARINI & S.M. LANIER. 1997. Localization of the imidazoline binding domain on monoamine oxidase B. Mol. Pharmacol. **52:** 549–553.
6. WISHART, M.J., G.S. TAYLOR & J.E. DIXON. 2001. Phoxy lipids: revealing PX domains as phosphoinositide binding modules. Cell **105:** 817–820.
7. IVANOV, T.R., J.C. JONES, M. DONTENWILL, *et al.* 1998. Characterization of a partial cDNA clone detected by imidazoline receptor-selective antisera. J. Auton. Nerv. Syst. **72:** 98–110.

8. DONTENWILL M., G. PASCAL, J. PILETZ, et al. 2003. IRAS, the human homologue of Nischarin, prolongs survival of transfected PC12 cells. Cell Death Differ. **10**: 933–935.
9. ALAHARI, S.K., J.W. LEE & R.L. JULIANO. 2000. Nischarin, a novel protein that interacts with the integrin alpha5 subunit and inhibits cell migration. J. Cell. Biol. **151**: 1141–1154.
10. SANO, H., S.C. LIU, W.S. LANE, et al. 2002. Insulin receptor substrate 4 associates with the protein IRAS. J. Biol. Chem. **277**: 19439–19447.
11. VONTHRON, C., F. HEEMSKERK, H. GRENEY, et al. 1998. Molecular characterization of human cerebral I_1 imdazoline receptor. Naunyn Schmiedeberg's Arch. Pharmacol. **358**: R69.
12. IVANOV, T.R., H. ZHU, S. REGUNATHAN, et al. 1998. Co-detection by two imidazoline receptor protein antisera of a novel 85 kilodalton protein. Biochem. Pharmacol. **55**: 649–655.
13. GARCIA-SEVILLA, J.A., P.V. ESCRIBA, M. SASTRE, et al. 1996. Immunodetection and quantitation of imidazoline receptor proteins in platelets of patients with major depression and in brains of suicide victims. Arch. Gen. Psychiatry **53**: 803–810.
14. PILETZ, J.E., H. ZHU, G. ORDWAY, et al. 2000. Imidazoline receptor proteins are decreased in the hippocampus of individuals with major depression. Biol. Psychiatry **48**: 910–919.
15. GAO, H., M. MOURTADA & N. MORGAN. 2003. Effects of the imidazoline binding site ligands, idazoxan and efaroxan, on the viability of insulin-secreting BRIN-BD11 cells. JOP **4**: 117–124.
16. ALAHARI, S. 2003. Nischarin inhibits Rac induced migration and invasion of epithelial cells by affecting signaling cascades involving PAK. Exp. Cell Res. **288**: 415–424.
17. HYNDS, D.L & D.M. SNOW. 2001. Fibronectin and laminin elicit differential behaviors from SH-SY5Y growth cones contacting inhibitory chondroitin sulfate proteoglycans. J. Neurosci. Res. **66**: 630–642.
18. ZHANG, Z., K. VUORI, J.C. REED, et al. 1995. The alpha5 beta1 integrin supports survival of cells on fibronectin and up-regulates Bcl-2 expression. Proc. Natl. Acad. Sci. U. S. A. **92**: 6161–6165.
19. VAUDRY, D., P.J. STORK, P. LAZAROVICI, et al. 2002. Signaling pathways for PC12 cell differentiation: making the right connections. Science **296**: 1648–1649.
20. GUILHERME, A., K. TORRES & M.P. CZECH. 1998. Cross-talk between insulin receptor and integrin alpha5 beta1 signaling pathways. J. Biol. Chem. **273**: 22899–22903.
21. IVANKOVIC-DIKIC, I., E. GRONROOS, A. BLAUKAT, et al. 2000. Pyk2 and FAK regulate neurite outgrowth induced by growth factors and integrins. Nat. Cell Biol. **2**: 574–581.
22. WILDERING, W.C., P.M. HERMANN & A.G. BULLOCH. 2002. Rapid neuromodulatory actions of integrin ligands. J. Neurosci. **22**: 2419–2426.
23. EDWARDS, L. & P. ERNSBERGER. 2003. The I(1)-imidazoline receptor in PC-12 pheochromocytoma cells reverses NGF-induced ERK activation and induces MKP-2 phosphatase. Brain Res. **980**: 71–79.

IRAS Is an Anti-Apoptotic Protein

MONIQUE DONTENWILL,[a] JOHN E. PILETZ,[b,c] MICHAEL CHEN,[c]
JAMES BALDWIN,[c] GÉRALDINE PASCAL,[d] PHILIPPE RONDÉ,[a]
LAURENCE DUPUY,[d] HUGUES GRENEY,[d] KEN TAKEDA,[a]
AND PASCAL BOUSQUET[d]

[a]*Pharmacologie et Physicochimie des Interactions Cellulaires et Moléculaires, UMR CNRS 7034, Faculté de Pharmacie, Université Louis Pasteur de Strasbourg, Illkirch, France*

[b]*Department of Biology, Jackson State University, Jackson, Mississippi 39217, USA*

[c]*Department of Psychiatry, University of Mississippi Medical Center, Jackson, Mississippi 39216, USA*

[d]*Laboratoire de Neurobiologie et Pharmacologie Cardiovasculaire, Faculté de Medecine, 11 rue Humann, 67000 Strasbourg, France*

ABSTRACT: Active cell death, also known as apoptosis, has been implicated in the pathophysiology of diseases such as cancer, heart failure and neurodegenerative disorders. We report the anti-apoptotic function of IRAS, which was previously shown to bind imidazoline ligands. The amino acid sequence of human IRAS (hIRAS) is unrelated to known proteins, except for rat IRAS and a mouse homologue named nischarin, which binds the alpha5 integrin subunit of the fibronectin receptor. When stably transfected into PC12 cells, hIRAS localizes to the cytosol as a 167 kDa immunoreactive protein. Clonal PC12 cell lines expressing hIRAS displayed normal serum growth responses. However, hIRAS expression led to prolonged cell survival against known apoptotic stimuli: serum starvation or thapsigargin or staurosporine treatments. The apoptotic population of hIRAS-expressing cells was significantly reduced, and this protection was achieved by a decrease in caspase-3 activity, phosphatidylserine translocation, and nuclear fragmentation. Similar protective effect was obtained in COS7 cells transiently transfected with hIRAS. A partial activation of the PI3 kinase pathway is possibly implicated in the anti-apoptotic effect of IRAS. Thus, IRAS appears to represent a previously unknown anti-apoptotic protein involved in the regulation of cell survival.

KEYWORDS: IRAS; nischarin; apoptosis; PC12 cells

INTRODUCTION

Our line of research originated in studies on imidazoline receptors (IRs).[1] Endogenous IRs in PC12 cells have been shown to mediate the effects of imidazolines to dose-dependently decrease cellular cAMP content[2] and activate a phosphatidylcholine-specific phospholipase C.[3] Recently, imidazolines were also shown to activate MAP kinases,[4] leading to the hypothesis that IRs may be implicated in the control

Address for correspondence: Monique Dontenwill, Pharmacologie et Physicochimie des Interactions Cellulaires et Moléculaires, UMR CNRS 7034, Faculté de Pharmacie, Université Louis Pasteur de Strasbourg, Illkirch, France. Voice: (+33) 3 90244267; fax: (+33) 3 90244313.
e-mail: mdontenwill@aspirine.u-strasbg.fr

of cell proliferation. To clarify the signaling pathways of IRs, an imidazoline binding protein was cloned from human hippocampus.[5] This protein, named IRAS (imidazoline receptor antisera selected), was selected with two specific anti-imidazoline receptor antisera[6] obtained either against a purified imidazoline binding protein[7] or by the anti-idiotypic route.[8] The two antibodies were shown to inhibit the binding of imidazoline ligands to imidazoline receptors.[7,8]

The distribution of IRAS mRNA was shown to correlate with saturation (B_{max}) values for radioligand binding to the I_1 subtype of imidazoline receptors in the rat brain.[9] Transfection of IRAS leads to the appearance of plasma membrane high-affinity imidazoline binding sites in CHO cells, although in a host-cell specific manner.[5] Transfected IRAS was localized mainly in the cytosol of CHO cells as a 167 kDa immunoreactive protein. The suggested relationship between the 167 kDa IRAS protein and imidazoline receptors prompted us to investigate the impact of transfection of IRAS into PC12 cells, which endogenously express an imidazoline receptor.[2,3]

Herein, we have studied whether human IRAS (hIRAS) expression in PC12 cells has any effect on cell proliferation and/or apoptosis. Our results indicate that expression of hIRAS has no effect on cell proliferation under standard conditions, but leads to a protective anti-apoptotic effect in PC12 cells submitted to different pro-apoptotic triggers.

TRANSFECTION AND EXPRESSION OF hIRAS IN CELLS

Three clonal cell lines (IE10, 6E7, and 7D5) were selected by transfecting hIRAS cDNA into PC12 cells, isolating single cells, and propagating under geneticin selection. In addition, two empty-vector clonal cell lines (pcDNA3.1 and 7D5a) were isolated in parallel by the same procedure. Cytologically, the cell lines were indistinguishable. The IE10, 6E7, and 7D5 sublines expressed hIRAS protein as a band of ~167 kD on western blots probed with anti-IRAS antiserum mainly in the cytoplasmic fraction (FIG. 1A). In PC12 cells, a protein of 210 kDa is also recognized by anti-IRAS antibody, which may correspond to the rat IRAS homologue (rIRAS), the partial cDNA sequence of which has been published (EST106159) and which is 75% identical to the sequence of hIRAS. The cDNA for hIRAS also was confirmed to be present in IE10, 6E7, and 7D5 cell lines as a 1.5 kb PCR band (data not shown) by the use of specific human IRAS primers. By comparison, the hIRAS immunoreactive ~167 kD band was not present in wild-type (un-transfected) PC12 cells or in either empty-vector control cell line.[10] Likewise, no 1.5 kb PCR products were observed in the pcDNA3.1 or 7D5a cell lines (data not shown). If we assume that hIRAS and rIRAS play the same role in the cells, thus transfected PC12 cells look like an overexpression system of IRAS.

EFFECT OF IRAS ON CELL GROWTH CHARACTERISTICS

First, numbers of viable cells were assessed by counting trypan blue–excluding cells with an hemocytometer after different periods of time. The growth curves confirmed that hIRAS-expressing cells (IE10 clone) behaved similarly to control cells

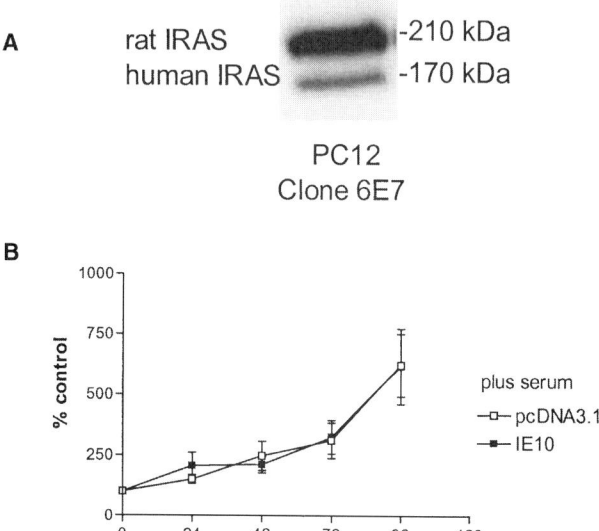

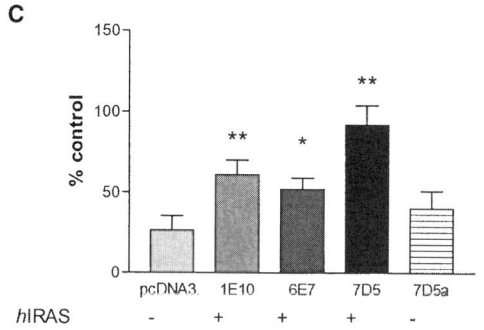

FIGURE 1. Effect of the expression of hIRAS in PC 12 cells on proliferation and survival. (**A**) Western blotting of one of the sublines (6E7) of hIRAS-transfected PC12 cells in the cytosolic fraction. Clonal subline 6E7 was grown to confluency in 12×75 mm^2 flasks, harvested, and the cytosolic fraction prepared. Ten µg of total protein were applied to an 8% SDS polyacrylamide gel. Following SDS-PAGE, proteins were electrotransferred to nitrocellulose blots, and standard Western blotting procedures used 1201 antiserum specific for human IRAS with enhanced chemiluminescence.[5] The full-length form of hIRAS is designated as human IRAS at ≈167 kD. (**B**) PC12 cells stably transfected with empty vector (pcDNA3.1 subclone) or hIRAS (IE10 subclone) were plated in suspension in 6-well plates (5×10^5 cells/well) in serum-containing medium. Cells were recovered after 24, 48, 72, and 96 hours and viable cells excluding trypan blue were counted. (**C**) The same experiment as in **B**, except that viable cells for each subclone were counted after 72 hours in serum-free medium.

(pcDNA3.1 clone) in serum-containing medium (FIG. 1B). However, serum deprivation resulted in a rapid death of control cells and after 72 hours of deprivation only 25% (pcDNA3.1 clone) to 40% (7D5a clone) of cells remained able to exclude trypan blue although hIRAS-expressing PC12 cells were more resistant to death (61, 52 and 92% of viable cells for IE10, 6E7 and 7D5 clones, respectively; FIG. 1C). Thus a main difference between control cells and hIRAS-expressing cells is the ability of the latter to survive longer in serum-free conditions.

IRAS AND APOPTOSIS

It is well known that serum deprivation of PC12 cells triggers cell death through programmed cell death or apoptosis.[11,12] This apoptotic stimulus activates a series of tightly regulated intracellular signaling events that in many cell lines induces the activation of cysteine proteases known as caspases. Caspases are classified into two main classes—the initiator (caspases 8 and 9) and the effector enzymes (in particular, caspase 3). This latter one is implicated in many different apoptotic paradigms and in many cell types. Therefore, we sought to determine whether overexpression of IRAS could be able to inhibit or delay cell apoptosis by inhibiting caspase-3 activity.

As we have shown elsewhere,[10] the hIRAS-expressing PC12 clones exhibited less caspase-3 activity after 6- or 24-h serum deprivation compared to control cells. In order to extend this result, we transiently expressed hIRAS in COS7 cells, which do not endogenously express IRAS (FIG. 2A). As can be seen in FIGURE 2B, 6-h serum deprivation of COS7 cells led to an increase in caspase-3 activity in non-transfected cells although this increase was significantly less evident in hIRAS-transfected cells. Thus, the inhibitory effect of IRAS on caspase-3 activation appears to not be restricted to the PC12 cell line.

A number of apoptotic stimuli proved able to increase caspase-3 activity in PC12 cells. In particular, we have confirmed that staurosporine, a protein kinase C inhibitor, triggers caspase-3 activity in the control cells (pcDNA3.1 and 7D5a clones), although markedly less activation of this enzyme could be recorded in hIRAS-transfected cells.[10] In addition, thapsigargin, another known pro-apoptotic stimulus, time-dependently increased caspase-3 activity in the control PC12 cells although hIRAS-transfected cells showed almost no increase in this enzyme activity at least until 24-h treatment (FIG. 2C). It is important to note that in this set of experiments, thapsigargin was added to 5% serum-containing medium (in place of 15% serum-containing growing medium) and that control cells do increase their caspase-3 activity even without addition of thapsigargin (FIG. 2C, open bars), in contrast to the hIRAS- expressing cells which do not (FIG. 2C, grey-filled bars). Thus, as far as caspase-3 activity is concerned, the overexpression of IRAS led to a decreased sensitivity of the cells to the impoverishment of the culture medium.

In the apoptotic process, cleavage of translocase by initiator caspases and /or activation of scramblase leads to a subsequent flip of phosphatidylserine from the inner to the outer leaflet of the plasma membrane. Surface-exposed phosphatidylserine can be detected by its affinity for annexin V, a phospholipid binding protein.[13] In order to confirm the anti-apoptotic effect of IRAS, we next used an annexin V-FITC flow cytometric sorting assay to determine the percent of the apoptotic cell population after 48-h serum-deprivation. As shown in FIGURE 3, all hIRAS-expressing PC12

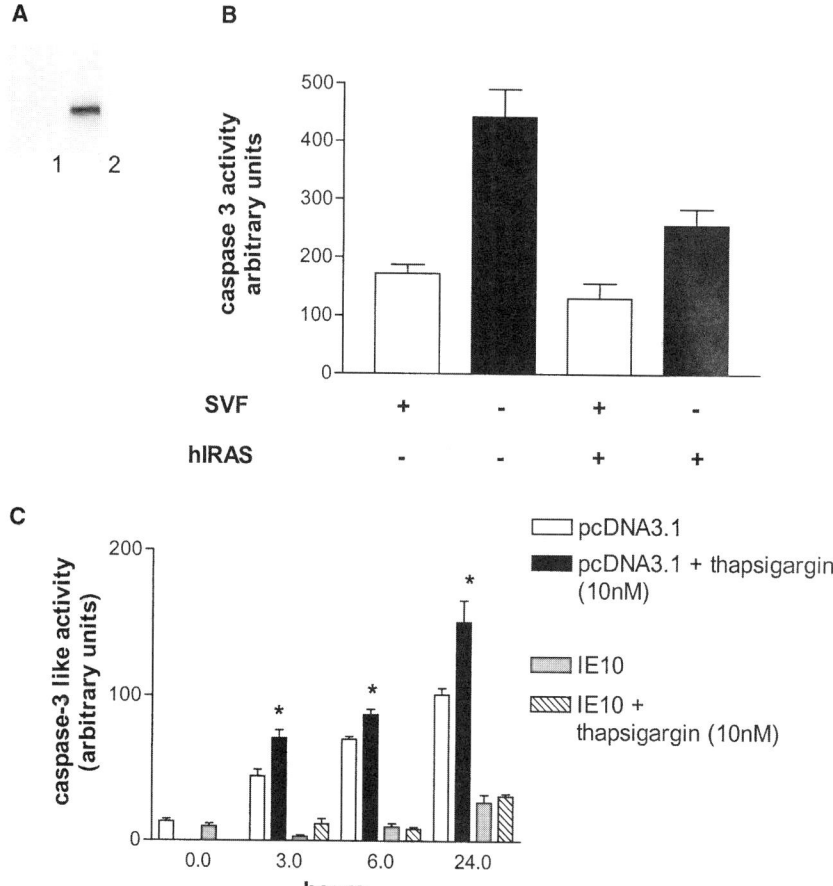

FIGURE 2. Effect of hIRAS expression on caspase-3 activity. (**A**) Western blotting of hIRAS in COS7 cells after transient transfection. Cytosolic fractions of either empty-vector (*lane* 1) or hIRAS-transfected cells (*lane* 2) were immunorevealed with antiserum 1201 three days after transfection. (**B**) COS7 cells transfected with empty vector or hIRAS-transfected cells were grown for 6 hours in 24-well plates (10^5 cells/well) in complete (*open bars*) or serum-free (*closed bars*) medium. Cell lysates were prepared and used to determine caspase enzymatic activities by measuring the release of the *para*-nitroaniline chromophore from peptide substrate (DEVD) selective for caspase-3-like protease. Background levels were determined by parallel incubations of samples in the presence of caspase-3-like inhibitor, Ac-DEVD-CHO (10 μM) and subtracted for each individual value. Enzymatic activity is expressed in arbitrary units as O.D. / μg protein for each sample. Data are the mean ± SEM of triplicate determinations from 7 experiments. (**C**) Caspase-3 activity determination after thapsigargin treatment in PC12 cells. PC12 cells transfected with empty vector (pcDNA3.1 subline) and IRAS-transfected cells (IE10 subline) were grown in suspension on 6-well plates (10^6 cells/well) in 5% serum-containing medium without or with thapsigargin (10 nM) for the indicated lengths of time. Caspase-3 activities were measured as described in **B**. Results are expressed as the mean ± SEM of two independent experiments each performed in sextuplicate. * $P < 0.01$ as compared to the cells grown for the same time without thapsigargin.

with serum

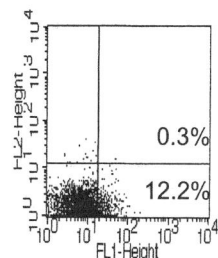

Control cells in serum-free medium

hIRAS expressing cells in serum-free medium

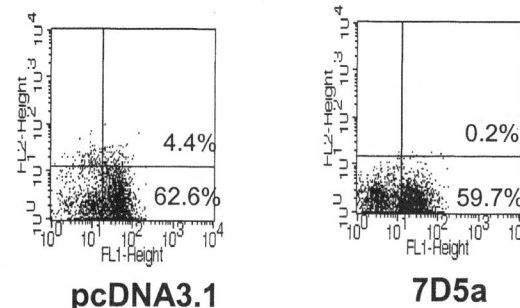
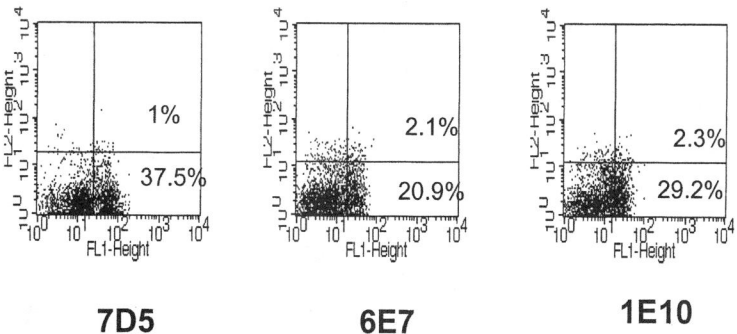

FIGURE 3. hIRAS-mediated protection of apoptosis measured by annexin V staining and flow cytometry. PC12 cells either expressing hIRAS (IE10, 7D5 and 6E7 sublines) or not-expressing hIRAS (pcDNA3.1 and 7D5a sublines) were grown for 48 hours before harvesting and analysis by annexin V-FITC staining. The upper panel show results with the pcDNA3.1 subline grown in serum. For simplicity, only results in the absence of serum are shown for the other sublines. Percentage values represent late apoptosis (*upper right quadrant*) and early apoptosis (*lower right quadrant*) populations of cells. In each case a representative experiment out of three is shown.

clones exhibited markedly less annexin V-FITC–positive cells as compared to control cell lines in serum-free medium. The activation of caspase-3 enzyme led also to nuclear condensation and fragmentation. Hoechst 33342 DNA binding dye was used to visualize the nuclear morphology. As shown in FIGURE 4, hIRAS-expressing PC12 cells also exhibited less apoptotic nuclei as compared to control cells after 6-h treat-

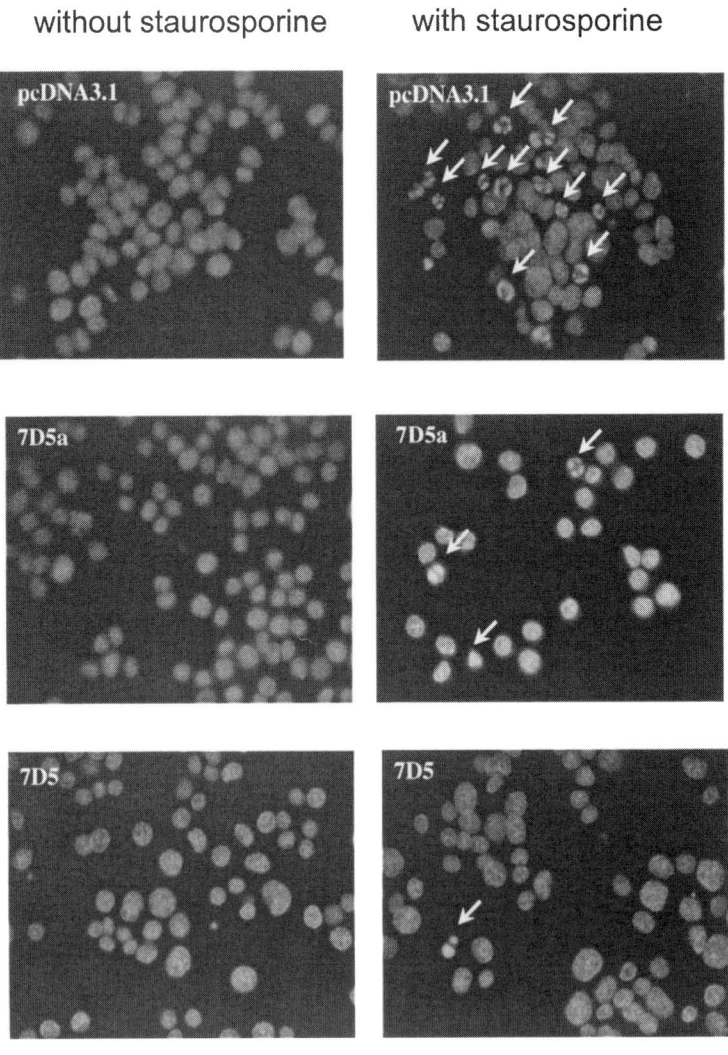

FIGURE 4. Nuclear fragmentation in hIRAS-transfected sublines in the absence or presence of staurosporine. Photomicrographs of nuclear fragmentation: Cells were incubated with staurosporine (1 μM) in 15% serum-containing medium. After 6 hours, the cells were processed for staining with Hoechst dye 33342 and microscopic observations made (×40 objective).

ment with 1 μM staurosporine, which may be related to the decrease in caspase-3 activity in these cells.

Mitochondria also play a crucial role in initiating the cascade of activation in response to different apoptotic stimuli. To measure mitochondrial activity in transfected and non-transfected cells, we used an assay based on the reduction of the tetrazolium salt 3,[4,5-dimethylthiazol-2-yl]-2,5-diphenyltetrazolium bromide (MTT). Transformation of MTT into an insoluble formazan by mitochondrial deshydrogenases may be used as an index of viable cells and is linearly related to the number of cells in culture. Numbers of viable hIRAS-transfected PC12 cells and control cells were found to correlate differentially with formazan production when MTT transformation was measured directly after seeding the cells in the wells (Fig. 5A). IRAS-transfected cells were better able to metabolize MTT than control cells in complete medium in a cell concentration-dependent manner. Thus IRAS over-expression led to higher MTT-reducing activity, suggesting an enhanced mitochondrial function in hIRAS-expressing PC12 cells. In addition, the metabolic activity of IRAS-transfected cells (5×10^5 cell/well) was compared after 24 and 48 hours in culture with or without serum-containing medium. In Figure 5B and C, IRAS-transfected cells (clone 1E10) are shown to have higher metabolic activity compared to empty-vector control cells after 24 h in complete as well as in serum-free medium and after 48 h only in serum-free medium. Similar results were obtained for the three hIRAS-expressing clones when tested after 24 h in serum-free medium (Figure 5D). Thus IRAS appears to enhance cellular mitochondrial activity, which may be correlated with its anti-apoptotic effect.

In summary, these results suggest that IRAS is able to protect PC12 cells against apoptosis. The overexpression of IRAS decreases many parameters involved in the programmed cell death: caspase activity, phosphatidylserine translocation, nuclear fragmentation, and inhibition of mitochondrial activity.

SIGNALING PATHWAYS OF IRAS

PI3-kinase activation is often involved in anti-apoptotic effects.[15] Therefore, the effects of two specific PI3 kinase inhibitors, LY294002 and wortmannin, were tested on serum deprivation-induced caspase-3 activities in control and hIRAS-transfected cells. As shown in Figure 6A, although no significant effect of LY294002 on caspase-3-like activity was recorded in empty-vector control PC12 cells after 24-h serum withdrawal (273 ± 34 units versus 266 ± 29 units with and without LY294002 respectively, $P = 0.79$, $n = 8$), this inhibitor was able to increase partly but significantly (162 ± 28 units versus 129 ± 9 units with and without LY294002 respectively; 125% increase, $P = 0.014$; $n = 7$) the caspase-3 activity in serum-deprived hIRAS transfected cells. This partial reversal of hIRAS's anti-apoptotic effect was also seen with wortmannin (500 nM), another PI3-kinase inhibitor (data not shown). For comparative purposes, we also treated cells with insulin (500 ng/mL), which is known to protect against serum withdrawal–induced cell death through a PI3 kinase–dependent pathway.[16] When added at the start of serum deprivation, insulin decreased dose-dependently caspase-3 activity in control cells as well as the residual caspase-3 activity in hIRAS-transfected cells (Fig. 6B). Insulin inhibited caspase-3 activity to $52 \pm 5\%$ ($n = 13$) in pcDNA3.1 control cells and to $59 \pm 7\%$ ($n = 12$) in hIRAS-transfected

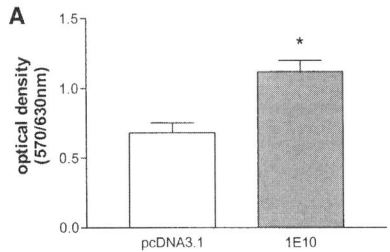
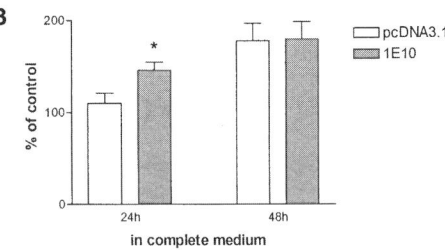
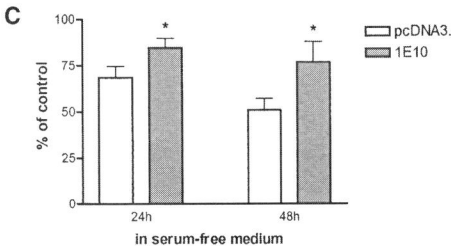
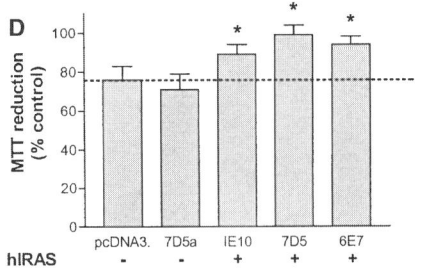

FIGURE 5. Metabolic activity of hIRAS transfectants. (**A**) PC12 cells stably transfected with empty vector (pcDNA3.1 subclone) or hIRAS (IE10 subclone) were plated in complete medium on 24-well plates at 5×10^5 cell/well. MTT was immediately added to the wells (300 μl, 5 mg/ml solution) and blue formazan product optical density recorded after 3 hours at 37°C. (**B**) Cells (5×10^5/well) were plated on 24-well plates in complete medium, and MTT was added at 0, 24, and 48 hours of culture for 3 hours at 37°C, and blue formazan product density recorded. Results are expressed as percent optical density obtained at 0 hour. (**C**) Same experiment as in **B** except that cells were grown in serum-free medium. Data are expressed as mean ± SEM of 8 experiments, each performed in triplicate. (**D**) Same experiment as in C for each PC12 subline grown 24 hours in serum-free medium.

cells compared to activities obtained with serum-free/insulin-free growing conditions (FIG. 6B). As expected, the effect of insulin on caspase-3 activity was also partially reversed by LY294002 (20 μM) in pcDNA3.1 control cells (165% reversal; FIG. 6B). This was also true in hIRAS-transfected (IE10) cells with insulin and LY294002 (216% reversal; FIG. 6B). These findings showed that the PI3-kinase pathway is functional in control cells as well as in hIRAS-transfected cells. These

FIGURE 6. Effect of PI3-kinase inhibitor LY294002 on caspase-3-like activity in control and IRAS-transfected IE10 cell lines. (**A**) PC12 cells stably transfected with empty vector (pcDNA3.1 subline) and IRAS-transfected cells (IE10 subline) were plated on 6-well plates (10^6 cells/well) in serum-free DMEM for 16–18 hours after two cycles of centrifugation in serum-free medium. LY294002 (20 μM) was included in the culture medium at the time of plating. Mean ± SEM of 7–8 independent experiments each performed in sextuplicate. * $P < 0.05$ as compared to control values (cells grown in the serum-free medium). (**B**) PC12 cells stably transfected with empty vector (pcDNA3.1 subline) and IRAS transfected cells (IE10 subline) were plated on 6-well plates (10^6 cells/well) in serum-free DMEM for 16–18 hours after two cycles of centrifugation in serum-free medium. Insulin (500 ng/mL) and LY294002 (20 μM) were added at the plating time and caspase-3-like activity recorded as described. Results are expressed as the mean ± SEM of 2–4 experiments each performed in sextuplicate. * $P < 0.05$ compared to control values (pcDNA3.1 or IE10 cells grown in the absence of drugs in serum-free medium). #$P < 0.05$ compared to values obtained in the presence of 500 ng/mL insulin. (**C**) Percent of apoptotic cell population after 24 h in serum-free medium detected with the annexinV-FITC assay in the absence or presence of wortmannin (1 μM) or PD98059 (30 μM). The hIRAS-expressing clones were 7D5 and 6E7.

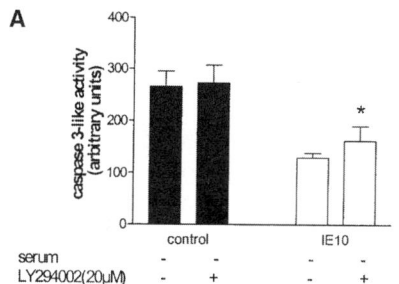
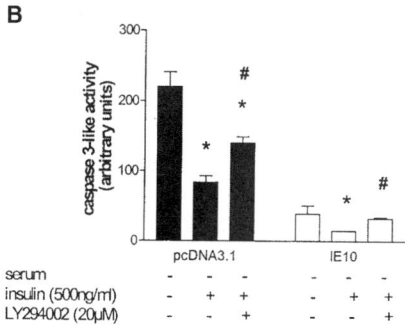
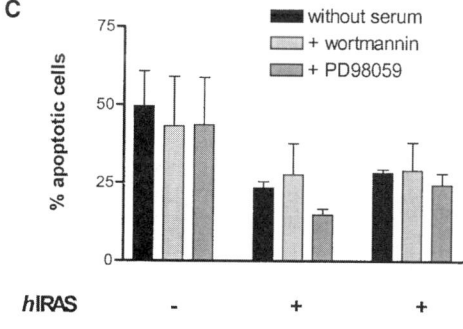

results suggest a role for PI3-kinase activation in the anti-apoptotic effects of hIRAS and confirm this role for insulin anti-apoptotic effect in PC12 cells.

We also tested the effect of LY294002 inhibitor on the apoptotic population as determined by the annexinV-FITC binding assay followed by flow cytometry. As shown in FIGURE 6C, no increase in the apoptotic population was obtained with this inhibitor neither in hIRAS-expressing cells nor in control cells. Similar results were obtained with PD98059, a MEK inhibitor (FIG. 6C). These results do not support a major role of these pathways in the anti-apoptotic effect of IRAS, at least in PC12 cells.

IRAS INTERACTS WITH OTHER PROTEINS

The mechanism by which IRAS exerts its anti-apoptotic effect is not clear, but our preliminary studies point to a new mechanism. Until recently, IRAS was not thought to belong to any known family of proteins implicated in cell growth or survival pathways. However, Juliano and colleagues[17] described a mouse homologue of IRAS, which they named nischarin. Nischarin was reported[17] to interact specifically with the cytoplasmic tail of the integrin α5 subunit of the fibronectin receptor, and to inhibit cell migration and lamellipodia formation in transfected NIH3T3 cells. The amino acid sequence of nischarin is about 80% homologous with IRAS except that nischarin lacks the N-terminal 244 amino acids of IRAS.[5,17] Amazingly, the α5 binding domain of nischarin (amino acids #435–581) is 100% identical with IRAS (amino acids #679–826). Furthermore, the integrin α5β1 dimer, which forms the fibronectin receptor, is known to protect HT29 cells and intestinal epithelial cells (RIE1 cells) from apoptosis through a PI3-kinase and PKB-dependent pathway.[18,19] Overexpression of integrin α5 subunits in RIE1 cells does not influence growth curves in the presence of serum, but enhances cell survival time when apoptosis is triggered by serum deprivation.[19] This, of course, is very similar to our results with IRAS in PC12 cells. Moreover, the cytoplasmic tail of the α5 subunit protein has been suggested to play a key role in elevating the expression of bcl-2, a well known anti-apoptotic protein.[20,21] It is therefore tempting to hypothesize that an interaction between integrins and IRAS may be involved in promoting cell survival in transfected cells. On the other hand, insulin has been reported to decrease caspase-3 activity in PC12 cells, which was partly reversed by a PI3 kinase inhibitor, LY294002.[22] In line with this, the human protein IRAS was also recently shown to interact with

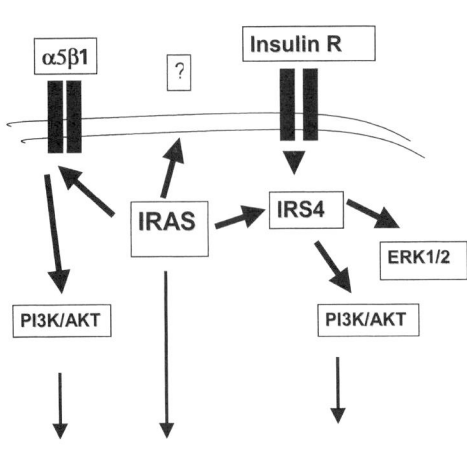

FIGURE 7. Hypothetical model of IRAS-mediated crosstalk between integrin α5β1 and insulin receptor.

insulin receptor substrates (IRS), particularly with IRS4 in HEK293 cells.[23] In transfected HEK293 cells, overexpression of hIRAS enhances IRS-4 dependent insulin activation of extracellularly regulated kinase, ERK1/2, without any effect on the PI3 kinase pathway. Thus, it is also tempting to hypothesize that IRAS may participate in integrin-growth factor receptor crosstalk, which has been already described[24] as giving rise to cell protection against apoptosis (FIG. 7).

In conclusion, we have identified a new cellular role for the recently cloned human protein IRAS. We demonstrate that hIRAS expression in PC12 cells results in protection against apoptosis induced by various stimuli. In the future it will be important to address the question of the mechanism of IRAS's protective effect. Additional regulatory mechanisms of cell death and growth will perhaps be identified, allowing the characterization of new therapeutic targets.

ACKNOWLEDGMENTS

We thank Dr. See Violaine for her help in the Hoechst dye 33342 experiments. This research was also partially funded by NIH grant MH49248 (to J.E.P.).

REFERENCES

1. DONTENWILL M., C. VONTHRON, H. GRENEY, et al. 1999. Identification of human I1 receptors and their relationship to α2-adrenoceptors. Ann. N.Y. Acad. Sci. **881:** 123–134.
2. GRENEY, H., P. RONDE, C. MAGNIER, et al. 2000. Coupling of I(1) imidazoline receptors to the cAMP pathway: studies with a highly selective ligand, benazoline. Mol. Pharm. **57:** 1142–1151.
3. SEPAROVIC D., M. KESTER & P. ERNSBERGER. 1996. Coupling of I_1-imidazoline receptors to diacylglyceride accumulation in PC12 rat pheochromocytoma cells. Mol. Pharm. **49:** 668–675.
4. EDWARDS L, D. FISHMAN, P HOROWITZ, et al. 2001. The I1-imidazoline receptor in PC12 pheochromocytoma cells activates protein kinases C, extracellular signa-regulated kinase (ERK) and c-jun N-terminal kinase (JNK). J. Neurochem. **79:** 931–940.
5. PILETZ J., T. IVANOV, J.D. SHARP, et al. 2000. Imidazoline antisera selected (IRAS) cDNA: cloning and characterization. DNA & Cell Biol. **19:** 319–329.
6. IVANOV T.R., J.C. JONES, M. DONTENWILL, et al. 1998. Characterization of a partial cDNA clone detected by imidazoline receptor-selective antisera. J. Auton. Nerv. Sys. **72:** 98–110.
7. WANG H., S. REGUNATHAN, D.A. RUGGIERO & D.J. REIS. 1993. Production and characterisation of antibodies specific for the imidazoline receptor protein. Mol. Pharmacol. **43:** 509–515.
8. BENNAI F., H. GRENEY, C. VONTHRON, et al. 1996. Polyclonal antiidiotypic antibodies to idazoxan and their interaction with human brain imidazoline binding sites. Eur. J. Pharmacol. **306:** 211–218.
9. PILETZ, J.E., J.C. JONES, H. ZHU, et al. 1999. Imidazoline receptor antisera-selected cDNA clone and mRNA distribution. Ann. N.Y. Acad. Sci. **881:** 1–7.
10. DONTENWILL M., G. PASCAL, J.E. PILETZ, et al. 2003. IRAS the human homologue of Nischarin, prolongs survival of transfected PC12 cells. Cell Death Diff. **10:** 933–935.
11. LAMBENG N., P.P. MICHEL, B.Y. BRUGGAGID & M.RUBERG. 1999. Mechanisms of apoptosis in PC12 cells irreversibly differentiated with nerve growth factor and cyclic AMP. Brain Res. **821:** 60–68.
12. KUMMER J.L., P.K. RAO & K.A. HEIDENREICH. 1997. Apoptosis induced by withdrawal of trophic factors is mediated by p38 mitogen-activated protein kinase. J. Biol. Chem. **272:** 20490–20494.

13. VAN ENGELAND M., L.J.W. NIELAND, F.C.S. RAMAEKERS, et al. 1998. AnnexinV-affinity assay: a review on an apoptosis detection system based on phosphatidylserine exposure. Cytometry **31:** 1–9.
14. WADIA J.S., R.M.E. CHALMERS-REDMAN, W.J.H. JU, et al. 1998. Mitochondrial membrane potential and nuclear changes in apoptosis caused by serum and nerve growth factor withdrawal: time course and modification by deprenyl. J. Neuroscience **18:** 932–947.
15. STAM J.C., W.J.C GEERTS, H.H. VERSTEEG, et al. 2001. The v-Crk oncogene enhances cell survival and induces activation of protein kinase B/Akt. J. Biol. Chem. **276:** 25176–25183.
16. BARBER A.J., M NAKAMURA., E.B WOLPERT, et al. 2001. Insulin rescues retinal neurons from apoptosis by a phosphatidylinositol 3-kinase/Akt-mediated mechanism that reduces the activation of caspase-3. J. Biol. Chem. **276:** 32814–32821.
17. ALAHARI, S.K., J.W. LEE & R.L JULIANO. 2000. Nischarin, a novel protein that interacts with the integrin alpha5 subunit and inhibits cell migration. J. Cell Biol. **151:** 1141–1154.
18. O'BRIEN, V., S.M. FRISCH & R.L JULIANO. 1996. Expression of the integrin alpha 5 subunit in HT29 colon carcinoma cells suppresses apoptosis triggered by serum deprivation. Exp. Cell Res. **224:** 208–213.
19. LEE, J.W. & R.L JULIANO. 2000. alpha5beta1 integrin protects intestinal epithelial cells from apoptosis through a phosphatidylinositol 3-kinase and protein kinase B-dependent pathway. Mol. Biol. Cell **11:** 1973–1987.
20. ZHANG, Z., C. VUORI, J. REED & E. RUOSLAHTI. 1995. The alpha 5 beta 1 integrin supports survival of cells on fibronectin and up-regulates Bcl-2 expression. Proc. Natl. Acad. Sci. U. S. A. **92:** 6161–6165.
21. MATTER, M.L. & E. RUOSLAHTI 2001. A signaling pathway from the alpha5beta1 and alpha(v)beta3 integrins that elevates bcl-2 transcription. J. Biol. Chem. **276:** 27757–27763.
22. BERTRAND, F., A ATFI, A. CADORET, et al. 1998 A role for nuclear factor kappaB in the antiapoptotic function of insulin. J. Biol. Chem. **273:** 2931–2938 .
23. SANO H., S.C.H LIU, W.S LANE, et al. 2002. Insulin receptor substrate 4 associates with the protein IRAS. J. Biol. Chem. **277:** 19439–19447.
24. GUILHERME A., K. TORRES & M.P. CZECH. 1998. Cross-talk between insulin receptor and integrin $\alpha 5 \beta 1$ signalling pathways. J. Biol. Chem. **273:** 22899–22903.

Assembly of PRR-Containing Receptors on Scaffolds

A Model for Imidazoline I_1-Receptor Action

I.F. MUSGRAVE,[a] F.C. DEHLE,[a] AND J. PILETZ[b]

[a]*Department of Clinical and Experimental Pharmacology, University of Adelaide, Adelaide, Australia*

[b]*Department of Biology, Jackson State University, Jackson, Mississippi 39216, USA*

> ABSTRACT: IRAS, a putative clone of the I_1-imidazoline receptor, possesses a proline-rich region (PRR) motif, which might interact with SH3 regions on tyrosine kinases, and an integrin-binding motif. Receptors with a PRR motif can generally assemble onto multi-element signaling complexes (eg., the β_3-receptor on the EGF receptor) and thereby modulate signal transduction. Integrins serve as scaffolds for multi-element signaling complexes, similar to that assembled with the EGF receptor. It is therefore possible that IRAS signals through a complex with other receptors.
>
> KEYWORDS: imidazoline receptors; signal transduction; integrin; scaffold; tyrosine kinase; Nischarin

INTRODUCTION

The cloning of an imidazoline-binding protein, IRAS, has not ended the controversy over the identity and actions of the I_1-receptor. Surprisingly, IRAS has little overall similarity to conventional receptors.[1,2] Although its structure has features that hint at a mode of action (e.g., IRAS possesses a proline-rich region [PRR] that might interact with SH3 regions on tyrosine kinases), it has not been clear how imidazoline ligand binding to IRAS might activate signal transduction pathways. When IRAS was found to have sequence identity with an integrin-binding domain of a related protein, Nischarin, the surprise was further compounded. How could a protein that binds to structural elements be responsible for the neurotransmission properties expected of an I_1-receptor in the CNS?

IRAS cDNA encodes a 1,504–amino acid protein that binds the I_1-receptor–selective compounds rilmenidine and moxonidine when expressed in Chinese hamster ovary (CHO) cells.[1] IRAS mRNA expression correlates with I_1-receptor density in various tissues, with most being in the brain.[1] Regional localization of IRAS protein has also shown its distribution generally parallels I_1-radioligand binding

---

Address for correspondence: Ian F. Musgrave, Department of Clinical and Experimental Pharmacology, University of Adelaide, Adelaide 5005, Australia. Voice: (+61) 8 8303 3905; fax (+61) 8 8224 0685.
  e-mail: ian.musgrave@adelaide.edu.au

distribution.[2] These results suggest that IRAS represents an I_1-receptor. Structurally, the IRAS protein seems to be unique. Although it is predicted to have a number of transmembrane domains, IRAS is clearly not a member of the G protein–coupled receptor family, consistent with studies that show the I_1-receptor is not a site on the α_2-adrenoceptor. Aside from some similarity to cytokine receptors, the IRAS protein does not seem to match any class of known receptors.[1,2]

I_1-receptors have been proposed to modulate several signal transduction systems. Stimulation of phosphatidyl-choline–specific phospholipase C (PC-PLC),[3] inhibition of nicotinic receptors,[4] and inhibition of K_{ATP} receptors[5] has been implicated in various systems. A key question then is how could IRAS stimulate signal transduction systems such as PC-PLC when it is not a G protein–coupled receptor and is not in itself a kinase/phosphatase enzyme or ion channel? The answer to this question may come from the fact that IRAS is an integrin-binding protein.

INTEGRINS: A KEY TO UNDERSTANDING IRAS SIGNALING

Recently, IRAS was shown to have greater than 93% similarity to an integrin-binding protein, Nischarin.[6] Indeed, Genbank now lists IRAS under the title "human Nischarin" (see Genbank accession number NM_007184). Nischarin modulates cell motility by binding to integrin, which in turn reorganizes the actin cytoskeleton that is anchored to the integrin scaffold.[6]

The integrin-binding motif of Nischarin is paralleled by an identical amino acid sequence in IRAS. Nischarin's integrin-binding motif[6] occupies residues 434–581 (Genbank accession number AF315344), whereas the identical motif in IRAS occupies residues 673 through 834 (Genbank accession number AF082516). This integrin-binding motif plus the presence of the PRR domain (SH3 interacting domain) and a PX domain (which is important in binding to cytoskeleton elements)[1] suggest that IRAS, and hence I_1-receptors generally, may modulate integrin signaling complexes.

IRAS REORGANIZES ACTIN CYTOSKELETON

We sought to determine if IRAS could reorganize the actin cytoskeleton in the same manner as Nischarin. To test this possibility, PC-12 cells (as characterized elsewhere[1,2]) were stably transfected with full-length IRAS, or with plasmid vector. Cells were then plated onto laminin-coated cover slips in six well plates at a density of 30,000 cells per well. After 48 hours in serum-containing RMPI medium, the cells were washed three times with cold phosphate-buffered saline (PBS), fixed for 10 minutes in 3.7% formaldehyde, and permeabilized in 1% Triton X-100 (Sigma-Aldrich, Sydney, NSW) for 10 minutes. The cells then were washed several times and blocked in 2% bovine serum albumin for 1 hour at room temperature. After rinsing in PBS, cover slips were incubated with fluorescent TRITC-phalloidin (1.5 μM Sigma-Aldrich) for 15 minutes to stain actin. Cells were observed with a fluorescence microscope using a 40× objective. Images were recorded using a CCD camera and a computer with SPOT image analysis software. Vector-transfected cells showed actin staining predominantly on the cell membrane, with a small amount of uniform binding over the rest of the cytoplasm (FIG. 1B). In contrast, the IRAS-transfected

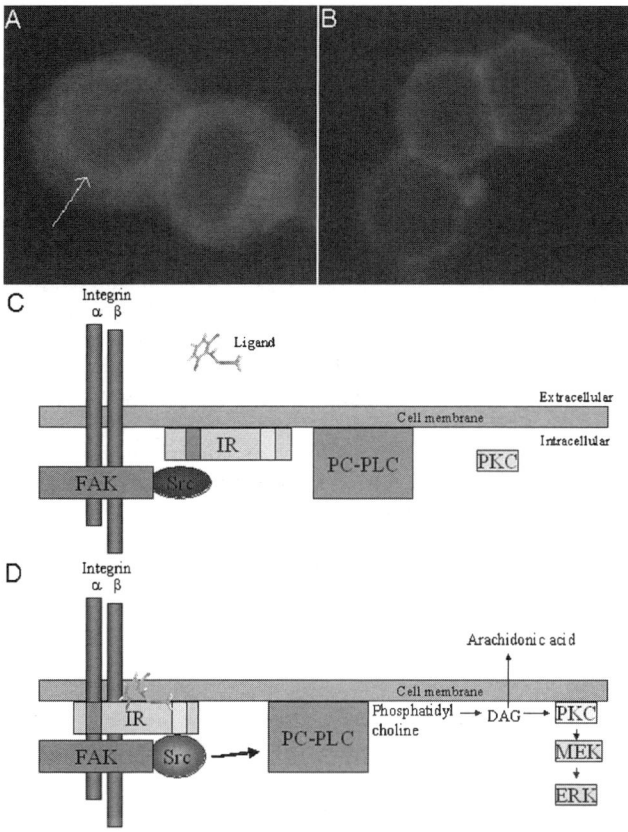

FIGURE 1. IRAS as an integrin binding protein, and its possible role in signal transduction. (**A, B**) Effects of IRAS (designated IR) on cytoskeletal organization. PC-12 cells were stably transfected with a plasmid-expressing full-length IRAS or an empty plasmid. Transfected cells were plated on integrin-coated cover slips and grown for 48 hours, then processed for TRITC-phalloidin staining of the actin cytoskeleton. (**A**) IRAS transfectants show dense staining of actin with prominent rings around the nucleus (*marked with arrow*). (**B**) Control cells transfected only with the vector show a sparse distribution of actin, with most staining concentrated at the cell membrane. (**C, D**) Action of I_1 receptors. Binding of a ligand to the receptor (IR) causes binding of the integrin-binding motif (*dark-shaded bar*) to α5 integrin, with subsequent binding of the proline rich region (*light-shaded bar*) in IR to a tyrosine kinase such as Src. Activated Src in turn activates PC-PLC with subsequent activation of protein kinase C and the mitogen-activated kinase pathway. DAG, diacylglycerol; ERK, extracellular signal-regulated kinase; FAK, focal adhesion kinase; IR, imidazoline receptor; MEK, mitogen-activated protein kinase/extracellular signal-regulated kinase; PC-PLC, phosphatidylcholine-specific phospholipase C; PKC, protein kinase C.

cells showed little actin staining in the membrane and bright staining concentrated in the cytoplasm (FIG. 1A), often with a high-intensity ring around the nucleus (*arrowed structure*, FIG. 1A). Analysis of pixel density showed that the perinuclear area was twice as bright in IRAS-transfected cells as in vector-transfected cells (69 ± 9 versus 35 ± 11 arbitrary units per pixel, $P < 0.05$, $N = 4$). Thus, IRAS seems to function like its close homologue Nischarin, probably as an integrin-binding protein.

Integrins are the main cell-surface receptors for extracellular matrix proteins such as fibronectin, laminin, and collagen.[7,8] Integrins have a two roles. They participate in cell adhesion as well as transmembrane signaling through assembly of signaling complexes onto the integrin scaffold. Kinases such as focal adhesion kinase (FAK) and integrin linked kinase (ILK) assembled onto the integrin scaffold activate tyrosine kinases such as Src, which in turn lead to the activation of multiple signal transduction pathways including cytosolic phospholipases.[7,8]

Our proposed model for IRAS signal transduction is shown in FIGURE 1 (*lower panel*). On activation, IRAS binds to the integrin-signaling complex through the integrin-binding domain (and possibly the PX domain) and binds to a tyrosine kinase (such as Src) in this complex through the PRR, activating the kinase and stimulating a cascade of events leading to activation of phospholipase C (FIG. 1C, D). This preliminary model attempts to unify the findings of Ernsberger *et al*.[3] showing activation of phosphatidyl-choline specific phospholipase C with our own preliminary results showing that I_1-receptors stimulate tyrosine phosphorylation (Musgrave and Meyer, unpublished observations).

SIGNALING SCAFFOLDS: A GENERAL MODULATORY MECHANISM

There is precedent for our model. Assembly of PRR-containing proteins onto signaling scaffolds is a recently recognized signaling modality, whereby proteins that by themselves do not contain signaling systems can activate or modulate signaling pathways. An example of this modality is the Shank family of proteins.[9] Other receptors are known to act through tyrosine kinase–signaling complexes by means of PRR domains and assembly onto scaffolds. For instance, β-adrenoceptors activate Src by assembling with the epidermal growth factor (EGF) receptor and then interacting with Src bound to the signaling complex on the scaffold.[10] c-Src is activated by direct interaction of a PRR in the third intracellular loop of the β_3-adrenoceptor with the SH3 region of Src.[11] The lysophosphatidic acid receptor also activates the MAP kinase pathway through interaction with FAK assembled on an integrin scaffold.[12] IRAS has also been found to associate with insulin receptor substrate,[13] which forms part of an integrin-signaling complex.[14] Thus the concept that imidazolines may modulate signal transduction by altering IRAS linkage to integrin signaling complexes is reasonable.

INTEGRINS AND NEUROTRANSMISSION

Integrins are well known to be important for many aspects of neuronal growth[15] and survival.[16] As such, these proteins could feasibly underlie imidazoline ligand effects on neuronal survival. In addition, the actin cytoskeleton also plays a critical role in maintaining neurotransmission, and it is therefore possible that modulation of integrin-signaling complexes through IRAS could also alter actin interactions with the reserve vesicle pool, and hence the availability of vesicles for release during nerve stimulation.[17] This process could occur by activation of protein kinase C leading to alteration of the actin cytoskeleton (FIG. 1D)[17] or by alteration of the actin cytoskeleton directly through its links to the integrin-signaling complex. Furthermore, there is evidence that integrins play a role in minute-to-minute neurotransmission (ie., integrin ligands can rapidly modulate long-term potentiation in mammalian and *Drosophila* neurons[18] and rapidly modulate neuronal calcium currents and neuronal calcium levels in snail neurons[19]). Thus, the fact that IRAS binds to and probably signals through integrin-signaling complexes similar to other PRR-containing proteins suggests a role in neuronal survival as well as rapid neuromodulatory actions.

CONCLUSION

A hypothesis is presented that IRAS signals through assembly onto an integrin scaffold where it may stimulate tyrosine kinases associated with the integrin scaffold through its PRR domain. The hypothesis is strengthened by our finding that IRAS reorganizes the actin cyoskeleton of PC-12 cells. It is also consistent with structural, biochemical, and functional information about I_1-receptors. We hope that this hypothesis will allow more focused investigation of these receptors and their interaction with endogenous ligands.

ACKNOWLEDGMENTS

This research was supported by the Australian National Health and Medical Research Council grant 981113 (I.M.), a University of Adelaide Faculty of Health Sciences B1 establishment grant (I.M.), and grant MH49248 from the National Institutes of Health in the United States (J.P.).

REFERENCES

1. PILETZ, J.E., *et al.* 2000. Imidazoline receptor antisera-selected (IRAS) cDNA: cloning and characterization. DNA Cell Biol. **19:** 319–329.
2. PILETZ, J.E., *et al.* 1999. Imidazoline receptor antisera-selected cDNA clone and mRNA distribution. Ann. N. Y. Acad. Sci. **881:** 1–7.
3. ERNSBERGER, P. 1999. The I_1-imidazoline receptor and its cellular signaling pathways. Ann. N. Y. Acad. Sci. **881:** 35–53.
4. MUSGRAVE, I.F. & R.A. HUGHES. 1999. Novel targets and techniques in imidazoline receptor research. Ann. N. Y. Acad. Sci. **881:** 301–312.
5. MORGAN, N.G., *et al.* 1999. Imidazolines and pancreatic hormone secretion. Ann. N. Y. Acad. Sci. **881:** 217–228.
6. ALAHARI, S.K., *et al.* 2000. Nischarin, a novel protein that interacts with the integrin alpha5 subunit and inhibits cell migration. J. Cell Biol. **151:** 1141–1154.
7. JULIANO, R.L. 2002. Signal transduction by cell adhesion receptors and the cytoskeleton: functions of integrins, cadherins, selectins, and immunoglobulin-superfamily members. Annu. Rev. Pharmacol. Toxicol. **42:** 283–323.

8. WU, C. & S. DEDHAR. 2001. Integrin-linked kinase (ILK) and its interactors: a new paradigm for the coupling of extracellular matrix to actin cytoskeleton and signaling complexes. J. Cell Biol. **155:** 505–510.
9. SHENG, M. & E. KIM. 2000. The Shank family of scaffold proteins. J. Cell Sci. **113:** 1851–1856.
10. MAUDSLEY, S., et al. 2000. The β_2-adrenergic receptor mediates extracellular signal-regulated kinase activation via assembly of a multi-receptor complex with the epidermal growth factor receptor. J. Biol. Chem. **275:** 9572–9580.
11. CAO, W., et al. 2000. Direct binding of activated c-Src to the β_3-adrenergic receptor is required for MAP kinase activation. J. Biol. Chem. **275:** 38131–38134.
12. DELLA ROCCA, G.J., et al. 1999. Pleiotropic coupling of G protein-coupled receptors to the mitogen-activated protein kinase cascade. Role of focal adhesions and receptor tyrosine kinases. J. Biol. Chem. **274:** 13978–13984.
13. SANO, H., et al. 2002. Insulin receptor substrate 4 associates with the protein IRAS. J. Biol. Chem. **277:** 19439–19447.
14. REISS, K., et al. 2001. Mechanisms of regulation of cell adhesion and motility by insulin receptor substrate-1 in prostate cancer cells. Oncogene **20:** 490–500.
15. GARY, D.S. & M.P. MATTSON. 2001. Integrin signaling via the PI3-kinase-Akt pathway increases neuronal resistance to glutamate-induced apoptosis. J. Neurochem. **76:** 1485–1496.
16. ISHII, T., et al. 2001. Integrin-linked kinase controls neurite outgrowth in N1E-115 neuroblastoma cells. J. Biol. Chem. **276:** 42994–43003.
17. IANNAZZO, L. 2001. Involvement of B-50 (GAP-43) phosphorylation in the modulation of transmitter release by protein kinase C. Clin. Exp. Pharmacol. Physiol. **28:** 901–904.
18. ROHRBOUGH, J., et al. 2000. Integrin-mediated regulation of synaptic morphology, transmission, and plasticity. J. Neurosci. **20:** 6868–6878.
19. WILDERING, W.C., et al. 2002. Rapid neuromodulatory actions of integrin ligands. J. Neurosci. **22:** 2419–2426.

IRAS Splice Variants

J.E. PILETZ,[a,b] W. DELEERSNIJDER,[c] B.L. ROTH,[d] P. ERNSBERGER,[e] H. ZHU,[a] AND D. ZIEGLER[e]

[a]*Department of Psychiatry, University of Mississippi Medical Center, Jackson, Mississippi 39216, USA*

[b]*Jackson State University, Jackson, Mississippi 39217, USA*

[c]*Innogenetics, Ghent, Belgium*

[d]*Case Western Reserve University, Cleveland, Ohio 44106, USA*

[e]*Solvay Pharma, Hannover, Germany*

ABSTRACT: The human I_1-imidazoline receptor candidate gene, *iras*, has previously been cloned and mapped to locus 3p21.1-9 (also known as *Nischarin;* accession #AC006208). By comparison to a database of expressed sequence tags (ESTs), three alternatively spliced transcripts have been deduced. A map of 21 exons was constructed for the medium-length transcript (IRAS-M) containing 5,232 base pairs (bp) and encoding 1,504 amino acids (aas). Introns 13B and 13C are inserted into the two alternative transcripts, forming IRAS-S and IRAS-L mRNA (short and long isoforms). Northern blots confirmed the existence of these mRNA isoforms. In most brain regions the order of mRNA abundance was IRAS-M > IRAS-L > IRAS-S mRNA. Although aas 1 through 510 are theoretically identical, truncated proteins could be derived from IRAS-S (2,678 bp transcript yields 515 aas) and IRAS–L (9,457 bp transcript yields 583 aas). Because exon-16 of the *iras* gene has been proposed to encode the functional domains of imidazoline and α-5 integrin binding, only IRAS-M is expected to possess I_1 receptor properties. Subtype-selective cDNA expression constructs were therefore generated and used to transfect CHO cells. High-affinity I_1 binding was endowed by IRAS-M and IRAS-L, but not by IRAS-S transfection.

KEYWORDS: IRAS; Nischarin; imidazoline receptors; introns; splicing; chromosome 3

INTRODUCTION

Two major subtypes of imidazoline receptors (I_1R and I_2R) have been extensively characterized by pharmacologic and biochemical means, but elucidating their molecular identities remains an area of active research. The pharmacologic definition of an I_1-binding site includes high affinity for clonidinelike compounds relative to the more planar idazoxanlike compounds, without affinity for known monoamines.[1] I_1-binding sites are associated with plasma membranes, whereas I_2 sites are associated with mitochondrial membranes.[2]

Address for correspondence: He Zhu, M.D., Department of Psychiatry, University of Mississippi Medical Center, 2500 North State Street, Jackson, MS 39216-4505, USA. Voice: 601-984-5798; fax: 601-984-5899.
    e-mail: HZhu@psychiatry.umsmed.edu

Ann. N.Y. Acad. Sci. 1009: 419–426 (2003). © 2003 New York Academy of Sciences.
doi: 10.1196/annals.1304.056

A candidate I_1 receptor named IRAS has been cloned from human hippocampus.[3] The mouse homologue of IRAS has also been cloned and named Nischarin.[4] Northern blots have revealed two isoforms of IRAS mRNA, at 5.5 and 9.5 kilobases (kb), which differ in tissue distribution.[5,6] The 5.5 kb transcript, formerly called IRAS-1,[3] has been sequenced and used to transfect I_1-binding sites into Chinese hamster ovary (CHO) cells.[3] In the present study, this transcript is called IRAS-M. We now also report the nature of the 9.5-kb isoform of IRAS mRNA (called IRAS-L) as well as that of a previously unrecognized alternative transcript at 3.0 kb (IRAS-S).

MATERIALS AND METHODS

Genomic Sequencing

A genomic library of human placental DNA was purchased from Stratagene (La Jolla, CA, USA) to screen for the *iras* gene by hybridization. The library was constructed in Stratagene's vector λ FIX II, and was grown in XL-1 Blue MRA (P2) host bacteria. The titer was approximately 50,000 plaques per 137-mm plate. Lifts from six plates were screened in duplicate by hybridization. The DNA probe used for screening was a 1.85-kb unique EcoR1 fragment from IRAS cDNA (expressed sequence tag [EST]04033) radiolabeled with [α-^{32}P]d-CTP according to Stratagene's Prime-It II random primer labeling kit. Plaques were lifted onto Duralon-UV membranes (Stratagene), denatured, and cross-linked under UV light. Hybridization was conducted under high stringency according to Stratagene's vector λ FIX II instruction manual. Two positive genomic clones of identical size (≈17-kb insert) were retained through three rounds of screening. One of the clones, JEP-1A, was tested by high-stringency Southern blotting with a radiolabeled 1,110-bp ApaI-EcoRI fragment from IRAS cDNA, and it revealed fragments identical with human blood DNA: a 14.1-kb EcoR1 fragment and a 7.7-kb SacI fragment. Clone JEP-1A was then deposited with the American Tissue Culture Collection (ATCC) under accession #ATCC 209216. Genomic sequencing of JEP-1A was also done on an ABI automated sequencer (Applied Biosystems, Foster City, CA) using ABI dye-terminator kits (contracted to Cadus Pharmaceuticals, Tarrytown, NY). A total of 15,202 bp was sequenced in JEP-1A, with the remaining 1.8 kb unidentified in the untranscribed 3' region. After confirming its identity with our published sequence of IRAS cDNA,[3] two supplemental sources of sequence were obtained. (1) 5' end primer walking was performed using custom oligonucleotides (Gibco-BRL, Gaithersburg, MD, USA) and Marathon RACE PCR from Clontech (Palo Alto, CA, USA). This addition raised the total sequence to 20,534 bp, which encoded aas #194 to 1,504 in IRAS-M. (2) The full sequence was then acquired from the DNA sequence of human chromosome 3, which at that time became available on the Internet (National Center for Biotechnology Information [NCBI] accession #AC006208). Clone AC006208 revealed the additional first 5 exons of *iras* (TABLE 1). The *iras* gene can also be viewed on the Web site of the NCBI, listed on human chromosome 3 region 52,876K–52,932K.

RNA Studies and Subtype-Selective Expression Vectors

Northern blotting was carried out on RNA from different regions of human brain (Clontech blot #7755-1) as previously described.[6] For the hybridizations, 25 ng of

TABLE 1. Position of 21 exons of IRAS-M from genomic sequence AC006208

Exon #	Start	End
1	First A.A. encoded at bp 64,082	64,176
2	66,283	66,366
3	67,102	67,284
4	79,299	79,347
5	80,254	80,417
6	80,743	80,838
7	82,174	82,269
8	84,887	85,039
9	86,014	86,082
10	86,537	86,722
11	86,889	87,017
12	88,189	88,302
13	88,624	88,735[a]
14	92,953[a]	93,077
15	94,218	94,267
16	95,636	97,045
17	97,776	98,118
18	98,515	98,671
19	99,145	99,273
20	99,792	99,953
21	100,312	Last A.A. (#1504) encoded at bp 100,917

[a] Intron where alternatively spliced stop codons exist (for IRAS-S and IRAS-L).

probe was radiolabeled using the random-primed incorporation of [^{32}P]dCTP. Hybridizations were conducted under high stringency as recommended by the vendor.

Subtype-selective expression vectors were prepared by PCR primer design. All PCR reactions were carried out in a Perkin-Elmer 9700 thermocycler (with heated lid) (Perkin Elmer, Boston, MA) using Taq polymerase (Boehringer, Mannheim, Germany).

(1) The following primer pair was designed for the PCR-cloning of IRAS-M coding area:
sense 5'-ACGGATCCGGCGGAGACCCGAACATGGC-3'
antisense 5'-ACTCTAGAGAACACAAAAGCCTGCTGCCC-3'
Using Marathon-Ready cDNA from human cerebellum (Clontech #7401-1; Clontech, Franklin Lakes, NJ) a major 4,580-bp DNA fragment was generated. It was first ligated into pGEM-T and transformed into *Escherichia coli*

strain DH5αF' for sequencing. After the sequence was ascertained to be 100% identical to the coding portion of IRAS-M, the insert was gel-purified and ligated into pcDNA3.1(+) for transfection studies. It was in the right direction as shown by sequencing. This vector was called IRM.

(2) The following primer pair was designed for the PCR-cloning of the IRAS-S coding region:
sense 5'-ACGGATCCGGCGGAGACCCGAACATGGC-3'
antisense 5'-ACTCTAGAGGCACACCCTCCCCTCCTCCG-3'
Using Marathon-Ready cDNA from human cerebellum (Clontech #7401-1) a major DNA fragment of 1,627 bp was generated. It was handled as described for primer pair 1 and was found to be 100% identical to the coding region of IRAS-S. This vector was named IRS.

(3) The following primer pair was then designed for the PCR-cloning of the IRAS-L coding region:
sense 5'-ACGGATCCGGCGGAGACCCGAACATGGC-3'
antisense 5'-ACTCTAGAGGAGCTGGATGTGGGC-3'
In this case we used a minor fragment generated from the IRAS-S PCR reaction that was 2,200 bp long. The PCR material was nested with the aforementioned IRAS-L primers. A major PCR-fragment of 1,830 bp was generated. We constructed the expression clone by assembling the correct part of this fragment (the 3' end) with the correct part of IRS. It was found to be 100% identical to the coding region of IRAS-L. It was shown to be properly inserted into pcDNA3.1(+) by restriction enzyme analysis. This vector was named IRL.

Transfection and Protein Studies

CHO cells were grown in RPMI 1640 medium (Sigma, St. Louis, MO) supplemented with 10% (v/v) heat-inactivated horse serum, 5% (v/v) heat-inactivated fetal bovine serum, penicillin 50 U/mL, and streptomycin 50 μg/mL. Cells were transiently transfected according to our previous report[3] with IRM, IRL, IRS, or the pDNA3.1(+) vector only. Cellular preparations were analyzed in two ways. (1) Radioligand binding was performed as previously described.[3] [^{3}H]Clonidine (58-65 Ci/mmol) and [^{125}I]p-iodoclonidine (final 440 Ci/mmol) were purchased from New England Nuclear (Boston, MA, USA). Four transfection batches were analyzed from each vector: two binding assays with each radioligand. The LIGAND curve-fitting program (Biosoft, MO, USA) was used to merge the data analysis.[7] Protein concentrations were 0.8 mg/mL for [^{3}H]clonidine and 0.2 mg/mL for [^{125}I]p-iodoclonidine binding. Moxonidine (gift from Lilly Pharmaceuticals) was used as the displacing agent. (2) Denatured protein samples were electrophoresed in SDS-polyacrylamide gels (SDS-PAGE), and Western blots were prepared. Blots were probed with anti-idiotypic antiserum$_{227-241}$ for IRAS. This antiserum is described in detail in a companion article by Zhu *et al.* in this volume.

RESULTS

By homology cloning, we obtained a 17-kb genomic clone (JEP-1A) which assisted us in ascertaining the complete sequence of the human *iras* gene. The sequence of JEP-1A (20,534 bp) was 99% identical to a region of chromosome 3. The human *iras* gene is now known to cover 36,835 bp in length from first to last codon and is located on chromosome 3 (at 3p21.1–9) (TABLE 1). IRAS-M is the new name for IRAS-1, which we previously identified as a 5,131-bp cDNA clone from human hippocampus.[3,6] The new sequence adds 101 nucleotides of 5′ untranslated sequence, making the full size of the IRAS-M transcript at least 5,232-bp long (not counting the poly-A+ tail). Five new 5′ RACE PCR–generated sequences from different cDNA clones were also isolated using primers in the 5′ area of the already known IRAS-1 cDNA, but none of them extended the IRAS-M sequence further upstream, indicating nearness to the 5′ end. Apart from the last two nucleotides before its poly-A tail, IRAS-M is completely identical to our previous report on the cDNA called IRAS-1.[3] Moreover, the predicted protein sequences are completely identical.

EST database information, publicly available from the NCBI, led us to predict the existence of alternatively spliced IRAS transcripts. By aligning more than 92 ESTs from IRAS, three alternative transcripts (IRAS-L, IRAS-M, and IRAS-S) could be accounted for by alternative splicing between exon 13 and exon 14 in *iras* (TABLES 1 and 2) and by an internal polyadenylation site discovered in the intervening intron. No other evidence was found for alternative splicing outside of exon 13. On the basis of these different EST clones, three types of transcripts were postulated: transcripts that contain a merger of exons 13A, 13B, 13C, and 14 (IRAS-L); transcripts that contain exon 13A merged to exon 13C (IRAS-S); and transcripts that have exon 13A merged to exon 14 (IRAS-M). In addition, at least 10 EST sequences were found to be indicative of an internal polyadenylation signal sequence in exon 13C. This finding makes IRAS-S a shorter transcript (2,768 bp). Because no ESTs were found with the internal polyadenylation signal sequence of exon 13C after a 13A-13B-13C merger, the presence of exon 13B in IRAS-L may be hypothesized to suppress this internal polyadenylation signal. Because IRAS-L does not use this internal polyadenylation site, its length is predicted to be 9,457 bp. To confirm these predictions, a number of relevant EST cDNA clones were obtained and fully sequenced on both strands, so that all three exon patterns were represented by at least three independent cDNA clones. The sequences from these EST clones completely confirmed the predicted splice variations in the three IRAS isoforms.

Northern blots of human brain tissues were also analyzed to verify the existence of differentially spliced mRNA isoforms of IRAS. Firstly, a 900-bp probe derived from exon 1 (an SpeI/NcoI fragment) was used to reveal mRNA bands of 9.5, 5.5,

TABLE 2. Molecular description of IRAS isoforms in humans

Alternative Transcripts	Transcript Sizes	Protein Sizes[a]
IRAS-S	2,678 bp plus alternate polyA+ tail (3-kb size)	Protein of 515 amino acids (57-kD size on SDS gels)
IRAS-M	5,232 bp plus polyA+ tail (5.5-kb size)	Protein of 1,504 amino acids (167-kD size on SDS gels)
IRAS-L	9,457 bp plus same polyA+ tail as IRAS-M (9.5-kb size)	Protein of 583 amino acids (65-kD on SDS gels)

[a] The three proteins are identical up to amino acid #510.

and 3 kb in all brain regions tested (plus spinal cord). The 5.5-kb band was more intense than the other bands except in cerebellum where the 5.5- and 9.5-kb bands were equally intense. The 3-kb band was weaker than the other bands. Secondly, a 380-bp NcoI/PstI fragment was obtained specific for exon 13B. This probe produced a band of 9.5 kb in all lanes, as well as a much weaker band of 3.5 kb. The 5.5-kb band (IRAS-M) was not detectable with this probe, as expected. Finally, when compared with our previous report[6] in which a 1,117-bp probe was used from exon 16 (Apa/EcoRI fragment), it is noteworthy that the earlier study showed only the 9.5-kb and 5.5-kb bands in brain, as expected. Collectively, these three selective probes confirmed the existence of three IRAS transcripts in brain. Their abundance in brain regions was generally IRAS-M > IRAS-L > IRAS-S. Their overall distribution was cerebellum > cerebral cortex > frontal lobe > temporal lobe > occipital lobe > putamen > medulla > spinal cord.

A comparison of the proteins was next undertaken. IRAS-M contains a long open-reading frame of 1,504 aas. By contrast, IRAS-S and IRAS-L transcripts encode proteins of 515 and 583 aas respectively. The N-terminal 510 aas of all three predicted proteins are identical. After residue #510, the C-terminal sequence of IRAS-S is ILGDE. By comparison, the unique C-terminal sequence of IRAS-L protein is NRVCILLLVE PHSPAWAPWL GWGWGRGAST CFQQGTQGG QCLLQAGPRG GTHGRGAWPD ASCCLLGEDS QLL. These alternative sequences bear no obvious similarity to any other protein sequences in public databases.

It was next of interest to compare the properties of the isoforms of IRAS. Plasmid expression vectors for IRAS-S, -M, and -L were prepared and used to transfect CHO cells. Western blots were probed with antiserum against an N-terminal epitope of IRAS (aas #227–241); the epitope is common to all three isoforms. Bands of appropriate sizes were enriched on the Western blots of the transfected CHO cells (TABLE 2). The levels of enrichment of these protein bands in the transfected cells was two- to threefold. Furthermore, the transfection of IRAS-M or IRAS-L led to more than twofold increases in the level of I_1 binding sites (TABLE 3). Their affinity constants were also significantly higher than in the vector-only control cells (TABLE 3). This

TABLE 3. Radioligand binding to imidazoline sites of IRAS isoforms transfected into CHO cells

Alternative Forms of Human IRAS	I_1-like Affinity (K_D) for Clonidine Binding[a] (nM)	I_1-like Density (B_{max}) for Clonidine Binding[a] (fmoles/mg protein)
Vector-only control	3.5 ± 0.9	41 ± 6.6
IRAS-S	1.3 ± 0.3^b	65 ± 8.9
IRAS-M	1.5 ± 0.5^b	90 ± 17^b
IRAS-L	2.3 ± 1.1	87 ± 26^b

[a] LIGAND curve-fitting analysis[7] was used to combine the results with [^{3}H]clonidine (n = 2/group) and [^{125}I]p-iodoclonidine (n = 2/group). Values represent the means ± SE of the estimates from the four experiments per category.

[b] Significantly different vertical comparisons between experimental groups and the vector-only control group ($P < 0.05$).

finding was accounted for by the appearance of high-affinity sites over a low-affinity background present in parent CHO cells, similar to that previously reported with the former IRAS-1.[3] Transfection of IRAS-S failed to yield I_1 binding sites, however (TABLE 3).

DISCUSSION

The human *iras* gene encompasses 37 kb on chromosome 3 at locus 3p21.1-9. Only 5.6 kb of this gene is transcribed into mRNA capable of encoding the full-length 1,504-aa protein that we named IRAS-M. The map of the human *iras* gene includes 20 introns and 21 exons for IRAS-M (TABLE 1). Transfection of IRAS-M cDNA into CHO cells yields I_1 binding capacity, making it an I_1R candidate gene.[3]

Alternative splicing events between exons 13 and 14 of *iras* were found to expose stop codons in two of the three alternative IRAS mRNA forms, yielding truncated proteins. The three main *iras* gene products are listed in TABLE 2. It is noteworthy that most of the functional domains of IRAS-M, including the proposed domains for IRAS-M to bind imidazoline drugs (from aas #622–698[3]), the α5-integrin protein (from aas #679–826[4]), and the insulin receptor substrate proteins (from aas #685–1,504[8]), are encoded downstream of aa #510 (the splice site). Therefore, the IRAS-S and IRAS-L isoforms would be expected to be inactive truncated isoforms. Nevertheless, these truncated forms would be expected to compete with IRAS-M for membrane anchoring and protein-protein assembly, because the respective PX and leucine-rich repeat domains of IRAS-M are encoded within the first 510 aas.[9,10]

Because only transfections with IRAS-M and IRAS-L led to I_1 binding sites in CHO cells (TABLE 3), it seems that the most severely truncated form of IRAS (IRAS-S) lacks the aas necessary to encode an imidazoline binding site. The binding domain for imidazolines has previously been suggested to require acidic aas—specifically those in region #622 through 698 of IRAS-M.[3] IRAS-L also lacks this acidic region but still has imidazoline binding capacity (TABLE 3). Therefore, we are obliged to postulate that the novel aas #511 through 583 in IRAS-L may substitute for the acidic aas #622 through 698 in IRAS-M. In this regard, previous transfection data from our laboratory in other cell lines led us earlier to speculate that the imidazoline binding site of IRAS requires interaction with another cell type specific protein for its expression,[3] because IRAS-M transfection does not produce any imidazoline binding sites in some cell lines even though the protein is overexpressed.[3] Given these facts, it may be that the length of aas after residue #510 is more critical than the exact sequence for interaction with another protein in CHO cells to take place and form an imidazoline-binding site. This possibility will require further study.

The human 3p21 chromosomal region has been implicated as having a role in cancer, because this region is deleted or rearranged in various cancers.[10] The importance of this region of chromosome 3 in tumor suppression nicely correlates with data by Dontenwill et al.[11] showing a role for IRAS in cell survival. Alahari et al.[4] have also shown that the mouse homologue, Nischarin, plays a role in inhibiting cell migration. The gene for mouse Nischarin, however, may not be the exact homologue of human *iras* because it has been mapped to the opposite side of the mouse chromosome (corresponding to 3q).[12] A paper by Piletz in this volume also shows that IRAS functions to regulate cell growth through a mitogen-activated pathway cascade.

Therefore, the *iras* gene may regulate important functions in neuronal growth and differentiation.

ACKNOWLEDGMENTS

This research was supported by NIH Grant MH49248 and a grant from Solvay Pharmaceuticals.

REFERENCES

1. ERNSBERGER, P., M.E. GRAVES, L.M. GRAFF, *et al.* 1995. I_1-imidazoline receptors: definition, characterization, distribution and transmembrane signalling. Ann. N. Y. Acad. Sci. **763:** 22–42.
2. RADDATZ, R. & S.M. LANIER. 1997. Relationship between imidazoline/guanidinium receptive sites and monoamine oxidase A and B. Neurochem. Int. **30:** 109–117.
3. PILETZ, J.E., T.R. IVANOV, J.D. SHARP, *et al.* 2000. Imidazoline receptor antisera-selected (IRAS) cDNA: cloning and characterization. DNA Cell Biol. **19:** 319–329.
4. ALAHARI, S.K.K., J.W. LEE, & R.L. JULIANO. 2000. Nischarin, a novel protein that interacts with the integrin α5 subunit and inhibits cell migration. J. Cell Biol. **151:** 1141–1154.
5. PILETZ, J.E., J.C. JONES, H. ZHU, *et al.* 1999. Imidazoline receptor antisera-selected cDNA clone and mRNA distribution. Ann. N. Y. Acad. Sci. **881:** 1–7.
6. IVANOV, T.R., J.C. JONES, M. DONTENWILL, *et al.* 1998. Characterization of a partial cDNA clone detected by imidazoline receptor-selective antisera. J. Auton. Nerv. Syst. **72:** 98–110.
7. MCPHERSON, C.A. 1985. Analysis of radioligand binding experiments. A collection of computer programs for the IBM PC. J. Pharmacol. Methods **14:** 213–228.
8. SANO, H., S.C. LIU, W.S. LANE, *et al.* 2002. Insulin receptor substrate 4 associates with the protein IRAS. J. Biol. Chem. **23:** 23.
9. XU, Y., L.-F. SEET, B. HANSON, *et al.* 2001. The Phox homology (PX) domain, a new player in phosphoinositide signalling. Biochem. J. **360:** 513–530.
10. TIMMER, T., P. TERPSTRA, A. VAN DEN BERG, *et al.* 1999. A comparison of genomic structures and expression patterns of two closely related flanking genes in a critical lung cancer region at 3p21.3. Eur. J. Hum. Genet. **7:** 478–486.
11. DONTENWILL, M., G. PASCAL, J.E. PILETZ, *et al.* 2003. IRAS, the human homologue of Nischarin, prolongs survival of transfected PC12 cells. Cell Death Differ. **10:** 933–935.
12. ALAHARI, S.K. 2001. Mapping of the gene for Nischarin, a novel integrin binding protein, to chromosome 3 by fluorescence in situ hybridization. Int. J. Human Genet. **1**(4): 271–274.

Intracellular Effect of Imidazoline Receptor on α_{2A}-Noradrenergic Receptor

MICHAEL J. CHEN,[a] HE ZHU,[b] AND JOHN E. PILETZ[c]

[a]*California State University, Los Angeles, California 90032, USA*
[b]*University of Mississippi Medical Center, Jackson, Mississippi 39216, USA*
[c]*Jackson State University, Jackson, Mississippi 39217, USA*

ABSTRACT: Imidazoline-1 receptors (I_1R) and α_2-noradrenergic receptors (α_2AR) are known to coexist in many cell types and bind many of the same imidazoline ligands. Herein, the possibility of an interaction between these receptors was explored using a cloned cDNA that encodes a protein with I_1R-like binding properties, designated imidazoline receptor antisera-selected (IRAS). Chinese hamster ovary (CHO) sublines permanently expressing the human subtype $\alpha_{2A}AR$ cDNA were transiently cotransfected with the human IRAS cDNA (*pIRAS*). Saturation radioligand binding experiments on membranes isolated from the various sublines allowed distinction between I_1R and $\alpha_{2A}AR$. Transfection of *pIRAS* into either subline led to a rise in membrane I_1R-binding sites. Immunoblotting revealed that IRAS was enriched in membranes more than in cytosolic fractions. Transfection of *pIRAS* in CHO cells harboring the $\alpha_{2A}AR$ cDNA resulted in a twofold increase in $\alpha_{2A}AR$ binding sites with no change in $\alpha_{2A}AR$ binding affinity, compared with controls. Immunoblotting also revealed increased expression of membranous $\alpha_{2A}AR$ by IRAS. Thus, *pIRAS* transfection led to I_1 binding sites and to an increase in $\alpha_{2A}AR$ binding sites in CHO cells expressing the human $\alpha_{2A}AR$. Although the mechanism is unclear, this increase in binding sites may explain previous imidazoline drug effects suggestive of interactions between these two receptors.

KEYWORDS: imidazoline receptors; alpha$_2$ adrenoceptor; IRAS; Nischarin; coincidence detection

INTRODUCTION

An oft-cited explanation for the nonadrenergic properties of clonidine invokes the existence of nonadrenergic receptors that bind imidazoline compounds.[1–4] In terms of new drug discovery, the α_2AR subtypes and imidazoline$_1$ receptors (I_1Rs) have generally been considered separate entities that do not interact. The predominant subtype of α_2AR in the brain is the $\alpha_{2A}AR$ subtype. $\alpha_{2A}ARs$ play a dominant vasodepressor role through the nucleus of the solitary tract[5–7] and also act in the rostral ventrolateral medulla (RVLM)[5,7,8] in response to endogenous norepinephrine (NE) or drugs such as clonidine. Furthermore, I_1Rs are implicated in stress mediation through

---

Address for correspondence: He Zhu, M.D., Department of Psychiatry, University of Mississippi Medical Center, 2500 North State Street, Jackson, MS 39216-4505, USA. Voice: 601-984-5898; fax: 601-984-5899.
e-mail: HeZhu@psychiatry.umsmed.edu

afferents on the locus coeruleus,[2,9] perhaps linked to facilitation of exploratory behavior in mice.[10] Facilitation of chemosensory afferent firing in the carotid body,[11] modulation of insulin action,[12–14] and regulation of sodium excretion from the kidney[15] are all considered at least partly I_1R-mediated. Because many tissues contain α_2AR and I_1R, the possibility that α_2AR and I_1R may interact should be considered.

Coincidence detection is the integration of separate neurotransmitter stimuli into a unified response system.[16] This phenomenon exists at many levels, including cross-talk between receptors within a single cell. Other neurotransmitter receptors that have been shown to interact directly in the same cells[17] include gamma aminobutyric acid–A ($GABA_A$) and D_5 dopamine receptors,[18] A_1 and A_{2A} adenosine receptors,[19] A_1 adenosine and glutamate receptors,[20] D_1 dopamine and A_1 adenosine receptors,[21] muscarinic m_3 and β_2-adrenergic receptors,[22] D_2 dopamine and somatostatin-5 receptors,[23] and calcyon and dopamine D_1 receptors.[24]

Given the large number of studies suggesting a pharmacologic synergism between $\alpha_{2A}AR$ and I_1R,[25,29] we postulated these receptors might interact intracellularly. Herein, we report radioligand binding and Western blotting evidence of an effect of I_1R on $\alpha_{2A}AR$ in cotransfected Chinese hamster ovary (CHO) cells.

EXPERIMENTAL PROCEDURES

Cell Lines

CHO cells permanently transfected with the human $\alpha_{2A}AR$ cDNA (designated CHO-$\alpha_{2A}AR$ subline) and the parent line of wild-type CHO cells (WT line) were kindly given to us by Dr. Marc Caron (Duke University, Durham, NC). The CHO-$\alpha_{2A}AR$ subline has been called AUA-C_{10} in previous reports.[26] All cells were maintained at 37°C with 5% CO_2 in RPMI-1640 media (Gibco, Grand Island, NY) containing 8.4% horse serum, 4.2% fetal calf serum, 3.3 µM glutamine, and 85 µg mL^{-1} penicillin/streptomycin. The CHO-$\alpha_{2A}AR$ cells also had 31 µg mL^{-1} geneticin added as a selection agent.

Transfection

Both lines of CHO cells (WT and CHO-$\alpha_{2A}AR$) were plated to reach approximately 60% confluency by the day after plating. These were then transiently transfected with *pIRAS*[27] or vector only using Gene Porter Transfection reagent (GeneTherapy Systems, San Diego, CA, USA) at a ratio of 8 µg DNA to 40 µL Gene Porter in 100-mm plates. When the plates reached 100% confluency (48–72 hours after transfection), cells were harvested, centrifuged, and the pellets stored at −80°C until subcellular fractionation was performed.

Subcellular Fractionation

Cells were homogenized in 25 mM Tris, pH 7.4, 250 mM sucrose, 2 mM $MgCl_2$, containing 4 mM Pefabloc protease inhibitor (Boehringer Mannheim, Indianapolis, IN), centrifuged at 1,400 rpm (900 gravity) twice to remove any remaining intact cells as well as nuclear fractions, and centrifuged at 105,000 gravity for 2 hours to collect the membranes (pellet) and cytosol (supernatant) fractions. This total membrane fraction was tested for radioligand binding. For Western blotting studies, the homogenates were prepared in a cocktail of eight protease inhibitors[28] and were centrifuged at 20,000 gravity for 20 minutes, yielding internal membranes. The supernatant with plasma membranes was recentrifuged at 105,000 gravity for 2 hours to yield plasma membrane and cytosolic fractions for Western blotting.

Western Blotting

Equal amounts of protein were added to each lane of 8.5% polyacrylamide gels for denaturing gel electrophoresis SDS-PAGE.[28] The proteins were then electrotransferred to nitrocellulose membranes. Standard Western blotting procedures were performed on the blots using anti-IRAS 1209 antiserum produced and characterized in our laboratory.[27] The blots were stripped and reprobed with anti-α_{2A}AR antiserum (kindly provided by H. Kurose, University of Tokyo, Toyko, Japan[29]). To ensure equal lane loads on the gels, the blots were stripped once again and probed with anti-α-tubulin (Chemicon International, Temecula, CA, USA). In each case, the blots were then detected by an enhanced chemiluminescence (ECL) (Amersham Bioscience Corp., Piscataway, NJ, USA) and exposed to Kodak Hyperfilm (Amersham). A standard curve of each protein was included in each gel and blot.

Densitometry

Optical densities (ODs) of the relevant bands for IRAS, α_{2A}AR, and α-tubulin were measured from lightly exposed films using a Gel-doc 2000 system (Bio-Rad Inc., Hercules, CA, USA). Relative optical densities of IRAS and α_{2A}AR were computed from the standard curve on each blot and by adjusting for the α-tubulin intensity in each lane. For human IRAS immunoreactivity, the relevant band had a relative mobility equivalent to approximately 170 kD[27]; for human α_{2A}AR, the relevant band had a relative mobility of approximately 66 kD,[29] and α-tubulin was revealed, as expected, as 43 kD.[30]

Radioligand Binding

Full-saturation binding curves were implemented as previously described.[31]

RESULTS

As a point of reference, only a low level of endogenous IRAS immunoreactivity (170-kD band) was observed on Western blots probed with anti-IRAS-1209 serum in untransfected or vector-only CHO cells (FIG. 1A). As previously reported,[27] this low level of endogenous IRAS in CHO cells does not impart high-affinity I_1R radioligand binding capacity.[27] By comparison, human IRAS immunoreactivity (170 kD) was clearly increased in CHO cells transfected with human *pIRAS* compared with sublines not transfected with *pIRAS* (FIG. 1A).

Quantitative Western blotting revealed that IRAS exists in both plasma membranes and cytosolic fractions (FIG. 1A). A first level of comparison was between the two CHO sublines without human *pIRAS* transfection: that is, between WT and α_{2A}AR sublines. Levels of endogenous IRAS were determined by densitometry in

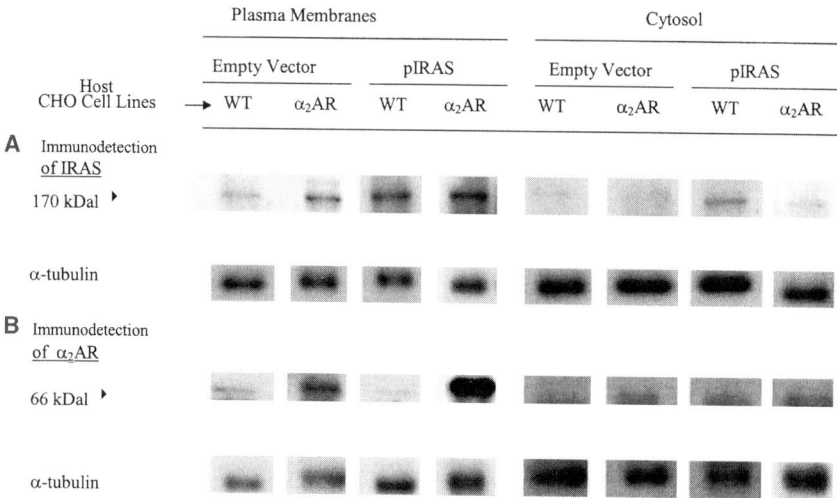

FIGURE 1. Representative Western blot bands of human IRAS and human $\alpha_{2A}AR$ proteins in plasma membranes and cytoplasmic fractions of CHO lines. Duplicate blots were probed separately with antiserum selective for (**A**) the 170-kD IRAS protein band (using IRAS-1209 antiserum), or (**B**) the 66-kD $\alpha_{2A}AR$ protein band detected by anti-$\alpha_{2A}AR$ serum. Both blots were stripped and reprobed with antiserum for a reference protein of 44-kD, α-tubulin (*lanes 2 and 4*). The four main conditions shown are wild-type parent CHO cells transiently transfected with empty vector *pcDNA3.1* (empty vector/ WT); CHO-$\alpha_{2A}AR$ subline transiently transfected with empty vector *pcDNA3.1* (empty vector/ $\alpha_{2A}AR$); wild-type parent CHO cells transiently transfected with human *pIRAS* (*pIRAS*/WT); and the CHO-$\alpha_{2A}AR$ subline transiently transfected with human *pIRAS* (*pIRAS*/ $\alpha_{2A}AR$). Bands are shown from films exposed identically to representative blots of the same samples.

plasma membranes and cytosolic fractions of the two lines. It can be seen that for transfection with the empty vector (FIG. 2), the distribution between plasma membranes and cytoplasm was the same for endogenous IRAS immunoreactivity in WT CHO cells and in the CHO-$\alpha_{2A}AR$ cell line. Even when the α-tubulin bias in favor of plasma membranes (because α-tubulin is mainly cytoplasmic) is taken into consideration, IRAS was still more abundant in plasma membranes than in cytosolic fractions (see FIG. 1A, FIG. 2). This finding indicated that the presence of transfected human $\alpha_{2A}AR$ protein did little to change the subcellular distribution of endogenous CHO IRAS immunoreactivity.

Transient transfection of WT CHO cells with *pIRAS* led to a rise in IRAS immunoreactivity (170-kD band, see FIG. 1A, FIG. 2). The level of human IRAS in *pIRAS*-transfected WT CHO cells was estimated by subtraction of endogenous 170-kD immunoreactivity in each subline. The overall IRAS level in transfected WT CHO cells was thus calculated to be two times higher than in vector-only or untransfected controls. Approximately half the rise was associated with plasma membranes and half with the cytosolic fraction in WT CHO cells (FIG. 2). Compared with WT CHO cells transiently transfected with *pcDNA3.1* (vector only), *pIRAS*-transfected WT CHO

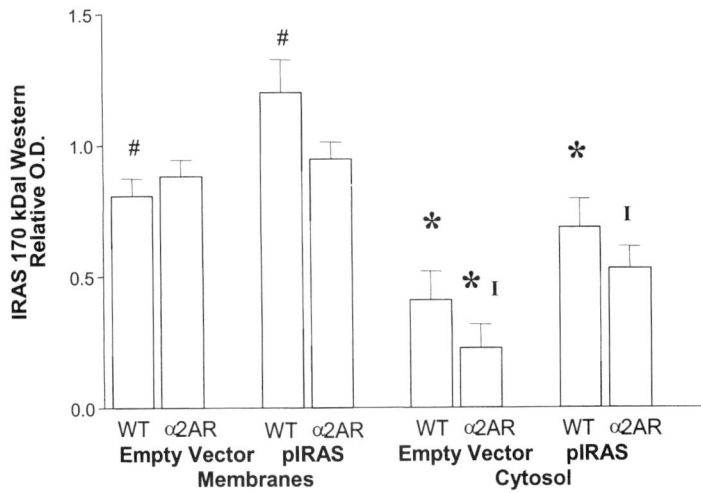

FIGURE 2. Relative ODs of 170-kD IRAS band (putative I_1R) as revealed by Western blotting in transfected CHO lines. Each condition was repeated at least three times and statistically compared by two-tailed unpaired t-tests. Values are expressed as IRAS band OD per α-tubulin 44-kD band OD in each lane. Bars superscripted by common typographic symbols denote means that are significantly different (minimum $P < 0.05$) from each other. The four comparisons on the left are among membrane fractions (e.g., # denotes that *pIRAS*-transfected WT CHO cells had more membranous 170-kD immunodensity than WT CHO cells transfected with empty vector). The four comparisons on the right are among cytosolic fractions (e.g., ∗ denotes that *pIRAS*-transfected WT CHO had more cytosolic 170-kD immunodensity than wild-type CHO cells transfected with empty vector; **I** denotes that *pIRAS*-transfected CHO-$α_{2A}$AR had more cytosolic 170-kD immunodensity than CHO-$α_{2A}$AR-transfected with only the empty vector).

cells thus showed elevations of 40% and 55% in the 170-kD bands of plasma membrane and cytosolic fractions, respectively.

IRAS immunoreactivity comparisons were also made in *pIRAS*-transfected CHO-$α_{2A}$AR cells. Only a small difference was found in comparison to the results in *pIRAS*-transfected WT CHO cells. IRAS immunoreactivity in *pIRAS*-transfected CHO-$α_{2A}$AR cells was more cytosolic rather than equal between fractions (FIG. 2). That is, WT CHO cells transfected with *pIRAS* displayed a clear rise in both membranous and cytosolic 170-kD bands, but only in the cytosolic fraction was the transfection of IRAS apparent in CHO-$α_{2A}$AR cells (FIG. 2).

Additional studies were performed on endogenous $α_2$AR immunoreactivity. Again, focus was first on the CHO-$α_{2A}$AR subline compared with WT CHO cells (see FIG. 1B, FIG. 3). Using antiserum selective for human $α_{2A}$AR,[29] the CHO-$α_{2A}$AR cell line was found to possess at least twice the immunoreactivity in the 66-kD range relative to untransfected WT CHO cells (see FIG. 1B, FIG. 3). Nonetheless, a low level of unidentified immunoreactivity was detected in the 66-kD range on Western blots of untransfected WT CHO or vector-only CHO plasma membranes (see FIG. 1B, FIG. 3). Because WT CHO cells lack $α_2$AR binding sites, this immunoreactivity is assumed to be background material.

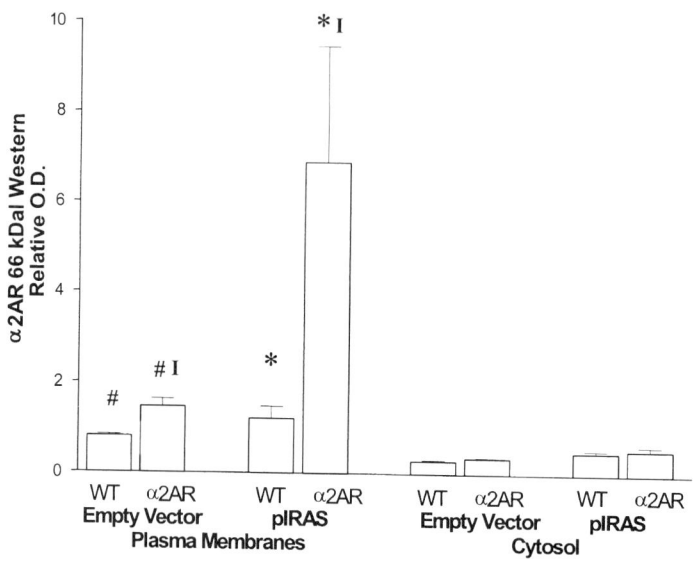

FIGURE 3. Relative ODs of 66-kD $\alpha_{2A}AR$ band as revealed by Western blotting in transfected CHO sublines. Values are expressed as $\alpha_{2A}AR$ band OD per α-tubulin 44-kD band OD in each lane. Background film immunostaining is shown in cytosol fractions. Bars linked by common typographic symbols denote means that are significantly different (minimum $P < 0.05$). Each condition was repeated at least three times and statistically compared by two-tailed unpaired t-tests. No effects of empty vector transfection alone were observed. # denotes that CHO-$\alpha_{2A}AR$ cells showed statistically more 66-kD immunoreactivity compared with WT CHO cells (the latter considered as background staining). * denotes that level of 66-kD band was greater in CHO-α_{2A} AR cells transfected with *pIRAS* relative to WT CHO cells transfected with *pIRAS* (the latter also considered background). **I** denotes that the level of 66-kD band was 4-fold greater in CHO-$\alpha_{2A}AR$ cells transfected with *pIRAS* relative to CHO-$\alpha_{2A}AR$ cells transfected with only the empty vector.

The effect of transiently expressed human IRAS on human $\alpha_{2A}AR$ was next studied by Western blotting in the cotransfected CHO-$\alpha_{2A}AR$ cell line. Unexpectedly, Western blots of CHO-$\alpha_{2A}AR$ cells cotransfected with *pIRAS* showed a large increase in membranous $\alpha_{2A}AR$ immunoreactivity relative to untransfected CHO-$\alpha_{2A}AR$ cells or to CHO-$\alpha_{2A}AR$ cells transfected with only *pcDNA3.1* (intense band of FIG. 1B). Following normalization to α-tubulin, this increase represented about a fivefold increase in $\alpha_{2A}AR$ resulting from IRAS (FIG. 3). Thus, a twofold increase mostly in the cytoplasmic form of human IRAS (see FIG. 2) was associated with a fivefold increase in the membrane form of human $\alpha_{2A}AR$ immunoreactivity in cotransfected cells (FIG. 3). No effect of *pIRAS* transfection was found in cytosolic fractions (i.e., cytoplasmic background staining of α_2AR did not change under any conditions).

Saturation radioligand binding measurements of I_1R and $\alpha_{2A}AR$ in the two CHO lines were next obtained to confirm the Western blotting data. Transfection of *pIRAS* into WT CHO cells resulted in a twofold increase in I_1R density (B_{max}) values in plasma membranes compared with background levels in control cells transfected

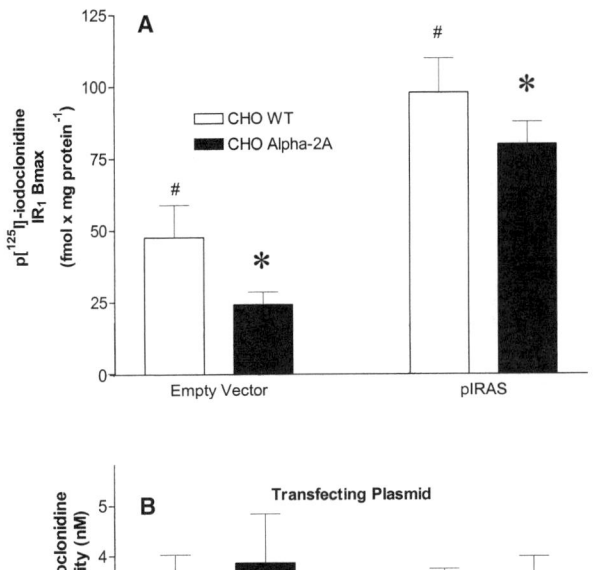

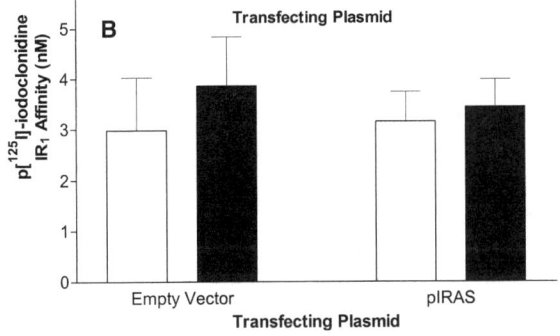

FIGURE 4. Radioligand binding data for I_1R sites in transfected CHO cell membranes from two CHO lines: CHO-α_{2A}AR (*solid bars*) versus CHO WT (*open bars*). Saturation-binding experiments of nonadrenergic sites were performed with [^{125}I]-*p*-iodoclonidine under masking concentrations using NE to eliminate α_2AR sites. The *upper panel* (**A**) displays I_1R-like binding site density (B_{max}), and the *lower panel* (**B**) displays affinity (K_D). The main comparison is between transfection of *pIRAS* and the transfection of empty vector. Bars linked by common typographic symbols denote means that are significantly different ($P < 0.05$). Each condition was repeated at least three times and statistically compared by two-tailed unpaired *t*-tests.

with vector only, *pcDNA3.1* (FIG. 4A, *open bars*). In similar manner, a threefold increase in I_1R B_{max} was found in CHO-α_{2A}AR membranes transfected with *pIRAS* relative to those cells transfected with the empty vector, *pcDNA3.1* (FIG. 4A, *solid bars*). There were no changes in the K_D affinity constants observed for I_1R binding in either of the CHO lines transfected with either *pcDNA3.1* or with *pIRAS* (FIG. 4B). The higher levels of I_1R expression in transfected WT CHO cells (FIG. 4A) were similar to those seen by IRAS Western blotting (see FIG. 2).

Similar to earlier Western blot evidence for IRAS enhancement of membrane α_{2A}AR immunoreactivity (see FIG. 1, FIG. 3), there was a clear increase in the B_{max}

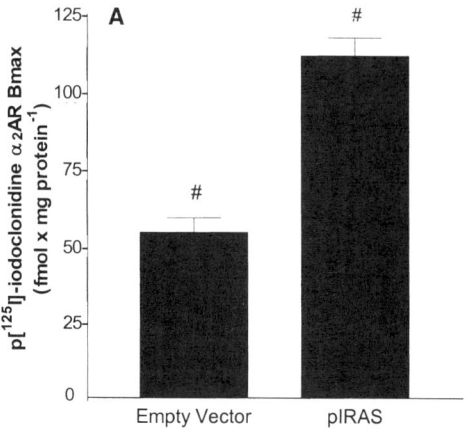

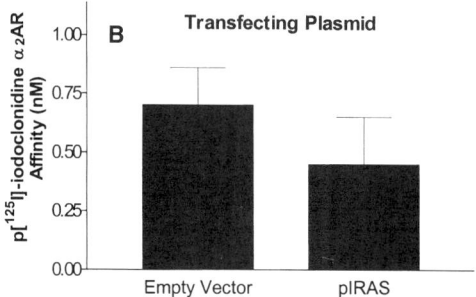

FIGURE 5. Radioligand binding data for α_2AR in transfected cell membranes from the lines of CHO cells expressing human α_{2A}AR (CHO-α_{2A}AR) without or with human IRAS (empty vector versus pIRAS co-transfection). Saturation binding experiments were performed with [^{125}I]-p-iodoclonidine, without masking. Norepinephrine was used to define selectively the nonspecific binding of α_2AR sites. The *upper panel* (**A**) displays α_2AR binding site density (B_{max}), and the *lower panel* (**B**) displays affinity (K_D). Comparing transfection of pIRAS to that of empty vector revealed that for α_{2A}AR the density increased about twofold. The $B_{max} \pm$ SE were vector-only, 54.9 ± 4.9 fmol $\times$ mg protein^{-1}; plus *pIRAS*, 113.5 ± 6.1 fmol $\times$ mg protein^{-1} ($^\# P < 0.05$). No change was seen in the affinity ($K_D \pm$ standard errors: vector only, 0.70 ± 0.16 nM; plus *pIRAS*, 0.45 ± 0.20 nM). Results with empty-vector CHO-α_{2A}AR cells were the same as in untransfected CHO-α_{2A}AR cells (the latter not shown). No α_2AR sites were detected in wild-type parent CHO cells with or without *pIRAS*-transfection (not shown). Each condition was repeated at least three times and statistically compared by two-tailed unpaired t-tests.

of α_2AR in *pIRAS*-transfected CHO-α_AAR plasma membranes compared with vector-only controls (FIG. 5A).

There was, however, no significant change in α_{2A}AR affinity (FIG. 5B) with respect to untransfected or vector-only controls. The WT CHO cells transiently transfected with either empty vector (*pcDNA3.1*) or *pIRAS*, continued to show low levels of background α_2AR binding sites (data not shown). Thus, transfection of human IRAS in the CHO-α_AAR subline seemed to have induced an increase in α_2AR binding sites.

DISCUSSION

The present findings indicate that transfection of human IRAS into CHO cells leads to I_1R-like radiolabeled clonidine binding (with nanomolar affinity similar to cotransfected human $\alpha_{2A}AR^{32,29,3}$), and causes increased expression of $\alpha_{2A}AR$ in plasma membranes of the same cells. These findings are the first evidence for an intracellular interaction between $\alpha_{2A}AR$ and IRAS.

There are no known bodily tissues in which I_1R and α_2AR binding sites do not coexist to some extent;[33] with certain cultured cell types excluded.[34] Both receptors coexist in many cells[35–37] and mediate some of the same physiologic responses.[1,37] From a cardiovascular perspective, both $\alpha_{2A}AR$ and I_1R seem to be involved in the central inhibition of sympathetic drive,[1,38] although their respective central sites of action seem to be different.[7,29,39] Treatments in the peripheral nervous system with imidazoline compounds also can mediate inhibitions of NE release in both adrenergic and nonadrenergic manners,[40,41] suggesting that $\alpha_{2A}AR$ and a subtype of IR reside on the same sympathetic nerve endings.[42] Correlations have also been established for receptor densities (B_{max}) between $\alpha_{2A}AR$ and I_1R on human platelet purified plasma membranes[43] as well as across multiple brain regions,[44] suggesting that these sites may be coregulated. Moreover, I_1R platelet density (B_{max}) has been reported[45] to be positively correlated with plasma NE concentrations. α_2AR and I_1R have been proposed to act synergistically based on several functional studies.[25,29]

At least four lines of evidence predating our findings support functional interactions between α_2AR and imidazoline receptors in vivo. (1) Göthert and colleagues[42] have provided evidence for cofunctional α_2AR and "non I_1R /non I_2R" within postganglionic sympathetic nerve terminals. By measuring electrically evoked NE release in response to treatments with various imidazoline and guanidine agents, these investigators showed that the two presynaptic receptors responded coincidently as imidazoline-mediated α_2AR antagonism and IR agonism, respectively.[42] (2) Head and colleagues[46] have also performed dose–response experiments by microinjecting imidazolines and other specific α_2AR antagonists into the RVLM of conscious rabbits to quantify hypotensive effects. They found evidence for α_2AR and I_1R interactions "in series" in the RVLM.[46] From this finding, they proposed that I_1Rs exist upstream on presynaptic neurons that synapse with the cell bodies of sympathoinhibitory neurons that in turn process α_2AR signals.[7] (3) Bousquet and colleagues[25,29] have taken further advantage of newer selective I_1R agents (e.g., LP509) to demonstrate synergistic effects of combined I_1R and α_2AR stimulation. The synergism they reported[29,30] between α-methy-NE (a non-hydrolyzable α_2AR agonist) and LP509 was not observed in D79N mutant mice lacking functional α_2AR.[29,39] (4) Evidence for cross-talk between I_1R and α_2AR also comes from clinical studies. It has been reported that positive correlations exist between the receptor densities of α_2AR and I_1R sites in platelets of blood donors[43] and in different human brain regions after autopsy.[44] Thus, several types of interactions between α_2AR and I_1R have long been suspected.

In what manner might IRAS exert its effect on membranous $\alpha_{2A}AR$ density? Both the Western blotting data (see FIGS. 1–3) and the radioligand binding data (see FIGS. 3 and 4) indicated that on transfection of WT CHO cells with human IRAS cDNA the level of IRAS in plasma membranes and cytosols was increased severalfold.[27] By comparison, in the CHO-$\alpha_{2A}AR$ cells co-transfected with human IRAS cDNA, only the level of cytosolic IRAS immunoreactivity (not membranous IRAS immunoreactivity) was statistically increased, as compared with that of CHO- $\alpha_{2A}AR$ cells transfected with empty vector only (see FIG. 2). This increase in cytosolic IRAS immunoreactivity was about twofold above the endogenous IRAS level (see FIG. 2) and was concordant with a twofold rise in I_1 B_{max} values (see FIG. 4A). The membrane preparations used for radiolgand binding experiments were purified plasma membranes (internal membranes excluded), whereas total membrane preparations were used for Western blotting. In any case, the results suggest that the greater increase in cytosolic IRAS, as compared with membranous IRAS, may actually be linked to an increased expression of $\alpha_{2A}AR$ in membranes. This effect may result from the interaction of cytosolic IRAS with the intracellular side of the $\alpha_{2A}AR$ in membranes. Future studies will be required to test this hypothesis.

In summary, co-transfection studies have revealed that human IRAS binds radiolabeled clonidine with nanomolar affinity similar to that of $\alpha_{2A}AR$ and also in some manner causes increased expression of $\alpha_{2A}AR$ in plasma membranes. Future studies will be required to determine if the $\alpha_{2A}AR$ and IRAS make physical contact. Alternatively, they may interact through a secondary signaling mechanism (e.g., phosphorylation). The present finding of an intracellular effect of IRAS on $\alpha_{2A}AR$ may be relevant to the long-standing controversy concerning the role of I_1R in the action of clonidine and other imidazoline compounds in hypotension. Therefore, coincidence activation of both targets may best explain clonidine's properties.

ACKNOWLEDGMENT

This project was supported by a grant from the National Institute of Mental Health (R01 MH49248).

REFERENCES

1. BOUSQUET, P., J. FELDMAN, E. TIBIRICA, et al. 1989. New concepts on the central regulation of blood pressure. Alpha 2-adrenoceptors and "imidazoline receptors." Am. J. Med. **87:** 10S–13S.
2. PILETZ, J.E., A. HALARIS & P.R. ERNSBERGER. 1994. Psychopharmacology of imidazoline and alpha 2-adrenergic receptors: implications for depression. Crit. Rev. Neurobiol. **9:** 29–66.
3. ERNSBERGER, P., M.E. GRAVES, L.M. GRAFF, et al. 1995. I1-Imidazoline receptors: definition, characterization, distribution and transmembrane signalling. Ann. N. Y. Acad. Sci. **763:** 22–42.
4. MOLDERINGS, G.J. 1997. Imidazoline receptors: basic knowledge, recent advances and future prospects for therapy. Drugs of the Future **22:** 757–772.
5. ERNSBERGER, P. & M.A. HAXHIU. 1997. The I1-imidazoline-binding site is a functional receptor mediating vasodepression via the ventral medulla. Am. J. Physiol. **42:** R1572–R1579.
6. ALTMAN, J.D., A.U. TRENDELENBURG, L. MACMILLAN, et al. 1999. Abnormal regulation of the sympathetic nervous system in alpha2A-adrenergic receptor knockout mice. Mol. Pharmacol. **56:** 154–161.
7. HEAD, G.A. 1999. Central imidazoline- and alpha 2-receptors involved in the cardiovascular actions of centrally acting antihypertensive agents. Ann. N. Y. Acad. Sci. **881:** 279–286.
8. REIS, D.J. 1996. Neurons and receptors in the rostroventrolateral medulla mediating the antihypertensive actions of drugs acting at imidazoline receptors. J. Cardiovasc. Pharmacol. **27**(Suppl 3): S11–S18.

9. RUIZ-ORTEGA, J.A., L. UGEDO, J. PINEDA, et al. 1995. The stimulatory effect of clonidine through imidazoline receptors on locus coeruleus noradrenergic neurones is mediated by excitatory amino acids and modulated by serotonin. Naunyn Schmiedeberg's Arch. Pharmacol. **352:** 121–126.
10. ZHU, H., I.A. PAUL, D.E. STEC, et al. 2003. Non-adrenergic exploratory behavior induced by moxonidine at mildly hypotensive doses in mice. Brain Res. **964:** 9–20.
11. ERNSBERGER, P., Y.R. KOU & N.R. PRABHAKAR. 1998. Carotid body I1-imidazoline receptors: binding, visualization and modulatory function. Respir. Physiol. **112:** 239–251.
12. TSOLI, E., S.L. CHAN & N.G. MORGAN. 1995. The imidazoline I1 receptor agonist, moxonidine, inhibits insulin secretion from isolated rat islets of Langerhans. Eur. J. Pharmacol. **284:** 199–203.
13. ROSEN, P., P. OHLY & H. GLEICHMANN. 1997. Experimental benefit of moxonidine on glucose metabolism and insulin secretion in the fructose-fed rat. J. Hypertens. Suppl. **15:** S31–S38.
14. SANO, H., S.C. LIU, W.S. LANE, et al. 2002. Insulin receptor substrate 4 associates with the protein IRAS. J. Biol. Chem. **23:** 23.
15. SMYTH, D.D. & S.B. PENNER. 1998. Imidazoline receptor mediated natriuresis: central and/or peripheral effect? J. Auton. Nerv. Sys. **72:** 155–162.
16. KONNERTH, A., R. TSIEN, K. MIKOSHIBA, et al. 1996. Coincidence Detection in the Nervous System: 175. Human Frontiers Science Program. Strasbourg, France.
17. SCHLICKER, E. & M. GÖTHERT. 1998. Interactions between the presynaptic alpha2-autoreceptor and presynaptic inhibitory heteroreceptors on noradrenergic neurones. Brain Res. Bull. **47:** 129–132.
18. LIU, F., Q. WAN, Z.B. PRISTUPA, et al. 2000. Direct protein-protein coupling enables cross-talk between dopamine D5 and gamma-aminobutyric acid A receptors. Nature **403:** 274–280.
19. LOPES, L.V., R.A. CUNHA & J.A. RIBEIRO. 1999. Cross talk between A(1) and A(2A) adenosine receptors in the hippocampus and cortex of young adult and old rats. J. Neurophysiol. **82:** 3196–3203.
20. CIRUELA, F., M. ESCRICHE, J. BURGUENO, et al. 2001. Metabotropic glutamate 1alpha and adenosine A1 receptors assemble into functionally interacting complexes. J. Biol. Chem. **276:** 18345–18351.
21. MAYFIELD, R.D., B.A. JONES, H.A. MILLER, et al. 1999. Modulation of endogenous GABA release by an antagonistic adenosine A1/dopamineD1 receptor interaction in rat brain limbic regions but not basal ganglia. Synapse **33:** 274–281.
22. BUDD, D.C., R.A. CHALLISS, K.W. YOUNG, et al. 1999. Cross talk between m3-muscarinic and beta(2)-adrenergic receptors at the level of receptor phosphorylation and desensitization. Mol. Pharmacol. **56:** 813–823.
23. ROCHEVILLE, M., D.C. LANGE, U. KUMAR, et al. 2000. Receptors for dopamine and somatostatin: formation of hetero-oligomers with enhanced functional activity. Science **288:** 154–157.
24. LEZCANO, N., L. MRZLJAK, S. EUBANKS, et al. 2000. Dual signaling regulated by calcyon, a D1 dopamine receptor interacting protein. Science **287:** 1660–1664.
25. BRUBAN, V., J. FELDMAN, H. GRENEY, et al. 2001. Respective contributions of alpha-adrenergic and non-adrenergic mechanisms in the hypotensive effect of imidazoline-like drugs. Br. J. Pharmacol. **133:** 261–266.
26. COTECCHIA, S., B.K. KOBILKA, K.W. DANIEL, et al. 1990. Multiple second messenger pathways of alpha-adrenergic receptor subtypes expressed in eukaryotic cells. J. Biol. Chem. **265:** 63–69.
27. PILETZ, J.E., T.R. IVANOV, J.D. SHARP, et al. 2000. Imidazoline receptor antisera-selected (IRAS) cDNA: cloning and characterization. DNA Cell Biol. **19:** 319–329.
28. IVANOV, T.R., H. ZHU, S. REGUNATHAN, et al. 1998. Co-detection by two imidazoline receptor protein antisera of a novel 85 kilodalton protein. Biochem. Pharmacol. **55:** 649–655.
29. KUROSE, H., J.L. ARRIZA & R.J. LEFKOWITZ. 1993. Characterization of alpha-2-adrenergic receptor subtype-specific antibodies. Mol. Pharmacol. **43:** 444–450.
30. PILETZ, J.E., H. ZHU, G. ORDWAY, et al. 2000. Imidazoline receptor proteins are decreased in the hippocampus of individuals with major depression. Biol. Psychiatry **48:** 910–919.

31. PILETZ, J.E. & K. SLETTEN. 1993. Nonadrenergic imidazoline binding sites on human platelets. J. Pharmacol. Exp. Ther. **267:** 1493–1502.
32. BUCCAFUSCO, J.J. 1992. Neuropharmacologic and behavioral actions of clonidine: interactions with central neurotransmitters. *In* International Review of Neurobiology: 55–107. Academic Press, San Diego, CA.
33. PILETZ, J.E., J.C. JONES, H. ZHU, *et al.* 1999. Imidazoline receptor antisera-selected cDNA clone and mRNA distribution. Ann. N. Y. Acad. Sci. **881:** 1–7.
34. ORDENER, C., H. GRENEY, J. DEVEDJIAN, *et al.* 1999. Transfected cells expressing the three subtypes of alpha 2-adrenergic receptors lack I1-imidazoline binding sites. Ann. N. Y. Acad. Sci. **881:** 59–60.
35. PILETZ, J.E., A.C. ANDORN, J.R. UNNERSTALL, *et al.* 1991. Binding of [3H]-p-aminoclonidine to a2-adrenoceptor states plus a non-adrenergic site on human platelet plasma membranes. Biochem. Pharmacol. **42:** 569–584.
36. IVANOV, T.R., Y. FENG, H. WANG, *et al.* 1998. Imidazoline receptor proteins are regulated in platelet-precursor MEG-01 cells by agonists and antagonists. J. Psychiatr. Res. **32:** 65–79.
37. MOLDERINGS, G.J., H. BONISCH, R. HAMMERMANN, *et al.* 2002. Noradrenaline release-inhibiting receptors on PC12 cells devoid of alpha(2(-)) and CB(1) receptors: similarities to presynaptic imidazoline and edg receptors. Neurochem. Int. **40:** 157–167.
38. ERNSBERGER, P., R. GIULIANO, R.N. WILLETTE, *et al.* 1990. Role of imidazole receptors in the vasopressor response to clonidine analogs in the rostral ventrolateral medulla. J. Pharmacol. Exp. Ther. **253:** 408–418.
39. TOLENTINO-SILVA, F.P., M.A. HAXHIU, S. WALDBAUM, *et al.* 2000. Alpha(2) adrenergic receptors are not required for central anti-hypertensive action of moxonidine in mice. Brain Res. **862:** 26–35.
40. FUDER, H. & P. SCHWARZ. 1993. Desensitization of inhibitory prejunctional alpha 2-adrenoceptors and putative imidazoline receptors on rabbit heart sympathetic nerves. Naunyn Schmiedeberg's Arch. Pharmacol. **348:** 127–133.
41. GÖTHERT, M. & G.J. MOLDERINGS. 1991. Involvement of presynaptic imidazoline receptors in the alpha 2-adrenoceptor-independent inhibition of noradrenaline release by imidazoline derivatives. Naunyn Schmiedeberg's Arch. Pharmacol. **343:** 271–282.
42. GÖTHERT, M., G.J. MOLDERINGS, K. FINK, *et al.* 1995. Alpha 2-adrenoceptor-independent inhibition by imidazolines and guanidines of noradrenaline release from peripheral, but not central noradrenergic neurons. Ann. N. Y. Acad. Sci. **763:** 405–419.
43. PILETZ, J.E. & A. HALARIS. 1995. Involvement of I1-imidazoline receptors in mood disorders. Ann. N. Y. Acad. Sci. **763:** 510–519.
44. PILETZ, J.E., G.A. ORDWAY, H. ZHU, *et al.* 2000. Autoradiographic comparison of [3H]-clonidine binding to non-adrenergic sites and alpha2-adrenergic receptors in human brain. Neuropsychopharmacology **23:** 697–708.
45. PILETZ, J.E., M. ANDREW, H. ZHU, *et al.* 1998. Alpha 2-adrenoceptors and I1-imidazoline binding sites: relationship with catecholamines in women of reproductive age. J. Psychiatr. Res. **32:** 55–64.
46. HEAD, G.A., C.K.S. CHAN & S.L. BURKE. 1998. Relationship between imidazoline and α2-adrenoreceptors involved in the sympatho-inhibitory actions of centrally acting antihypertensive agents. J. Auton. Nerv. Sys. **72:** 163–169.

Relationship between Platelet Imidazoline Receptor-Binding Peptides and Candidate Imidazoline-1 Receptor, IRAS

HE ZHU,[a] JONATHAN HAYES,[b] MICHAEL CHEN,[a] JAMES BALDWIN,[a] AND JOHN E. PILETZ[a,b]

[a]*Department of Psychiatry, University of Mississippi Medical Center, Jackson, Mississippi 39216, USA*

[b]*Department of Biology, Jackson State University, Jackson, Mississippi 39217, USA*

> ABSTRACT: A candidate human imidazoline-1 receptor, designated imidazoline receptor antisera-selected (IRAS) protein, was cloned based on immunoreactivity with antiserum against a purified imidazoline receptor binding peptide (IRBP antiserum). Human IRAS is 167 kD in size, different from 33- to 85-kD IRBP bands previously linked to the human platelet I_1 receptor. To explore the possible relationship between IRAS and these smaller proteins, seven different epitope-specific antisera against IRAS were raised in rabbits for comparison with IRBP antiserum. Focus was on antiserum$_{227-241}$, corresponding to amino acids #227 to 241 in IRAS, because this antiserum was found uniquely able to immunoprecipitate non-denatured 85-kD and 170-kD forms of IRAS from a human megakaryoblastoma cell line (MEG01), a model of platelet-producing cells. Human platelets lacked the 170-kD form of IRAS, but 33-kD and 85-kD bands were detectable and seemed to be possible fragments of full-length IRAS. The intensity of the 85-kD band detected by antiserum$_{227-241}$ was significantly correlated ($r = 0.62$, $P = 0.04$) with the intensity of the 33-kD band across 11 human platelet samples. A positive correlation between the intensities of the 33-kD and 85-kD bands is consistent with both being fragments of IRAS.
>
> KEYWORDS: imidazoline receptors; platelets; IRAS, Nischarin; antiserum

INTRODUCTION

IRAS, the candidate imidazoline-1 receptor protein, was cloned from a human hippocampal $\lambda\lambda$gt11 cDNA expression library[1,2] using antiserum developed by Reis and coworkers,[3] which has been designated imidazoline receptor binding peptide (IRBP) antiserum.[3] Transfection of human IRAS cDNA into Chinese Hamster ovary (CHO) cells led to the appearance of radioligand binding sites consistent with I_1 receptor pharmacology.[2] Transfection of the 5,131 base pair (bp) cDNA of IRAS encoded a surprisingly large protein (1504 amino acids), however.[2] Furthermore, the sequence of IRAS bears little similarity to other families of neurotransmitter receptors.[2]

Address for correspondence: He Zhu, M.D., Department of Psychiatry, University of Mississippi Medical Center, 2500 North State Street, Jackson, MS 39216-4505, USA. Voice: 601-984-5798; fax: 601-984-5899.

e-mail: HZhu@psychiatry.umsmed.edu

The size of transfected human IRAS (170 kD) after denaturing SDS polyacrylamide gel electrophoresis (SDS-PAGE), is different from 33- to 35-kD, 43- to 45-kD, or 85-kD candidate proteins previously reported[4–6] as candidates for the human I_1 receptor. To better understand better the possible relationship between these molecules, we describe in this report seven epitope-selective antisera to various domains of human IRAS. The amino acid (aa) sequence of epitopic peptide #227-241 in IRAS is unique, not found in other public databases. Herein, the antiserum to this peptide is also shown to be unique in detecting appropriately-sized bands on Western blots (i.e., 85-kD, 33-kD, and 170-kD bands) as known I_1-receptor candidates. Additional studies are presented to indicate that antiserum$_{227\text{-}241}$ can immunoprecipitate native 170-kD and 85-kD IRAS proteins. Furthermore, a comparison is made between the proteins detected proportionately in antiserum$_{227\text{-}241}$ and in the original IRBP antiserum.

MATERIALS AND METHODS

Preparation of Antisera

Two epitope-selective antisera, directed at mid-regions of IRAS, have already been described.[2] They were formerly known as 1201 and 1209 antisera, respectively.[2] Herein, we renamed them antiserum$_{648\text{-}671}$ and antiserum$_{783\text{-}809}$ based on the aa sequences they target within IRAS. To supplement these antisera, five new 14-mer peptides and their associated epitope-selective antisera were produced by Genosys (The Woodlands, TX, USA). The design of the peptides was based on their uniqueness in public databases, ease of chemical synthesis, likelihood of being immunogenic, and to cover three N-terminal domains (aas #8–22, #79–92, and #227–241) and two C-terminal domains (aas #1113–1126 and #1444–1458). Each peptide was conjugated with Keyhole limpet hemocyanin (KLH), the unconjugated end was amidated, and an emulsion was injected into two rabbits (six immunizations/animal). The rabbits were injected six times over a 70-day period and bled at 0, 7, 9, 11, and 15 weeks (the final bleed). Each antiserum differed in titer by ELISA against its antigen (the peptide). A range was found from the fourth bleed of antiserum$_{227\text{-}241}$ at 1:75,000 dilution being equivalent to the second bleed at 1:20,000 dilution. For comparative Western blotting, dilutions were made so that all titers were the same.

Immunoprecipitation

The human megakaryoblastoma cell line, MEG01, was grown as previously described.[7] This cell line has been shown to possess I_1 radioligand binding sites.[7] Solubilized membrane proteins were prepared according to Amersham protocols RPN 2202 and 2203 (Piscataway, NJ, USA). The method involved suspension of cells in isotonic buffer containing 1% NP-40 and protease inhibitors without mechanical lysis. The immunoprecipitation procedure employed protein G as per Amersham RPN 2202 and 2203.

Subjects

Eleven adult human subjects were recruited through local advertisements. They signed consent forms approved by the Institutional Review Board. The female:male ratio was 9:2. The overall mean age was 38.9 years ± 12.9 SD). All subjects passed a physical examination and were unmedicated at the time of blood drawing.

Western Blotting

The seven epitope-selective antisera to IRAS were compared as probes against two Western blots containing (1) a common batch of authentic human IRAS expressed in Sf9 cell membranes as previously described,[2] and (2) a common batch of purified plasma membranes from human platelets. Antiserum$_{227-241}$ and IRBP antiserum were subsequently used to study 11 fresh samples of platelet plasma membranes from the same subjects. Fresh blood platelets were prepared as previously described.[8] Samples (7.5 μg protein in 15 μL) were denatured and electrophoresed through 13.7% denaturing polyacrylamide gels (SDS-PAGE) and then electrotransferred onto nitrocellulose membranes. Prestained molecular weight *(MW)* markers were included in each gel (Bio-Rad, Laboratories, Hercules, CA, USA; low range). The blots were incubated 2 hours either with antiserum$_{227-241}$ plus saturating KLP (1 mg) to obscure any reactivity with carrier protein, or with antiserum to IRBP (1:3,000 dilution) at 21°C. Detection involved horseradish peroxidase-conjugated donkey anti-rabbit IgG antiserum (1:3,000 dilution) and Amersham's Enhanced Chemiluminesence (ECL) detection system followed by film exposure (Hyperfilm, Amersham, Arlington Heights, IL, USA). The nitrocellulose membranes were subsequently stripped and integrin β3 chain subunit (CD 61 antigen) was also assessed as a protein reference. Integrin β3 was also detected by ECL using a monoclonal antibody (clone RUU-PL 7F12) from Becton Dickinson (San Jose, CA, USA) diluted 1:3,000, and sheep anti-mouse IgG at 1:3,000 dilution. Densitometry was performed with the Image Quant program (Molecular Dynamics, Sunnyvale, CA, USA). Optical density (OD) values from different blots were compared based on a standard curve within each blot (composed of 3.5, 7.5, and 11.5 μg protein from a common batch of platelet purified membranes obtained from Mississippi Blood Services). Samples were analyzed at least twice on different gel blots, and the results were averaged.

RESULTS

Anti-IRAS sera were first compared on Western blots against authentic human IRAS expressed in membranes from transfected Sf9 insect cells. The results are summarized in TABLE 1. The results were obtained with at least three separate bleeds from two rabbits per targeted epitope, not seen in control lanes against untransfected Sf9 cells, and none of the bands were detectable when pre-immune antisera was used to probe. As indicated, multiple bands were seen with most antisera, except at the C-terminal end of IRAS where antiserum$_{1444-1458}$ reacted with a single band, which was 38 kD in size. Unfortunately, neither of the two C-terminal epitopes was detectable within full-length IRAS on Western blots (TABLE 1). Another two antisera directed at mid regions of IRAS (aas #648–671 and #783–809) reacted strongly with the 170-kD band of IRAS, but neither of these antisera reacted with band sizes of 85 kD or smaller. Then, the three N-terminal antisera reacted similarly with bands in a size range (33–85 kD) previously suggested to be imidazoline-1 receptor proteins. Among the N-terminal antisera, antiserum$_{227-241}$ reacted strongest with the full-

TABLE 1. Antigenicity against human IRAS in transfected Sf9 membranes as revealed by Western blotting

Peptide Epitope	Amino Acid Sequence on IRAS (Nos.)	Approximate Molecular Weights	
		Strong Sites (kD)	Weak Sites (kD)
NTP-1	GPEREAEPAKEARV (8–22)	120, **85**, 80, 75, (doublet at ~45), 38, 36, **33**	**170**, 25
NTP-2	KNSRSLVEKREKDL (79–92)	120, **85**, 80, 75, 65, (doublet at ~45), 38, 36, **33**	**170**, 25
NTP-3	DAKHIRGLVASKPT (227–241)	**170**, 75, 70, 65, 60, 45	120, **85**, 38, 36, **33**
1201	DVAENRYFEMGPPD VEEEEGGGQG (648–671)	**170**	150
1209	KVRHSENTLFIISDAA NLHEFHADLRS (783–809)	**170**, 150, 120	150
CTP-1	QATSEENQIPSHLP (1,113–1,126)	120, 90, 80	45
CTP-2	GSVTLDHFGEVPGGP (1,444–1,458)		38*

Inclusion criteria required bands to be revealed with postimmune antisera, and they had to be reproducibly revealed when probed with replicate rabbits' antisera. Exclusion criteria were any bands that appeared in untransfected Sf9 membranes (unless markedly enhanced) or that appeared in the pre-immune sera as well as in the postimmune antisera. Numbers in bold indicate appropriately sized bands based on the full-length size of IRAS (170 kD) and the bands from human platelets under investigation in this study (85 kD and 33 kD).

* A weak approximately 38-kD band in CTP-2 appeared in both rabbits that were immunized with this peptide, but it was not detected by the pre-immune sera nor present in untransfected Sf9 membranes. One rabbit immunized with CTP-2 revealed a strong doublet band at approximately 65 kD, which was completely absent in the other rabbit's antisera for the same peptide.

length form of IRAS (170 kD) on Western blots. Thus, antiserum$_{227-241}$ had the strongest immunoreactivity for the bands of interest.

The second level of analysis involved screening all antisera for ability to immunoprecipitate human IRAS from solubilized cells. Membranes from human MEG01 cells were solubilized with 1% NP-40 detergent, and a series of immunoprecipitations were analyzed on Western blots. The first step involved incubation for 3 hours with pre-immune antiserum (the clearing pellet: 1P). Supernatant from this step was then incubated with the epitopic antiserum of choice (antiserum$_{227-241}$). After another 3-hour incubation, the mixture was centrifuged, and comparisons were made of equal protein loads of thrice-washed immunoprecipitate-1 (2P), its supernatant (SN), and the thrice-washed pre-immune antiserum's pellet (1P). To determine specificity further, the blots were probed with a different anti-IRAS serum than that used for the immunoprecipitations (antiserum$_{783-809}$). Results were considered positive

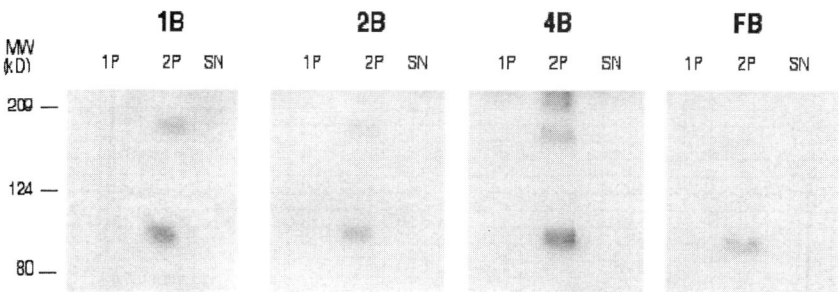

FIGURE 1. Immunoprecipitation of IRAS from human MEG01 cells using rabbit antiserum$_{227-241}$ against IRAS. The procedure was a standardized one following Amersham RPN 2202 and 2203 protocols. Cells (10^9) were gently incubated for 20 minutes at 4°C in hypotonic medium with 1% NP-40 plus protease inhibitors.[6] The supernatant from these cells was cleared by incubation for 3 hours with pre-immune antiserum plus protein G, which gave rise to the first pellet, 1P. The remaining cleared supernatant was incubated for 3 hours with one of several bleeds from a single rabbit immunized against epitope 227–241 of human IRAS. This gave rise to two more fractions, 2P and SN. Equal protein loads from all fractions were suspended 1:1 with 40 uL loading buffer, boiled to denature, and loaded onto a 7.5% acrylamide gel for SDS-PAGE and subsequent Western blotting onto nitrocellulose filters. Western blots were probed with antiserum$_{783-809}$ against a different epitope in the center of IRAS. Films were exposed to 15 minutes of ECL. An immunoprecipitated band corresponding to full-length IRAS ran between MW markers of 124 and 209 kD, and a second band ran between MW markers of 80 and 124 kD, only in the 2P fractions with antiserum$_{227-241}$. 1B, precipitated with first bleed antiserum$_{227-241}$; 2B, precipitated with second bleed antiserum$_{227-241}$; 4B, precipitated with fourth bleed antiserum$_{227-241}$; FB, precipitated with final bleed antiserum$_{227-241}$; 1P, pre-immune precipitant after 3× washing with lysis buffer; 2P, immune precipitants following 3× washing with lysis buffer, and SN, supernatants remaining after two immunoprecipitations.

only if obtained with multiple bleeds of duplicate antisera (two rabbits per targeted epitope) and never seen in the pellet of the pre-immune antiserum or the final supernatant. By these criteria, only antiserum$_{227-241}$ was capable of immunoprecipitating native forms of IRAS from MEG01 cells. The immunoprecipitated full-length form of IRAS ran between MW markers of 124 and 209 kD on the blots (FIG. 1). Thus, the 170-kD IRAS band was seen with all bleeds of antiserum$_{227-241}$ (the first, second, and fourth bleeds are shown in FIGS. 1B, 2B, and 4B, respectively). A band of approximately 85 kD was also immunoprecipitated in all bleeds of antiserum$_{227-241}$. This finding suggested that an 85-kD peptide fragment of IRAS might contain aas #227 to 241.

A long-standing question has been whether the 33- to 35-kD protein detected in human platelets by IRBP antiserum is a breakdown fragment of IRAS. This has often been assumed to be the case, because antiserum to IRBP was the tool used to clone IRAS. We further tested this assumption by comparing IRBP antiserum with antiserum$_{227-241}$ in terms of bands detected on Western blots of human platelet plasma membranes. We found that IRBP antiserum revealed a clear band of 33 kD on Western blots of purified plasma membranes.[7] Two faint bands of MW = 95 kD and 45 kD were also detected with antiserum to IRBP, but these appeared only after

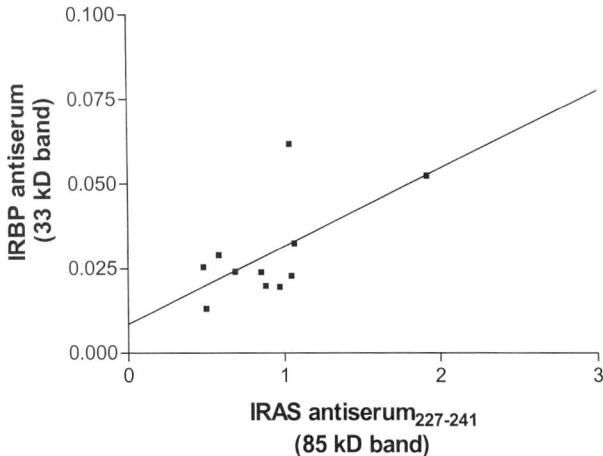

FIGURE 2. Correlation between the immunoreactive bands detected by IRAS antiserum$_{227\text{-}241}$ (85-kD band) and IRBP antiserum (33-kD band): r = 0.62, P = 0.04. Points are individual values taken from samples from different subjects.

extended film exposure times (i.e., 1 hour). By comparison, in the same samples, the major band revealed by antiserum$_{227\text{-}241}$ was found to be 85 kD in size. A weak 33-kD band was also seen by probing with antiserum$_{227\text{-}241}$ after extended film exposures. In a few subjects, antiserum$_{227\text{-}241}$ also revealed weak bands of 66 kD and 120 kD. Because the OD values of 33-kD, 66-kD, and 120-kD minor bands detected by antiserum$_{227\text{-}241}$ were below the linear range of the standard curve, they were deemed unreliable for quantitative study.

Densitometry of all prominent platelet bands on Western blots revealed a positive correlation (r = 0.62, P = 0.04) between the intensity of the 33-kD protein detected with IRBP antiserum versus the intensity of the 85-kD protein detected with antiserum$_{227\text{-}241}$ (FIG. 2). Correlational studies do not establish cause and effect, but a lack of correlation between IRBP and IRAS would certainly have minimized any precursor–product relationship. Therefore, the present result is consistent with the possibility that 85-kD and 33-kD platelet proteins are related in a product–precursor relationship with IRAS, or they may somehow simply share common epitopes and be co-regulated.

DISCUSSION

We found that three antisera targeting the N-terminus of IRAS were capable of detecting the full-length form of IRAS (170 kD) plus at least three other bands on Western blots (85, 45, and 33 kD; TABLE 1). None of the other antisera were able to detect all four of these bands in IRAS-expressing Sf9 membrane preparations or other cells. Of course, claim can be made that all the bands listed in TABLE 1 are IRAS peptides because they were observed only from transfected cells and were not detected by pre-immune antisera. This paper focuses on the 85-kD and 33-kD peptides because they are the sizes that have been reported[7] to be IRBP in megakayoblastoma MEG01 cells and platelets, respectively.[7] The fact that all three of the N-terminal antisera gave comparable results (TABLE 1) further argues that the 85-, 45-, and 33-kD peptides are N-terminal fragments of IRAS.

With fresh human platelet samples none of the seven anti-IRAS sera were capable of detecting the full-length form of IRAS (170 kD). Thus, we conclude that full-length IRAS does not exist in platelet membranes. On the other hand, two of the N-terminal antisera, corresponding to aas #79 to 92 and #227 to 241, were well able to detect 85-kD and 33-kD bands in human platelet membranes. We might speculate that because platelets are a terminal cell type, the full-length form of IRAS may be rapidly and more extensively fragmented in platelets than in other cell types.

Antiserum$_{227-241}$ was found to be unique in being able to immunoprecipitate IRAS proteins from detergent-solubilized human MEG01 cells (see FIG. 1). Our procedure required that the antibody recognize its target in a nondenatured protein state. The two proteins that were immunoprecipitated from MEG01 cells ran at 170 kD (full-length IRAS) and 85 kD (apparent IRAS N-terminal fragment). Aas #227 through 241 reside with a domain of IRAS called PX.[9] In other proteins, PX domains are known to bind to phosphoinositide triphosphate (PI3), which anchors the protein to the plasma membrane. Therefore, antigenicity at aas #227 through 241 in the nondenatured state of IRAS may represent a potent tool for future studies of PI3 interactions with IRAS in cells.

In summary, the main focus of this study was to determine whether bands detected by antiserum against IRBP on Western blots are actually peptide fragments of IRAS. The original IRBP antiserum as well as the new antiserum$_{227-241}$ against IRAS were both capable of detecting a 33-kD band on Western blots of human platelet membranes. In addition, the intensity of the 85-kD band detected on Western blots by antiserum$_{227-241}$ was significantly correlated with the intensity of the 33-kD band detected by IRBP antiserum (FIG. 2). These results suggest that the 33-kD and 85-kD bands in platelets are actually two N-terminal breakdown fragments of IRAS, containing aas #227 through 241.

ACKNOWLEDGMENT

This research was supported by Grant RO1 MH049248 from the National Institute of Mental Health.

REFERENCES

1. IVANOV, T.R., J.C. JONES, M. DONTENWILL, et al. 1998. Characterization of a partial cDNA clone detected by imidazoline receptor-selective antisera. J. Auton. Nerv. Syst. **72:** 98–110.
2. PILETZ, J.E., T.R. IVANOV, J.D. SHARP, et al. 2000. Imidazoline receptor antisera-selected (IRAS) cDNA: cloning and characterization. DNA Cell Biol. **19:** 319–329.
3. WANG, H., S. REGUNATHAN, D.A. RUGGIERO, et al. 1993. Production and characterization of antibodies specific for the imidazoline receptor protein. Mol. Pharmacol. **43:** 509–515.
4. ESCRIBA, P.V., M. SASTRE, H. WANG, et al. 1994. Immunodetection of putative imidazoline receptor proteins in the human and rat brain and other tissues. Neurosci. Lett. **178:** 81–84.

5. BENNAI, F., H. GRENEY, C. VONTHRON, et al. 1996. Polyclonal anti-idiotypic antibodies to idazoxan and their interaction with human brain imidazoline binding sites. Eur. J. Pharmacol. **306:** 211–218.
6. IVANOV, T.R., H. ZHU, S. REGUNATHAN, et al. 1998. Co-detection by two imidazoline receptor protein antisera of a novel 85 kilodalton protein. Biochem. Pharmacol. **55:** 649–655.
7. IVANOV, T.R., Y. FENG, H. WANG, et al. 1998. Imidazoline receptor proteins are regulated in platelet-precursor MEG01 cells by agonists and antagonists. Psychiatr. Res. **32:** 65–79.
8. PILETZ, J., A. HALARIS, A. SARAN, et al. 1990. Elevated ^{3}H-para-aminoclonidine binding to platelet purified plasma membranes from depressed patients. Neuropsychopharmacology **3:** 201–210.
9. WISHART, M.J., G.S. TAYLOR & J.E. DIXON. 2001. Phoxy lipids: revealing PX domains as phosphoinositide binding modules. Cell **105:** 817–820.

Index of Contributors

Altunbas, H., 136, 196
Anderson, N.J., 157, 175
Andrade, C.A.F., 262
Aricioglu, F., 106, 127, 136, 141, 147, 180, 185, 190, 196

Baker, G.B., 309
Baldwin, J., 400, 439
Barrow, C.J., 222
Berkman, K., 141, 190
Berkowitz, D.B., 52
Bokvist, K., 332
Bönisch, H., 75, 279
Botta, M., 52
Bousquet, P., 228, 400
Bozkurt, A., 106
Brenner, M.B., 332
Bruban, V., 228
Brüss, M., 75, 279
Burgdorf, C., 265
Burke, S.L., 234

Chan, S.L., 386
Chen, M., 400, 439
Chen, M.J., 427
Cooper, E.J., 167
Crosby, J., 157

Davies, N., 302
De Luca, L.A., Jr., 262
Dehle, F.C., 413
Delagrange, P., 175
Deleersnijder, W., 419
Dominiak, P., 270
Dontenwill, M., 400
Dulger, G., 147
Dunn, W.R., 386
Dupuy, L., 400

Efanov, A.M., 332
Eglen, R.M., 201
Ehrhardt, J.D., 228
El-Ayoubi, R., 244, 274
Engelhardt, A., 265
Ercil, E., 147
Ernsberger, P., 244, 251, 419

Fairbanks, C.A., 82, 378
Feldman, J., 228
Feng, Y., 152
Ferrer-Alcon, M., 323
Finn, D.P., 302
Forzley, B., 288

Garcia-Sevilla, J.A., 323
Garfield, B., 386
Glennon, R.A., 361
Goracke-Postle, C.J., 82
Göthert, M., 44, 75, 279
Grella, B., 361
Greney, H., 228, 400
Grigg, M., 222
Gromada, J., 332
Grosse-Lackmann, T., 371
Gutkowska, J., 244, 274

Halaris, A., 1, 296
Häuser, W., 270
Hayes, J., 439
Head, G.A., 234
Heinen, A., 44
Hills, C.E., 167
Holt, A., 309
Homann, J., 44
Huang, M.-J., 52

Hudson, A.L., 157, 167, 175, 283, 302, 353, 357, 361, 364, 367
Husbands, S., 302
Husbands, S.M., 175

Jankowski, M., 244
Jungbluth, B., 270

Kaminski, L.L., 82
Kan, B., 141
Kendall, D.A., 201, 216
Kimura, A., 302, 364
Koletsky, R.J., 251
Korcegez, E., 106, 141, 180, 190
Kurz, T., 265

Lalies, M.D., 302
Lau, A., 361
LeBlanc, M.H., 152
Lee, K., 52
Llorente, J., 133
Lübbecke, F., 44

Ma, J.K., 341
MacLennan, S.J., 201
Martí, O., 302
Martinez, G., 262
May, P.J., 64
McClendon, E., 52
Menani, J.V., 262
Menaouar, A., 244, 274
Menzel, S., 44
Mest, H.-J., 332
Minchin, M.C.W., 302, 364
Molderings, G.J., 44, 75, 279
Monassier, L., 228
Morgan, A.D., 82
Morgan, N.G., 167
Morris, S.M., Jr., 30
Mukaddam-Daher, S., 244, 274
Musgrave, I.F., 222, 413

Nguyen, H.O.X., 82
Nutt, D.J., 157, 175, 283, 302, 353, 357, 361, 364, 367

Oliveira, L.B., 262
Overland, A.C., 82
Ozyalcin, S., 106, 180

Parker, C.A., 167
Pascal, G., 400
Paterson, L.M., 353, 367
Pedersen, M.L., 52
Penner, S.B., 288
Piletz, J., 413
Piletz, J.E., 1, 20, 52, 64, 127, 296, 341, 347, 392, 400, 413, 419, 427, 439
Pineda, J., 133
Pinthong, D., 201, 216
Pirnat, D., 288
Price, R.E., 283

Raasch, W., 265, 270
Regunathan, S., 20, 52, 127
Richardt, G., 265
Robinson, E., 302
Robinson, E.S.J., 157, 175, 283, 367
Roerig, S.C., 116
Rondé, P., 400
Roth, B.L., 419
Ruiz-Durántez, E., 133
Rustenbeck, I., 371

Saczewski, F., 357
Saczewski, J., 357
Satriano, J., 34
Schäfer, U., 265, 270
Schann, S., 228
Silva, D.C.F., 262
Smyth, D.D., 288
Squires, P.E., 167
Stone, L.S., 378

INDEX OF CONTRIBUTORS

Tabin, P., 357
Takeda, K., 400
Todd, K.G., 309
Travagli, M., 52
Tyacke, R.J., 302, 353, 357, 361, 364

Ugedo, L., 133
Ulibarri, I., 133
Utkan, T., 185

Van Der Zypp, A., 222
Velliquette, R.A., 244, 251

Wang, G., 52, 64, 392
Wang, M., 386
Wilcox, G.L., 378
Wilson, V.G., 201, 216, 386

Yi, G.B., 52
Yillar, O., 141, 190

Zhu, H., 64, 296, 341, 347, 392, 419, 427, 439
Ziegler, D., 419
Zünkler, B.J., 371

OHIO UNIVERSITY LIBRARY

Please return this book as soon as you have finished with it. In order to avoid a fine it must be returned by the latest date stamped below. All books are subject to recall after two weeks or immediately if needed for reserve.

CF